Cardiopulmonary Anatomy & Physiology

Essentials of Respiratory Care

Sixth Edition

Terry Des Jardins, MEd, RRT

Professor Emeritus
Former Director
Department of Respiratory Care
Parkland College
Champaign, Illinois

Faculty/Staff Member
University of Illinois College of Medicine at Urbana-Champaign

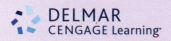
DELMAR
CENGAGE Learning·

Australia • Brazil • Japan • Korea • Mexico • Singapore • Spain • United Kingdom • United States

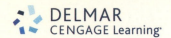

**Cardiopulmonary Anatomy & Physiology:
Essentials of Respiratory Care, Sixth Edition**
Terry Des Jardins, MEd, RRT

Vice President, Careers and Computing:
Dave Garza

Director of Learning Solutions: Matthew Kane

Associate Acquisitions Editor: Christina Gifford

Managing Editor: Marah Bellegarde

Senior Product Manager: Laura J. Wood

Editorial Assistant: Anthony Souza

Vice President, Marketing: Jennifer Ann Baker

Marketing Director: Wendy E. Mapstone

Associate Marketing Manager:
Jonathan Sheehan

Senior Production Director: Wendy A. Troeger

Production Manager: Andrew Crouth

Content Project Manager: Allyson Bozeth

Senior Art Director: David Arsenault

Library of Congress Control Number: 2012933334

ISBN-13: 978-0-8400-2258-5

ISBN-10: 0-8400-2258-1

Delmar
5 Maxwell Drive
Clifton Park, NY 12065-2919
USA

Cengage Learning is a leading provider of customized learning solutions with office locations around the globe, including Singapore, the United Kingdom, Australia, Mexico, Brazil, and Japan. Locate your local office at:
international.cengage.com/region

Cengage Learning products are represented in Canada by Nelson Education, Ltd.

To learn more about Delmar, visit **www.cengage.com/delmar**

Purchase any of our products at your local college store or at our preferred online store **www.cengagebrain.com**

Notice to the Reader

Printed in the United States of America
1 2 3 4 5 6 7 15 14 13 12

Cardiopulmonary Anatomy & Physiology

Essentials of Respiratory Care

Sixth Edition

To
Katherine, Alexander, Destinee, and Ashley
The Next Generation

Grandpa T

Contents

Section One

The Cardiopulmonary System—The Essentials   1

Chapter 1

The Anatomy and Physiology of the Respiratory System   3

Chapter 2

Ventilation   77

Section Two

Advanced Cardiopulmonary Concepts and Related Areas—The Essentials 425

Chapter 17

Sleep Physiology and Its Relationship to the Cardiopulmonary System 523

Section Three

The Cardiopulmonary System During Unusual Environmental Conditions   555

Chapter 18

Exercise and Its Effects on the Cardiopulmonary System   557

Chapter 19

High Altitude and Its Effects on the Cardiopulmonary System   575

Chapter 20

High-Pressure Environments and Their Effects on the Cardiopulmonary System   587

List of Tables

List of Clinical Connections

Chapter 3

Chapter 4

Foreword
To the Sixth Edition

The sixth edition of Des Jardins' *Cardiopulmonary Anatomy & Physiology—Essentials of Respiratory Care* picks up with a reiteration of the apparent—namely, that form and function are inextricably tied together, from the submicroscopic forms to those visible with the naked eye. It continues with a more in-depth explanation of the notion of "mission criticality," using the new Clinical Connection feature, which links form and function to the clinical day-to-day practice of cardiopulmonary and sleep medicine.

In the interval between the fifth and sixth editions, the virtually irreplaceable nature of the original forms of the body system design have become ever clearer to me. Mechanical cardiac assist devices, cardiopulmonary bypass, and renal dialysis are short-term "fixes" at best, as is the modern ventilator (with a few exceptions). The system redundancies that have been built in to our "original equipment" (think of secondary polycythemia and acid–base compensating mechanisms, for example) are without peer. Virtually NO "replacement" for the central nervous system has yet been developed, let alone made operational, and probably never will be.

This said, we must preserve and, if possible, improve the "original equipment," damaged though it may be by disease, and to do that, we must be able to visualize it as clearly as possible from the bedside.

The secret to learning anatomy and physiology is not memorization. It is *visualization!* The best of success as you look ahead!

George G. Burton, MD, FACP, FCCP, FAARC
Associate Dean for Medial Affairs
Kettering College of Medical Arts
Kettering, Ohio
Clinical Professor of Medicine and Anesthesiology
Wright State University School of Medicine
Dayton, Ohio

Preface

Overview

It is important to emphasize that knowledge of an anatomic *structure* is essential to the understanding of the *function* of that structure. It therefore makes little sense to present students with physiologic details without first establishing a solid foundation in anatomy. Because most college-level anatomy courses spend only a limited amount of time on the cardiopulmonary system, respiratory care educators generally need to cover this subject themselves. With regard to a textbook, however, educators usually find the cardiopulmonary section of college-level anatomy and physiology texts too introductory in nature. On the other hand, textbooks concentrating solely on the respiratory system are too complex or esoteric.

As a solution to this problem, this book is designed to provide students of cardiopulmonary anatomy and physiology with the most accurate and complete information essential for respiratory care. It is assumed that the student has no previous knowledge of respiratory anatomy or physiology. Great efforts have been made to present a comprehensive overview of the subject matter in an organized, interesting, and readable manner. The organization of this book is based on my experiences as an educator of respiratory anatomy and physiology since 1973—and the countless things I have learned from my students and fellow colleagues. In response to these personal experiences and helpful suggestions, the following pedagogic approach is used in this book.

Organization

The sixth edition of this book is divided into three major sections. **Section I, The Cardiopulmonary System—The Essentials,** consists of Chapters 1 through 11. Chapter 1 provides the student with a thorough discussion of anatomic structures associated with the respiratory system. This chapter also features a large number of colorful illustrations. The visual impact of this chapter is intended to (1) stimulate interest in the subject under discussion, (2) facilitate the rapid visualization of anatomic structures, and (3) help the student relate classroom knowledge to clinical experiences.

Chapters 2 through 9 cover the major concepts and mechanisms of respiratory physiology. The discussions are comprehensive, logically organized, and, most importantly, presented at a level suitable for the average college student. When appropriate, anatomic and physiologic principles are applied to common clinical situations to enhance understanding and retention (e.g., the gas transport calculations and their clinical application to the patient's hemodynamic status). In addition, a large number of colorful line drawings and tables appear throughout these chapters to assist in the understanding of various concepts and principles.

Chapters 2, 3, 6, 7, and 8 feature several unique line drawings that relate familiar visual concepts to standard graphs and nomograms. While I have found that the types of graphs and nomograms presented in this book are often (at first) difficult for students to understand, it is important to stress that the "physiology literature" uses these items extensively. **The student must understand how to read every graph and nomogram in this book to comprehend its contents fully!**

Chapter 10 covers the major anatomic structures and physiologic mechanisms associated with fetal and newborn gas exchange and circulation. It presents the basic cardiopulmonary foundation required to understand fetal and neonatal respiratory disorders. Chapter 11 describes changes that occur in the cardiopulmonary system with age. Because the older age groups are expected to increase each year until about the year 2050, basic knowledge of this material will become increasingly important to respiratory care practitioners.

Section II, *Advanced Cardiopulmonary Concepts and Related Areas— The Essentials,* consists of Chapters 12 through 17. Chapter 12 covers the essential electrophysiology of the heart required for ECG interpretation, Chapter 13 presents the major components of the standard 12-ECG lead system, and Chapter 14 provides a systematic approach to ECG interpretation and the major cardiac dysrhythmias seen by the respiratory care practitioner. Chapter 15 gives the reader the essential knowledge foundation required for hemodynamic measurements and interpretations. Chapter 16 presents the structure and function of the renal system and the major cardiopulmonary problems that develop when the renal system fails. This chapter is particularly important for respiratory care practitioners working with patients in the critical care unit. Chapter 17—which has been extensively updated—presents sleep physiology and its relationship to the cardiopulmonary system. During the past few years, there has been a tremendous increase in the demand for sleep medicine care services. Many of these sleep care centers are staffed with respiratory care practitioners who work routinely with patients who have various sleep-related disorders that adversely impact the cardiopulmonary system, such as obstructive sleep apnea.

Section III, *The Cardiopulmonary System during Unusual Environmental Conditions,* consists of Chapters 18, 19, and 20. Chapter 18 presents the effects of exercise on the cardiopulmonary system. During heavy exercise, the components of the cardiopulmonary system may be stressed to their limits. Cardiac patients involved in exercise training after myocardial infarction demonstrate a significant reduction in mortality and major cardiac mishaps. As our older population increases, cardiovascular rehabilitation programs will become increasingly more important to respiratory care practitioners. Chapter 19 describes the effects of high altitude on the cardiopulmonary system. It provides a better understanding of chronic oxygen deprivation, which can then be applied to the treatment of chronic hypoxia caused by lung disease. Chapter 20 provides an overview of high-pressure environments and their profound effect on the cardiopulmonary system. The therapeutic administration of oxygen at increased ambient pressures (hyperbaric medicine) is commonly used to treat a number of pathologic conditions.

Finally, at the end of each chapter there is a set of review questions designed to facilitate learning and retention. In addition, at the end of Chapters 2 through 10 and 15, 16, and 17, the reader is provided with a clinical application section. In this part of the chapters, one or two clinical scenarios are presented that apply several of the concepts, principles, or formulas that are presented in the chapter to actual clinical situations. These clinical scenarios are flagged throughout the chapters—in the form of abbreviated Clinical Connections (see description of Clinical Connections below)—to help highlight important points or concepts as they appear in the chapter. This feature further facilitates the transfer of classroom material to the clinical setting. Following the clinical applications are related questions to facilitate the development of critical thinking skills.

A glossary is included at the end of the text, followed by appendices that cover symbols, abbreviations, and units of measurement commonly used in respiratory physiology. Also included is a nomogram that can be copied and laminated for use as a handy clinical reference tool in the interpretation of specific arterial blood gas abnormalities. Finally, the answers to the chapter review questions appear in the last appendix.

New to the Sixth Edition

Clinical Connections

A new—and very useful—feature to the sixth edition is the addition of 128 **Clinical Connections.** The Clinical Connections—which are interspersed throughout each chapter—provide the reader with a direct link between the topics being discussed and, importantly, how they may be applied to the clinical setting—to "real-life" situations. In addition to enhancing the transfer of classroom material to the clinical setting, the Clinical Connections are designed to (1) further stimulate classroom discussions; (2) provide a brief preview (i.e., coming attractions) of more advanced cardiopulmonary topics—such as, respiratory disorders, pharmacology, and the benefits and hazards or mechanical ventilation; (3) help in clarifying important cardiopulmonary concepts; and (4) further stimulate the student's excitement—and anticipation—of ultimately working and caring for patients in the profession of respiratory care.

The Clinical Connections are also intended to help the student—the early apprentice of respiratory care—answer the following types of commonly asked questions:

- "Why am I learning this material?"
- "When will I ever see this information in the clinical setting?"
- "How will this material ever be used in my 'real life'—when I am working as a licensed respiratory therapist?"

With the addition of the Clinical Connections, these types of questions are appropriately addressed—the student is now provided with commonly seen relationships between what is being studied in the classroom and how this material may be used in clinical setting.

Chapter 1: The Anatomy and Physiology of the Respiratory System

- Thirty two new full color figures illustrating important features associated with the anatomy of the cardiopulmonary system. Two new photographs and five new chest x-rays have also been added.
- 21 Clinical Connections providing a direct link to the chapter content and the clinical setting.
- Revised and new discussions over several topics, including the nose, oral cavity, nasal pharynx, oral pharynx, alveolar epithelium, and the muscles of ventilation.

Chapter 2: Ventilation

- 5 new full color figures illustrating important features associated with the mechanics of ventilation. Two new photographs and two new chest x-rays have also been added.
- 18 Clinical Connections providing a direct link to the chapter content and the clinical setting.
- New content and extensive updates covering the mechanisms of pulmonary ventilation, ventilation, pressure gradients, and Boyle's law and its relationship to pressure gradients in ventilation.
- Revised and updated Tables 2–1 and 2–2.

Chapter 3: Pulmonary Function Measurements

- 2 new full color figures illustrating important concepts related to pulmonary function measurements
- 10 Clinical Connections providing a direct link to the chapter content and the clinical setting.
- Updated and simplified content discussion covering lung volumes and capacities and lung volumes and capacities in obstructive and restrictive lung disorders.
- New section covering the factors affecting predicted normal values.
- New section covering the rapid shallow breathing index ratio (RSBI).
- Updated and restructured Table 3–1.
- New Table 3–2.

Chapter 4: The Diffusion of Pulmonary Gases

- 1 new full color illustration of atmospheric gases
- 6 Clinical Connections providing a direct link to the chapter content and the clinical setting.
- Clarified and updated content covering Dalton's law, the partial pressures of atmospheric gases, and gas diffusion—pressure gradients versus diffusion gradients.

Chapter 5: The Anatomy and Physiology of the Circulatory System

- 1 new full color figure illustrating the composition of whole blood. Two new photographs, two x-rays, and 1 angiogram have also been added.

- 11 Clinical Connections providing a direct link to the chapter content and the clinical setting.
- Revised section clarifying and updating the discussion of blood, red blood cells, white cells, platelets, and plasma.
- Updated and restructured Table 5–1.

Chapter 6: Oxygen and Carbon Dioxide Transport

- 1 new photograph of a radial-arterial blood gas stick.
- 7 Clinical Connections providing a direct link to the chapter content and the clinical setting.
- The addition of the section regarding how carbon dioxide is transported from the tissues to the lungs.
- Updated and restructured Table 6–12.

Chapter 7: Acid–Base Balance and Regulation

- 11 Clinical Connections providing a direct link to the chapter content and the clinical setting—especially arterial blood gas interpretations.

Chapter 8: Ventilation-Perfusion Relationships

- 1 new full color figure illustrating important features associated with ventilation-perfusion relationships
- 3 Clinical Connections providing a direct link to the chapter content and ventilation-perfusion relationships.

Chapter 9: Control of Ventilation

- 1 new x-ray showing the site at which the phrenic nerve emerges from the spinal cord at level C3 through C5
- 1 new photograph illustrating a sneeze reflex.
- 6 Clinical Connections providing a direct link to the chapter content.
- Updated section covering the medullary respiratory centers—including the ventral respiratory group (VRG), the dorsal respiratory group (DGR), the pontine respiratory center, and their influence on the medullary respiratory centers—and factors that influence the rate and depth of breathing.

Chapter 10: Fetal Development and the Cardiopulmonary System

- 3 new full color figures illustrating important features associated with fetal development and the cardiopulmonary system.
- 6 Clinical Connections providing a direct link to the chapter content.
- A restructured and simplified discussion covering the circulatory changes at birth.

Chapter 11: Aging and the Cardiopulmonary System

- 1 Clinical Connection providing a direct link to the chapter content.

Chapter 12: Electrophysiology of the Heart

- 1 Clinical Connection providing a direct link to the chapter content.

Chapter 13: The Standard 12-ECG Lead System

- 1 Clinical Connection providing a direct link to the chapter content.

Chapter 14: ECG Interpretation

- 4 Clinical Connections providing a direct link to the chapter content.

Chapter 15: Hemodynamic Measurements

- 8 Clinical Connections providing a direct link to the chapter content.

Chapter 16: Renal Failure and Its Effects on the Cardiopulmonary System

- 5 new full color figures illustrating important features associated with renal failure and its effects on the cardiopulmonary system.
- 2 Clinical Connections providing a direct link to the chapter content.

Chapter 17: Sleep Physiology and Its Relationship to the Cardiopulmonary System

- 1 new full color figure illustrating important features associated with sleep apnea. Three new photographs depict a sleep disorder specialist at work, a nocturnal polysomnography (sleep study), and a CPAP device.
- 8 Clinical Connections providing a direct link to the chapter content.
- Updated discussion on non-REM sleep, including stages N1, N2, and N3.
- Updated and revised figures and tables to match sleep stages according to the current American Academy of Sleep Medicine standards.
- The addition of a case study at the end of the chapter.
- 3 new photographs

Chapter 18: Exercise and Its Effects on the Cardiopulmonary System

- 1 Clinical Connection providing a direct link to the chapter content.
- New Table 18–1.
- New Table 18–2.

Chapter 19: High Altitude and Its Effects on the Cardiopulmonary System

- 1 Clinical Connection providing a direct link to the chapter content.
- Clarified and updated content covering pulmonary function and mechanics as an individual ascends.
- Updated content covering oxygen diffusion capacity at high altitudes.
- Revised and simplified content covering ventilation-perfusion relationships at high altitudes.
- New Table 19–1.

Chapter 20: High-Pressure Environments and Their Effects on the Cardiopulmonary System

- 2 Clinical Connections providing a direct link to the chapter content.
- 1 new photograph illustrating breath-holding.

Also Available

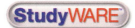

Online StudyWARE™

Free with purchase of a new textbook, **StudyWARE™ software** is **now online** and includes helpful activities for each chapter:

- Labeling exercises
- Hangman game
- Word Search game
- Concentration game
- Matching quizzes
- Multiple choice and true/false quizzing

Redeeming an Access Code:

1. Go to www.CengageBrain.com.

2. Enter the Access code in the Prepaid Code or Access Key field, **Redeem**.

3. Register as a new user, or log in as an existing user if you already have an account with Cengage Learning or CengageBrain.com, **Redeem**.

4. Select **Go to My Account**.

5. Open the product from the My Account page.

PRINTED ACCESS CARD Premium Website to accompany Cardiopulmonary Anatomy & Physiology ISBN-13: 978-1-1337-8874-4

INSTANT ACCESS CODE Premium Website to accompany Cardiopulmonary Anatomy & Physiology ISBN-13: 978-1-1337-8873-7

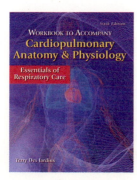

Workbook

In the **Student Workbook** (ISBN-13: 978-0-8400-2261-5), additional exercises and questions are organized by major topic headings. This organization allows students to concentrate on specific topics, if necessary. The workbook is designed to enhance learning, understanding, retention, and clinical application of the content presented in the textbook. Completed sections provide an excellent study resource for quiz and test preparation. The workbook has been fully updated to correspond to the new content discussed in the textbook and includes:

- New! Key terms lists provide students with a list of the important terminology discussed in each chapter.

- Written exercises and problems that parallel the content presented in the textbook:
  - Image labeling and coloring illustrations.
  - Fill-in questions.
  - Matching.
  - Short answer.
  - Terminology review.
  - Calculations.
  - An answer key provides answers to all exercises to help facilitate study and review of materials.

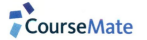

CourseMate

CourseMate with eBook for Cardiopulmonary Anatomy & Physiology: Essentials of Respiratory Care, 6th Edition.

CourseMate includes:

- An interactive eBook, with highlighting, note taking and search capabilities.
- Interactive learning tools including:
  - Quizzes
  - Flashcards
  - Animations
  - Case studies
  - Web links
  - And more!
- Engagement Tracker, a first-of-its-kind tool that monitors student engagement in the course.

Go to www.cengagebrain.com to access these resources, and look for this icon

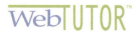 to find resources related to your text.

INSTANT ACCESS CODE CourseMate with eBook for Cardiopulmonary Anatomy & Physiology ISBN-13: 978-0-8400-2266-0

PRINTED ACCESS CARD CourseMate with eBook for Cardiopulmonary Anatomy & Physiology ISBN-13: 978-0-8400-2265-3

Webtutor™ Advantage

WebTUTOR™ Advantage is an eLearning software solution that turns everyone in your classroom or training center into a front-row learner using a learning management system. The Webtutor™Advantage includes chapter learning objectives, online course preparation, study sheets, FAQs documents, glossary flashcards, discussion topics, web links, animations and video, and an online forum to exchange notes and questions. In addition, online chapter quizzes are provided in various formats, including matching exercises, true-false questions, short-answer, and multiple-choice questions with immediate feedback for correct and incorrect answers. Whether you want to Web-enhance your class, or offer an entire course online, **WebTUTOR**™ allows you to focus on what you do best, Teaching.

PRINTED ACCESS CARD: Cardiopulmonary Anatomy & Physiology Webtutor™ Advantage on Blackboard ISBN-13: 978-0-8400-2260-8

PRINTED ACCESS CARD: Cardiopulmonary Anatomy & Physiology Webtutor™ Advantage on Angel ISBN-13: 978-0-8400-2271-4

Instructor Resources CD-ROM
Spend Less Time Planning and More Time Teaching!

With Delmar, Cengage Learning's Instructor Resources to Accompany *Cardiopulmonary Anatomy & Physiology,* preparing for class and evaluating students has never been easier! As an instructor, you will find this tool offers invaluable assistance by giving you access to all of your resources—anywhere and at any time.

Features:

- Each chapter in the **Instructor's Manual** provides (1) an overview of the content of the chapter; (2) instructional objectives; (3) key terms; (4) instructor and student resources; and (5) a chapter lesson plan and overview—which includes each instructional objective, where in the textbook it is discussed, and what PowerPoint® slides can be used to facilitate the presentation and discussion of the material.
- The **Computerized Testbank** in **ExamView®** makes generating tests and quizzes a snap. With over 1000 questions and different styles to choose from, including multiple choice, true/false, completion, and short answer, you can create customized assessments for your students with the click of a button. Add your own unique questions and print answers for easy class preparation. All questions have been thoroughly updated to reflect content updates made to the sixth edition. Questions have also been edited to provide more correlation to the NBRC exam format.
- Customizable instructor support slide presentations in **PowerPoint®** format focus on key points for each chapter; these include photos where appropriate. Approximately 1500 slides have been fully updated to correlate to the content updates made to the sixth edition.
- Use the hundreds of images from the **Image Library** to enhance your instructor support slide presentations, insert art into test questions, or add visuals wherever you need them. These valuable images, which are pulled from the accompanying textbook, are organized by chapter and are easily searchable.
- New! **Animations** related to important respiratory care topics such as normal body system function and common respiratory ailments offer enhanced visual aids to help students comprehend important concepts.

ExamView® is a registered trademark of eInstruction Corp.

PowerPoint® is a registered trademark of the Microsoft Corporation.

INSTRUCTOR RESOURCES CD-ROM TO ACCOMPANY CARDIOPULMONARY ANATOMY & PHYSIOLOGY ISBN-13: 978-0-8400-2268-4

Instructor Companion Website

The Instructor Companion Website contains the same resources as the Instructor Resources CD-ROM in an online format. To access these resources, contact your sales representative, or go to http://login.cengage.com.

ISBN-13: 978-0-8400-2263-9

Concept Media Video Series

Explore the pathophysiology, risk factors, symptoms, and diagnostics of various respiratory disorders and acute respiratory disorders. Topics include Allergies and Anaphylaxis and Pulmonary Embolism.

Respiratory Disorders: Complete Series
CD: 978-0-495-81886-1
DVD: 978-0-495-81884-7

Acute Respiratory Disorders: Complete Series
CD: 978-1-6023-2300-1
DVD: 978-1-6023-2124-3

Acknowledgments

A number of people have provided important contributions to the development of the sixth edition of this textbook. First, I extend a very special thank you to Dr. George Burton for the hours he spent editing the clinical connections. In addition, Dr. Burton provided many important updates to Chapter 17, Sleep Physiology and Its Relationship to the Cardiopulmonary System. For the 49 pieces of new artwork generated for this book, an extended thank you goes to Joe Chovan. The excellent colored illustrations Joe provided undoubtedly enhance the visualization—and, importantly, the understanding—of the material presented throughout the textbook. Joe's artistic work in Chapters 1, 5, 10, and 16 is especially outstanding.

For all their help, suggestions, and guidance for the Clinical Connections added to the this new edition, a special thank you goes to James R. Sills, MEd, CPFT, RRT; and David Zobeck, MBA, CPFT, RRT For her outstanding work in writing—in NBRC format—the student website review questions, and the instructor website test and quiz questions, my sincere gratitude goes out to Trudy Watson, BS, RRT, AE-C, FAARC. A special thank you also goes to Chad Goveia, RRT, Director of Respiratory Care, BroMenn Health Care Center, Bloomington, Illinois, for providing radiology images of the epiglottis.

For his help in obtaining a number of important radiology images—including the chest X-ray and CT scan of a 2-year-old little boy who was accidently shot in the right ventricle with a nail gun, renal arteriogram, and the lateral view of the spinal cord at level C3 through C5—my gratefulness goes to Joseph C. Barkmeier, MD, Radiology, Carle Clinic Association, Urbana, Illinois. For obtaining a colored image of the vocal cords during a bronchoscopy and the chest X-ray of a tracheoesophageal fistula, my thanks goes out to Maury Topolosky, MD, Pulmonologist, Christie Clinic, Champaign, Illinois.

For their extensive and comprehensive reviews and suggestions regarding the overall depth, breadth, and accuracy of the material presented in this textbook, I offer an individual thank you to each of the following outstanding respiratory care educators:

Stacia E. Biddle, RRT
Assistant Professor of Respiratory Therapy
The University of Akron
Akron, Ohio

Lisa M. Johnson, MS, RRT-NPS
Vice Chair, Clinical Assistant Professor
Respiratory Care Program
Stony Brook University
Stony Brook

Paul LaMere, MS, RRT
Director of Clinical Education
Respiratory Care Department
St. Catherine University
St. Paul, MN

Robert Langenderfer, MEd, RRT-NPS
Associate Professor and Program Director
Respiratory Care Program
Northern Kentucky University
Highland Heights, KY

Kathryn Patterson BS, RRT
Faculty
GateWay Community College
Phoenix, AZ

James R. Sills, MEd, CPFT, RRT
Professor Emeritus
Former Director, Respiratory Care Program
Rock Valley College
Rockford, Illinois

Meg Trumpp, MEd, RRT, AE-C
Program Director
Respiratory Care Newman University
Wichita, KS

David Zobeck, Masters of Management, RRT, CPRT
Chair of the Respiratory Care Program, Health Sciences
Lancaster General College of Nursing and Health Sciences
Lancaster, PA

Finally, I am very grateful to Tari Broderick, Laura Wood, Allyson Bozeth, and Manoj Kumar. Their work and helpful coordination during the development of this textbook, and the supplemental student and instructor packages associated with this book, has been most appreciated.

Terry Des Jardins, MEd, RRT

How to Use the Text and Software

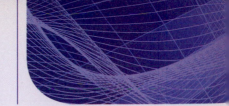

Objectives at the beginning of each chapter list in detail the theoretical and practical goals of the chapter.

Objectives

By the end of this chapter, the student should be able to:

1. Describe the following three major components of the upper airway:
   —Nose
   —Oral cavity
   —Pharynx
   —Larynx
2. List the primary functions of the upper airway:
   —Conductor of air
   —Humidify air
   —Prevent aspiration
   —Area for speech and smell
3. Describe the following three primary functions of the nose:
   —Filter
   —Humidify
   —Condition (warm or cool air)
4. Identify the following structures that form the outer portion of the nose:
   —Nasal bones
   —Frontal process of the maxilla
   —Lateral nasal cartilage
   —Greater alar cartilage
   —Lesser alar cartilages
   —Septal cartilage
   —Fibrous fatty tissue
5. Explain the clinical connection associated with flaring nostrils (or nasal flaring).
   —Frontal process of the maxilla
   —Cribriform plate of the ethmoid
   —Palatine process of the maxilla
   —Palatine bones
   —Soft palate
   —Nares
   —Vestibule
   —Vibrissae
   —Stratified squamous epithelium
   —Pseudostratified ciliated columnar epithelium
   —Turbinates (conchae)
   • Superior
   • Middle
   • Inferior
   —Paranasal sinuses
   • Maxillary
   • Frontal
   • Ethmoid
   • Sphenoid
   —Olfactory region
   —Choanae
7. Describe the clinical connection associated with the nose as an excellent route of administration for topical agents.
8. Discuss the clinical connection associated with nosebleeds (epistaxis).
9. Describe the clinical connection associated with rhinitis.

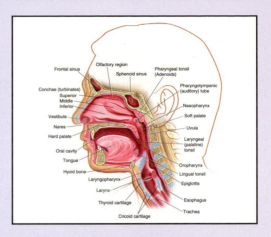

49 new figures assist in understanding the various concepts and principles of anatomy, physiology, and pathophysiology.

New! 128 Clinical Connections provide the reader with a direct link between the topics being discussed and how they may be applied to "real-life" in the clinical setting.

Clinical Connection—2-8

Pulmonary Surfactant Deficiency

The respiratory therapist will encounter a number of pulmonary disorders that are associated with a pulmonary surfactant deficiency. For example, this problem is commonly seen in premature infants who are diagnosed with **respiratory distress syndrome (RDS)**. These babies are born before their type II alveolar cells are mature enough to produce a sufficient amount of pulmonary surfactant. Low levels of pulmonary surfactant increase the surface tension forces in the lungs and, in severe cases, cause the alveoli to collapse (atelectasis). Alveolar collapse shifts the baby's volume–pressure curve to the right, decreases lung compliance, decreases the baby's oxygenation level, and increases the work of breathing.

The treatment of choice during the early stages of RDS is **continuous positive airway pressure (CPAP)**. CPAP works to (1) re-inflate the lungs, (2) decrease the work of breathing, and (3) return the baby's oxygenation level to normal. Mechanical ventilation, in these cases, is avoided as long as possible. Because of the pulmonary surfactant deficiency associated with RDS, the administration of exogenous surfactant preparations such as **beractant** (Survanta®), **calfactant** (Infasurf®), and **poractant alfa** (Curosurf®) is often helpful.

Clinical Application Cases provide opportunities to use critical thinking skills to reflect on the material and relate the concepts to real-life situations.

1 Clinical Application Case

A 22-year-old male who had been in a motorcycle crash was brought to the emergency department with several facial, neck, and shoulder abrasions and lacerations, and multiple broken ribs. During each breath, the patient's right anterior chest moved inward during inspiration and outward during exhalation (clinically this is called a *flail chest*). The patient was alert, in pain, and stated, "I can't breathe. Am I going to die?"

The patient's skin was pale and blue. His vital signs were blood pressure—166/93 mm Hg, heart rate—135 beats/min, and respiratory rate—26 breaths/min and shallow. While on a simple oxygen mask, the

Four hours later, the patient appeared comfortable and his skin color was normal. The ventilator was set at a rate of 12 breaths/min, an inspired oxygen concentration ($F_{I_O_2}$) of 0.3, and a PEEP of +5 cm H_2O. No spontaneous breaths were generated between each mechanical ventilation. During each mechanical breath, both the right and left side of the patient's chest expanded symmetrically. His blood pressure was 127/83 mm Hg and heart rate was 76 beats/min. A second chest X-ray revealed that his right lung had re-expanded. His peripheral oxygen saturation level was 97 percent.

XXXV

Chapter Summary

Review Questions

Clinical Application Questions

At the end of each chapter, reinforce your understanding of the concepts covered through the **Chapter Summary**, **Review Questions**, and **Clinical Application Questions**.

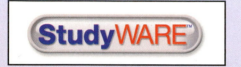

StudyWARE™ is interactive software with learning activities and quizzes to help you study key concepts and test your comprehension. The activities and quiz content correspond with each chapter of the book.

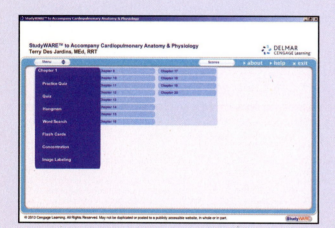

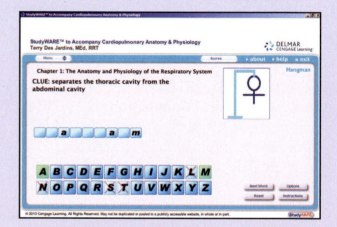

The activities include Labeling exercises, Hangman game, Word Search game, Concentration game, and Matching quizzes.

Supplements At-a-Glance

Supplement:	What It is:	What's In It:
Online StudyWARE **StudyWARE**	Software program (Available online via www.cengagebrain.com)	Labeling exercises Hangman game Word search game Concentration game Matching quizzes
Workbook	Print	Written exercises and problems that parallel the content presented in the textbook Image labeling, fill-in questions, matching, short answer, and terminology review

CourseMate **CourseMate**	Web access via www. cengagebrain.com	• An interactive eBook, with highlighting, note taking and search capabilities
		• Interactive learning tools including:
		  ○ Quizzes
		  ○ Flashcards
		  ○ Animations
		  ○ Case studies
		  ○ Web links
		  ○ and more!
		• Engagement Tracker, a first-of-its-kind tool that monitors student engagement in the course

WebTutor™ Advantage **WebTUTOR**	eLearning software solution; Web access	Available for various learning management systems, including Blackboard and Angel Content and quizzes corresponding to each chapter Animations and case studies
Instructor Resources CD-ROM	CD-ROM	Instructor's Manual Computerized test bank Slide presentations in PowerPoint® Image library Animations
Instructor Companion Website	Web access via http://login.cengage.com	Same components as available on the Instructor Resources CD-ROM

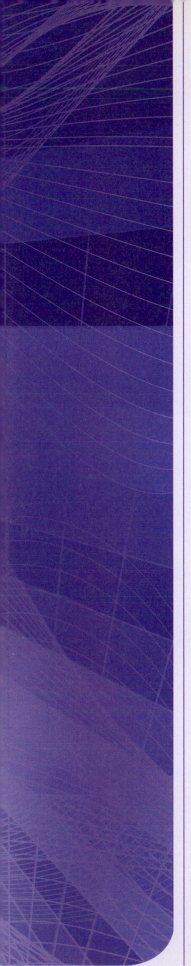

1

The Anatomy and Physiology of the Respiratory System

Objectives

By the end of this chapter, the student should be able to:

1. Describe the following three major components of the upper airway:
   —Nose
   —Oral cavity
   —Pharynx
   —Larynx
2. List the primary functions of the upper airway:
   —Conductor of air
   —Humidify air
   —Prevent aspiration
   —Area for speech and smell
3. Describe the following three primary functions of the nose:
   —Filter
   —Humidify
   —Condition (warm or cool air)
4. Identify the following structures that form the outer portion of the nose:
   —Nasal bones
   —Frontal process of the maxilla
   —Lateral nasal cartilage
   —Greater alar cartilage
   —Lesser alar cartilages
   —Septal cartilage
   —Fibrous fatty tissue
5. Explain the clinical connection associated with flaring nostrils (or nasal flaring).
6. Identify the following structures that form the internal portion of the nose:
   —Nasal septum
     • Perpendicular plate of the ethmoid
     • Vomer
     • Septal cartilage
   —Nasal bones

   —Frontal process of the maxilla
   —Cribriform plate of the ethmoid
   —Palatine process of the maxilla
   —Palatine bones
   —Soft palate
   —Nares
   —Vestibule
   —Vibrissae
   —Stratified squamous epithelium
   —Pseudostratified ciliated columnar epithelium
   —Turbinates (conchae)
     • Superior
     • Middle
     • Inferior
   —Paranasal sinuses
     • Maxillary
     • Frontal
     • Ethmoid
     • Sphenoid
   —Olfactory region
   —Choanae
7. Describe the clinical connection associated with the nose as an excellent route of administration for topical agents.
8. Discuss the clinical connection associated with nosebleeds (epistaxis).
9. Describe the clinical connection associated with rhinitis.
10. Describe the clinical connection associated with nasal congestion and its influence on taste.
11. Describe the clinical connection associated with sinusitis.
12. Identify the following structures of the oral cavity:
   —Vestibule
   —Tongue

(continues)

3

—Hard palate
  • Palatine process of the maxilla
  • Palatine bones
—Soft palate
—Uvula
—Levator veli palatinum muscle
—Palatopharyngeal muscles
—Stratified squamous epithelium
—Palatine arches
  • Palatoglossal arch
  • Palatopharyngeal arch
—Palatine tonsils

13. Identify the location and structure of the following:
—Nasopharynx
  • Pseudostratified ciliated columnar epithelium
  • Pharyngeal tonsils (adenoids)
  • Pharyngotympanic (auditory) tubes (eustachian tubes)
—Oropharynx
  • Lingual tonsil
  • Stratified squamous epithelium
  • Vallecula epiglottica
—Laryngopharynx
  • Esophagus
  • Epiglottis
  • Aryepiglottic folds
  • Stratified squamous epithelium

14. Explain the clinical connection associated with infected and swollen pharyngeal tonsils (adenoids).

15. Describe the clinical connection associated with otitis media.

16. Describe the clinical connection associated with the importance of the anatomic landmarks of the laryngopharynx and larynx when inserting an endotracheal tube.

17. Identify the following cartilages of the larynx:
—Thyroid cartilage
—Cricoid cartilage
—Epiglottis
—Arytenoid cartilages
—Corniculate cartilages
—Cuneiform cartilages

18. Identify the structure and function of the following components of the interior portion of the larynx:
—False vocal folds
—True vocal folds
—Vocal ligament
—Glottis (rima glottidis)
—Epithelial lining above and below the vocal cords

19. Discuss the clinical connection associated with laryngitis.

20. Describe the clinical connection associated with the croup syndrome.

21. Identify the structure and function of the following laryngeal muscles:
—Extrinsic muscles
  • Infrahyoid group
    ○ Sternohyoid
    ○ Sternothyroid
    ○ Thyrohyoid
    ○ Omohyoid
  • Suprahyoid group
    ○ Stylohyoid
    ○ Mylohyoid
    ○ Digastric
    ○ Geniohyoid
    ○ Stylopharyngeus
—Intrinsic muscles
  • Posterior cricoarytenoid
  • Lateral cricoarytenoid
  • Transverse arytenoid
  • Thyroarytenoid
  • Cricothyroid

22. Describe the following ventilatory functions of the larynx:
—Primary function: free flow of air
—Secondary function: Valsalva's maneuver

23. Describe the histology of the tracheobronchial tree, including the following components:
—Components of the epithelial lining (upper and lower airways)
  • Pseudostratified ciliated columnar epithelium
  • Basement membrane
  • Basal cells
  • Mucous blanket
    ○ Sol layer
    ○ Gel layer
  • Goblet cells
  • Bronchial glands (submucosal glands)
  • Mucociliary transport mechanism
—Components of the lamina propria
  • Blood vessels
  • Lymphatic vessels
  • Branches of the vagus nerve
  • Smooth-muscle fibers
  • Peribronchial sheath
  • Mast cells
    ○ Immunologic mechanism
—Cartilaginous layer

24. Describe the clinical connection associated with excessive airway secretions.
25. Describe the clinical connection associated with an abnormal mucociliary transport mechanism.
26. Identify the location (generation) and structure of the following cartilaginous airways:
   —Trachea
   —Carina
   —Main stem bronchi
   —Lobar bronchi
   —Segmental bronchi
   —Subsegmental bronchi
27. Describe the clinical connection associated with the hazards of endotracheal tubes.
28. Describe the clinical connection associated with inadvertent intubation of the right main stem bronchus.
29. Identify the location (generation) and structure of the following noncartilaginous airways:
   —Bronchioles
   —Terminal bronchioles
     • Canals of Lambert
     • Clara cells
30. Describe how the cross-sectional area of the tracheobronchial tree changes from the trachea to the terminal bronchioles.
31. Describe the structure and function of the following components of the bronchial blood supply:
   —Bronchial arteries
   —Azygos veins
   —Hemiazygos veins
   —Intercostal veins
32. Describe the structure and function of the following sites of gas exchange:
   —Respiratory bronchioles
   —Alveolar ducts
   —Alveolar sacs
   —Primary lobule
     • Acinus
     • Terminal respiratory unit
     • Lung parenchyma
     • Functional units
33. Discuss the structure and function of the following components of the alveolar epithelium:
   —Alveolar cell types
     • Type I cell (squamous pneumocyte)
     • Type II cell (granular pneumocyte)
   —Pulmonary surfactant
   —Pores of Kohn
   —Alveolar macrophages (Type III alveolar cells)

34. Describe the structure and function of the interstitium, including the:
   —Tight space
   —Loose space
35. Describe the structure and function of the following components of the pulmonary vascular system:
   —Arteries
     • Tunica intima
     • Tunica media
     • Tunica adventitia
   —Arterioles (resistance vessels)
     • Endothelial layer
     • Elastic layer
     • Smooth-muscle fibers
   —Capillaries
     • Single squamous epithelial layer
   —Venules and veins (capacitance vessels)
36. Describe the structure and function of the following components of the lymphatic system:
   —Lymphatic vessels
   —Lymphatic nodes
   —Juxta-alveolar lymphatic vessels
37. Describe how the following components of the autonomic nervous system relate to the neural control of the lungs:
   —Sympathetic nervous system
     • Neural transmitters
     • Epinephrine
     • Norepinephrine
     • Receptors
       ○ Beta$_2$ receptors
       ○ Alpha receptors
   —Parasympathetic nervous system
     • Neural transmitters
       ○ Acetylcholine
38. Identify the effects the sympathetic and parasympathetic nervous systems have on the following:
   —Heart
   —Bronchial smooth muscle
   —Bronchial glands
   —Salivary glands
   —Stomach
   —Intestines
   —Eye
39. Describe the clinical connection associated with the role of neural control agents in respiratory care.
40. Discuss the clinical connection associated with an asthmatic episode and the role of bronchodilator and anti-inflammatory drugs.

(continues)

41. Identify the following structures of the lungs:
—Apex
—Base
—Mediastinal border
—Hilum
—Specific right lung structures
  • Upper lobe
  • Middle lobe
  • Lower lobe
  • Oblique fissure
  • Horizontal fissure
—Specific left lung structures
  • Upper lobe
  • Lower lobe
  • Oblique fissure

42. Identify the following lung segments from the anterior, posterior, lateral, and medial views:
—Right lung segments
  • Upper lobe
    ○ Apical
    ○ Posterior
    ○ Anterior
  • Middle lobe
    ○ Lateral
    ○ Medial
  • Lower lobe
    ○ Superior
    ○ Medial basal
    ○ Anterior basal
    ○ Lateral basal
    ○ Posterior basal
—Left lung segments
  • Upper lobe
    ○ Upper division
      1) Apical-posterior
      2) Anterior
    ○ Lower division (lingular)
      1) Superior lingula
      2) Inferior lingula
  • Lower lobe
    ○ Superior
    ○ Anterior medial basal
    ○ Lateral basal
    ○ Posterior basal

43. Describe the clinical connection associated with postural drainage therapy.

44. Identify the following components of the mediastinum:
—Trachea
—Heart
—Major blood vessels
—Nerves
—Esophagus
—Thymus gland
—Lymph nodes

45. Identify the following components of the pleural membranes:
—Parietal pleurae
—Visceral pleurae
—Pleural cavity

46. Describe the clinical connection associated with abnormal conditions of the pleural membrane, and include:
—Pleurisy
—Friction rub
—Pleural effusion
—Empyema
—Thoracentesis

47. Describe the clinical connection associated with a pneumothorax.

48. Identify the following components of the bony thorax:
—Thoracic vertebrae
—Sternum
  • Manubrium
  • Body
  • Xiphoid process
—True ribs
—False ribs
—Floating ribs

49. Describe the clinical connection associated with the puncture site for a thoracentesis.

50. Describe the structure and function of the diaphragm and include the following:
—Hemidiaphragms
—Central tendon
—Phrenic nerves
—Lower thoracic nerves

51. Describe the structure and function of the following accessory muscles of inspiration:
—External intercostal muscles
—Scalene muscles
—Sternocleidomastoid muscles
—Pectoralis major muscles
—Trapezius muscles

52. Describe the structure and function of the following accessory muscles of expiration:
—Rectus abdominis muscles
—External abdominis obliquus muscles
—Internal abdominis obliquus muscles
—Transversus abdominis muscles
—Internal intercostal muscles

53. Complete the review questions at the end of this chapter.

The Airways

The passageways between the ambient environment and the gas exchange units of the lungs (the alveoli) are called the **conducting airways**. Although no gas exchange occurs in the conducting airways, they are, nevertheless, important to the overall process of ventilation. The conducting airways are divided into the **upper airway** and the **lower airways**.

The Upper Airway

The upper airway consists of the **nose**, **oral cavity**, **pharynx**, and **larynx** (Figure 1–1). The primary functions of the upper airway are (1) to act as a conductor of air, (2) to humidify and warm or cool the inspired air, (3) to prevent foreign materials from entering the tracheobronchial tree, and (4) to serve as an important area involved in speech and smell.

Figure 1–1

Sagittal section of human head, showing the upper airway.

© Cengage Learning 2013

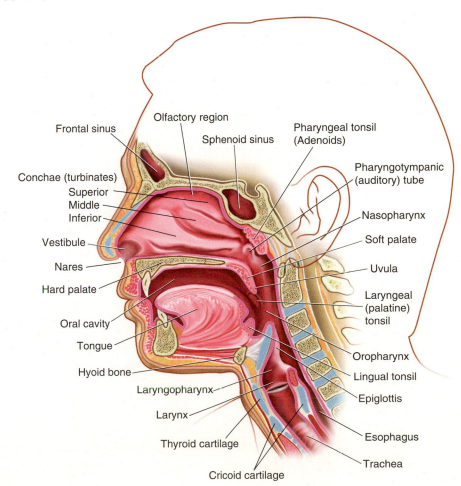

The Nose

The primary functions of the nose are to *filter*, *humidify*, and *condition (warm or cool)* inspired air. The nose is also important as the site for the sense of smell and to generate resonance in phonation.

The outer portion of the nose is composed of bone and cartilage. The upper third of the nose (the bridge) is formed by the **nasal bones** and the **frontal process** of the **maxilla**. The lower two-thirds consist of the **lateral nasal cartilage**, the **greater alar cartilage**, the **lesser alar cartilages**, the **septal cartilage**, and some **fibrous fatty tissue** (Figure 1–2).

In the internal portion of the nose a partition, the **nasal septum**, separates the nasal cavity into two approximately equal chambers. Posteriorly, the nasal septum is formed by the **perpendicular plate** of the **ethmoid bone** and by the **vomer**. Anteriorly, the septum is formed by the **septal cartilage**. The roof of the nasal cavity is formed by the **nasal bones**, the **frontal process of the maxilla**, and the **cribriform plate of the ethmoid bone**. The floor is formed by the **palatine process of the maxilla** and by the **palatine bones**—the same bones that form the hard palate of the roof of the mouth. The posterior section of the nasal cavity floor is formed by the superior portion of the **soft palate** of the oral cavity, which consists of a flexible mass of densely packed collagen fibers (Figure 1–3).

Figure 1–2

Structure of the nose.

© Cengage Learning 2013

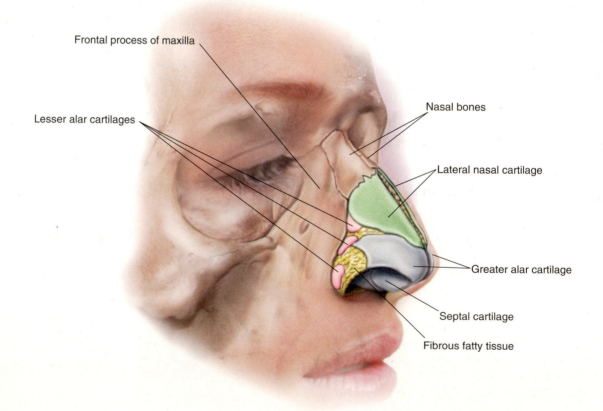

Frontal process of maxilla

Lesser alar cartilages

Nasal bones

Lateral nasal cartilage

Greater alar cartilage

Septal cartilage

Fibrous fatty tissue

Figure 1–3

Sagittal section through the nose, showing the parts of the nasal septum.

© Cengage Learning 2013

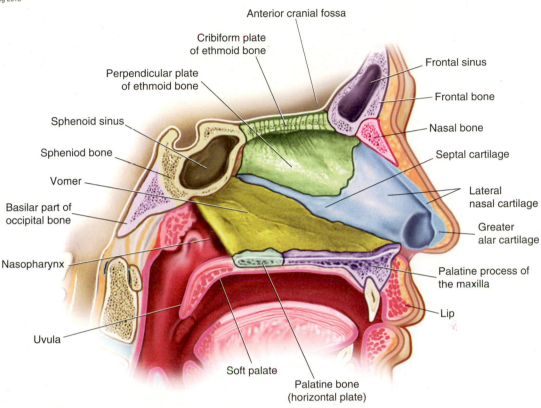

Anterior cranial fossa

Cribiform plate
of ethmoid bone

Perpendicular plate
of ethmoid bone

Sphenoid sinus

Sphenoid bone

Vomer

Basilar part of
occipital bone

Nasopharynx

Uvula

Soft palate

Palatine bone
(horizontal plate)

Frontal sinus

Frontal bone

Nasal bone

Septal cartilage

Lateral
nasal cartilage

Greater
alar cartilage

Palatine process of
the maxilla

Lip

Clinical Connection—1-1

Nasal Flaring and Alar Collapse

Nasal flaring is the widening of the nostrils during periods of respiratory difficulty. The identification of nasal flaring is considered a classic sign of respiratory discomfort—especially in the newborn infant. During periods of respiratory distress—caused by (1) increased airway resistance (e.g., asthma) or (2) lungs that are stiffer than normal (e.g., pneumonia)—the patient commonly generates a greater than normal negative pressure during each inspiration to pull air into the airways more rapidly. The widening of the nostrils further augments the movement of gas flow into the nasal passage during each inspiration (Figure 1–4A and B). Common respiratory disorders associated with nasal flaring include respiratory distress syndrome of the newborn infant, pneumonia, acute asthma, and any airway obstruction. Clinically, aggressive respiratory

Figure 1–4

A. Normal nostrils. B. Nasal flaring. C. Patient with alar collapse during exhalation. D. Patient with alar collapse during inspiration.

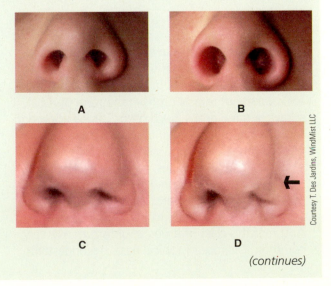

A

B

C

D

Courtesy T. Des Jardins, WindMist LLC

(continues)

Clinical Connection—1-1, continued

therapy modalities should be activated to increase the patient's arterial blood oxygen level.

The reverse of nasal flaring is called **alar collapse** and is an important sign of nasal obstruction (Figure 1–4C and D). Nasal obstruction causes the victim to be an obligate mouth breather, and is one of the causes of snoring and obstructive sleep apnea (refer to Chapter 17).

Air enters the nasal cavity through the two openings formed by the septal cartilage and the alae nasi, called the nares, or nostrils. Initially, the air passes through a slightly dilated area called the vestibule (see Figure 1–1), which contains hair follicles called vibrissae. The vibrissae function as a filter and are the tracheobronchial tree's first line of defense. Stratified squamous epithelium (nonciliated) lines the anterior one-third of the nasal cavity (Figure 1–5A). The posterior two-thirds of the nasal cavity are lined with pseudostratified ciliated columnar epithelium (Figure 1–5B). The cilia propel mucus toward the nasopharynx.

There are three bony protrusions on the lateral walls of the nasal cavity called the superior, middle, and inferior nasal turbinates, or conchae (see Figure 1-1). The turbinates separate inspired gas into several different airstreams—this action increases the contact area between the inspired air and the warm, moist surface of the nasal mucosa. The nasal mucosa has a rich supply of blood vessels and nerve endings. When the inspired air is cold, the vascular system becomes engorged with blood and warms the air. The turbinates play a major role in the humidification and warming of inspired air. The receptors for the sense of smell are located in the olfactory region, which is near the superior and middle turbinates. When the nasal mucosa nerve endings are irritated with particles—such as powder, dust, or pollen—a sneeze reflex is triggered. The two nasal passageways between the nares and the nasopharynx are also called the choanae.

Clinical Connection—1-2

The Nose—A Route of Administration for Topical Agents

Because of the large quantity of blood vessels located near the surface of the nasal mucosa, the nose serves as an excellent route of administration for a variety of topical drugs in the form of nasal sprays or nasal drops. Such drugs can be applied directly to the mucous membranes to produce a local effect, with little or no systemic absorption. For example, in cold remedies, medications like Neo-Synephrine® (phenyleprine) are commonly applied for their sympathomimetic, alpha-stimulating, and vasoconstriction effects, to treat nasal congestion. Abuse of this class of drugs is, unfortunately, very common. Overuse of topical nasal decongestants can result in the undesired effect of engorgement of the nasal membranes.

Synthetic corticosteroids—such as fluticasone, budesonide, ciclesonide, mometasone, triamcinolone, and fluticasone—are used to treat nasal mucosa inflammation. Ipratropium bromide, an anticholinergic agent, and cromolyn sodium, a mast cell stabilizing agent, are used to treat nasal congestion, sneezing, and itchy, runny nose. In addition, other medications, including influenza vaccines, can be delivered by intranasal administration.

Figure 1–5

Epithelium of the conducting airways. **A. Stratified squamous epithelium** consists of several layers of cells. This tissue is found in the anterior portion of the nasal cavity, oral cavity, oropharynx, and laryngopharynx. **B. Pseudostratified ciliated columnar epithelium** appears stratified because the nuclei of the cells are located at different levels. These cells have microscopic hairlike projections called cilia that extend from the outer surface. Mucous-producing goblet cells are also found throughout this tissue. Pseudostratified columnar ciliated epithelium lines the posterior two-thirds of the nasal cavity and the tracheobronchial tree. **C. Simple cuboidal epithelium** consists of a single layer of cube-shaped cells. These cells are found in the bronchioles. **D. Simple squamous epithelium** consists of a single layer of thin, flattened cells with broad and thin nuclei. Substances such as oxygen and carbon dioxide readily pass through this type of tissue. These cells form the walls of the alveoli and the pulmonary capillaries that surround the alveoli.

© Cengage Learning 2013

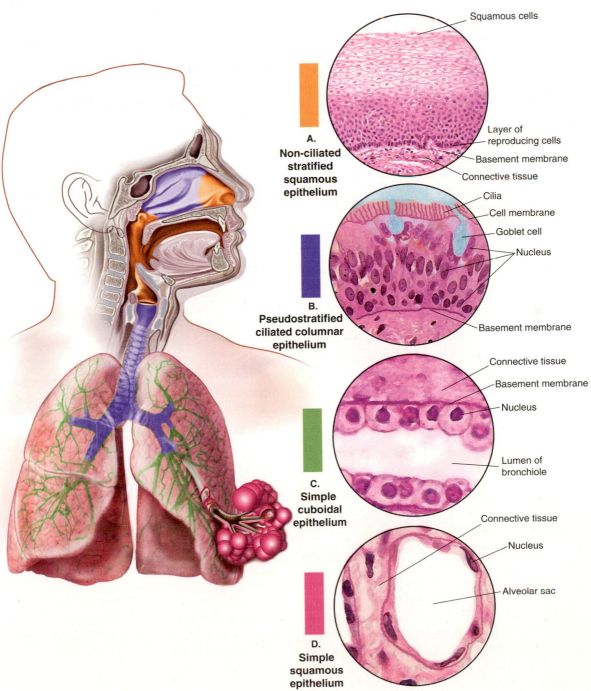

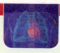

Clinical Connection—1-3

Nosebleeds (Epistaxis)

Because of the abundance and superficial location of the vascular system throughout the mucosa of the nasal cavity—especially the anterior septum area—nosebleeds are commonly seen both in and out of the hospital setting. The nosebleed may be profuse or merely a minor complication. Nosebleeds tend to occur more often during the winter months, when the air is dry and warmed from household heaters. Nosebleeds can also occur in a hot and dry climate with low humidity. In other words, nosebleeds tend to occur during periods of low humidity. Although nosebleeds may occur at any age, they are most commonly seen in children between 2 and 10 years of age and in adults between 50 and 80 years of age.

Nosebleeds are classified as either *anterior*, originating from the highly vascularized anterior septum of the nose, or *posterior*, originating from the back of the nose. **Anterior nosebleeds** make up more than 90 percent of nosebleeds and are usually stopped at home by simply pinching the nostrils closed or packing them with cotton. **Posterior nosebleeds** are much less common. The bleeding usually originates from an artery located in the back of the nasal cavity. Blood usually flows down the back of the pharynx—even when the person is sitting or standing. Posterior nosebleeds tend to occur more often in the elderly and are usually more complicated. Posterior nosebleeds can be very serious and may require hospitalization for management.

Common causes of anterior nosebleeds include trauma (e.g., a hard blow or smack to the nose), nose-picking and trauma from foreign bodies (very common in children), a difficult nasal intubation, exposure to cold and dry climates with low humidity, exposure to a hot and dry climate with low humidity, high altitudes, head colds and allergies, and certain medications. For example, individuals are more susceptible to nosebleeds when they are taking the anti-blood-clotting medication warfarin (Coumadin® or Panwarfarin®), aspirin, or any anti-inflammatory medications. Significant nosebleeds can result in these cases.

When the nosebleed is caused by dry nasal mucosa, a little water-soluble jelly, applied about 0.5 inch into the nose using a Q-tip, two to four times a day, may be helpful. Although a room humidifier may be helpful, caution must be taken to prevent the growth of molds and other allergens. Do not use a petroleum-based product (e.g., Vaseline). A petroleum-based product will dry, not moisten the nose. In the hospital setting, the respiratory therapist adds humidity to oxygen therapy when flow rates exceed 4 liters per minute.

Common causes of posterior nosebleeds include serious nose trauma (e.g., displaced broken nose from a motor vehicle accident or fall), nasal mucosal infections, high blood pressure, nasal tumors, atherosclerosis, drug abuse (e.g., cocaine), and leukemia. Treatment includes packing the nose with cotton or inserting an inflatable balloon to stop the bleeding. Cauterization of the ruptured blood vessels may be required.

Clinical Connection—1-4

Nasal Congestion and Its Influence on Taste

An individual's taste is strongly influenced by olfactory sensations. It is estimated that more than 80 percent of our taste sensation depends on the sense of smell. When the olfactory receptors in the nasal cavity are blocked by nasal congestion, the taste of food is bland. Without the sense of smell, our morning coffee would lack its richness and taste bitter. Bacon, eggs, and hot cinnamon rolls would taste bland. This is why individuals with a head cold often complain that they cannot taste their food. This phenomenon can easily be experienced by pinching one's nose to close off the nasal passages, while trying to taste a particular type of food.

Clinical Connection—1-5

Rhinitis

Rhinitis is the inflammation of the mucous membranes of the nasal cavity and is usually accompanied by swelling of the mucosa, excessive mucus production, nasal congestion, and postnasal drip. Cold viruses, streptococcal bacteria, and various allergens commonly cause rhinitis. Because the nasal mucosa extends into the nasolacrimal (tear) ducts and the passageways leading to the paranasal sinuses, a nasal cavity infection often spreads to these areas—resulting in sinusitis (see Clinical Connection 1–6: Sinusitis). When the passageways connecting the paranasal sinuses to the nasal cavity are blocked by mucus or infection—without any sinus involvement—the air in the sinus cavities is absorbed; this, in turn, results in a partial vacuum and a sinus headache.

Immediately below the superior and middle turbinates are the openings of the paranasal sinuses, which are air-filled cavities in the bones of the skull that communicate with the nasal cavity. The paranasal sinuses include the maxillary, frontal, ethmoid, and sphenoid sinuses (Figure 1–6). The paranasal sinuses produce mucus for the nasal cavity and act as resonating chambers for the production of sound.

Figure 1–6

Lateral view of the head, showing sinuses.

© Cengage Learning 2013

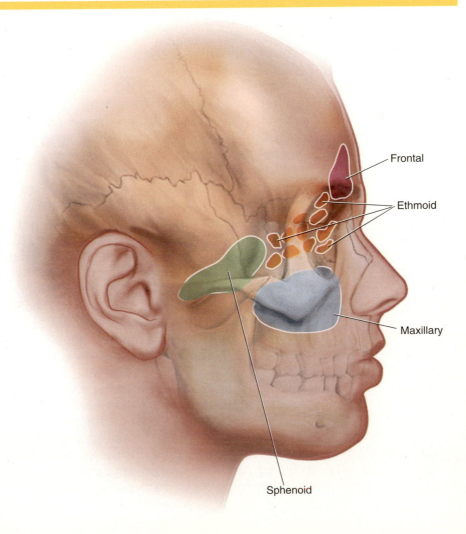

Frontal

Ethmoid

Maxillary

Sphenoid

Clinical Connection—1-6

Sinusitis

An inflammation of the mucous membrane of one or more of the paranasal sinuses is called **sinusitis**. Sinusitis can be caused by an upper respiratory infection, dental infection, atmospheric pressure changes (e.g., air travel or underwater swimming), placement of a nasal endotracheal tube, or a structural defect of the nasal cavity. When the mucous membranes become inflamed, they swell and produce excess mucus. As the swelling and mucus production intensifies, the passageways leading to the nasal cavity become partially or completely obstructed, resulting in sinus secretion accumulation. The mucus accumulation within the paranasal sinuses further promotes the development of bacterial infections. The mucus accumulation causes pressure, pain, headaches, fever, and local tenderness. Treatment consists of antibiotics to treat bacterial infections and various therapeutic modalities designed to enhance sinus drainage, such as, decongestants, hydration, and steam inhalation.

Oral Cavity

The **oral cavity** is considered an accessory respiratory passage. It consists of the **vestibule**, which is the small outer portion between the teeth (and gums) and lips, and a larger section behind the teeth and gums that extends back to the oropharynx (Figure 1–7). The **tongue** is located on the floor of the oral cavity and fills most of the oral cavity when the mouth is closed. The tongue is composed of interlacing bundles of skeletal muscles and fibers. When chewing food, the tongue holds the food and continuously repositions it between the teeth. In addition, the tongue mixes the food with saliva and forms a compact mass called a **bolus**, and then initiates swallowing by moving the bolus posteriorly into the pharynx. During speech, the tongue is used to help form consonants such as *k*, *d*, and *t*.

The tongue consists of both intrinsic and extrinsic skeletal muscle fibers. The **intrinsic muscles** are only located in the tongue and are not attached to bone. The intrinsic muscle fibers allow the tongue to change its shape—e.g., to become thinner, thicker, longer, or shorter. The intrinsic muscles are also used during speech and swallowing. The extrinsic muscles of the tongue extend from their points of origin on bones of the skull or of the soft palate. The extrinsic muscles allow the tongue to change position—e.g., protrude outward, retract inward, or to move it from side to side.

The tongue is secured to the floor of the mouth by a fold of mucosa called **lingual frenulum**. The lingual frenulum also limits posterior movements of the tongue. Taste buds are found in papillae, peg-like projections of the tongue mucosa, which give the tongue surface a slightly abrasive feel. The taste buds can be grouped into one of the following basic qualities: sweet, sour, salty, bitter, and umami (a savory taste produced by several amino acids).

The roof of the mouth is formed by the **hard** and **soft palate**. The hard palate is composed of the **palatine process of the maxilla** and the **palatine bones** (see Figure 1–3). The soft palate consists of a flexible mass of densely packed collagen fiber that projects backward and downward, ending in the soft, fleshy structure called the **uvula** (see Figure 1–7). The soft palate closes off the opening between the nasal and oral pharynx by moving upward and

Figure 1–7

Oral cavity.

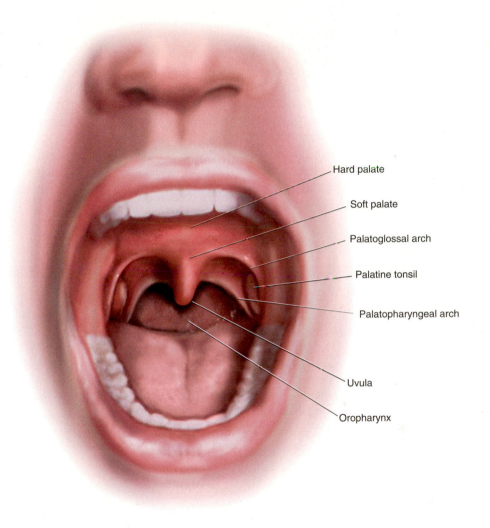

Hard palate

Soft palate

Palatoglossal arch

Palatine tonsil

Palatopharyngeal arch

Uvula

Oropharynx

backward during swallowing, sucking, and blowing and during the production of certain speech sounds. The **levator veli palatinum muscle** elevates the soft palate, and the **palatopharyngeal muscles** draw the soft palate forward and downward. The oral cavity is lined with nonciliated **stratified squamous epithelium** (see Figure 1–5A).

Two folds of mucous membrane pass along the lateral borders of the posterior portion of the oral cavity. These folds form the **palatoglossal arch** and the **palatopharyngeal arch**, named for the muscles they cover. Collectively, these arches are called the **palatine arches**. The **palatine tonsils** (faucial) are located between the palatine arches on each side of the oral cavity (see Figure 1–7). The palatine tonsils, like the pharyngeal tonsils or nasopharynx adenoids, are lymphoid tissues and are believed to serve certain immunologic defense functions.

The Pharynx

After the inspired air passes through the nasal cavity, it enters the pharynx. The **pharynx** is divided into three parts: nasopharynx, oropharynx, and laryngopharynx (see Figure 1–1).

Nasopharynx

The nasopharynx is located between the posterior portion of the nasal cavity (posterior nares) and the superior portion of the soft palate. The nasopharynx is lined with pseudostratified ciliated columnar epithelium (see Figure 1–5B). The **pharyngeal tonsil** (also call the **adenoid**) is located in the posterior nasopharynx. A tonsil is a large mass of lymphatic nodules and diffuse lymphatic tissue that protect against bacteria and other harmful substances that enter the nasopharynx. When the pharyngeal tonsil is inflamed and swollen, it may completely block the passage of air between the nose and throat (see Figure 1–1).

Clinical Connection—1-7

Infected and Swollen Pharyngeal Tonsils (Adenoids)

When the pharyngeal tonsil is infected and swollen, inspired air through the nose becomes partially or completely blocked—making it necessary to breathe through the mouth. As a result, the inspired air is not adequately humidified, warmed, or filtered before entering the lungs. A chronically enlarged pharyngeal tonsil can adversely affect speech and sleep and may require surgical removal.

The openings of the **pharyngotympanic (auditory) tubes**, formerly called the *eustachian tubes*, are located on the lateral surface of the nasopharynx. The pharyngotympanic tubes run downward to connect the middle ears to the nasopharynx and serve to equalize the pressure in the middle ear. The mucosa of the middle ear is continuous with the mucosa that lines the pharynx (throat). Normally, the pharynogotympanic tubes are flattened and closed. However, when swallowing or yawning, the tubes open briefly to equalize pressure in the middle ear cavity with internal air pressure. The ear-popping sensation of pressures equalizing is familiar to anyone who has flown in an airplane or traveled through a mountainous terrain. Inflammation and excessive mucus production in the pharyngotympanic tube may disrupt the pressure-equalizing process and impair hearing. This problem is frequently seen in young children with **otitis media** (i.e., ear infection).

Oropharynx

The oropharynx lies between the soft palate superiorly and the base of the tongue inferiorly (at the level of the hyoid bone) (see Figure 1–1). Two groups of tonsils are located in the oropharynx. The **palatine tonsils**—which are

Clinical Connection—1-8

Otitis Media

Otitis media, or **middle ear infection**, is fairly common in young children with a recent history of a sore throat. These infections usually develop from an infection of mucous membranes of the pharynx that spreads through the pharyngotympanic (auditory) tubes to the mucous lining of the middle ear. In young children, the pharyngotympanic tubes are shorter and run more horizontally. This is because the head of a young child is usually more round in shape. This round shape of the head causes the pharyngotympanic tubes to be more horizontal—which cannot always drain adequately when they become infected. As the child grows older, the head becomes more oval in shape and the auditory tubes shift downward, or become more vertical in the upright position.

The symptoms of otitis media consist of a low-grade fever, lethargy, and irritability—symptoms that are often not easily recognized by a parent as being a middle ear infection. Otitis media is the most frequent cause of hearing loss in young children and is a result of fluid buildup that dampens the tympanic membrane, or eardrum. During an acute middle ear infection, the eardrum bulges and becomes inflamed and red. Most cases of otitis media are treated with antibiotics. When large amounts of fluid or pus accumulate in the middle ear, a *myringotomy* (lancing of the eardrum) may be performed to relieve the pressure. A tiny tube inserted in the eardrum permits drainage into the external ear. The tube usually falls out on its own within a year.

usually referred to as "the tonsils"—are relatively large, oval in shape, located on each side of the oral cavity between the palatopharyngeal arch and the palatoglossal arch (see Figure 1–6).

The **lingual tonsil** is a loosely associated collection of lymphatic nodules located on the posterior, base of the tongue. The mucosa of the oropharynx is composed of nonciliated stratified squamous epithelium (see Figure 1–5A). The **vallecula epiglottica** is located between the glossoepiglottic folds on each side of the posterior oropharynx. It appears as a depression or crevice that runs from the base of the tongue to the epiglottis (Figure 1–8 on page 18). The vallecula epiglottica is an important anatomic landmark during the insertion of an endotracheal tube into the trachea (see next section for more information about endotracheal tubes).

Laryngopharynx

The **laryngopharynx** (also called the hypopharynx) lies between the base of the tongue and the entrance of the **esophagus**. The laryngopharynx is lined with noncilated stratified squamous epithelium (see Figure 1–5A). The epiglottis, the upper part of the larynx, is positioned directly anterior to the laryngopharynx (see Figure 1–1). The **aryepiglottic folds** are mucous membrane folds that extend around the margins of the larynx from the epiglottis. They function as a sphincter during swallowing. Clinically, the major structures associated with the laryngopharynx are often viewed from above using a laryngoscope while the patient is supine—especially note the close proximity of the epiglottis, vocal cords, and esophagus (see Figure 1–8).

Image A © Cengage Learning 2013

Figure 1–8

A. View of the base of the tongue, vallecula epiglottica, epiglottis, and vocal cords. **B.** Photo of the vocal cords.

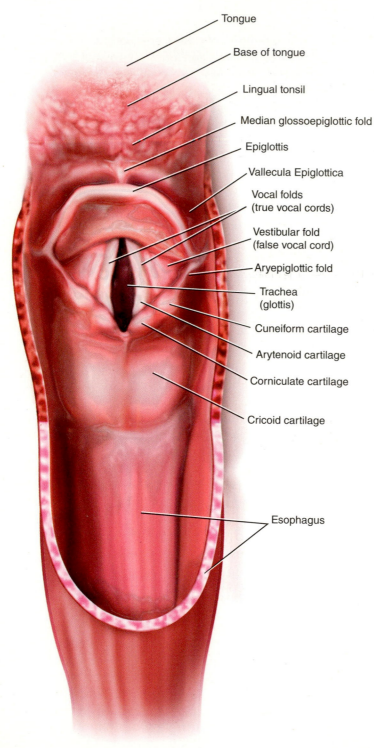

Tongue

Base of tongue

Lingual tonsil

Median glossoepiglottic fold

Epiglottis

Vallecula Epiglottica

Vocal folds
(true vocal cords)

Vestibular fold
(false vocal cord)

Aryepiglottic fold

Trachea
(glottis)

Cuneiform cartilage

Arytenoid cartilage

Corniculate cartilage

Cricoid cartilage

Esophagus

A

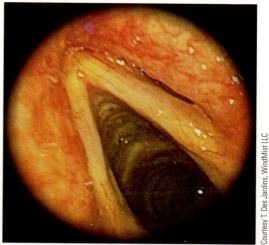

B

Courtesy T. Des Jardins, WindMist LLC

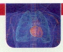

Clinical Connection—1-9

Endotracheal Tubes

In the clinical setting, the respiratory therapist frequently bypasses the entire upper airway to better *ventilate* and *oxygenate* the patient. A **nasal endotracheal tube**, an **oral endotracheal tube**, or a **tracheostomy tube** can be used to by-pass the patient's upper airway (Figure 1–9). When an endotracheal tube is in place, the gas being delivered to the patient must be appropriately *warmed* and *humidified*. Failure to do so dehydrates the mucous layer of the tracheobronchial tree, which in turn causes the mucous layer to become thick and immobile and the mucous itself to become thick and sticky.

The respiratory therapist must learn—and differentiate—the major anatomic landmarks of the laryngopharynx and larynx (e.g., vallecula, epiglottis, esophagus, vocal folds, and trachea), especially when inserting an endotracheal tube. An endotracheal tube can easily be inserted into the patient's esophagus rather than into the trachea, especially during an emergency situation. When this occurs, the patient's stomach—rather than lungs—is ventilated. A misplaced endotracheal tube in the esophagus can be fatal (Figure 1–10 on page 20).

Figure 1–9

An oral endotracheal tube placed in proper position in the trachea. The inflated cuff at the tip of the tube separates the lower airways from the upper airway.

© Cengage Learning 2013

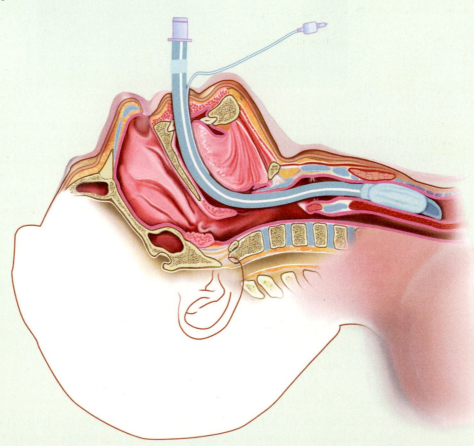

(continues)

Clinical Connection—1-9, continued

Figure 1–10

A. An endotracheal tube misplaced in patient's esophagus. Note that the endotracheal tube is positioned to the right (patient's left) of the spinal column. Clinically, this is an excellent sign that the tube is in the esophagus. **B.** Stomach inflated with air.

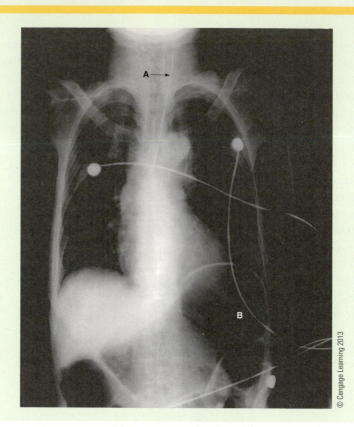

© Cengage Learning 2013

The laryngopharyngeal musculature receives its sensory innervation from the ninth cranial (glossopharyngeal) nerve and its motor innervation from the tenth cranial (vagus) nerve. When stimulated, these muscles and nerves work together to produce the **pharyngeal reflex** (also called the "gag" or "swallowing" reflex), which helps to prevent the aspiration of foods and liquids. It also helps to prevent the base of the tongue from falling back and obstructing the laryngopharynx, even in the person who is asleep in the supine position.

The Larynx

The **larynx**, or voice box, is located between the base of the tongue and the upper end of the trachea (see Figure 1–1). The larynx is commonly described as a vestibule opening into the trachea from the pharynx. The larynx serves three functions: (1) it acts as a passageway of air between the pharynx and the trachea, (2) it serves as a protective mechanism against the aspiration of solids and liquids, and (3) it generates sounds for speech.

Cartilages of the Larynx

The larynx consists of a framework of nine cartilages (Figure 1–11). Three are single cartilages: **thyroid cartilage**, **cricoid cartilage**, and the **epiglottis**. Three are paired cartilages: **arytenoid**, **corniculate**, and **cuneiform cartilages** (see Figure 1–11A, B). The cartilages of the larynx are held in position by ligaments, membranes, and **intrinsic** and **extrinsic muscles**. The interior of the larynx is lined with mucous membrane.

Figure 1–11

Cartilages and intrinsic muscles of the larynx.

LARYNGEAL CARTILAGES

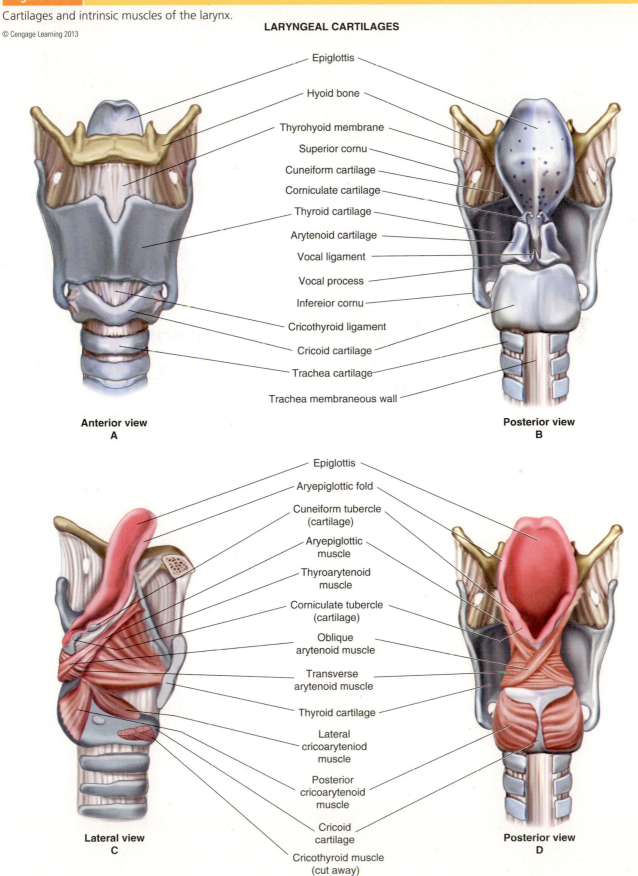

Epiglottis

Hyoid bone

Thyrohyoid membrane

Superior cornu

Cuneiform cartilage

Corniculate cartilage

Thyroid cartilage

Arytenoid cartilage

Vocal ligament

Vocal process

Infereior cornu

Cricothyroid ligament

Cricoid cartilage

Trachea cartilage

Trachea membraneous wall

Anterior view
A

Posterior view
B

Epiglottis

Aryepiglottic fold

Cuneiform tubercle
(cartilage)

Aryepiglottic
muscle

Thyroarytenoid
muscle

Corniculate tubercle
(cartilage)

Oblique
arytenoid muscle

Transverse
arytenoid muscle

Thyroid cartilage

Lateral
cricoaryteniod
muscle

Posterior
cricoarytenoid
muscle

Cricoid
cartilage

Cricothyroid muscle
(cut away)

Lateral view
C

Posterior view
D

INTRINSIC MUSCLES OF THE LARYNX

The thyroid cartilage (commonly called the Adam's apple) is the largest cartilage of the larynx. It is a double-winged structure that spreads over the anterior portion of the larynx. Along its superior border is a V-shaped notch, the **thyroid notch**. The upper portion of the thyroid cartilage is suspended from the horseshoe-shaped hyoid bone by the **thyro-hyoid membrane**. Technically, the hyoid bone is not a part of the larynx.

The epiglottis is a broad, spoon-shaped fibrocartilaginous structure. Normally, it prevents the aspiration of foods and liquids by covering the opening of the larynx during swallowing. The epiglottis and the base of the tongue are connected by folds of mucous membranes, which form a small space (the vallecula) between the epiglottis and the base of the tongue. Clinically, the vallecula serves as an important anatomic landmark when inserting an endotracheal tube (see Figure 1–8).

The cricoid cartilage is shaped like a signet ring. It is located inferior to the thyroid cartilage and forms a large portion of the posterior wall of the larynx. The inferior border of the cricoid cartilage is attached to the first C-shaped cartilage of the trachea (see Figure 1–11).

The paired arytenoid cartilages are shaped like a three-sided pyramid. The base of each arytenoid cartilage rests on the superior surface of the posterior portion of the cricoid cartilage. The apex of each arytenoid cartilage curves posteriorly and medially and flattens for articulation with the corniculate cartilages. At the base of each arytenoid cartilage is a projection called the **vocal process**. The **vocal ligaments**, which form the medial portion of the vocal folds, attach to the vocal process.

The paired cuneiform cartilages and corniculate cartilages are small accessory cartilages that are closely associated with the arytenoid cartilages. The cuneiform cartilages are embedded within the aryepiglottic folds that extend from the apices of the arytenoid cartilages to the epiglottis. They probably act to stiffen the folds. The two corniculate cartilages lie superior to the arytenoid cartilages.

Interior of the Larynx

The interior portion of the larynx is lined by a mucous membrane that forms two pairs of folds that protrude inward. The upper pair are called the **false vocal folds** because they play no role in vocalization. The lower pair functions as the **true vocal folds** (vocal cords). The medial border of each vocal fold is composed of a strong band of elastic tissue called the **vocal ligament**. Anteriorly, the vocal cords attach to the posterior surface of the thyroid cartilage. Posteriorly, the vocal folds attach to the vocal process of the arytenoid cartilage. The arytenoid cartilages can rotate about a vertical axis through the cricoarytenoid joint, allowing the medial border to move anteriorly or posteriorly. This action, in turn, loosens or tightens the true vocal cords.

The space between the true vocal cords is termed the **rima glottidis** or, for ease of reference, the **glottis** (see Figure 1–8). In the adult, the glottis is the narrowest point in the larynx. In the infant, the cricoid cartilage is the narrowest point. Glottic and subglottic swelling (edema) secondary to viral or bacterial infection is commonly seen in infants and young children, and is known as the **croup syndrome**.

Clinical Connection—1-10

Laryngitis

Laryngitis is an inflammation of the mucous membrane lining the larynx, accompanied by swelling and edema of the vocal cords. This condition causes hoarseness or complete loss of voice. Laryngitis can be caused by a number of things, including heavy smoking, bacterial infections, very dry air, inhalation of irritating fumes, sudden temperature changes, overuse of the voice, and tumors. Of particular importance to the respiratory therapist is the laryngitis caused by **post-extubation laryngeal edema**. Because the endotracheal tube is placed between the vocal cords of the larynx for extended periods of time, the vocal cords often have some degree of trauma, edema, and swelling.

In response to acute laryngitis, the patient may have a cough or may complain of a sore, scratchy throat. In young children, acute laryngitis may cause severe respiratory distress. This is because the relatively small vocal cords of the young child have a tendency to spasm when they become irritated, inflamed, or infected. In these cases, partial or complete airway obstruction can occur. Treatment consists of an aerosolized alpha-adrenergic drug, such as racemic epinephrine—the treatment of choice for post-extubation laryngeal edema—high humidification (vaporized cool mists and steam inhalation), avoidance of any irritants (e.g., smoke, fumes, dust), voice rest, cough medication, and antiseptic throat sprays.

Clinical Connection—1-11

Croup Syndrome

A common clinical manifestation seen in children is **croup** (also called **inspiratory stridor**). The term croup is a general term used to describe the inspiratory, barking or brassy sound associated with a partial upper airway obstruction—in short, a croup sound is a "clinical sign." The two major causes of croup—that is, a barking or brassy inspiratory sound—are **laryngotracheobronchitis** (LTB) and **acute epiglottitis**.

Acute epiglottitis is a supraglottic airway obstruction resulting from inflammation of the epiglottitis, aryepiglottic folds, and false vocal folds—**and is a life-threatening emergency!** Acute epiglottitis is almost always caused by a bacterial infection of **Haemophilus influenzae type B** (Figure 1–12A on page 24). Figure 1–12B shows a lateral X-ray of a 27-year-old man with severe epiglottitis.

LTB is a subglottic airway obstruction; acute epiglottitis is a supraglottic airway obstruction (see Figure 1–13A on page 24). Pathologically, LTB is an inflammatory process that causes edema and swelling of the mucous membranes below the glottis. Figure 1–13B shows a chest X-ray of a 3-year-old patient with a LTB obstruction. The **parainfluenza virus** causes most LTB cases.

Aerosolized **racemic epinephrine** is commonly used to treat LTB for its alpha-adrenergic stimulation—which causes mucosal vascular constriction. This action, in turn, reduces the edema and swelling of the airway—in short, racemic epinephrine widens the subglottic airway. Racemic epinephrine has long been recognized as an effective and safe aerosol decongestant. In patients with a suspected acute epiglottitis, an examination of the pharynx and larynx is absolutely contraindicated, except in the operating room with a fully trained team in attendance.

(continues)

Clinical Connection—1-11, continued

Figure 1–12

A. Acute epiglottitis (swollen epiglottis). **B.** A 27-year-old male with severe epiglottis (arrow) caused by crack cocaine abuse and upper neck and head trauma from a motorcycle accident.

Image A © Cengage Learning 2013

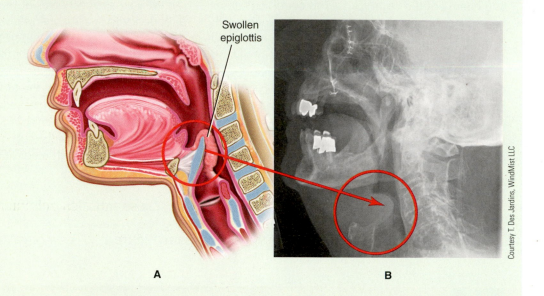

Swollen epiglottis

A   B

Courtesy T. Des Jardins, WindMist LLC

Figure 1–13

A. LTB, swollen trachea tissue below the vocal cords. **B.** Close-up of neck on a chest X-ray of a 3-year-old patient with a subglottic airway narrowing.

© Cengage Learning 2013

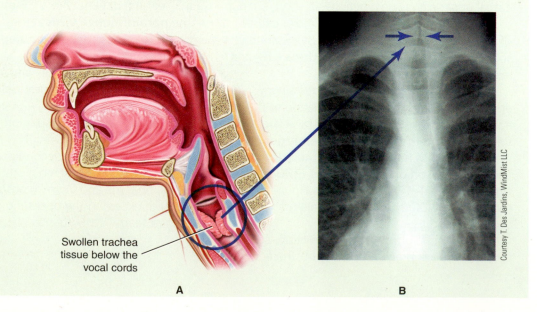

Swollen trachea tissue below the vocal cords

A   B

Courtesy T. Des Jardins, WindMist LLC

Above the vocal cords, the laryngeal mucosa is composed of (noncilated) stratified squamous epithelium (see Figure 1–5A). Below the vocal cords, the laryngeal mucosa is covered by pseudostratified ciliated columnar epithelium (see Figure 1–5B).

Laryngeal Musculature

The muscles of the larynx consist of the extrinsic and intrinsic muscle groups. The extrinsic muscles are subdivided into an infrahyoid and a suprahyoid group. The infrahyoid group consists of the sternohyoid, sternothyroid, thyrohyoid, and omohyoid muscles (Figure 1–14). These muscles pull the larynx and hyoid bone down to a lower position in the neck. The suprahyoid group consists of the stylohyoid, mylohyoid, digastric, geniohyoid, and stylopharyngeus muscles. These muscles pull the hyoid bone forward, upward, and backward—which can be seen when a person swallows (see Figure 1–14). The major intrinsic muscles that control the movement of the vocal folds are illustrated in Figure 1–11C, D. The action(s) of these muscles are described next.

Posterior Cricoarytenoid Muscles. These muscles pull inferiorly on the lateral angles of the arytenoids, causing the vocal folds to move apart (abduct) and thus allowing air to pass through (Figure 1–15A on page 26).

Figure 1–14

Extrinsic laryngeal muscles.

© Cengage Learning 2013

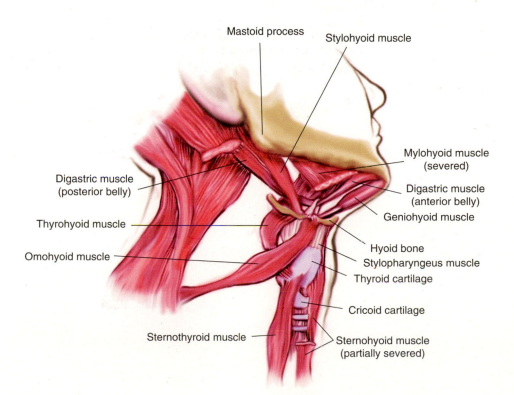

© Cengage Learning 2013

Figure 1–15

Intrinsic laryngeal muscles.

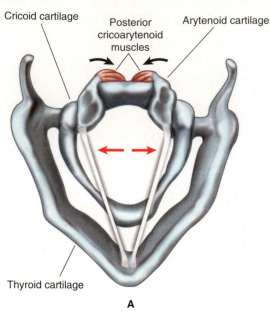

Cricoid cartilage

Posterior cricoarytenoid muscles

Arytenoid cartilage

Thyroid cartilage

A

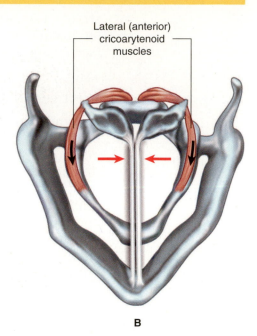

Lateral (anterior) cricoarytenoid muscles

B

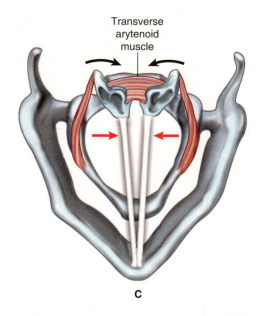

Transverse arytenoid muscle

C

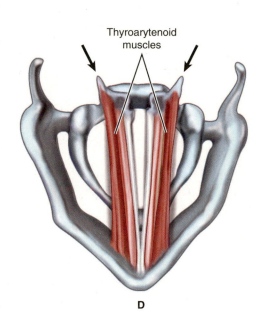

Thyroarytenoid muscles

D

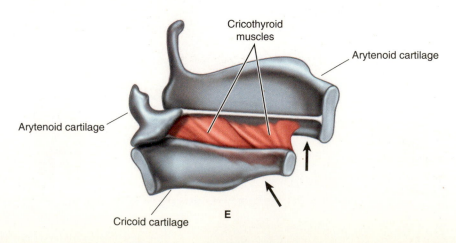

Cricothyroid muscles

Arytenoid cartilage

Arytenoid cartilage

Cricoid cartilage

E

Lateral Cricoarytenoid Muscles. The action of these muscles opposes that of the posterior cricoarytenoid muscles. These muscles pull laterally on the lateral angles of the arytenoids, causing the vocal folds to move together (adduct) (Figure 1–15B).

Transverse Arytenoid Muscles. These muscles pull the arytenoid cartilages together and thereby position the two vocal folds so that they vibrate as air passes between them during exhalation, thus generating the sounds for speech or singing (Figure 1–15C).

Thyroarytenoid Muscles. These muscles lie in the vocal folds lateral to the vocal ligaments. Contraction of the thyroarytenoid muscles pulls the arytenoid cartilages forward. This action loosens the vocal ligaments and allows a lower frequency of phonation (Figure 1–15D).

Cricothyroid Muscles. These muscles, which are located on the anterior surface of the larynx, can swing the entire thyroid cartilage anteriorly. This action provides an additional way to tense the vocal folds and thereby change the frequency of phonation (Figure 1–15E).

Ventilatory Function of the Larynx

A primary function of the larynx is to ensure a free flow of air to and from the lungs. During a quiet inspiration, the vocal folds move apart (abduct) and widen the glottis. During exhalation, the vocal folds move slightly toward the midline (adduct) but always maintain an open glottal airway.

A second vital function of the larynx is effort closure during exhalation, also known as Valsalva's maneuver. During this maneuver, there is a massive undifferentiated adduction of the laryngeal walls, including both the true and false vocal folds. As a result, the lumen of the larynx is tightly sealed, preventing air from escaping during physical work such as lifting, pushing, coughing, throat-clearing, vomiting, urination, defecation, and parturition.

The Lower Airways

The Tracheobronchial Tree

After passing through the larynx, inspired air enters the tracheobronchial tree, which consists of a series of branching airways commonly referred to as generations, or orders. These airways become progressively narrower, shorter, and more numerous as they branch throughout the lungs (Figure 1–16 on page 28). Table 1–1 on page 28 lists the major subdivisions of the tracheobronchial tree.

In general, the airways exist in two major forms: (1) cartilaginous airways and (2) noncartilaginous airways. (The main structures of these airways are discussed in detail on pages 27–42.) The cartilaginous airways serve only to conduct air between the external environment and the sites of gas exchange. The noncartilaginous airways serve both as conductors of air and as sites of gas exchange. These will be discussed in detail later.

Histology of the Tracheobronchial Tree

The tracheobronchial tree is composed of three layers: an epithelial lining, the lamina propria, and a cartilaginous layer (Figure 1–17 on page 29).

Figure 1–16

Tracheobronchial tree.

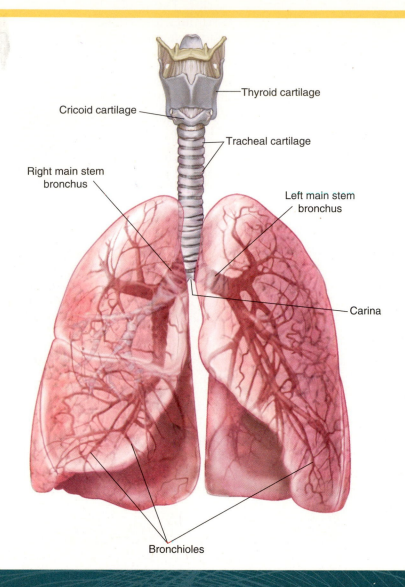

- Thyroid cartilage
- Cricoid cartilage
- Tracheal cartilage
- Right main stem bronchus
- Left main stem bronchus
- Carina
- Bronchioles

Table 1–1

Major Structures and Corresponding Generations of the Tracheobronchial Tree

	Structures of the Lungs	Generations*	
Conducting Zone	Trachea	0	Cartilaginous airways
	Main stem bronchi	1	
	Lobar bronchi	2	
	Segmental bronchi	3	
	Subsegmental bronchi	4–9	
	Bronchioles	10–15	Noncartilaginous airways
	Terminal bronchioles	16–19	
Respiratory Zone	Respiratory bronchioles†	20–23	Sites of gas exchange
	Alveolar ducts†	24–27	
	Alveolar sacs†	28	

* NOTE: The precise number of generations between the subsegmental bronchi and the alveolar sacs is not known.

† These structures collectively are referred to as a primary lobule (see pages 42–45) or lung parenchyma; they are also called terminal respiratory units and functional units.

Figure 1–17

Histology of the tracheobronchial tree.

© Cengage Learning 2013

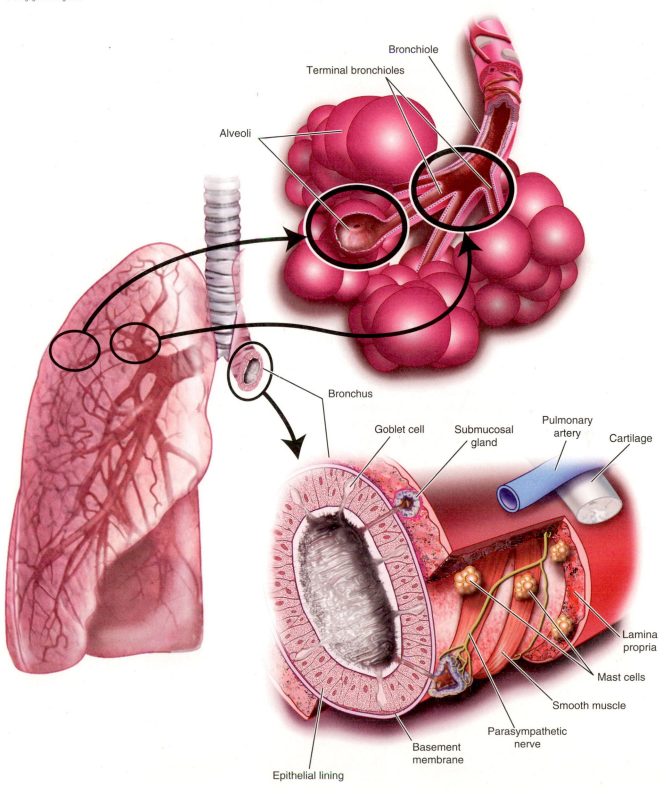

The Epithelial Lining. The epithelial lining is predominantly composed of pseudostratified ciliated columnar epithelium interspersed with numerous mucous glands and separated from the lamina propria by a basement membrane (see Figure 1–17). Along the basement membrane of the epithelial lining are oval-shaped basal cells. These cells serve as a reserve supply of cells and replenish the superficial ciliated cells and mucous cells as needed.

The pseudostratified ciliated columnar epithelium extends from the trachea to the respiratory bronchioles. There are about 200 cilia per ciliated cell. The length of each cilium is about 5 to 7 mm (microns). As the bronchioles become progressively smaller, the columnar structure of the epithelium decreases in height and appears more cuboidal than columnar (see Figure 1–5C). The cilia progressively disappear in the terminal bronchioles and are completely absent in the respiratory bronchioles.

A mucous layer, commonly referred to as the mucous blanket, covers the epithelial lining of the tracheobronchial tree (Figure 1–18).

In general, the mucous blanket is composed of 95 percent water, with the remaining 5 percent consisting of glycoproteins, carbohydrates, lipids, DNA, some cellular debris, and foreign particles. The mucous is produced by (1) the goblet cells, and (2) the submucosal, or bronchial, glands (see Figure 1–17). The goblet cells are located intermittently between the pseudostratified ciliated columnar cells and have been identified down to, and including, the terminal bronchioles. They empty when stimulated by infection or inhaled smoke or dust. The submucosal glands, which produce most of the mucous blanket, extend deep into the lamina propria. These glands are innervated by the vagal parasympathetic nerve fibers (the tenth cranial nerve) and produce about 100 mL of bronchial secretions per day. Increased sympathetic activity decreases glandular secretions. The submucosal glands are particularly numerous in the medium-sized bronchi and disappear in the distal terminal bronchioles (see Figure 1–18).

Figure 1–18

Epithelial lining of the tracheobronchial tree.

© Cengage Learning 2013

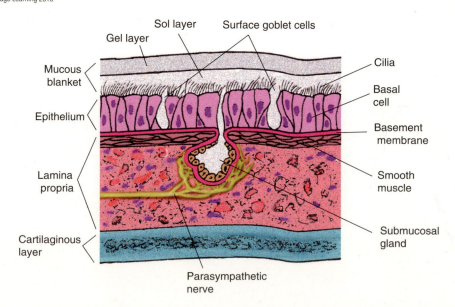

Clinical Connection—1-12

Excessive Airway Secretions

Bronchial irritation, inflammation, and excessive bronchial secretions commonly develop in a number of respiratory disorders—such as cystic fibrosis (Figure 1–19). If left untreated, thick and immobile secretions rapidly lead to (1) excessive accumulation, (2) partial airway obstruction and air trapping, (3) alveolar hyperinflation, or (4) complete airway obstruction and airway collapse. The respiratory therapist must always be aware that excessive bronchial secretions can adversely affect—or completely block—alveolar gas exchange. Various respiratory therapy modalities—such as postural drainage and chest percussion—should be activated as soon as

possible to correct any of the problems associated with excessive airway secretions.

Excessive airway secretions also increase the patient's airway resistance to gas flow and, therefore, diminish the cough effectiveness. In addition, bacterial infections of the airways are more likely when excessive bronchial secretions are chronically present. When a bacterial infection is present, the patient's secretions will appear green and yellow. At the bedside, patients with excessive airway secretions commonly demonstrate a noisy, moist-sounding cough. The cough usually produces secretions. When listening to the patient's chest

---

Figure 1–19

Cystic fibrosis. Pathology includes (1) excessive production and accumulation of thick bronchial secretions, (2) partial bronchial obstruction and air trapping, (3) alveolar hyperinflation, and (4) complete airway obstruction and alveolar collapse.

© Cengage Learning 2013

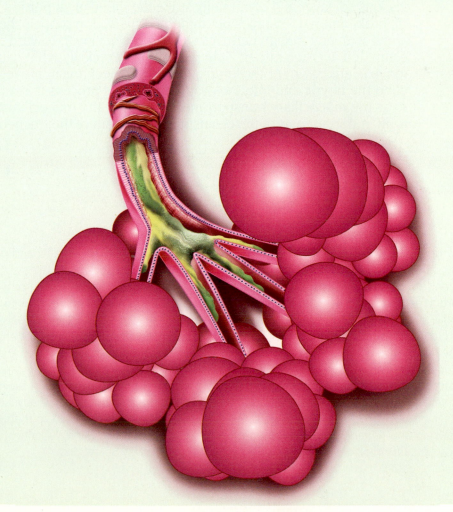

(continues)

Clinical Connection—1-12, continued

with a stethoscope, coarse, "bubbly" sounds (called rhonchi) are often heard over large airways during exhalation. In addition, over the small and medium-sized airways, fine and crackling wet sounds (called crackles) are typically heard during inspiration.

Depending on the nature and severity of the disorder, the bronchial secretions may take several forms. For example, during the early stages of bronchitis, the secretions usually appear clear, thin, and odorless. During the late stages, the secretions are often copious, thick, and yellow and green in appearance—the classic sign of bacterial infection.

Clinically, there are many good therapeutic approaches used to mobilize excessive bronchial secretions. These therapies include (1) postural drainage therapy (the use of patient positioning to enhance gravitational drainage, may also be accompanied with chest percussion or vibration), (2) cough and deep breathing techniques, (3) positive airway pressure therapies (e.g., positive airway pressure [PAP] or continuous positive airway pressure [CPAP]), (4) high-frequency compression/oscillation mechanical ventilation procedures, (5) mobilization and exercise techniques, and (6) tracheobronchial tree suctioning.

The viscosity of the mucous blanket progressively increases from the epithelial lining to the inner luminal surface. The blanket has two distinct layers: (1) the sol layer, which is adjacent to the epithelial lining, and (2) the gel layer, which is the more viscous layer adjacent to the inner luminal surface. Under normal circumstances, the cilia move in a wavelike fashion through the less viscous sol layer and continually strike the inner-most portion of the gel layer (approximately 1500 times per minute). This action propels the mucous layer, along with any foreign particles stuck to the gel layer, toward the larynx at an estimated average rate of 2 cm per minute. Precisely what causes the cilia to move is unknown. At the larynx, the cough mechanism moves secretions beyond the larynx and into the oropharynx. This process is commonly referred to as the mucociliary transport mechanism, or the mucociliary escalator, and is an important part of the cleansing mechanism of the tracheobronchial tree.

Clinical Connection—1-13

Abnormal Mucociliary Transport Mechanism

There are a number of abnormal conditions that can significantly slow the rate of the mucociliary transport mechanisms. Such conditions include the excessive bronchial secretions associated with chronic bronchitis, emphysema, bronchiectasis, and cystic fibrosis. Additional risk factors known to irritate and inflame the bronchial airways are tobacco smoke, dehydration, positive-pressure ventilation, endotracheal suctioning, high inspired oxygen concentrations, hypoxia, occupational dusts, irritating chemical vapors, indoor air pollution (e.g., biomass fuel used for cooking and heating), outdoor air pollution (e.g., silicates, sulfur dioxide, nitrogen oxides, and ozone), general anesthetic, and parasympatholytic drugs (e.g., atropine).

When the mucociliary escalator is compromised, coughing is the only means to mobilize secretions. For this reason, individuals with a depressed mucociliary transport—for any reason—should avoid medications that depress the cough reflex. In addition, the respiratory care practitioner will likely need to activate and/or up-regulate the patient's bronchial hygiene therapy (see common therapeutic approaches used to mobilize excessive bronchial secretions, Clinical Connection 1-12: Excessive Airway Secretions).

The Lamina Propria. The lamina propria is the submucosal layer of the tracheobronchial tree. Within the lamina propria there is a loose, fibrous tissue that contains tiny blood vessels, lymphatic vessels, and branches of the vagus nerve. Also found within the lamina propria are two sets of smooth-muscle fibers. These sets of muscles wrap around the tracheobronchial tree in fairly close spirals, one clockwise and the other counterclockwise. The smooth-muscle fibers extend down to, and include, the alveolar ducts (see the section on sites of gas exchange in this chapter). The outer portion of the lamina propria is surrounded by a thin connective tissue layer called the peribronchial sheath.

Immune Response. Mast cells play an important role in the immunologic mechanism. Mast cells are found in the lamina propria—near the branches of the vagus nerve and blood vessels and scattered throughout the smooth-muscle bundles, in the intra-alveolar septa, and as one of the cell constituents of the submucosal glands (Figure 1–20). Outside of the lungs, mast cells are found in the loose connective tissue of the skin and intestinal submucosa.

When they are activated, numerous substances are released from the mast cells that can significantly alter the diameter of the bronchial airways. Because of this fact, a basic understanding of how the mast cells function in the immunologic system is essential for the respiratory care practitioner.

Figure 1–20

Cross-section of a bronchus showing the mast cells in the lamina propria.

© Cengage Learning 2013

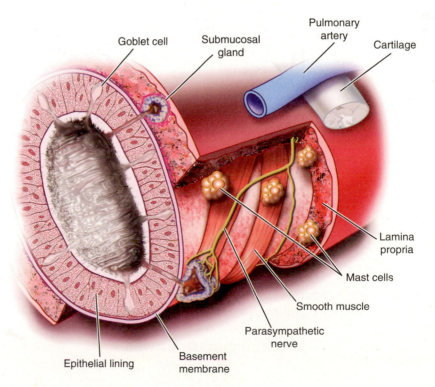

There are two major immune responses: cellular immunity and humoral immunity. The cellular immune response involves the sensitized lymphocytes that are responsible for tissue rejection in transplants. This immune response is also termed a type IV, or delayed, type of hypersensitivity.

The humoral immune response involves the circulating antibodies that are involved in allergic responses such as allergic asthma. Antibodies (also called immunoglobulins) are serum globulins, or proteins, that defend against invading environmental antigens such as pollen, animal dander, and feathers. Although five different immunoglobulins (IgG, IgA, IgM, IgD, and IgE) have been identified, the IgE (reaginic) antibody is basic to the allergic response. The mechanism of the IgE antibody-antigen reaction is as follows:

1. When a susceptible individual is exposed to a certain antigen, the lymphoid tissues release specific IgE antibodies. The newly formed IgE antibodies travel through the bloodstream and attach to surface receptors on the mast cells. It is estimated that there are between 100,000 and 500,000 IgE receptor sites on the surface of each mast cell. Once the IgE antibodies attach to the mast cell, the individual (or more specifically, the mast cell) is said to be sensitive to the specific antigen (Figure 1–21A).

2. Each mast cell also has about 1000 secretory granules that contain several chemical mediators of inflammation. Continued exposure, or reexposure, to the same antigen creates an IgE antibody–antigen reaction on the surface of the mast cell, which works to destroy or inactivate the antigen. This response, however, causes the mast cell to degranulate (break down) and to release the following chemical mediators (Figure 1–21B):
   a. Histamine
   b. Heparin
   c. Platelet-activating factor (PAF)
   d. Eosinophilic chemotactic factor of anaphylaxis (ECF-A)
   e. Leukotrienes.

3. The release of these chemical mediators causes increased vascular permeability, smooth-muscle contraction, increased mucous secretion, and vasodilation with edema.

Such a reaction in the lungs can be extremely dangerous and is seen in individuals during an allergic asthmatic episode. The production of IgE antibodies may be 20 times greater than normal in some patients with asthma (the normal IgE antibody level in the serum is about 200 ng/mL). During an asthmatic attack, the patient demonstrates bronchial edema, bronchospasms and wheezing, increased mucous production, mucous plugging, air trapping, and lung hyperinflation (Figure 1–21C).

The Cartilaginous Layer. The cartilaginous layer, which is the outer-most layer of the tracheobronchial tree, progressively diminishes in size as the airways extend into the lungs. Cartilage is completely absent in bronchioles less than 1 mm in diameter (see Figure 1–17).

The Cartilaginous Airways

As shown in Table 1–1, the cartilaginous airways consist of the trachea, main stem bronchi, lobar bronchi, segmental bronchi, and subsegmental bronchi. Collectively, the cartilaginous airways are referred to as the conducting zone.

Figure 1–21

Immunologic mechanisms.

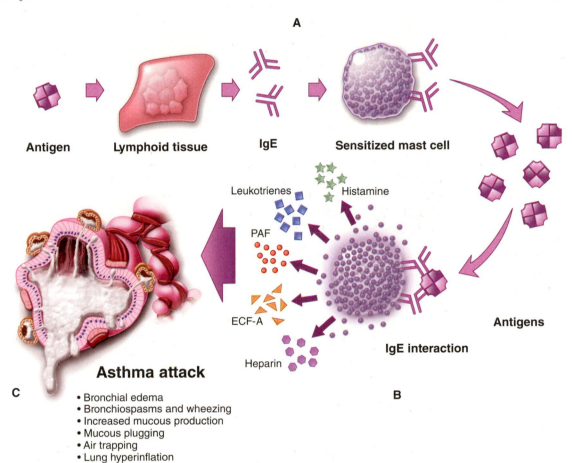

A

Antigen Lymphoid tissue IgE Sensitized mast cell

Leukotrienes Histamine

PAF

ECF-A Antigens

IgE interaction

Heparin

Asthma attack

C **B**

• Bronchial edema
• Bronchiospasms and wheezing
• Increased mucous production
• Mucous plugging
• Air trapping
• Lung hyperinflation

Trachea. The adult trachea is about 11 to 13 cm long and 1.5 to 2.5 cm in diameter (Figure 1–22 on page 36). It extends vertically from the cricoid cartilage of the larynx to about the level of the second costal cartilage, or fifth thoracic vertebra. At this point, the trachea divides into the right and left main stem bronchi. The bifurcation of the trachea is known as the carina. Approximately 15 to 20 C-shaped cartilages support the trachea. These cartilages are incomplete posteriorly where the trachea and the esophagus share a fibroelastic membrane (Figure 1–23 on page 36).

Main Stem Bronchi. The right main stem bronchus branches off the trachea at about a 25-degree angle; the left main stem bronchus forms an angle of 40 to 60 degrees with the trachea. The right main stem bronchus is wider, more vertical, and about 5 cm shorter than the left main stem bronchus. It should be noted that because the right main stem bronchus is wider—and more vertical—than the left main stem bronchus, the respiratory care practitioner must always make certain that the endotracheal tube has not been over-advanced into the right main stem bronchus during intubation. Similar to the trachea, the main stem bronchi are supported by C-shaped cartilages. In the newborn, both the right and left main stem bronchi form about a 55-degree angle with the trachea. The main stem bronchi are the tracheobronchial tree's first generation.

Figure 1–22

Tracheobronchial tree.

Trachea

Peribronchial sheath

Cricoid cartilage

Cartilage

Right main stem bronchus

Left main stem bronchus

To upper lobe

To upper lobe

Carina

To median lobe

To lower lobe

To lower lobe

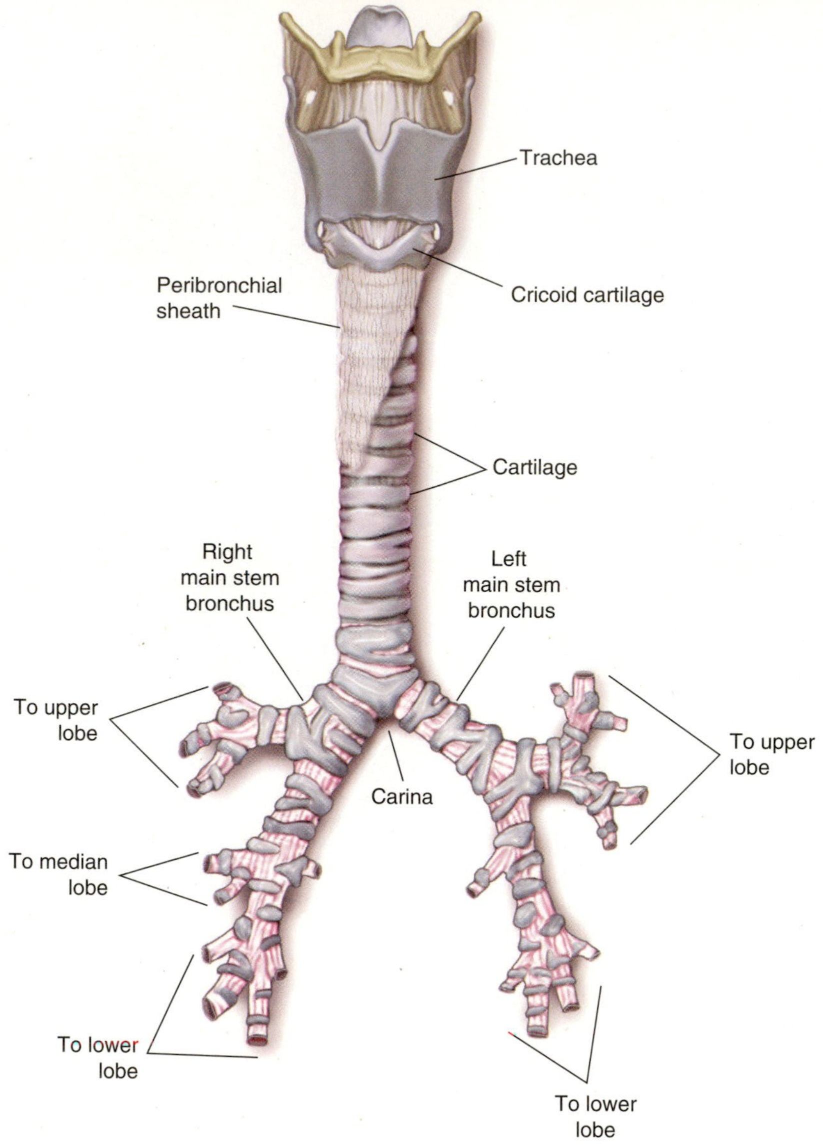

Figure 1–23

Cross-section of the trachea.

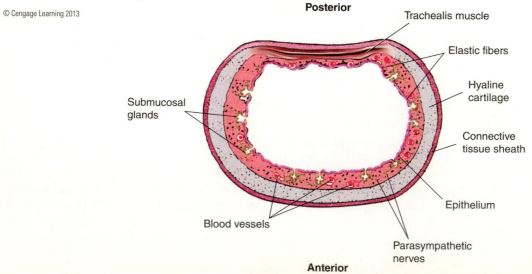

Posterior

Trachealis muscle

Elastic fibers

Hyaline cartilage

Connective tissue sheath

Submucosal glands

Epithelium

Blood vessels

Parasympathetic nerves

Anterior

Clinical Connection—1-14

Hazards Associated with Endotracheal Tubes

Endotracheal tube cuffs are used to seal the airway to (1) adequately apply positive pressure mechanical ventilation and (2) to prevent aspiration. The respiratory therapist must carefully monitor and maintain the cuff pressure below the tracheal mucosal capillary blood pressure—estimated to range between 25 and 30 mm Hg under normal conditions. Clinically, the recommended "safe range" is a cuff pressure between 20 and 25 mm Hg. Should the lateral cuff pressure exceed the tracheal blood pressure, the tracheal mucosal blood supply—immediately adjacent to the tube cuff—will be inadequate, or completely blocked off. Prolonged and excessive cuff pressure can lead to tracheal mucosal ischemia, inflammation, necrosis, ulceration, and destruction of the tracheal wall cartilage.

When the preceding chain of events occurs, any number of additional harmful conditions can develop—including tracheal dilatation and erosion.

Tracheal erosion can ultimately lead to a **fistula**—that is, an abnormal communication between the trachea and a nearby structure. Common fistulas associated with tracheal cuff erosions are the **innominate artery** (tracheoinnominate fistula) and the **esophagus** (tracheoesophageal fistula). In fact, the innominate artery is the most common artery involved in massive hemorrhage associated with a tracheostomy.

Figure 1–24 shows a chest X-ray of a patient who managed—and, unfortunately, overinflated and overpressurized—her own tracheal tube cuff at home. At the time of this X-ray, the excessive cuff pressure had already significantly dilated the trachea and eroded into her esophagus, causing a tracheoesophageal fistula. Figure 1–25 on page 38 shows the close anatomic proximity of a tracheostomy tube cuff and the innominate artery and esophagus.

Figure 1–24

A. A 48-year-old female who managed—and, unfortunately, overinflated and overpressurized—her tracheal tube at home. **B.** Note the close-up of the dilated trachea (red arrows and dark area) around the tracheal tube. Note: Only the tracheal tube can be seen. The cuff does not appear on chest X-rays, because it is primarily composed on air.

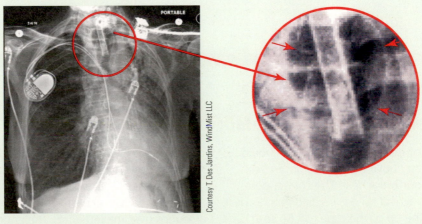

Courtesy T. Des Jardins, WindMist LLC

A   B

(continues)

Clinical Connection—1-14, continued

Figure 1–25

The close anatomic proximity of a tracheostomy tube cuff and the innominate artery and esophagus.

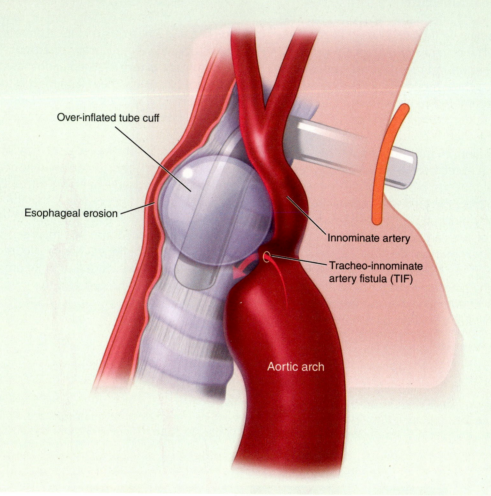

Clinical Connection—1-15

Inadvertent Intubation of Right Main Stem Bronchus

Clinically, the tip of the endotracheal tube should be about 4 to 6 cm above the carina, or between the second and fourth tracheal. The correct position of the endotracheal tube is verified with a chest radiograph (i.e., the tip of the tube can be seen about 4 to 6 cm above the carina). When an endotracheal tube is inserted too deeply (beyond the carina), it most commonly enters the right main stem bronchus. When this occurs, the left lung receives little or no ventilation and alveolar collapse (atelectasis) ensues (Figure 1–26A). When this condition is identified (via a chest X-ray or absence of breath sounds over the left lung), the endotracheal tube should be pulled back immediately (Figure 1–26B).

Clinical Connection—1-15, continued

Figure 1–26

Chest radiograph of 86-year-old post-open-heart surgical patient. **A.** The endotracheal tube tip in the right mainstem bronchus (see arrow). Because of the preferential ventilation to the right lung, atelectasis and volume "loss is" present in the patient's left lung (i.e., white fluffy areas in left lung). **B.** The same patient 20 minutes after the endotracheal tube was pulled back above the carina (see arrow). Note that the patient's left lung is now better ventilated (i.e., increased darker area in the left lung).

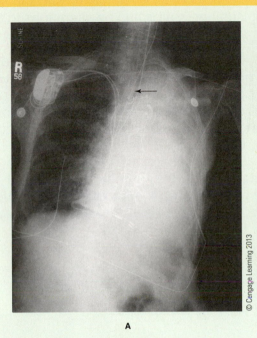
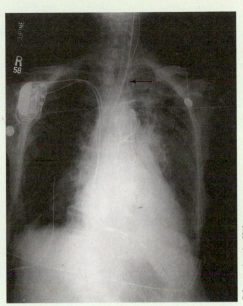

A

B

© Cengage Learning 2013

© Cengage Learning 2013

Lobar Bronchi. The right main stem bronchus divides into the upper, middle, and lower lobar bronchi. The left main stem bronchus branches into the upper and lower lobar bronchi. The lobar bronchi are the tracheobronchial tree's second generation. The C-shaped cartilages that support the trachea and the main stem bronchi progressively form cartilaginous plates around the lobar bronchi.

Segmental Bronchi. A third generation of bronchi branch off the lobar bronchi to form the segmental bronchi. There are 10 segmental bronchi in the right lung and 8 in the left lung. Each segmental bronchus is named according to its location within a particular lung lobe.

Subsegmental Bronchi. The tracheobronchial tree continues to subdivide between the fourth and approximately the ninth generation into progressively smaller airways called subsegmental bronchi. These bronchi range in diameter from 1 to 4 mm. Peribronchial connective tissue containing nerves, lymphatics, and bronchial arteries surround the subsegmental bronchi to about the 1-mm diameter level. Beyond this point, the connective tissue sheaths disappear.

The Noncartilaginous Airways

The noncartilaginous airways are composed of the bronchioles and the terminal bronchioles.

Bronchioles. When the bronchi decrease to less than 1 mm in diameter and are no longer surrounded by connective tissue sheaths, they are called bronchioles. The bronchioles are found between the tenth and fifteenth generations. At this level, cartilage is absent and the lamina propria is directly connected with the lung parenchyma (see lung parenchyma in the section on sites of gas exchange in this chapter). The bronchioles are surrounded by spiral muscle fibers and the epithelial cells are more cuboidal in shape (see Figure 1–17). The rigidity of the bronchioles is very low compared with the cartilaginous airways. Because of this, the airway patency at this level may be substantially affected by intra-alveolar and intrapleural pressures and by alterations in the size of the lungs. This lack of airway support often plays a major role in respiratory disease.

Terminal Bronchioles. The conducting tubes of the tracheobronchial tree end with the terminal bronchioles between the sixteenth and nineteenth generations. The average diameter of the terminal bronchioles is about 0.5 mm. At this point, the cilia and the mucous glands progressively disappear, and the epithelium flattens and becomes cuboidal in shape (see Figures 1–5C and 1–17).

As the wall of the terminal bronchioles progressively becomes thinner, small channels, called the canals of Lambert, begin to appear between the inner luminal surface of the terminal bronchioles and the adjacent alveoli that surround them (Figure 1–27). Although specific information as to their function is lacking, it is believed that these tiny pathways may be important

Figure 1–27

Canals of Lambert.

© Cengage Learning 2013

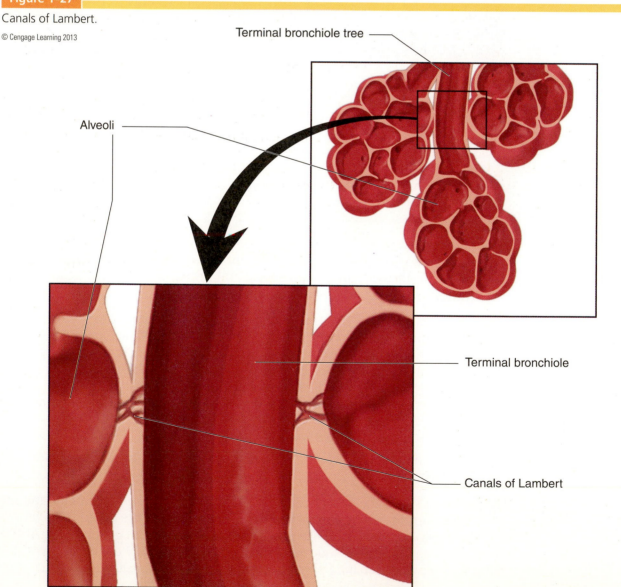

secondary avenues for collateral ventilation in patients with certain respiratory disorders (e.g., chronic obstructive pulmonary disease [COPD]).

Also unique to the terminal bronchioles is the presence of Clara cells. These cells have thick protoplasmic extensions that bulge into the lumen of the terminal bronchioles. The precise function of the Clara cells is not known. They may have secretory functions that contribute to the extracellular liquid lining the bronchioles and alveoli. They may also contain enzymes that work to detoxify inhaled toxic substances.

The structures beyond the terminal bronchioles are the sites of gas exchange and, although directly connected to it, are not considered part of the tracheobronchial tree.

Bronchial Cross-Sectional Area

The total cross-sectional area of the tracheobronchial tree steadily increases from the trachea to the terminal bronchioles. The total cross-sectional area increases significantly beyond the terminal bronchioles because of the many branches that occur at this level. The structures distal to the terminal bronchioles are collectively referred to as the respiratory zone (Figure 1–28).

Air flows down the tracheobronchial tree as a mass to about the level of the terminal bronchioles, like water flowing through a tube. Because the cross-sectional area becomes so great beyond this point, however, the forward motion essentially stops and the molecular movement of gas becomes the dominant mechanism of ventilation.

Bronchial Blood Supply

The bronchial arteries nourish the tracheobronchial tree. The arteries arise from the aorta and follow the tracheobronchial tree as far as the terminal

Figure 1–28

Cross-section of bronchial area. Note the rapid increase in the total cross-sectional area of the airways in the respiratory zone.

© Cengage Learning 2013

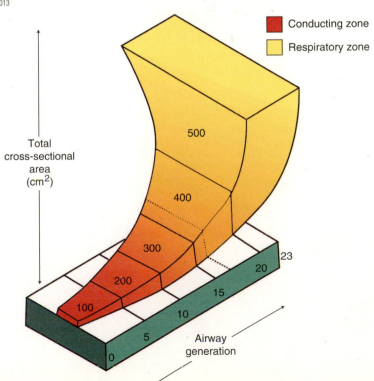

bronchioles. Beyond the terminal bronchioles, the bronchial arteries lose their identity and merge with the pulmonary arteries and capillaries, which are part of the pulmonary vascular system. The normal bronchial arterial blood flow is about 1 percent of the cardiac output. In addition to the tracheobronchial tree, the bronchial arteries nourish the mediastinal lymph nodes, the pulmonary nerves, a portion of the esophagus, and the visceral pleura.

About one-third of the bronchial venous blood returns to the right atrium by way of the azygos, hemiazygos, and intercostal veins. Most of this blood comes from the first two or three generations of the tracheobronchial tree. The remaining two-thirds of the bronchial venous blood drains into the pulmonary circulation, via bronchopulmonary anastomoses, and then flows to the left atrium by way of the pulmonary veins. In effect, the bronchial venous blood, which is low in oxygen and high in carbon dioxide, mixes with blood that has just passed through the alveolar-capillary system, which is high in oxygen and low in carbon dioxide. The mixing of venous blood and freshly oxygenated blood is known as venous admixture. (The effects of venous admixture are discussed in greater detail in Chapter 6.)

The Sites of Gas Exchange

The structures distal to the terminal bronchioles are the functional units of gas exchange. They are composed of about three generations of respiratory bronchioles, followed by about three generations of alveolar ducts and, finally, ending in 15 to 20 grapelike clusters, the alveolar sacs (Figure 1–29). The respiratory bronchioles are characterized by alveoli budding from their walls. The walls of the alveolar ducts that arise from the respiratory bronchioles

Figure 1–29

Schematic of the structures distal to the terminal bronchioles; collectively, these are referred to as the primary lobule.

© Cengage Learning 2013

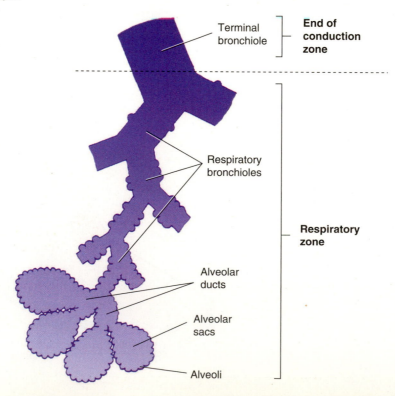

are completely composed of alveoli separated by septal walls that contain smooth-muscle fibers. Most gas exchange takes place at the alveolar-capillary membrane (Figure 1–30). In the lungs of the adult male, there are approximately 300 million alveoli between 75 and 300 μm in diameter, and small pulmonary capillaries cover about 85 to 95 percent of the alveoli. This arrangement provides an average surface area of 70 m² (about the size of a tennis court) available for gas exchange.

Collectively, the respiratory bronchioles, alveolar ducts, and alveolar clusters that originate from a single terminal bronchiole are referred to as a primary lobule. Each primary lobule is about 3.5 μm in diameter and contains about 2000 alveoli. It is estimated that there are approximately 130,000 primary lobules in the lung. Synonyms for primary lobule include acinus, terminal respiratory unit, lung parenchyma, and functional units (see Table 1–1).

Figure 1–30	

Alveolar-capillary network. The blow up of the alveolar-capillary network illustrates the (1) pulmonary capillaries, (2) alveolar type I cells (squamous alveolar cells), (3) alveolar type II cells (septal cells), (4) alveolar macrophage, and (5) alveolar pores of kohn.

© Cengage Learning 2013

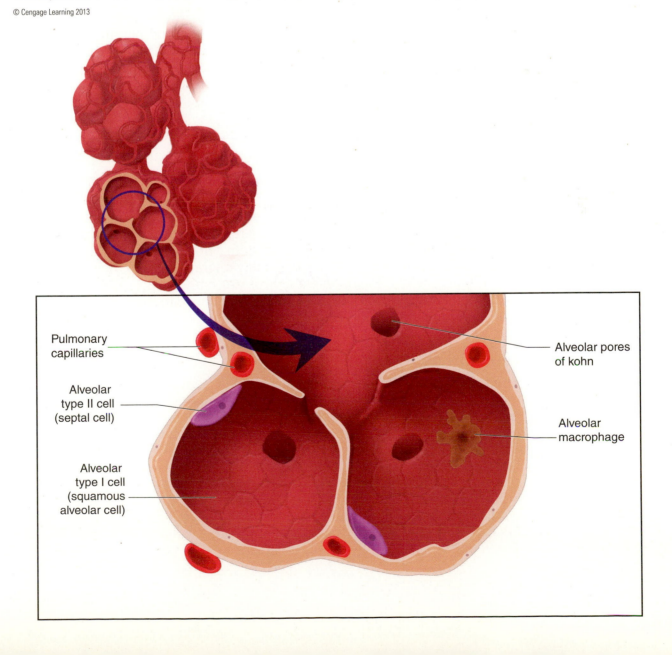

Pulmonary capillaries

Alveolar type II cell (septal cell)

Alveolar type I cell (squamous alveolar cell)

Alveolar pores of kohn

Alveolar macrophage

Alveolar Epithelium

The alveolar epithelium is composed of two principal cell types: the type I cell, or squamous pneumocyte, and the type II cell, or granular pneumocyte.

Type I cells are primarily composed of a cytoplasmic ground substance. They are broad, thin cells that form about 95 percent of the alveolar surface. They are 0.1 to 0.5 μm thick and are the major sites of alveolar gas exchange. Several type I cells connect edge to edge to form one or more alveoli. When type I cells die, they are replaced by type II cells that convert to type I cells. Type I cells are unable to reproduce, while type II cells can.

Type II cells form the remaining 5 percent of the total alveolar surface. They have microvilli and are cuboidal in shape. They are believed to be the primary source of pulmonary surfactant. Surfactant molecules are situated at the air–liquid interface of the alveoli and play a major role in decreasing the surface tension of the fluid that lines the alveoli (see Figure 1–30).

Pores of Kohn

The pores of Kohn are small holes in the walls of the interalveolar septa (see Figure 1–26). They are 3 to 13 μm in diameter and permit gas to move between adjacent alveoli. The formation of the pores may include one or more of the following processes: (1) the desquamation (i.e., shedding or peeling) of epithelial cells due to disease, (2) the normal degeneration of tissue cells as a result of age, and (3) the movement of macrophages, which may leave holes in the alveolar walls. Diseases involving the lung parenchyma accelerate the formation of alveolar pores of Kohn, and the number and size of the pores increase progressively with age.

Alveolar Macrophages

Alveolar macrophages, or type III alveolar cells, play a major role in removing bacteria and other foreign particles that are deposited within the acini. Macrophages are believed to originate from stem cell precursors in the bone marrow. Then, as monocytes, they presumably migrate through the bloodstream to the lungs, where they move about or are embedded in the extracellular lining of the alveolar surface. There is also evidence that the alveolar macrophages reproduce within the lung (see Figure 1–30).

Interstitium

The alveolar-capillary clusters are surrounded, supported, and shaped by the interstitium (Figure 1–31). The interstitium is a gel-like substance composed of hyaluronic acid molecules that are held together by a web-like network of collagen fibers. The interstitium has two major compartments: the tight space and the loose space. The tight space is the area between the alveolar epithelium and the endothelium of the pulmonary capillaries—the area where most gas exchange occurs. The loose space is primarily the area that surrounds the bronchioles, respiratory bronchioles, alveolar ducts, and alveolar sacs. Lymphatic vessels and neural fibers are found in this area. Water content in this area can increase more than 30 percent before a significant pressure change develops.

© Cengage Learning 2013

Figure 1–31

Pulmonary Interstitium. Most gas exchange occurs in the tight space area. The area around the respiratory bronchioles, alveolar ducts, and alveolar sacs is called the loose space.

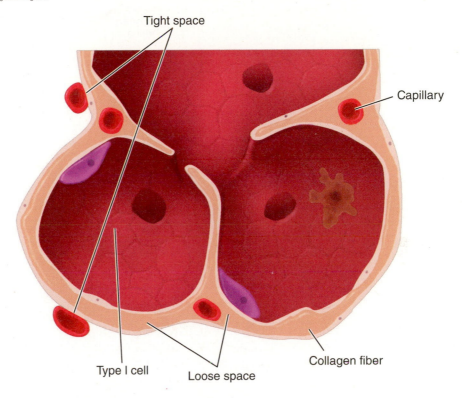

The collagen in the interstitium is believed to limit alveolar distensibility. Expansion of a lung unit beyond the limits of the interstitial collagen can (1) occlude the pulmonary capillaries or (2) damage the structural framework of the collagen fibers and, subsequently, the wall of the alveoli.

The Pulmonary Vascular System*

The pulmonary vascular system delivers blood to and from the lungs for gas exchange. In addition to gas exchange, the pulmonary vascular system provides nutritional substances to the structures distal to the terminal bronchioles. Similar to the systemic vascular system, the pulmonary vascular system is composed of arteries, arterioles, capillaries, venules, and veins.

Arteries

The right ventricle of the heart pumps deoxygenated blood into the pulmonary artery. Just beneath the aorta the pulmonary artery divides into the right and left branches (Figure 1–32 on page 46). The branches then penetrate

---

* Refer to Chapter 5 for a more comprehensive presentation of the pulmonary vascular system.

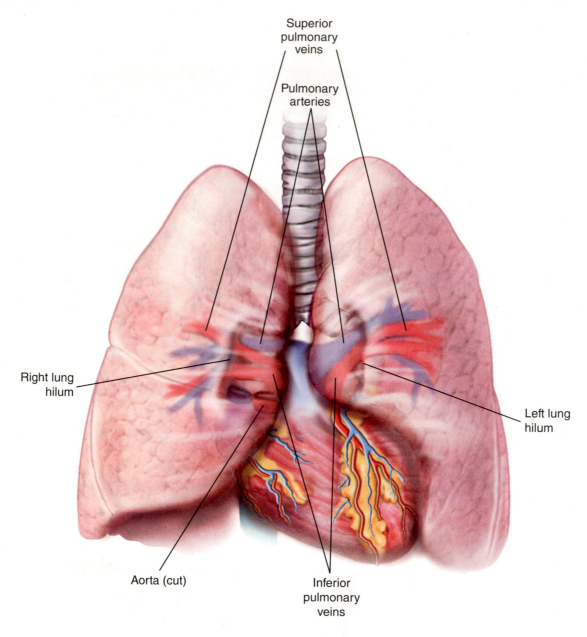

their respective lung through the hilum, which is that part of the lung where the main stem bronchi, vessels, and nerves enter. In general, the pulmonary artery follows the tracheobronchial tree in a posterolateral relationship branching or dividing as the tracheobronchial tree does.

The pulmonary arteries have three layers of tissue in their walls (Figure 1–33). The inner layer is called the tunica intima and is composed of endothelium and a thin layer of connective and elastic tissue. The middle layer is called the tunica

Figure 1–33

Schematic of the components of the pulmonary blood vessels.

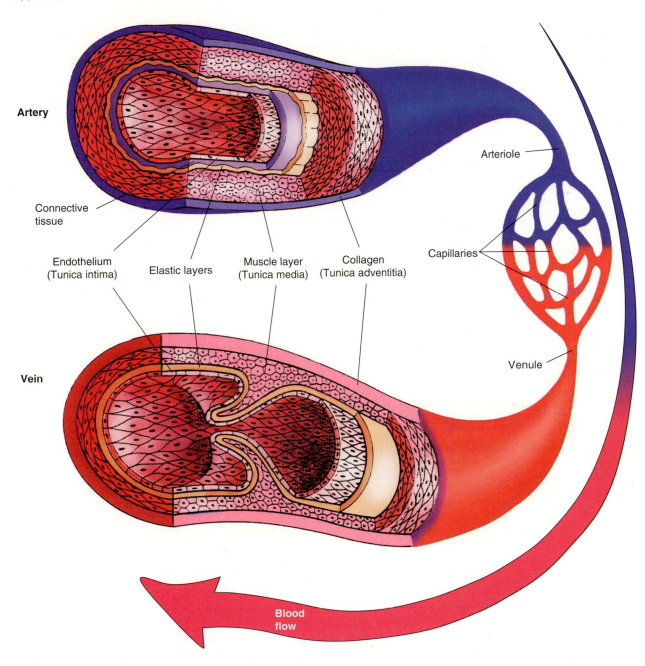

media and consists primarily of elastic connective tissue in large arteries and smooth muscle in medium-sized to small arteries. The tunica media is the thickest layer in the arteries. The outermost layer is called the tunica adventitia and is composed of connective tissue. This layer also contains small vessels that nourish all three layers. Because of the different layers, the arteries are relatively stiff vessels that are well suited for carrying blood under high pressures in the systemic system.

Arterioles

The walls of the pulmonary arterioles consist of an endothelial layer, an elastic layer, and a layer of smooth-muscle fibers (see Figure 1–33). The elastic and smooth-muscle fibers gradually disappear just before entering the alveolar-capillary system. The pulmonary arterioles supply nutrients to the respiratory bronchioles, alveolar ducts, and alveoli. By virtue of their smooth-muscle fibers, the arterioles play an important role in the distribution and regulation of blood and are called the resistance vessels.

Capillaries

The pulmonary arterioles give rise to a complex network of capillaries that surround the alveoli. The capillaries are composed of an endothelial layer (a single layer of squamous epithelial cells) (see Figure 1–33). The capillaries are essentially an extension of the inner lining of the larger vessels. The walls of the pulmonary capillaries are less than 0.1 µm thick, and the external diameter of each vessel is about 10 µm. The capillaries are where gas exchange occurs. The pulmonary capillary endothelium also has a selective permeability to substances such as water, electrolytes, and sugars.

In addition to gas and fluid exchange, the pulmonary capillaries play an important biochemical role in the production and destruction of a broad range of biologically active substances. For example, serotonin, norepinephrine, and some prostaglandins are destroyed by the pulmonary capillaries. Some prostaglandins are produced and synthesized by the pulmonary capillaries, and some circulating inactive peptides are converted to their active form; for example, the inactive angiotensin I is converted to the active angiotensin II.

Venules and Veins

After blood moves through the pulmonary capillaries, it enters the pulmonary venules, which are actually tiny veins continuous with the capillaries. The venules empty into the veins, which carry blood back to the heart. Similar to the arteries, the veins usually have three layers of tissue in their walls (see Figure 1–33).

The veins differ from the arteries, however, in that the middle layer is poorly developed. As a result, the veins have thinner walls and contain less smooth muscle and less elastic tissue than the arteries. There are only two layers in the smaller veins, lacking a layer comparable to the tunica adventitia. In the systemic circulation, many medium- and large-sized veins (particularly those in the legs) contain one-way, flaplike valves that aid blood flow back to the heart. The valves open as long as the flow is toward the heart but close if flow moves away from the heart.

The veins also differ from the arteries in that they are capable of collecting a large amount of blood with very little pressure change. Because of this unique feature, the veins are called capacitance vessels. Unlike the pulmonary arteries, which generally parallel the airways, the veins move away from the bronchi and take a more direct route out of the lungs. Ultimately, the veins in each lung merge into two large veins and exit through the lung hilum. The four pulmonary veins then empty into the left atrium of the heart (see Figure 1–32).

The Lymphatic System

Lymphatic vessels are found superficially around the lungs just beneath the visceral pleura and in the dense connective tissue wrapping of the bronchioles, bronchi, pulmonary arteries, and pulmonary veins. The primary function of the lymphatic vessels is to remove excess fluid and protein molecules that leak out of the pulmonary capillaries.

Deep within the lungs, the lymphatic vessels arise from the loose space of the interstitium. The vessels follow the bronchial airways, pulmonary arteries, and veins to the hilum of the lung (Figure 1–34). Single-leaf, funnel-shaped valves are found in the lymphatic channels. These one-way valves direct fluid toward the hilum. The larger lymphatic channels are surrounded by smooth-muscle bands that actively produce peristaltic movements regulated by the autonomic nervous system. Both the smooth-muscle activity and the normal, cyclic pressure changes generated in the thoracic cavity move lymphatic fluid toward the hilum. The vessels end in the pulmonary and bronchopulmonary lymph nodes located just inside and outside the lung parenchyma (Figure 1–35 on page 50).

Figure 1–34

Lymphatic vessels of the bronchial airways, pulmonary arteries, and veins.

© Cengage Learning 2013

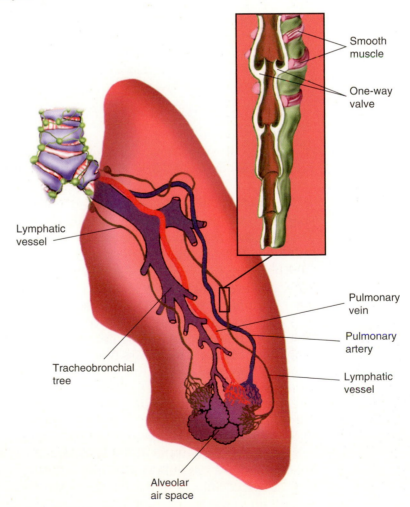

Lymph nodes associated with the trachea and the right and left main stem bronchi.

© Cengage Learning 2013

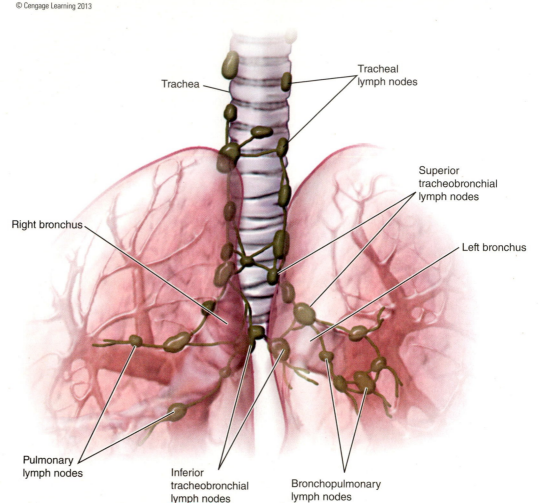

The lymph nodes are organized collections of lymphatic tissue interspersed along the course of the lymphatic stream. Lymph nodes produce lymphocytes and monocytes. The nodes act as filters, keeping particulate matter and bacteria from entering the bloodstream.

There are no lymphatic vessels in the walls of the alveoli. Some alveoli, however, are strategically located immediately adjacent to peribronchovascular lymphatic vessels. These vessels are called juxta-alveolar lymphatics and are thought to play an active role in the removal of excess fluid and other foreign material that gain entrance into the interstitial space of the lung parenchyma. The excess fluid and foreign substances move through the thoracic duct and empty into the left brachial vein just before the superior vena cava.

There are more lymphatic vessels on the surface of the lower lung lobes than on that of the upper or middle lobes. The lymphatic channels on the left lower lobe are more numerous and larger in diameter than the lymphatic vessels on the surface of the right lower lobe (Figure 1–36). This anatomic difference provides a possible explanation why patients with bilateral effusion (i.e., the escape of fluid from the blood vessels from both lungs) commonly have more fluid in the lower right lung than in the lower left.

Figure 1–36

Lymphatic vessels of
the visceral pleura of
the lungs.

© Cengage Learning 2013

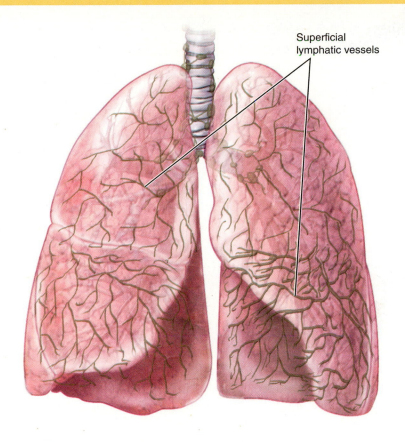

Superficial
lymphatic vessels

Neural Control of the Lungs

The balance, or tone, of the bronchial and arteriolar smooth muscle of the lungs is controlled by the autonomic nervous system. The autonomic nervous system is the part of the nervous system that regulates involuntary vital functions, including the activity of cardiac muscle, smooth muscle, and glands. It has two divisions: (1) the sympathetic nervous system, which accelerates the heart rate, constricts blood vessels, relaxes bronchial smooth muscles, and raises blood pressure, and (2) the parasympathetic nervous system, which slows the heart rate, constricts bronchial smooth muscles, and increases intestinal peristalsis and gland activity. Table 1–2 on page 52 lists some effects of the two divisions of the autonomic nervous system.

When the sympathetic nervous system is activated, neural transmitters, such as epinephrine and norepinephrine, are released. These agents stimulate (1) the beta$_2$ receptors in the bronchial smooth muscles, causing relaxation of the airway musculature, and (2) the alpha receptors of the smooth muscles of the arterioles, causing the pulmonary vascular system to constrict. When the parasympathetic nervous system is activated, the neutral transmitter acetylcholine is released, causing constriction of the bronchial smooth muscle.

Inactivity of either the sympathetic or the parasympathetic nervous system allows the action of the other to dominate the bronchial smooth-muscle response. For example, if a beta$_2$-blocking agent such as propranolol is administered to a patient, the parasympathetic nervous system becomes dominant and bronchial constriction ensues. In contrast, if a patient receives a parasympathetic blocking agent such as atropine, the sympathetic nervous system becomes dominant and bronchial relaxation occurs.

Table 1–2

Some Effects of Autonomic Nervous System Activity

Effector Site	Sympathetic Nervous System	Parasympathetic Nervous System
Heart	Increases rate	Decreases rate
	Increases strength of contraction	Decreases strength of contraction
Bronchial smooth muscle	Relaxation	Constriction
Bronchial glands	Decreases secretions	Increases secretions
Salivary glands	Decreases secretions	Increases secretions
Stomach	Decreases motility	Increases motility
Intestines	Decreases motility	Increases motility
Eyes	Widens pupils	Constricts pupils

© Cengage Learning 2013

Clinical Connection—1-16

The Role of Neural Control Agents in Respiratory Care

Clinically, the respiratory therapist commonly administers inhaled aerosolized medications that mirror the bronchodilator effects of the autonomic nervous system. In general, the bronchodilator drugs used to offset bronchial smooth muscle constriction (bronchospasm) either (1) mimic the sympathetic nervous system—that is, mimic the bronchial smooth muscle relaxation effects, or (2) block the parasympathetic nervous system—that is, block the bronchial smooth muscle constriction effects. In other words, drugs that mimic the sympathetic nervous system cause bronchial smooth muscle relaxation; drugs that block the parasympathetic nervous system prevent the activation of bronchial smooth muscle constriction—thereby, allowing bronchodilation to prevail.

Agents that mimic the sympathetic nervous system are called **sympathomimetic drugs**. In short,

sympathomimetic agents stimulate the same **adrenergic beta$_2$ receptors**—located in the bronchial smooth muscle—that are normally stimulated by the sympathetic nervous system to cause bronchodilation. This is why sympathomimetic agents—such as **albuterol**, **levalbuterol**, **salmeterol**, and **formoterol**—are often referred to as **beta$_2$ adrenergic drugs**. On the other hand, drugs that block the **cholinergic receptors** of the parasympathetic nervous system—that is, the receptors that cause the bronchial smooth muscle constriction effect—are called **parasympatholytic agents** (also called **anticholinergic drugs**). Common aerosolized parasympatholytic agents administered by the respiratory therapist include **ipratropium bromide**. Agents that include combinations of sympathomimetic and parasympatholytic agents (e.g., ipratropium and albuterol) are also available.

Clinical Connection—1-17

An Asthmatic Episode and the Role of Bronchodilator and Anti-Inflammatory Drugs

As shown in Figure 1–37, **asthma** is characterized by periodic episodes of (1) reversible bronchial smooth muscle constriction called bronchospasm; (2) airway inflammation which results in mucosal edema and airway swelling; (3) excessive production of thick, whitish bronchial secretions; (4) mucus

plugging; and (5) air trapping and hyperinflation of the alveoli. The risk factors for asthma can be divided into two groups: (1) the risk factors one is born with that cause the development of asthma (e.g., genetic traits or sex), and (2) the risk factors that trigger asthma symptoms (e.g., dust, pollens, fungi, molds,

Clinical Connection—1-17, continued

animal fur, or tobacco smoke). An asthmatic episode can develop rapidly with symptoms that include a cough, wheezing, excessive mucus production, a feeling of chest tightness, and shortness of breath.

During life-threatening asthmatic attacks, fast-acting bronchodilator drugs—called **quick relief medications**—are commonly administered by the respiratory therapist to relax constricted bronchial smooth muscles. Quick relief agents include **albuterol** or **levalbuterol**. **Controller medications** include long-acting beta agonists such as **salmeterol** or **formoterol**, and anti-inflammatory corticosteroids such as **beclomethasone**, **fluticasone**, or **budesonide**. In addition, asthma management may also include agents such as **leukotriene modifiers**, **mast cell stabilizers**, **methyxanthines**, and **immunomodulators**.

Figure 1–37

Asthma is characterized by periodic episodes of (1) reversible bronchial smooth muscle constriction, called bronchospasm; (2) airway inflammation, which results in mucosal edema and airway swelling; (3) excessive production of thick, whitish bronchial secretions; (4) mucus plugging; and (5) air trapping and hyperinflation of the alveoli.

© Cengage Learning 2013

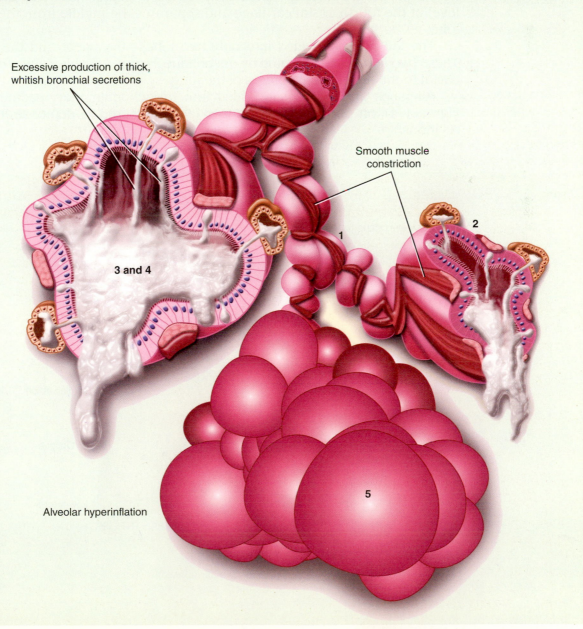

Excessive production of thick, whitish bronchial secretions

Smooth muscle constriction

3 and 4

1

2

Alveolar hyperinflation

5

The Lungs

The apex of each lung is somewhat pointed and the base is broad and concave to accommodate the convex diaphragm (Figures 1–38 and 1–39). As shown in Figure 1–40, the apices of the lungs rise to about the level of the first rib. In the normal adult at end exhalation, the base extends anteriorly to about the level of the sixth rib (xiphoid process level) and posteriorly to about the level of the eleventh rib (two ribs below the inferior angle of the scapula). The mediastinal border of each lung is concave to fit the heart and other mediastinal structures. At the center of the mediastinal border is the hilum, where the main stem bronchi, blood vessels, lymph vessels, and various nerves enter and exit the lungs.

The right lung is larger and heavier than the left. It is divided into the upper, middle, and lower lobes by the oblique and horizontal fissures. The oblique fissure extends from the costal to the mediastinal borders of the lung and separates the upper and middle lobes from the lower lobe. The horizontal fissure extends horizontally from the oblique fissure to about the level of the fourth costal cartilage and separates the middle from the upper lobe.

The left lung is divided into only two lobes—the upper and the lower. These two lobes are separated by the oblique fissure, which extends from the costal to the mediastinal borders of the lung.

All lobes are further subdivided into bronchopulmonary segments. In Figure 1–41 on page 56, the segments are numbered to demonstrate their relationship.

Figure 1–38

Anterior view of the lungs.

© Cengage Learning 2013

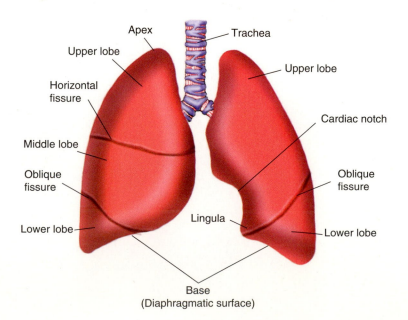

Figure 1–39

Medial view of the lungs.

© Cengage Learning 2013

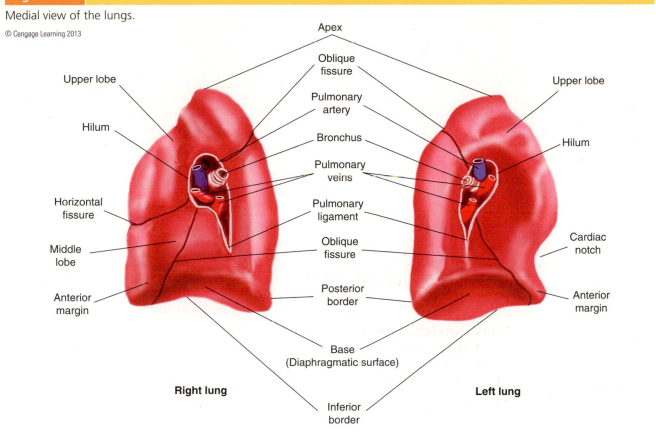

Right lung

Left lung

Figure 1–40

Anatomic relationship of the lungs and the thorax.

© Cengage Learning 2013

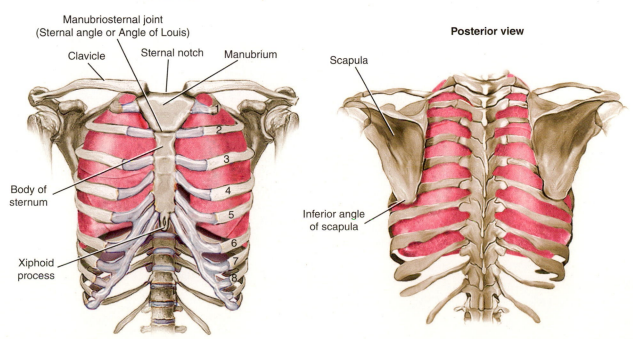

Figure 1–41

Lung segments. Although the segment subdivisions of the right and left lungs are similar, there are some slight anatomic differences, which are noted by combined names and numbers. Because of these slight variations, some researchers consider that, technically, there are only eight segments in the left lung: the **apical posterior segments** in the upper lobe are counted as a single segment, and the **anterior medial basal segments** of the lower lobe are counted as a single segment.

Right lung		Left lung	
Upper lobe		Upper lobe	
Apical	1	Upper division	
Posterior	2	Apical/Posterior	1 & 2
Anterior	3	Anterior	3
Middle lobe		Lower division (lingular)	
Lateral	4	Superior lingula	4
Medial	5	Inferior lingula	5
Lower lobe		Lower lobe	
Superior	6	Superior	6
Medial basal	7	Anterior medial basal	7 & 8
Anterior basal	8	Lateral basal	9
Lateral basal	9	Posterior basal	10
Posterior basal	10		

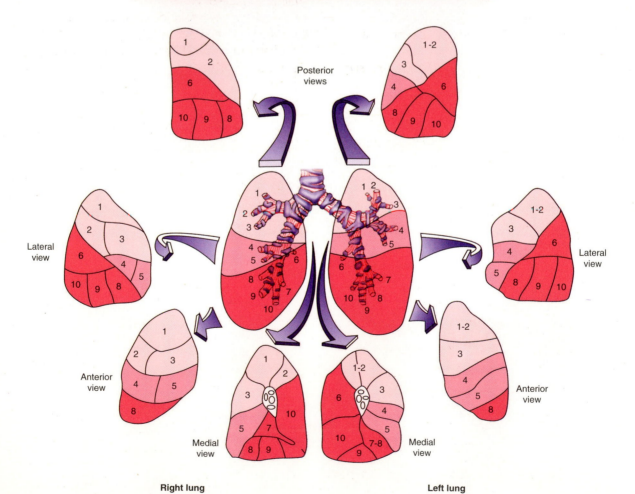

Clinical Connection—1-18

Postural Drainage Therapy

Postural drainage is commonly applied by the respiratory therapist to the patient with excessive airway secretions. Postural drainage therapy involves positioning the patient—with pillows and bed positions—to use gravity to help mobilize excessive bronchial secretions from bronchial lung segments. Depending on the specific locations and extent of the airway secretions, the patient may be placed in 1 to 12 different postural drainage positions. The indications for postural drainage therapy include patients who have (1) excessive bronchial secretions; (2) a weak or absent cough; (3) breath sounds with rhonchi (i.e., gurgling wet sounds), suggesting excessive airway secretions; and/or (4) an abnormal chest radiograph that indicates mucus plugging with alveolar collapse (atelectasis).

Clinically, the therapeutic values of postural drainage can be very helpful. For example, consider the patient with both a weak cough and excessive bronchial secretions in the **anterior segment** of the **right lower lobe**. In this case—and assuming there are no contraindications for postural drainage (such as a head or neck injury or a distended abdomen)—the patient would be positioned in the supine position (lying on back) with the foot of the bed raised 18 inches. Based on the anatomy of the anterior segment of the right lower lobe, this position generates the greatest gravitational pull on the secretions located in this region of the lung (Figure 1–42).

Postural drainage is often supplemented with **percussion** and **vibration** to enhance the mobilization of secretions. Percussion and vibration entail the application of mechanical energy to the chest wall by the use of either cupped hands or a variety of electric or pneumatic devices. Once the secretions have moved into the trachea, they are either coughed out by the patient or suctioned out by the health care practitioner.

Figure 1–42

Postural drainage position for the anterior basal segment of the right lower lobe. The patient is positioned in the supine position (lying on back) with the foot of the bed elevated 18 inches.

© Cengage Learning 2013

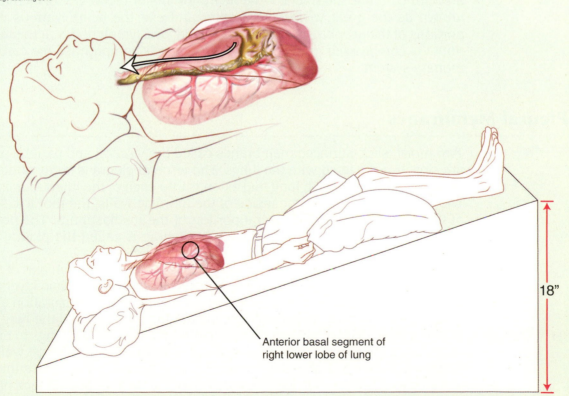

Anterior basal segment of right lower lobe of lung

18"

Figure 1–43

Major structures surrounding the lungs.

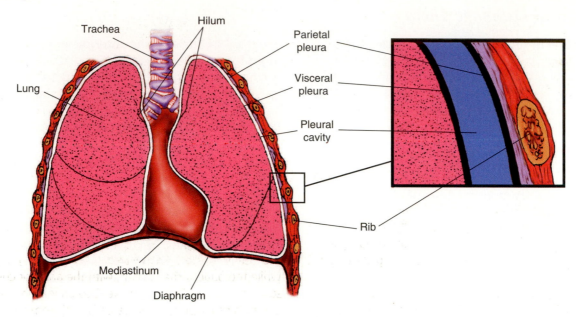

The Mediastinum

The mediastinum is a cavity that contains organs and tissues in the center of the thoracic cage between the right and left lungs (Figure 1–43). It is bordered anteriorly by the sternum and posteriorly by the thoracic vertebrae. The mediastinum contains the trachea, the heart, the major blood vessels (commonly known as the great vessels) that enter and exit the heart, various nerves, portions of the esophagus, the thymus gland, and lymph nodes. If the mediastinum is compressed or distorted, it can severely compromise the cardiopulmonary system.

The Pleural Membranes

Two moist, slick-surfaced membranes called the visceral and parietal pleurae are closely associated with the lungs. The visceral pleura is firmly attached to the outer surface of each lung and extends into each of the interlobar fissures. The parietal pleura lines the inside of the thoracic walls, the thoracic surface of the diaphragm, and the lateral portion of the mediastinum. The potential space between the visceral and parietal pleurae is called the pleural cavity (see Figure 1–43).

The visceral and parietal pleurae are held together by a thin film of serous fluid—somewhat like two flat, moistened pieces of glass. This fluid layer allows the two pleural membranes to glide over each other during inspiration and expiration. Thus, during inspiration, the pleural membranes hold the lung tissue to the inner surface of the thorax and diaphragm, causing the lungs to expand. Because the lungs have a natural tendency to collapse and the chest wall has a natural tendency to expand, a negative or subatmospheric pressure (negative intrapleural pressure) normally exists between the parietal and visceral pleurae.

Clinical Connection—1-19

Abnormal Conditions of the Pleural Membrane

Several respiratory disorders—such as congestive heart failure, bacterial pneumonia, tuberculosis, and fungal lung diseases—can adversely affect the pleural membranes. These pulmonary disorders can cause the pleural membranes to become inflamed—a condition called **pleurisy**. The inflamed pleurae become irritated and rough. This condition causes friction and a stabbing pain with each breath—especially during inspiration. Through a stethoscope, the patient's breath sounds are described as a **friction rub**, a "leather-like" creaking or grating sound, which is caused by the roughened, inflamed surfaces of the pleura rubbing together; these sounds are evident during inspiration, expiration, or both.

In more serious cases, fluid may accumulate in the pleural cavity. The general term for fluid accumulation in the pleural cavity is **pleural effusion**, or if infected, an **empyema** (Figure 1–44). Similar to the accumulation of free air in the pleural space (see Clinical Connection 1–20: Pneumothorax, page 60), fluid accumulation separates the visceral and parietal pleura. If untreated, the lung will collapse and the great veins may be compressed causing cardiac output to decrease. Pleural effusion and empyema cause a restrictive lung disorder.

Clinically, a pleural effusion is treated with a **thoracentesis**. A thoracentesis is a procedure in which excess fluid accumulation between the chest cavity and lungs (pleural space) is aspirated through a needle inserted through the chest wall. The fluid is examined for abnormal cells, white blood cells, red blood cells, glucose, and microorganisms. A thoracentesis is commonly performed at the bedside while the patient sits upright, with the anterior chest supported by a pillow or an over-bed table. When the patient's cardiopulmonary status is compromised—for example, because of a reoccurring fluid accumulation—the insertion of a large chest tube in the pleural space is secured for continual drainage.

Figure 1–44

A. Anterior-posterior chest X-ray of a right-sided pleural effusion. **B.** Lateral chest X-ray view of same patient.

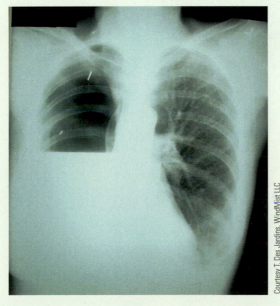

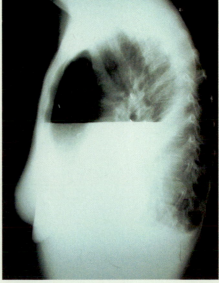

Courtesy T. Des Jardins, WindMist LLC

Courtesy T. Des Jardins, WindMist LLC

A

B

Clinical Connection—1-20

Pneumothorax

A **pneumothorax**, also known as *air in the chest cavity*, is the introduction of gas into the pleural cavity through an opening in the chest wall or a rupture of the lung. Gas accumulation in the pleural cavity causes the visceral and parietal pleural to separate and, subsequently, the lung to collapse (atelectasis). This is because when the lung's visceral and parietal pleura are separated, the **lung's natural inward recoil force** is no longer offset by the **chest wall's natural outward recoil force**—thus, allowing the lung to collapse.

Common causes of a pneumothorax include (1) a penetrating chest wound (e.g., knife, bullet, or fractured rib) and (2) a rupture of the lung (commonly caused by positive pressure mechanical ventilation). A pneumonthorax can be classified as either **closed** or **open**, based on the way in which gas gains entrance to the pleural space. In a **closed pneumothorax**, the gas in the intrapleural space is not in direct contact with the atmosphere (e.g., caused by rupture of the lung). In an **open pneumothorax**, the gas in the intrapleural space is in direct contact with the atmosphere and can move freely in and out (e.g., a penentrating chest wound). When the gas pressure in the intrapleural space exceeds the atmospheric pressure, the patient is said to have a **tension pneumothorax**. Figure 1–45 illustrates a right-sided tension pneumothorax.

In severe cases, the excessive gas pressure in the pleural cavity can (1) depress the diaphragm, (2) shift the mediastinum to the unaffected side of the chest, (3) compress the great veins and decrease cardiac output, and (4) diminish oxygen transport. The treatment for a pneumothorax is the insertion of a chest tube into the intrapleural space and the application of suction to draw out the air and re-expand the lung.

Figure 1–45

A right-side tension pneumothorax.

© Cengage Learning 2013

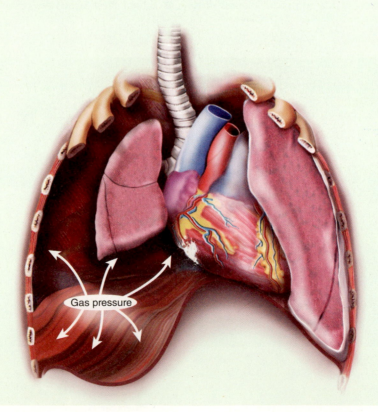

Gas pressure

The Thorax

The thorax houses and protects the organs of the cardiopulmonary system. Twelve thoracic vertebrae form the posterior midline border of the thoracic cage. The sternum forms the anterior border of the chest. The sternum is composed of the manubrium sterni, the body of the sternum, and the xiphoid process. The joint between the manubrium and the body of the sternum is called the **manubriosternal joint**, and is referred to as the **sternal angle** or **angle of Louis**. Clinically, the angle of Louis provides an important palpable landmark. It identifies (1) the approximate level of the second pair of costal cartilages, (2) the level of the intervertebral disc between T4 and T5, (3) the approximate beginning and end of the aortic arch, and (4) the bifurcation of the trachea into the left and right mainstem bronchi (Figure 1–46).

The 12 pairs of ribs form the lateral boundaries of the thorax. The ribs attach directly to the vertebral column posteriorly and indirectly by way of the costal cartilage anteriorly to the sternum. The first seven ribs are referred to as true ribs, because they are attached directly to the sternum by way of their costal cartilage. Because the cartilage of the eighth, ninth, and tenth ribs attaches to the cartilage of the ribs above, they are referred to as false ribs.

Figure 1–46

The thorax. The angle of Louis (the joint between the manubrium and the body of the sternum) is a palpable mark of the bifurcation of the right and left mainstem bronchi.

© Cengage Learning 2013

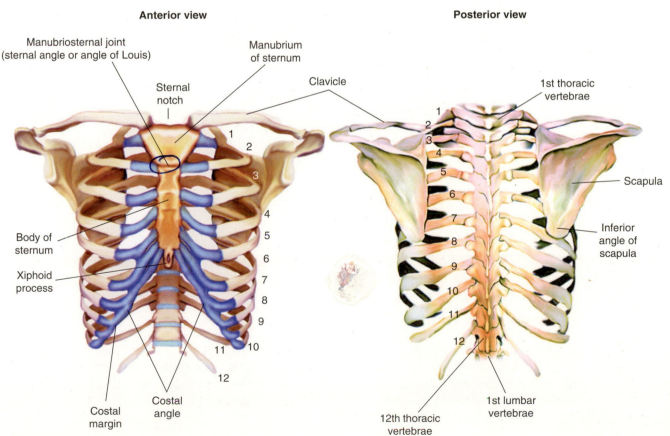

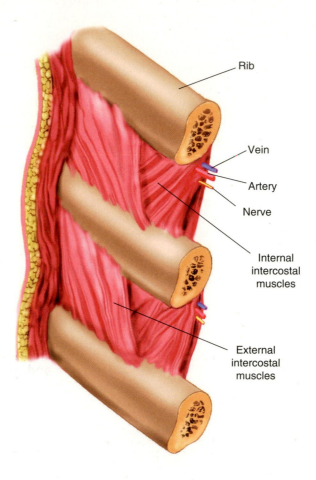

Figure 1–47

The intercostal space.

© Cengage Learning 2013

Rib

Vein

Artery

Nerve

Internal
intercostal
muscles

External
intercostal
muscles

Ribs eleven and twelve float freely anteriorly and are called floating ribs. There are 11 intercostal spaces between the ribs. Each intercostal space contains blood vessels, intercostal nerves, and the external and internal intercostal muscles. The veins, arteries, and nerves within each intercostal space run along the inferior margin of each rib (Figure 1–47).

Clinical Connection—1-21

Puncture Site for a Thoracentesis

Because the intercostal veins, arteries, and nerves course along the lower margin of each rib, the protocol for a thoracentesis entails the insertion of the needle slightly superior to the rib margin (Figure 1–48). Although bleeding from a thoracentesis is rare, a needle puncture is one of the most common causes of an **iatrogenic pneumothorax**—that is, a health complication caused by medical personnel or procedure.

Clinical Connection—1-21, continued

Figure 1–48

To safely miss the intercostal artery, vein, and nerve, a thoracentesis involves the insertion of the needle slightly superior to the rib margin.

© Cengage Learning 2013

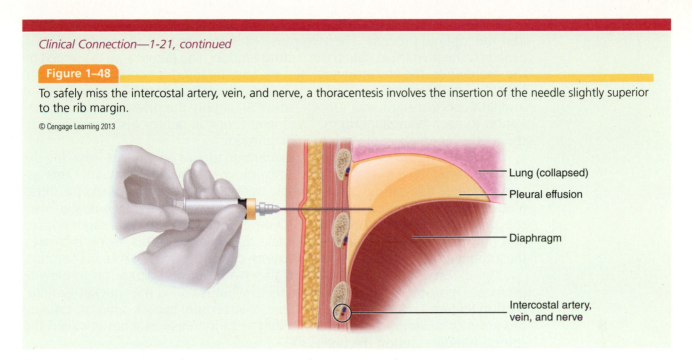

- Lung (collapsed)
- Pleural effusion
- Diaphragm
- Intercostal artery, vein, and nerve

The Muscles of Ventilation

During normal quiet breathing, contraction of the **diaphragm** alone, or contraction of both the diaphragm and **external intercostal muscles**, activate quiet inspiration. The diaphragm is the major muscle of ventilation (Figure 1–49). It is a dome-shaped musculofibrous partition located between the thoracic cavity and the abdominal cavity. Although the diaphragm is generally referred to as one muscle, it is actually composed of two separate muscles known as the right and left hemidiaphragms.

Figure 1–49

The diaphragm.

© Cengage Learning 2013

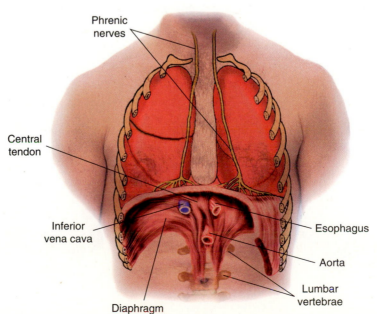

Phrenic nerves

Central tendon

Inferior vena cava

Esophagus

Aorta

Lumbar vertebrae

Diaphragm

Each hemidiaphragm arises from the lumbar vertebrae, the costal margin, and the xiphoid process. The two muscles then merge at the midline into a broad connective sheet called the central tendon. The diaphragm is pierced by the esophagus, the aorta, several nerves, and the inferior vena cava. Terminal branches of the phrenic nerves, which leave the spinal cord between the third and fifth cervical segments (C3, C4, and C5), supply the primary motor innervation to each hemidiaphragm. The lower thoracic nerves also contribute to the motor innervation of each hemidiaphragm.

When stimulated to contract, the diaphragm moves downward—making the thoracic cavity longer—and the lower ribs move upward and outward. This action increases the volume of the thoracic cavity, which, in turn, lowers the intrapleural and intra-alveolar pressures in the thoracic cavity. As a result, gas from the atmosphere flows into the lungs. During expiration, the diaphragm relaxes and moves upward—making the thoracic cavity smaller. This action increases the intrapleural and intra-alveolar pressures, causing gas to flow out of the lungs.

The external intercostal muscles also work during inspiration to elevate the lateral portion of the thoracic cavity in what is called the "bucket-handle" motion (Figure 1-50A). At the same time, the sternum moves upward, causing the anterior-posterior portion of the thorax to increase in what is called the "pump-handle" motion (Figure 1-50B).

Figure 1-50

The movement of the rib cage during breathing. **A.** "Bucket-handle" motion. **B.** "Pump-handle" motion.

© Cengage Learning 2013

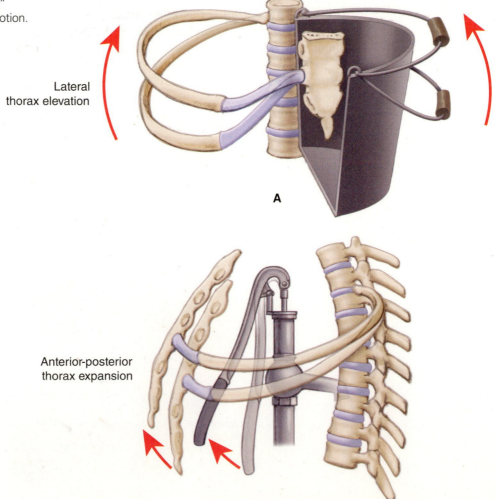

Lateral thorax elevation

A

Anterior-posterior thorax expansion

B

Finally, during periods of respiratory distress, the contraction of the accessory muscles of inspiration—the scalenus, sternocleidomastoid, pectoralis major, and trapezius muscles—are typically activated to aid in the elevation of the sternum and rib cage during inspiration.

The Accessory Muscles of Ventilation

During normal ventilation by a healthy person, the diaphragm alone can manage the task of moving gas in and out of the lungs. However, during vigorous exercise and the advanced stages of COPD, the accessory muscles of inspiration and expiration are activated to assist the diaphragm.

The Accessory Muscles of Inspiration

The accessory muscles of inspiration are those muscles that are recruited to assist the diaphragm in creating a subatmospheric pressure in the lungs to enable adequate inspiration. The major accessory muscles of inspiration are:

- External intercostal muscles
- Scalenus muscles
- Sternocleidomastoid muscles
- Pectoralis major muscles
- Trapezius muscles

External Intercostal Muscles

The external intercostal muscles arise from the lower border of each rib (the upper limit of an intercostal space) and insert into the upper border of the rib below. Anteriorly, the fibers run downward and medially. Posteriorly, the fibers run downward and laterally (Figure 1–51). The external intercostal muscles

---

Figure 1–51

Internal and external intercostal muscles.

© Cengage Learning 2013

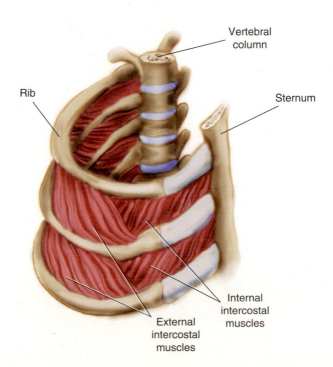

Figure 1–52

Scalenus muscles.

© Cengage Learning 2013

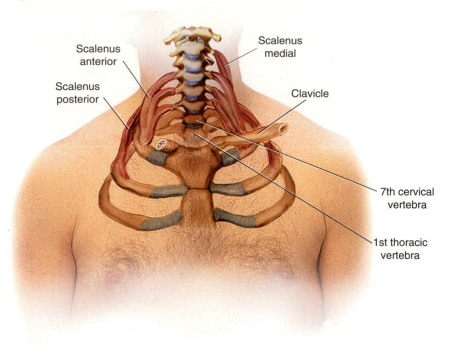

contract during inspiration and pull the ribs upward and outward, increasing both the lateral and anteroposterior diameter of the thorax (an antagonistic action to the internal intercostal muscles). This action increases lung volume and prevents retraction of the intercostal space during an excessively forceful inspiration.

Scalenus Muscles

The scalenus muscles are three separate muscles that function as a unit. They are known as the anterior, the medial, and the posterior scalene muscles. They originate on the transverse processes of the second to the sixth cervical vertebrae and insert into the first and second ribs (Figure 1–52).

The primary function of these muscles is to flex the neck. When used as accessory muscles for inspiration, they elevate the first and second ribs, an action that decreases the intrapleural pressure.

Sternocleidomastoid Muscles

The sternocleidomastoid muscles are located on each side of the neck (Figure 1–53). They originate from the sternum and the clavicle and insert into the mastoid process and occipital bone of the skull. Normally, the sternocleidomastoid muscles pull from their sternoclavicular origin and rotate the head to the opposite side and turn it upward. When the sternocleidomastoid muscles function as an accessory muscle of inspiration, the head and neck are fixed by other muscles and the sternocleidomastoid pulls from its insertion on the skull and elevates the sternum. This action increases the anteroposterior diameter of the chest.

Figure 1–53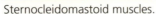

Sternocleidomastoid muscles.

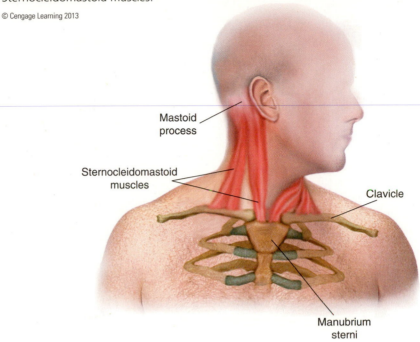

Mastoid process

Sternocleidomastoid muscles

Clavicle

Manubrium sterni

Pectoralis Major Muscles

The pectoralis major muscles are powerful, fan-shaped muscles located on each side of the upper chest. They originate from the clavicle and the sternum and insert into the upper part of the humerus.

Normally, the pectoralis majors pull from their sternoclavicular origin and bring the upper arm to the body in a hugging motion (Figure 1–54). When functioning as accessory muscles of inspiration, they pull from the humeral insertion and elevate the chest, resulting in an increased anteroposterior diameter. Patients with COPD frequently brace their arms against something stationary and use their pectoralis majors to increase the diameter of their chest (Figure 1–55 on page 68).

Figure 1–54

Pectoralis major muscles.

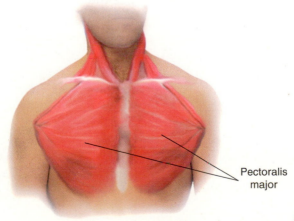

Pectoralis major

Figure 1–55

How an individual may appear when using the pectoralis major muscles for inspiration.

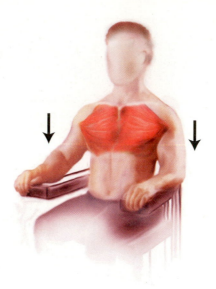

Trapezius Muscles

The trapezius muscles are large, flat, triangular muscles that are situated superficially in the upper back and the back of the neck. They originate from the occipital bone, the ligamentum nuchae, and the spinous processes of the seventh cervical vertebra and all the thoracic vertebrae. They insert into the spine of the scapula, the acromion process, and the lateral third of the clavicle (Figure 1–56).

Normally, the trapezius muscles rotate the scapula, raise the shoulders, and abduct and flex the arms. Their action is typified in shrugging of the shoulders (Figure 1–57). When used as accessory muscles of inspiration, the trapezius muscles help to elevate the thoracic cage.

Figure 1–56

Trapezius muscles.

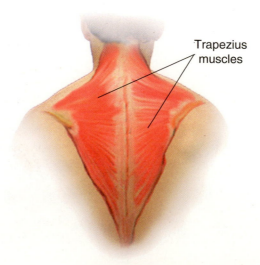

Trapezius
muscles

Figure 1–57

Shrugging of the shoulders typifies the action of the trapezius muscles.

© Cengage Learning 2013

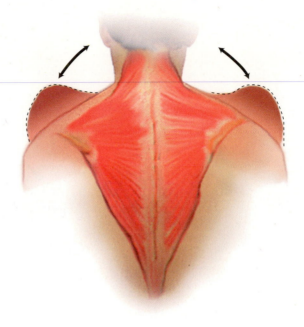

The Accessory Muscles of Expiration

The accessory muscles of expiration are the muscles recruited to assist in exhalation when airway resistance becomes significantly elevated. When these muscles contract, they increase the intrapleural pressure and offset the increased airway resistance. The major accessory muscles of exhalation are:

- Rectus abdominis muscles
- External abdominis obliquus muscles
- Internal abdominis obliquus muscles
- Transversus abdominis muscles
- Internal intercostal muscles

Rectus Abdominis Muscles

The rectus abdominis muscles are a pair of muscles that extend the entire length of the abdomen. Each muscle forms a vertical mass about 10 cm wide and is separated from the other by the linea alba. The muscles arise from the iliac crest and pubic symphysis and insert into the xiphoid process and the fifth, sixth, and seventh ribs.

When contracted, the rectus abdominis muscles assist in compressing the abdominal contents. This compression, in turn, pushes the diaphragm into the thoracic cage (Figure 1–58A on page 70), thereby assisting in exhalation.

External Abdominis Obliquus Muscles

The external abdominis obliquus muscles are broad, thin muscles located on the anterolateral sides of the abdomen. They are the longest and the most

Figure 1–58

Accessory muscles of expiration.

© Cengage Learning 2013

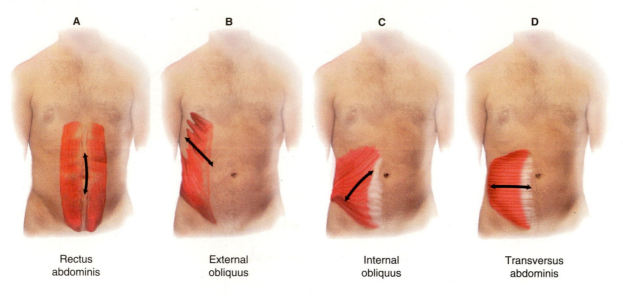

A	B	C	D
Rectus abdominis	External obliquus	Internal obliquus	Transversus abdominis

superficial of all the anterolateral abdominal muscles. They arise by eight digitations from the lower eight ribs and the abdominal aponeurosis and insert into the iliac crest and the linea alba.

When contracted, the external abdominis obliquus muscles assist in compressing the abdominal contents which, in turn, push the diaphragm into the thoracic cage (Figure 1–58B), thereby assisting in exhalation.

Internal Abdominis Obliquus Muscles

Smaller and thinner than the external abdominis obliquus, the internal abdominis obliquus muscles are located in the lateral and ventral parts of the abdominal wall directly under the external abdominis obliquus muscles. They arise from the inguinal ligament, the iliac crest, and the lower portion of the lumbar aponeurosis. They insert into the last four ribs and into the linea alba.

The internal abdominis obliquus muscles also assist in exhalation by compressing the abdominal contents and in pushing the diaphragm into the thoracic cage (Figure 1–58C).

Transversus Abdominis Muscles

The transversus abdominis muscles are found immediately under the internal abdominis obliquus muscles. These muscles arise from the inguinal ligament, the iliac crest, the thoracolumbar fascia, and the lower six ribs and insert into the linea alba. When activated, they also help to constrict the abdominal contents (Figure 1–58D).

When all four pairs of accessory muscles of exhalation contract, the abdominal pressure increases and drives the diaphragm into the thoracic cage. As the diaphragm moves into the thoracic cage during exhalation, the intrapleural pressure increases, thereby enhancing the amount of gas flow (Figure 1–59).

Figure 1–59

The collective action of the accessory muscles of expiration causes the intrapleural pressure to increase, the chest to move outward, and bronchial gas flow to increase.

© Cengage Learning 2013

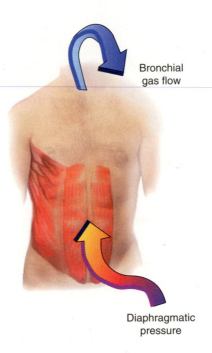

Bronchial gas flow

Diaphragmatic pressure

Internal Intercostal Muscles

The internal intercostal muscles run between the ribs immediately beneath the external intercostal muscles. The muscles arise from the inferior border of each rib and insert into the superior border of the rib below. Anteriorly, the fibers run in a downward and lateral direction. Posteriorly, the fibers run downward and in a medial direction (see Figure 1–51). The internal intercostal muscles contract during expiration and pull the ribs downward and inward, decreasing both the lateral and anteroposterior diameter of the thorax (an antagonistic action to the external intercostal muscles). This action decreases lung volume and offsets intercostal bulging during excessive expiration.

Chapter Summary

An essential cornerstone to the understanding of the practice of respiratory care is a strong knowledge base of the normal anatomy and physiology of the respiratory system. The major anatomic areas of the respiratory system can be divided into (1) the upper airway, (2) the lower airways, (3) the sites of gas exchange, (4) the pulmonary vascular system, (5) the lymphatic system, (6) the neural control of the lungs, (7) the lungs, (8) the mediastinum, (9) the pleural membranes, (10) the thorax, (11) the muscles of ventilation, and (12) the accessory muscles of ventilation. The upper airway includes the structures and functions associated with the nose, oral cavity, nasal pharynx, oropharynx, laryngopharynx and larynx. The lower airway includes the structures and functions related to the tracheobronchial tree and its histology.

Clinical connections associated with these topics include (1) flaring nostrils, (2) the nose as an excellent route of administration for topical agents, (3) rhinitis, (4) nosebleeds, (5) nasal congestion and its influence on taste, (6) sinusitis, (7) infected and swollen pharyngeal tonsils, (8) otitis media, (9) landmarks of the laryngopharynx and larynx when inserting an endotracheal tube, (10) laryngitis, (11) the croup syndrome, (12) excessive airway secretions, (13) an abnormal mucociliary transport mechanism, (14) the hazards of endotracheal tubes and tracheostomies, and (15) inadvertent intubation of the right main stem bronchus.

The anatomic structures associated with sites of gas exchange include the respiratory bronchioles, alveolar ducts, alveolar sacs, and the primary lobules. The alveolar epithelium consists of type I cells, type II cells, pulmonary surfactant, pores of Kohn, alveolar macrophages, and the intersitium. The structures of the pulmonary vascular system include the arteries, arterioles, capillaries, venules, and veins. The components of the lymphatic system include the lymph nodes and juxta-alveolar lymphatics. The neural control of the lungs consists of the autonomic nervous system, sympathetic nervous system, and parasympathetic nervous system. Clinical connections associated with the neural control of the lung include the role of neural control agents in respiratory care, an asthmatic episode, and the role of bronchodilator and anti-inflammatory drugs.

The key structures of the lung include the apex, base, mediastinal border, hilum, right lung (upper, middle, and lower lobes), left lung (upper and lower lobes), and the lung segments. A clinical connection associated with the lung segments includes the therapeutic effects of postural drainage therapy. Anatomic structures of the mediastinum are the trachea, heart, major blood vessels, nerves, esophagus, thymus gland, and lymph nodes. Anatomic components of the pleural membranes are the parietal pleura, visceral pleura, and pleural cavity. Clinical connections associated with the pleural membranes include pleurisy, friction rub, pleural effusion, empyema, thoracentesis, and pneumothorax.

The major parts of the thorax include the thoracic vertebrae, sternum, manubrium sterni, xyphoid process, true ribs, false ribs, and floating ribs. A clinical connection associated with the ribs of the thorax includes the puncture site for a thoracentesis. The major structures related to the diaphragm are the right and left hemidiaphragms, the central tendon, the phrenic nerve, and the lower thoracic nerves. The accessory muscles of ventilation are the external intercostal muscles, scalene muscles, sternocleidomastoid muscles, pectoralis major muscles, and trapezius muscles. The accessory muscles of expiration are the rectus abdominis muscles, external abdominis obliquus muscles, internal abdominis obliquus muscles, and the internal intercostal muscles.

For the respiratory care practitioner, a strong foundation of the normal anatomy and physiology of the respiratory system is an essential prerequisite to better understand the anatomic alterations of the lungs caused by specific respiratory disorders, the pathophysiologic mechanisms activated throughout the respiratory system as a result of the anatomic alterations, the clinical manifestations that develop as a result of the pathophysiologic mechanisms, and the basic respiratory therapies used to improve the anatomic alterations and pathophysiologic mechanisms caused by the disease. When the anatomic alterations and pathophysiologic mechanisms caused by the disorder are improved, the clinical manifestations also should improve.

Review Questions

1. Which of the following line the anterior one-third of the nasal cavity?
   - A. Stratified squamous epithelium
   - B. Simple cuboidal epithelium
   - C. Pseudostratified ciliated columnar epithelium
   - D. Simple squamous epithelium

2. Which of the following form(s) the nasal septum?
   1. Frontal process of the maxilla bone
   2. Ethmoid bone
   3. Nasal bones
   4. Vomer
      - A. 3 only
      - B. 4 only
      - C. 1 and 3 only
      - D. 2 and 4 only

3. Which of the following prevents the aspiration of foods and liquids?
   - A. Epiglottis
   - B. Cricoid cartilage
   - C. Arytenoid cartilages
   - D. Thyroid cartilages

4. The canals of Lambert are found in the
   - A. trachea
   - B. terminal bronchioles
   - C. alveoli
   - D. main stem bronchi

5. The pharyngotympanic (auditory) tubes are found in the
   - A. nasopharynx
   - B. oropharynx
   - C. laryngopharynx
   - D. oral cavity

6. The inferior portion of the larynx is composed of the
   - A. thyroid cartilage
   - B. hyoid bone
   - C. glottis
   - D. cricoid cartilage

7. Which of the following has the greatest combined cross-sectional area?
   - A. Terminal bronchioles
   - B. Lobar bronchi
   - C. Trachea
   - D. Segmental bronchi

8. The left main stem bronchus angles off from the carina at about
   - A. 10–20 degrees from the carina
   - B. 20–30 degrees from the carina
   - C. 30–40 degrees from the carina
   - D. 40–60 degrees from the carina

9. Ninety-five percent of the alveolar surface is composed of which of the following?
   1. Type I cells
   2. Granular pneumocytes
   3. Type II cells
   4. Squamous pneumocytes
      A. 1 only
      B. 2 only
      C. 2 and 3 only
      D. 1 and 4 only

10. Which of the following is (are) released when the parasympathetic nerve fibers are stimulated?
   1. Norepinephrine
   2. Atropine
   3. Epinephrine
   4. Acetylcholine
      A. 2 only
      B. 4 only
      C. 1 and 3 only
      D. 1, 2, and 3 only

11. Which of the following is (are) released when the sympathetic nerve fibers are stimulated?
   1. Norepinephrine
   2. Propranolol
   3. Acetylcholine
   4. Epinephrine
      A. 1 only
      B. 2 only
      C. 1 and 4 only
      D. 2, 3, and 4 only

12. Pseudostratified ciliated columnar epithelium lines which of the following?
   1. Oropharynx
   2. Trachea
   3. Nasopharynx
   4. Oral cavity
   5. Laryngopharynx
      A. 2 only
      B. 1 and 4 only
      C. 2 and 3 only
      D. 1, 2, 3, and 5 only

13. Which of the following is (are) accessory muscles of inspiration?
   1. Trapezius muscles
   2. Internal abdominis obliquus muscles
   3. Scalene muscles
   4. Transversus abdominis muscles
      A. 1 only
      B. 2 only
      C. 1 and 3 only
      D. 2 and 4 only

14. The horizontal fissure separates the
   A. middle and upper lobes of the right lung
   B. upper and lower lobes of the left lung
   C. middle and lower lobes of the right lung
   D. oblique fissure of the left lung

15. Which of the following supply the motor innervation of each hemidiaphragm?
   1. Vagus nerve (tenth cranial nerve)
   2. Phrenic nerve
   3. Lower thoracic nerves
   4. Glossopharyngeal nerve (ninth cranial nerve)
      A. 1 only
      B. 2 only
      C. 1 and 4 only
      D. 2 and 3 only

16. The lung segment called the superior lingula is found in the
   A. left lung, lower division of the upper lobe
   B. right lung, lower lobe
   C. left lung, upper division of the upper lobe
   D. right lung, upper lobe

17. Cartilage is found in which of the following structures of the tracheo-bronchial tree?
   1. Bronchioles
   2. Respiratory bronchioles
   3. Segmental bronchi
   4. Terminal bronchioles
      A. 1 only
      B. 3 only
      C. 2 and 3 only
      D. 1 and 4 only

18. The bronchial arteries nourish the tracheobronchial tree down to, and including, which of the following?
   A. Respiratory bronchioles
   B. Segmental bronchi
   C. Terminal bronchioles
   D. subsegmental bronchi

19. Which of the following elevates the soft palate?
   A. Palatoglossal muscle
   B. Levator veli palatine muscle
   C. Stylopharyngeus muscles
   D. Palatopharyngeal muscle

20. Which of the following are called the resistance vessels?
   A. Arterioles
   B. Veins
   C. Venules
   D. Arteries

Chapter 2

Ventilation

Objectives

By the end of this chapter, the student should be able to:

1. Define ventilation.
2. Explain the role of the following mechanisms of pulmonary ventilation:
   Atmospheric pressure (barometric pressure)
   —Pressure gradients
   —Boyle's law
3. Describe how the primary mechanisms of ventilation are applied to the human airways, and include the excursion of the diaphragm and the effects on pleural pressure, intra-alveolar pressure, and bronchial gas flow during
   —Inspiration
   —End-inspiration
   —Expiration
   —End-expiration
4. Describe the clinical connection associated with inspiratory intercostal retractions.
5. Differentiate between the following pressure gradients across the lungs:
   —Driving pressure
   —Transrespiratory pressure
   —Transmural pressure
   —Transpulmonary pressure
   —Transthoracic pressure
6. Describe the clinical connection associated with pulmonary disorders that force the patient to breathe at the top—flat portion—of the volume-pressure curve.
7. Describe the elastic properties of the lung and chest wall.
8. Define lung compliance.
9. Calculate lung compliance.
10. Describe the clinical connection associated with the harmful effects of pressure gradients when the thorax is unstable.
11. Discuss the clinical connection associated with pulmonary disorders that shift the volume-pressure curve to the right—decreased lung compliance conditions.
12. Explain how Hooke's law can be applied to the elastic properties of the lungs.
13. Describe the clinical connection associated with positive-pressure ventilation and include
    —Inspiration
    —End-inspiration
    —Expiration
    —End-expiration
14. Describe the clinical connection associated with the hazards of positive-pressure ventilation and include
    —Pneumothorax
    —Decreased cardiac output and blood pressure
15. Describe the clinical connection associated with negative-pressure ventilation and include
    —Inspiration
    —End-inspiration
    —Expiration
    —End-expiration
16. Define surface tension.
17. Describe Laplace's law.
18. Describe how Laplace's law can be applied to the alveolar fluid lining.
19. Explain how pulmonary surfactant offsets alveolar surface tension.
20. List respiratory disorders that cause a deficiency of pulmonary surfactant.
21. Describe the clinical connection associated with pulmonary surfactant deficiency in premature infants diagnosed with respiratory distress syndrome (RDS).
22. Define the term *dynamic*.

(continues)

23. Describe how Poiseuille's law arranged for flow relates to the radius of the bronchial airways.
24. Describe how Poiseuille's law arranged for pressure relates to the radius of the bronchial airways.
25. Describe how Poiseuille's law can be rearranged to simple proportionalities.
26. Describe the clinical connection associated with respiratory disorders that decrease the radius of the airways.
27. Define airway resistance and explain how it relates to
    —Laminar flow
    —Turbulent flow
    —Tracheobronchial or transitional flow
28. Calculate airway resistance.
29. Define time constants and explain how they relate to alveolar units with a/an
    —Increased airway resistance
    —Decreased compliance
30. Explain the meaning of dynamic compliance.
31. Describe the clinical connection associated with restrictive lung disorders, time constants, and breathing pattern relationships.
32. Describe the clinical connection associated with obstructive lung disorders, time constants, and breathing pattern relationships.
33. Discuss the clinical connection associated with auto-PEEP and its relationship to airway resistance during rapid ventilatory rates.
34. Describe how the following relate to the normal ventilatory pattern:
    —Tidal volume (V_T)
    —Ventilatory rate
    —I:E ratio
35. Discuss the clinical connection associated with the normal respiratory rates for different age groups.
36. Explain the clinical connection associated with the tidal volume and respiratory rate strategies for mechanical ventilation.
37. Differentiate between alveolar ventilation and dead space ventilation, and explain the following:
    —Anatomic dead space
    —Alveolar dead space
    —Physiologic dead space
38. Describe how the following affect alveolar ventilation:
    —Depth of breathing
    —Rate of breathing
39. Calculate an individual's alveolar ventilation when given the following information:
    —Alveolar ventilation
    —Dead space ventilation
    —Breaths per minute
40. Describe the clinical connection associated with a giraffe's neck and its relationship to alveolar ventilation, dead space ventilation, and include how this relationship may be applied to an endotracheal tube or the tubing circuitry on a mechanical ventilator.
41. Explain the clinical connection associated with pulmonary embolus and dead space ventilation.
42. Describe how the normal pleural pressure differences cause regional differences in normal lung ventilation.
43. Describe how the following alter the ventilatory pattern (i.e., the respiratory rate and tidal volume):
    —Decreased lung compliance
    —Increased airway resistance
44. Describe the clinical connection associated with how the adopted breathing pattern changes in chronic obstructive lung disorders when compromised by a restrictive lung disorder.
45. Compare and contrast the following types of ventilation:
    —Apnea
    —Eupnea
    —Biot's breathing
    —Hyperpnea
    —Hyperventilation
    —Hypoventilation
    —Tachypnea
    —Cheyne-Stokes breathing
    —Kussmaul's breathing
    —Orthopnea
    —Dyspnea
46. Discuss the clinical connection associated with the arterial carbon dioxide level and its relationship to the clinical verification of hyperventilation and hypoventilation.
47. Complete the review questions at the end of this chapter.

Introduction

The term **ventilation** is defined as the process that moves gases between the external environment and the alveoli. It is the mechanism by which oxygen is carried from the atmosphere to the alveoli and by which carbon dioxide (delivered to the lungs in mixed venous blood) is carried from the alveoli to the atmosphere.

To fully understand the process of ventilation, the respiratory therapist must understand (1) the **mechanisms of pulmonary ventilation**, (2) the **elastic properties of the lungs and chest wall**, (3) the **dynamic characteristics of the lungs** and **how they affect ventilation**, and (4) the **characteristics of normal and abnormal ventilatory patterns**.

Mechanisms of Pulmonary Ventilation

Before the primary mechanisms of pulmonary ventilation can be described, it is important to understand that the pulmonary pressures discussed throughout this textbook are always presented relative to the **atmospheric pressure (P_{atm})**—also called **the barometric pressure (P_B)**. The P_B is the force exerted by the air (gases) that surrounds the earth—and the body. As explained in Figure 2–1 on page 80, the P_B can be measured with a mercury barometer. At sea level under standard conditions, the P_B is 760 mm Hg.[1]

Although there are a number of measuring units used to quantify the P_B, pulmonary ventilating pressures are most commonly expressed as either (1) **millimeters of mercury (mm Hg—also called torr)**, or (2) **centimeters of water (cm H_2O)**. The respiratory therapist must be familiar with both of these pressure units and, importantly, know how to covert from one pressure unit to another. The conversion factors are as follows:

- **mm Hg (torr) to cm H_2O: 1 mm Hg ÷ 0.7355 (factor) = 1.36 cm H_2O**
- **cm H_2O to mm Hg: 1 cm H_2O × 1.36 (factor) = 1.36 mm Hg**

Thus, a normal P_B at sea level can be expressed as either of 760 mm Hg or 1033 cm H_2O (760 ÷ 0.7355 = 1033.31 cm H_2O)—depending on which pressure unit measurement is used.[2]

When the pulmonary pressures—mm Hg or cm H_2O—are used to describe ventilation pressures, they are always referenced to the atmospheric pressure and given a baseline value of zero. In other words, even though the atmospheric pressure at sea level is 760 mm Hg (or 1033 cm H_2O), it is designated as 0 mm Hg (or 0 cm H_2O). Thus, when the pulmonary pressure increases by +10 mm Hg (13.6 cm H_2O) during a positive-pressure breath, the pressure actually increases from 760 to 770 mm Hg (1033 to 1046.6 cm H_2O).

---

[1] Depending on the weather conditions, the atmospheric pressure (barometric pressure) can widely vary. The pressure of 760 mm Hg is an excellent reference point to discuss the mechanism of pulmonary ventilation. A P_B of 760 mm Hg is equal to 1033 cm H_2O, 14.7 psi, 29.9 in Hg, 101.3 kPa, or 1013.25 millibars.

[2] Although the mm Hg and cm H_2O are the most common pressure units used for pulmonary pressure changes, they do not represent the SI standard (International System of Units). The SI unit for pressure is the kilopascal (kPa); 1 kPa = 7.5 mm Hg or 10.2 cm H_2O.

Mercury barometer. The standard mercury barometer is composed of a vacuum-filled, glass tube of about 30 in. (76 cm) in height. The glass column is closed at one end, and open at the other. The open end of the tube is placed in a mercury-filled base that interfaces with the atmospheric pressure. Relative to (1) the weight of the mercury in the column, and (2) the atmospheric forces exerted on the mercury reservoir, the mercury moves up or down the column—similar to a liquid moving up a straw in a glass of water. In other words, the weight of the air pressing down on the surface of the mercury in the open dish pushes the mercury down into the dish and up the tube.

The greater the air pressure pushing down on the mercury surface, the higher up the tube the mercury will be forced. For example, during high barometric pressure periods, more force is exerted on the mercury reservoir—thus, forcing the mercury to climb higher up the glass column. On the other hand during low-pressure periods, less force is exerted on the mercury reservoir—thus allowing the mercury to move down the glass column. Under standard conditions at sea level, the barometric pressure (PB) causes the mercury to move up the glass column to a height of 760 mm (29.92 in.). This pressure can also be expressed in atmosphere units: atmospheric pressure = 760 mm Hg = 1 atm.

© Cengage Learning 2013

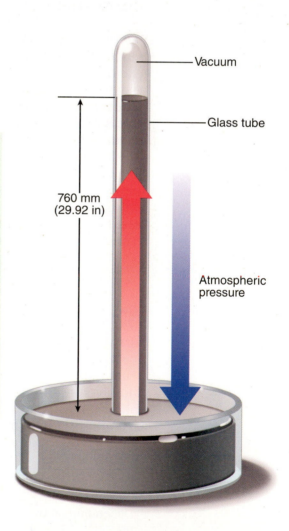

It should be noted that it is common to use either mm Hg or torr for gas pressure values (e.g., P_{O_2}, P_{CO_2}, N_2). The torr was named after Evangelista Torricelli, an Italian physicist and mathematician, who discovered the principe of the mercury barometer in 1644. In honor of Torricelli, the torr was defined as a unit of pressure equal to 1 mm Hg—i.e., 1 torr = 1 mm Hg.

The National Board for Respiratory Care (NBRC) uses the following on national board exams:

* torr is used for blood gas values (e.g., Pa_{O_2} or Pa_{CO_2}).
* mm Hg is used for blood pressure and barometric values.

Labels on figure: Vacuum; Glass tube; 760 mm (29.92 in); Atmospheric pressure

Or, stated three more ways to further drive this important pressure relationship home:

- A pressure of −5 mm Hg in the trachea, means the pressure in the trachea is lower than the atmospheric pressure by 5 mm Hg (760 − 5 = 755 mm Hg).
- Or, a positive pressure of +5 mm Hg in the alveoli, means the pressure in alveoli is higher than the atmosphere by 5 mm Hg (760 + 5 = 765 mm Hg).

- Or, a zero pressure in the trachea means the pressure in the trachea is equal to the atmospheric pressure (760 − 760 = 0 mm Hg).

With this fundamental understanding, the reader is prepared to examine the pressure relationships that normally exist throughout the thoracic cavity during a normal breathing cycle.

Pressure Gradients (Pressure Differences)

A gas or liquid always moves from an area of high pressure to an area of low pressure. In other words, in order for gas to flow from one point to another, there must be a "pressure difference" between the two points. In pulmonary physiology, a pressure difference is called a **pressure gradient**. Gas always moves "down" its pressure gradient—which means that gases always move from a high-pressure area to a low-pressure area. The mechanisms of pulmonary ventilation that create a pressure gradient are known as the **primary principles of ventilation**.

For example, when the atmospheric pressure is 760 mm Hg, the air pressure in the alveoli at **end-expiration**—and just before the beginning of another inspiration (pre-inspiration)—also exerts a pressure of 760 mm Hg. This explains why air is neither entering nor leaving the lungs at end-expiration and pre-inspiration. In other words, in order for pulmonary ventilation to occur, a mechanism must first be established that causes a pressure gradient between the atmosphere and the intra-alveoli.

As shown in Figure 2–2A, when the atmospheric pressure is higher than intra-alveoli pressure, air moves down the gas pressure gradient. In this case, gas moves from the atmosphere to the alveoli—and, inspiration occurs. On the other hand, when the intra-alveolar pressure is greater than the atmospheric pressure, air again moves down a pressure gradient. In this case, air flows from the alveoli to the atmosphere—and, expiration occurs.

The bottom line is this: in order for either inspiration or expiration to occur, the mechanisms of pulmonary ventilation must first establish a means to create (1) a pressure gradient for inspiration, in which the intra-alveolar pressure (P_{Alv}) is lower than the atmospheric pressure (or barometric pressure, P_B), and (2) a pressure gradient for expiration—in which the intra-alveolar pressure is greater than the atmospheric pressure (Figure 2–2B).

Figure 2–2

The primary principle of ventilation: Gas always moves down a pressure gradient—that is, gas always moves from a high-pressure area to a lower-pressure area. **A.** During inspiration, the barometric pressure (P_B) is greater than the alveolar pressure (P_A). **B.** During expiration, the alveolar pressure is higher than the barometric pressure.

© Cengage Learning 2013

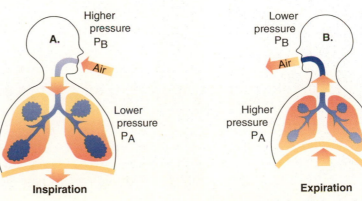

Boyle's Law and Its Relationship to Pressure Gradients in Ventilation

To fully comprehend how the pressure gradients for inspiration and expiration are produced, an understanding of how **Boyle's law** works to create pressure changes throughout the thoracic cavity during inspiration and expiration is absolutely essential.

Boyle's law ($P_1 \times V_1 = P_2 \times V_2$) states a volume of gas varies inversely proportional to its pressure at a constant temperature. For example, if an airtight container, which has a volume of 200 mL and a pressure of 10 cm H_2O, has its volume reduced 50 percent (100 mL), the new pressure in the container will double—that is, increase to 20 cm H_2O (Figure 2–3). This example can be computed as follows:

$$P_2 = \frac{P_1 \times V_1}{V_2}$$
$$= \frac{10 \text{ cm } H_2O \times 200 \text{ mL}}{100 \text{ mL}}$$
$$= 20 \text{ cm } H_2O$$

In applying Boyle's law to the mechanics of ventilation, therefore, it should be understood that when the thoracic cavity increases in size (increase in volume)—caused by the downward contraction of the diaphragm during inspiration—the pressure in the thoracic cavity decreases. This action causes air to move down the pressure gradient from the atmosphere to the alveoli. On the other hand, when the thoracic cavity decreases in size (decrease in volume)—caused by the relaxation of the diaphragm during expiration—the pressure in the thoracic cavity increases. This action causes air to move down the pressure gradient from the alveoli to the atmosphere.

Figure 2–3

Boyle's law states a volume of gas varies inversely proportional to its pressure at a constant temperature. For example, as shown in this figure, if the pressure on a gas increased from 10 cm H_2O to 20 cm H_2O, the gas volume would decrease from 200 mL to 100 mL. In other words, doubling the pressure reduces the volume by half.

© Cengage Learning 2013

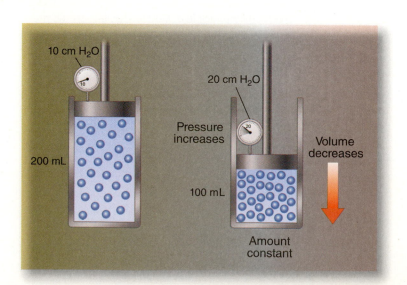

Balloon Model of Ventilation

The mechanisms of ventilation are often visually demonstrated by using a balloon in a bell-shaped jar (Figure 2–4). The bell-shaped jar represents the rib cage (thoracic cavity). The rubber sheet across the bottom of the jar represents the diaphragm. The balloon represents the lung. The space between the outside of the balloon and the inside of the jar represents the pleural space. The tube connected to the balloon and the cork at the top of the jar represents the trachea—which provides the only passageway between the inside of the balloon (lung) and the atmosphere.

To simulate **inspiration** the diaphragm is pulled downward, causing the size of the thoracic cavity to increase (increased volume)—which, in turn, causes the pleural pressure (P_{pl}) to decrease (remember, according to Boyle's law, as volume increases, pressure decreases). Because the balloon is composed of a thin stretchy, rubbery, material (similar to the elastic tissue of the normal lung), the decrease in the P_{pl} is transmitted to the inside of the balloon. This mechanism causes a pressure gradient between the inside of the balloon and the atmosphere. Because the atmospheric pressure is higher than the pressure inside of the balloon—that is, a pressure gradient exists—gas from the atmosphere moves down the tube into the balloon (Figure 2–4A).

The gas flow continues until the pressure inside the balloon "equals" the pressure in the atmosphere—the **equilibrium point** (zero pressure point).

Figure 2–4

Balloon model of ventilation. **A.** Inspiration, caused by downward movement of the rubber sheet (diaphragm). **B.** End-inspiration (equilibrium point, no gas flow). **C.** Expiration. Caused by the elastic recoil of the diaphragm upward movement. **D.** End-expiration (equilibrium point, no gas flow).

© Cengage Learning 2013

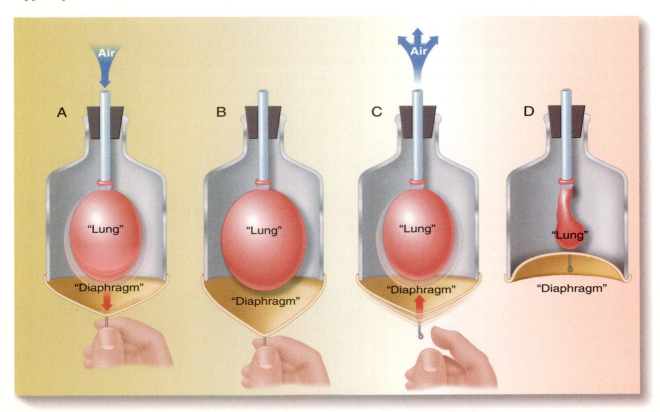

Once the *equilibrium point* is reached, gas flow stops. This period of no gas flow represents **end-inspiration** (Figure 2–4B).

To simulate **expiration**, the elastic diaphragm is allowed to recoil upward, causing the size of the thoracic cavity to decrease (decreased volume)—which, in turn, causes the intrapleural pressure to increase (remember, according to Boyle's law, as volume decreases, pressure increases). Again, because the balloon is composed of a thin rubbery material, the increase in P_{pl} is transmitted to the inside of the balloon. This mechanism causes a pressure gradient between the inside of the balloon and the atmosphere. Because the pressure is now higher inside the balloon than the atmosphere—that is, a pressure gradient exists—gas from inside the balloon flows through the tube into the atmosphere (Figure 2–4C).

The gas flow will continue until the pressure inside the balloon equals the pressure in the atmosphere. Once the equilibrium point is reached, gas flow stops. This period of no gas flow represents **end-expiration** (Figure 2–4D).

The entire simulated breathing sequence—that is, inspiration, end-inspiration, expiration, and end-expiration—represents one **respiratory cycle**.

The Primary Mechanisms of Ventilation Applied to the Human Airways

Figure 2–5 applies the same pressure gradient principle illustrated in the balloon model to the human thoracic cavity, lungs, diaphragm, and airways. During **inspiration**, the diaphragm contracts downward, causing the size of the thoracic cavity to increase (increased volume). This action causes the pleural pressure (P_{pl}) to decrease. Because the lung is composed of a thin elastic tissue, the decrease in the P_{pl} is transmitted to the inside of the alveoli—which, in turn, causes the intra-alveolar pressure to decrease. This mechanism causes a pressure gradient to develop between the intra-alveoli pressure and the atmospheric pressure. Because the atmospheric pressure is higher than the intra-alveolar pressure—that is, a pressure gradient exists—gas from the atmosphere moves through the tracheobronchial tree to the alveoli (Figure 2–5A).

The gas flow will continue until the intra-alveolar pressure and the atmospheric pressure are in equilibrium. Once the equilibrium point is reached, gas flow stops. This period of no gas flow is the **end-inspiration** (or pre-expiration) phase of the respiratory cycle (Figure 2–5B).

During **expiration**, the diaphragm relaxes and moves upward, causing the size of the thoracic cavity to decrease (decreased volume). This action causes the pleural pressure (P_{pl}) to increase. Again, because the lung is composed of a thin elastic tissue, the increase in the P_{pl} is transmitted to the inside of the alveoli—which, in turn, causes the intra-alveolar pressure to increase. This mechanism causes a pressure gradient between the intra-alveoli pressure and the atmospheric pressure. Because the intra-alveolar pressure is higher than the atmospheric pressure—that is, a pressure gradient exists—gas from the alveoli moves through the tracheobronchial tree to the atmosphere (Figure 2–5C).

The gas flow will continue until the intra-alveolar pressure and the atmospheric pressure are in equilibrium. Once equilibrium point is reached, gas flow stops. This period of no gas flow is the **end-expiration** (or pre-inspiration) phase of the respiratory cycle (Figure 2–5D).

Under normal conditions, the intrapleural pressure—during both inspiration and expiration—is always below the barometric pressure. This is because the lungs have a natural tendency to recoil inward, and the chest wall has a

Figure 2–5

How the excursion of the diaphragm affects the intrapleural pressure, intra-alveolar pressure, and bronchial gas flow during inspiration and expiration.

Normal Inspiration and Expiration

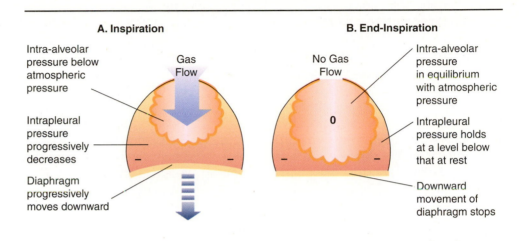

A. Inspiration

Intra-alveolar pressure below atmospheric pressure

Gas Flow

Intrapleural pressure progressively decreases

Diaphragm progressively moves downward

B. End-Inspiration

No Gas Flow

Intra-alveolar pressure in equilibrium with atmospheric pressure

0

Intrapleural pressure holds at a level below that at rest

Downward movement of diaphragm stops

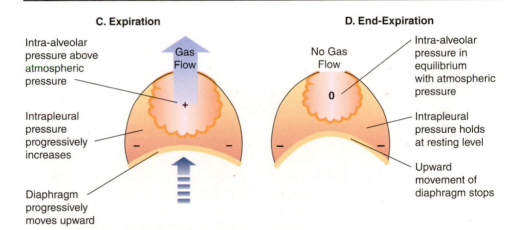

C. Expiration

Intra-alveolar pressure above atmospheric pressure

Gas Flow

Intrapleural pressure progressively increases

Diaphragm progressively moves upward

D. End-Expiration

No Gas Flow

Intra-alveolar pressure in equilibrium with atmospheric pressure

0

Intrapleural pressure holds at resting level

Upward movement of diaphragm stops

natural tendency to expand outward. These two opposing forces generate a subatmospheric pressure—that is, negative pleural pressure—between the parietal and visceral pleurae. With normal breathing at rest, the excursion of the diaphragm is about 1.5 cm, and the normal pleural pressure change is about 3 to 6 cm H_2O pressure (2 to 4 mm Hg). During a deep inspiration, however, the diaphragm may move as much as 6 to 10 cm—which can cause the pleural pressure to drop to as low as –50 cm H_2O subatmospheric pressure. During a forced expiration, the pleural pressure may climb to between +70 and 100 cm H_2O above atmospheric pressure.

To summarize, it should be clear that a complete understanding of Boyle's law and its relationship to pressure gradients during the respiratory cycle is essential to understanding the mechanisms of ventilation. In other words, the fundamental principle of ventilation is based on these two pressure gradient facts: (1) gas always flows from an area of high pressure to an area of low pressure—that is, a pressure gradient must exist (e.g., inspiration and expiration)—and (2) there is no gas movement when the pressure gradient is zero—that is, there is no gas flow when the pressure between two points is equal (e.g., end-inspiration and end-expiration).

Clinical Connection—2-1

Inspiratory Intercostal Retractions

At the bedside, the respiratory therapist (RT) will see **inspiratory intercostal retractions** as inward movements of the tissue between the ribs, above the clavicle, or below the rib cage. This is a key indicator of severe respiratory distress—especially in infants (Figure 2–6). These are commonly referred to as intercostal retractions, supraclavicular retractions, or subcostal retractions, respectively. Additionally, the chest of the newborn is composed of a large amount of cartilage and is very flexible. The RT can actually observe these flexible ribs move inward on inspiration. When this happens, the infant's inspiratory volume will be diminished.

The RT must be aware of any respiratory disorder that increases the work of breathing—for example, narrowing of the airway such as asthma or a stiff lung such as pneumonia—that

can activate the muscles of inspiration to contract forcefully in an effort to generate a greater negative intrapleural and intra-alveolar pressure to draw in more air. The inspiratory retractions overlying the chest wall are a direct result of the increased negative intrapleural pressure.

Clinically, intercostal retractions are an excellent warning sign that the patient is experiencing severe respiratory distress. Although intercostal retractions can be seen in most patients with respiratory distress, they are common in the newborn infant with stiff lung—for example, **respiratory distress syndrome**. This is because the chest of the newborn is composed of a large amount of cartilage and is very flexible. Retractions are often hard to see in the obese patient because of the extra tissue covering the chest.

Figure 2–6

Newborn infant showing intercostal retractions (black arrows) and substernal retractions (blue arrows).

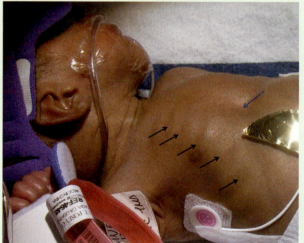

Courtesy T. Des Jardins, WindMist LLC

Finally, the respiratory care practitioner must also know and understand the following five different types of pressure measurements commonly used in pulmonary physiology: driving pressure, transrespiratory pressure, transmural pressure, transpulmonary pressure, and transthoracic pressure. Once these measurements are understood, and the idea of pressure gradients are mastered, the differences between normal spontaneous ventilation, positive-pressure ventilation, and negative-pressure ventilation become crystal clear.

Figure 2–7

Driving pressure. At point A, gas pressure is 20 mm Hg. At point B, gas pressure is 5 mm Hg. Thus, the driving pressure between point A and point B is 15 mm Hg.

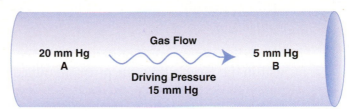

Driving pressure is the pressure difference between two points in a tube or vessel; it is the force moving gas or fluid through the tube or vessel. For example, if the gas pressure at the beginning of a tube is 20 mm Hg and the pressure at the end of the same tube is 5 mm Hg, then the driving pressure is 15 mm Hg. In other words, the force required to move the gas through the tube is 15 mm Hg (Figure 2–7).

Transrespiratory pressure (P_{rs}) (also called transairway pressure) is the difference between the barometric (atmospheric) pressure (P_B) and the alveolar pressure (P_{alv}). In other words, the P_{rs} is the pressure gradient difference between the mouth pressure (atmospheric pressure) and the alveolar pressure (P_{alv}).

$$P_{rs} = P_B - P_{alv}$$

For example, if the P_{alv} is 757 mm Hg and the P_B is 760 mm Hg during inspiration, then the P_{rs} is 3 mm Hg (Figure 2–8A).

$$P_{rs} = P_B - P_{alv}$$
$$= 760 \text{ mm Hg} - 757 \text{ mm Hg}$$
$$= 3 \text{ mm Hg}$$

Or, if the P_{alv} is 763 mm Hg and the P_B is 760 mm Hg during expiration, then the P_{rs} is –3 mm Hg. Gas in this example, however, is moving in the opposite direction (Figure 2–8B). The P_{rs} causes airflow in and out of the conducting

Figure 2–8

Transrespiratory pressure (P_{rs}): The difference between the body surface pressure (P_{bs})* and the alveolar pressure (P_{alv}). Even though gas is moving in opposite directions in A and B, the transrespiratory pressure is 3 mm Hg in both examples.
*Note: In this illustration, the body surface pressure (P_{bs}) is equal to the barometric pressure (P_B).

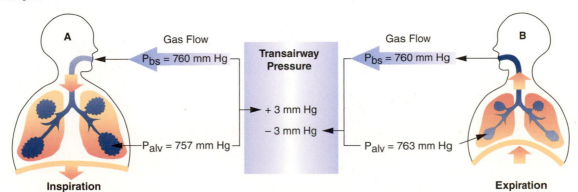

airways. In essence, the P_{rs} represents the driving pressure (the pressure difference between the mouth and the alveolus) that forces gas in or out of the lungs.

Transmural pressure (P_{tm}) is the pressure difference that occurs across the airway wall. The transmural pressure is calculated by subtracting the intra-airway pressure (P_{iaw}) from the pressure on the outside of the airway (P_{oaw}).

$$P_{tm} = P_{oaw} - P_{iaw}$$

Positive transmural pressure is said to exist when the pressure is greater within the airway than the pressure outside the airway. For example, if the P_{iaw} pressure is 765 mm Hg and the P_{oaw} is 760 mm Hg, there is a positive transmural pressure of 5 mm Hg (Figure 2–9A).

$$
\begin{aligned}
P_{tm} &= P_{oaw} - P_{iaw} \\
&= 765 \text{ mm Hg} - 760 \text{ mm Hg} \\
&= 5 \text{ mm Hg (positive transmural pressure)}
\end{aligned}
$$

Negative transmural pressure is said to exist when the pressure is greater outside the airway than the pressure inside the airway. For example, if the P_{iaw} pressure is 755 mm Hg and the P_{oaw} is 760 mm Hg, there is a negative transmural pressure of 5 mm Hg (Figure 2–9B).

Transpulmonary pressure (P_{tp}) is the difference between the alveolar pressure (P_{alv}) and the pleural pressure (P_{pl}).

$$P_{tp} = P_{alv} - P_{pl}$$

For example, if the P_{pl} is 755 mm Hg and the P_{alv} is 760 mm Hg (e.g., inspiration), then the P_{tp} is 5 mm Hg (Figure 2–10A).

$$
\begin{aligned}
P_{tp} &= P_{alv} - P_{pl} \\
&= 760 \text{ mm Hg} - 755 \text{ mm Hg} \\
&= 5 \text{ mm Hg}
\end{aligned}
$$

Or, if the P_{alv} is 763 mm Hg and the P_{pl} is 758 mm Hg (e.g., expiration), then the P_{tp} is 5 mm Hg (Figure 2–10B). In the normal lung, the P_{alv} is always greater than the P_{pl}, which, in turn, maintains the lungs in an inflated state.

Figure 2–9

Transmural pressure: the pressure difference that occurs across the wall of the airway. **A.** Airway with a positive transmural pressure. **B.** Airway with a negative transmural pressure.

© Cengage Learning 2013

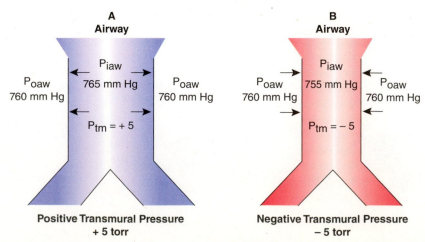

A Airway	B Airway
P_{oaw} 760 mm Hg — P_{iaw} 765 mm Hg — P_{oaw} 760 mm Hg — $P_{tm} = +5$	P_{oaw} 760 mm Hg — P_{iaw} 755 mm Hg — P_{oaw} 760 mm Hg — $P_{tm} = -5$
Positive Transmural Pressure + 5 torr	**Negative Transmural Pressure** − 5 torr

Figure 2–10

Transpulmonary pressure: The difference between the alveolar pressure (P_{alv}) and the pleural pressure (P_{pl}). This illustration assumes a barometric pressure (P_B) of 761 mm Hg.

© Cengage Learning 2013

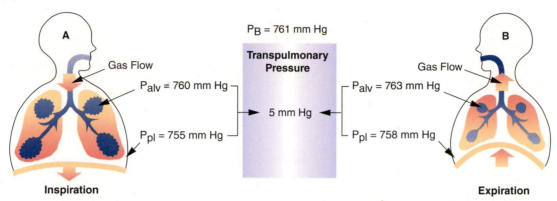

Transthoracic pressure (P_{tt}) is the difference between the alveolar pressure (P_{alv}) and the body surface pressure (P_{bs}).

$$P_{tt} = P_{alv} - P_{bs}$$

For example, if the P_{alv} is 757 mm Hg and the P_{bs} is 760 mm Hg (e.g., inspiration), then the P_{tt} is −3 mm Hg (Figure 2–11A).

$$
\begin{aligned}
P_{tt} &= P_{alv} - P_{bs} \\
&= 757 \text{ mm Hg} - 760 \text{ mm Hg} \\
&= -3 \text{ mm Hg}
\end{aligned}
$$

Or, if the P_{alv} is 763 mm Hg and the P_{bs} is 760 mm Hg (e.g., expiration), then the P_{tt} is 3 mm Hg (Figure 2–11B). The P_{tt} is the pressure responsible for expanding the lungs and chest wall in tandem.

Technically, there is no real difference between the transrespiratory pressure (P_{rs}) and the transthoracic pressure (P_{tt}). The P_{tt} is merely another way to view the pressure differences across the lungs.

Figure 2–11

Transthoracic pressure: The difference between the alveolar pressure (P_{alv}) and the body surface pressure (P_{bs}). Note: In this illustration, the body surface pressure (P_{bs}) is equal to the barometric pressure (P_B).

© Cengage Learning 2013

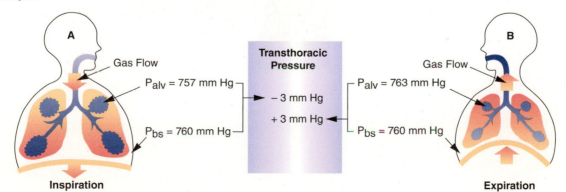

Clinical Connection—2-2

The Harmful Effects of Pressure Gradients When the Thorax Is Unstable

In the Clinical Application Section—Case 1 (page 138), the respiratory therapist is called to assist in the care of a 22-year-old male motorcycle crash victim who presents in the emergency room with numerous abrasions, lacerations, and a very serious chest injury—multiple broken ribs over the right anterior chest. In this case, the RT must be aware of how (1) the **negative intrapleural pressure**, (2) the **transpulmonary pressure**, and (3) the **transthoracic pressure** all profoundly affect the patient's ability to breathe when the chest wall is unstable.

For example, each time the patient inhales, the transpulmonary and transthoracic pressure gradients cause his broken ribs to sink inward. This condition is called a **flail chest** (Figure 2–12). This movement causes the patient's inspiratory volume to decrease. During each exhalation, the pressure gradients cause the patient's broken ribs to bulge outward. This action causes some of the exhaled air from the unaffected lung to move into the affected lung—the lung directly under the broken ribs—rather than being exhaled out. The movement of air from one lung to another is known as a **pendelluft**.

Case 1 also shows how the respiratory therapist must be aware of this inward movement of the chest—during each inspiration—and how it will work against the patient's ability to breathe. To correct this problem, the therapist must place the patient on a positive-pressure ventilator. The positive-pressure ventilator eliminates the negative intrapleural pressure changes during each inspiration—which, in turn, stops the adverse effects of the transpulmonary and transthoracic pressure gradients during inspiration. The respiratory therapist uses positive-pressure ventilation to prevent the flailed portion of the chest from affecting breathing and to provide time for the broken ribs to heal.

Figure 2–12

Right-sided flail chest. See red arrows for broken ribs. Note the **subcutaneous emphysema**—which is the presence of air in the subcutaneous tissues (green arrow). Subcutaneous emphysema is a common complication associated with chest trauma.

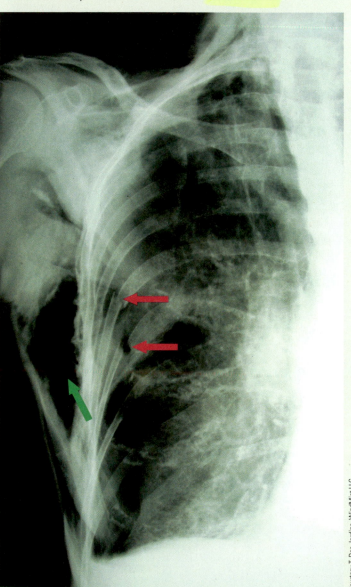

Courtesy T. Des Jardins, WindMist LLC

Elastic Properties of the Lung and Chest Wall

Both the lungs and the chest wall each have their own elastic properties—and, under normal conditions, each elastic system works against the other. That is, the chest wall has a natural tendency to move outward or to expand as a result of the bones of the thorax and surrounding muscles. The lungs have a natural tendency to move inward or collapse because of the natural elastic properties of the lung tissue. This lung–chest wall relationship is often compared to that of two springs working against each other—that is, the chest wall works to spring outward; the lungs work to recoil inward. Clinically, the elastic forces of the lungs are routinely evaluated by measuring the lung compliance.

Lung Compliance

How readily the elastic force of the lungs accepts a volume of inspired air is known as **lung compliance** (C_L); C_L is defined as the *change in lung volume* (ΔV) per *unit pressure change* (ΔP) Mathematically, C_L is expressed in liters per centimeter of water pressure (L/cm H_2O). In other words, C_L determines how much air, in liters, the lungs will accommodate for each centimeter of water pressure change (e.g., each transpulmonary pressure change).

For example, if an individual generates a negative pleural pressure change of 5 cm H_2O during inspiration, and the lungs accept a new volume of 0.5 L (500 mL) of gas, the C_L of the lungs would be expressed as 0.1 L/cm H_2O (100 mL/cm H_2O):

$$C_L = \frac{\Delta V \ (L)}{\Delta P \ (cm \ H_2O)}$$

$$= \frac{0.5 \ L \ of \ gas}{5 \ (cm \ H_2O)}$$

$$= 0.1 \ L/cm \ H_2O \ (or \ 100 \ mL/cm \ H_2O)$$

It is irrelevant whether the change in driving pressure is in the form of positive or negative pressure. In other words, a negative 5-cm H_2O pressure generated in the pleural space, around the lungs, will produce the same volume change as a positive 5-cm H_2O pressure delivered to the tracheobronchial tree (e.g., by means of a mechanical ventilator) (Figure 2–13 on page 92).

At rest, the average C_L for each breath is about 0.1 L/cm H_2O. In other words, approximately 100 mL of air is delivered into the lungs per 1-cm H_2O pressure change (see Figure 2–13). When lung compliance is increased, the lungs accept a greater volume of gas per unit of pressure change. When C_L is decreased, the lungs accept a smaller volume of gas per unit of pressure change. This relationship is also illustrated by the volume–pressure curve in Figure 2–14 on page 93.

Note that—both in the normal and abnormal lung—C_L progressively decreases as the alveoli approach their total filling capacity. This occurs because the elastic force of the alveoli steadily increases as the lungs expand, which, in turn, reduces the ability of the lungs to accept an additional volume of gas (see Figure 2–14).

Chest Wall Compliance

As discussed earlier, the chest wall has its own elastic properties, caused by the bones of the thorax and surrounding muscles. As a result, the chest wall works to offset the normal elastic properties of the lungs. If unopposed, the normal compliance of both the lungs and chest wall are about equal at

Figure 2–13

Normal volume–pressure curve. The curve shows that lung compliance progressively decreases as lungs expand in response to increased volume. For example, note the greater volume change between 5 and 10 cm H_2O (small/medium alveoli) than between 30 and 35 cm H_2O (large alveoli).

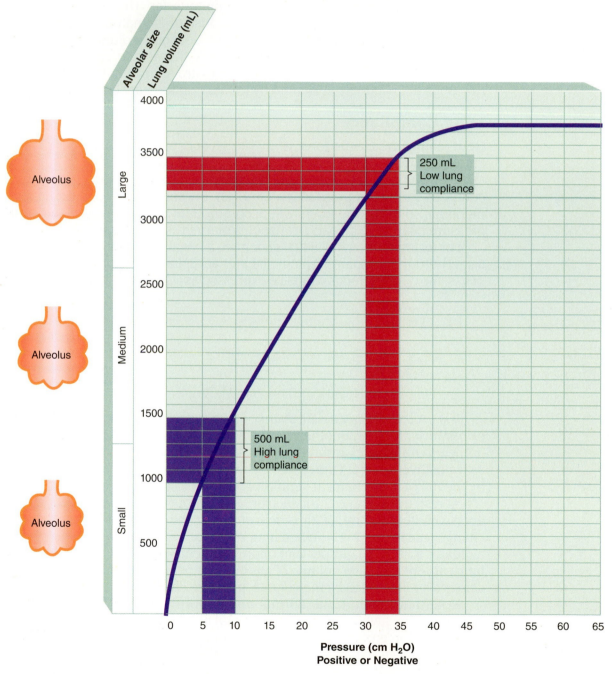

0.2 L/cm H_2O. However, because the lungs are enclosed within the thorax—and attached to the internal surface of the chest wall—the two elastic systems function as springs that naturally recoil away from each other. This action, in turn, decreases the compliance of each elastic system to about one-half of the individual components—or 0.1 L/cm H_2O. In other words, the normal lung compliance of 0.1 L/H_2O is actually the end result of the "combined" chest wall compliance and lung compliance.

Figure 2–14

How changes in lung compliance affect the volume–pressure curve. When lung compliance decreases, the volume–pressure curve shifts to the right. When lung compliance increases, the volume–pressure curve shifts to the left.

© Cengage Learning 2013

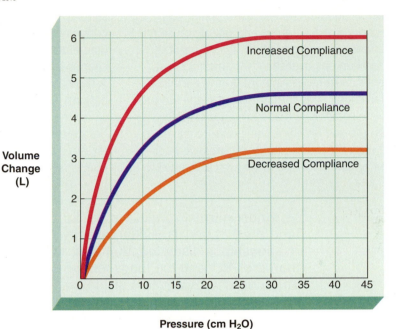

Clinical Connection—2-3

Pulmonary Disorders That Force the Patient to Breathe at the Top—Flat Portion—of the Volume–Pressure Curve

In the Clinical Application Section—Case 2 (page 139), the respiratory therapist is called to assist in the care of a 14-year-old girl with a long history of asthma. This clinical event illustrates how an obstructive lung disorder—an acute asthma attack, in this case—can quickly cause an acute decrease in the patient's lung compliance. During an asthmatic episode, the patient's bronchial airway obstruction progressively worsens—impeding the patient's ability to fully exhale. This condition causes air trapping and hyperinflation of the lungs. Sometimes, the respiratory therapist can see this plotted on the volume–pressure curve, which shows that as the lungs become overinflated, the patient's lung compliance moves to the top—upper right-hand portion—of the volume–pressure curve—that is, the flat, very low compliant, part of the curve.

When ventilating on this portion of the volume–pressure curve, the work of breathing is very high. In this case, the patient is forced to generate very high intrapleural pressure changes—with little, or no, volume change. This can be an extremely frightening experience for any patient! Common obstructive lung disorders that can cause air trapping, overinflation, and decreased lung compliance—because the patient is forced to breathe on the very top, flat part of the volume–pressure curve—include cystic fibrosis, chronic bronchitis, and emphysema.

To personally experience how a patient may feel during an asthma attack, try this activity: inhale as deep as possible—that is, to the very top of the volume–pressure curve—and then attempt to breathe in and out normally without fully exhaling. Can you feel how hard it is to inhale once your lungs are fully inflated? How long do you think you could breathe at this level of your volume–pressure curve? As a respiratory therapist, you will be treating many patients who have had this experience with every acute asthmatic episode.

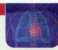

Clinical Connection—2-4

Pulmonary Disorders That Shift the Volume–Pressure Curve to the Right

Clinical Application Section—Case 1 (page 138), describes how a chest trauma can rapidly cause an acute decrease in lung compliance. As a result of multiple broken ribs over the right anterior chest, the patient's chest moves inward during each inspiration (flail chest). This condition causes the lung to collapse (atelectasis)—a restrictive lung disorder.

When plotted on a volume–pressure curve, it can be seen that as the lungs progressively collapse, the patient's volume–pressure curve quickly shifts to the right—lung compliance decreases. This condition forces the patient to generate high intrapleural pressure changes—with little or no volume change—and the work of breathing increases. A flail chest can be extremely frightening for any patient! Other restrictive lung disorders that can cause the volume–pressure curve to shift to the right include pneumonia, pneumothorax, pleural effusion, acute respiratory distress syndrome, pulmonary edema, and interstitial lung disease.

Under normal conditions, the lungs and chest wall recoil to a resting volume, the functional residual capacity (FRC).[3] When the normal lung–chest wall relationship is disrupted, the chest wall tend to expand to a volume greater than the FRC, and the lungs tend to collapse to a volume less than the FRC. This lung–chest wall relationship has many clinical implications. For example, pulmonary disorders that decrease a patient's lung compliance (e.g., pneumonia, atelectasis, or acute respiratory distress syndrome) not only hinder the patient's lung expansion, but also significantly decrease the patient's chest wall expansion. On the other hand, a pulmonary disorder that causes the lungs to break away from the chest wall (e.g., pneumothorax) can result in an over-expansion of the chest wall on the affected side (see Clinical Connection 2–6 and Figure 2–18 later in this chapter).

Hooke's Law

Hooke's law provides another way to explain compliance by describing the physical properties of an elastic substance. **Elastance** is the natural ability of matter to respond directly to force and to return to its original resting position or shape after the external force no longer exists. In pulmonary physiology, elastance is defined as the change in pressure per change in volume:

$$\text{Elastance} = \frac{\Delta P}{\Delta V}$$

Elastance is the reciprocal (opposite) of compliance. Thus, lungs with high compliance (greater ease of filling) have low elastance; lungs with low compliance (lower ease of filling) have high elastance. Note that elastance is the reciprocal of compliance for only a truly elastic body. Because the normal lung–chest wall is not a total, or absolute, elastic mechanism, it functions in a more *sigmoidal* than *linear* manner. Regardless of this point, it is still a satisfactory and practical approximation. Also, because of the viscous nature of the lungs and thorax, a mild degree of *hysteresis* is demonstrated on the volume–pressure curves when comparing inspiration to expiration (see Figure 2–27 later in this chapter).

---

[3] Read more on the functional residual capacity in Chapter 3.

Hooke's law states that when a truly elastic body, like a spring, is acted on by 1 unit of force, the elastic body will stretch 1 unit of length, and when acted on by 2 units of force it will stretch 2 units of length, and so forth. This phenomenon is only true, however, within the elastic body's normal functional range. When the force exceeds the elastic limits of the substance, the ability of length to increase in response to force rapidly decreases. Should the force continue to rise, the elastic substance will ultimately break (Figure 2–15).

| Figure 2–15 |

Hooke's law. When a truly elastic body—such as the spring in this illustration—is acted on by 1 unit of force, the elastic body will stretch 1 unit of length; when acted on by 2 units of force, it will stretch 2 units of length; and so forth. When the force goes beyond the elastic limit of the substance, however, the ability of length to increase in response to force quickly ceases.

© Cengage Learning 2013

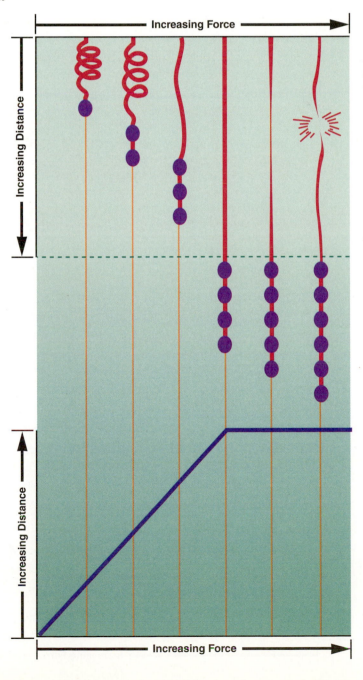

When Hooke's law is applied to the elastic properties of the lungs, *volume* is substituted for *length,* and *pressure* is substituted for *force.* Thus, over the normal physiologic range of the lungs, volume varies directly with pressure. The lungs behave in a manner similar to the spring, and once the elastic limits of the lung unit are reached, little or no volume change occurs in response to pressure changes. Should the change in pressure continue to rise, the elastic limits are exceeded and the lung unit will rupture (Figure 2–16).

Clinically, this phenomenon explains a hazard associated with mechanical ventilation. That is, if the pressure during mechanical ventilation (positive-pressure breath) causes the lung unit to expand beyond its elastic capability, the lung unit could rupture, allowing alveolar gas to move into the pleural space, and thus causing the lungs to collapse. This condition is called a **tension pneumothorax** (see Figure 2–18 on page 99).

Figure 2–16

Hooke's law applied to the elastic properties of the lungs. Over the physiologic range, volume changes vary directly with pressure changes. Once the elastic limits are reached, however, little or no volume change occurs in response to pressure change.

© Cengage Learning 2013

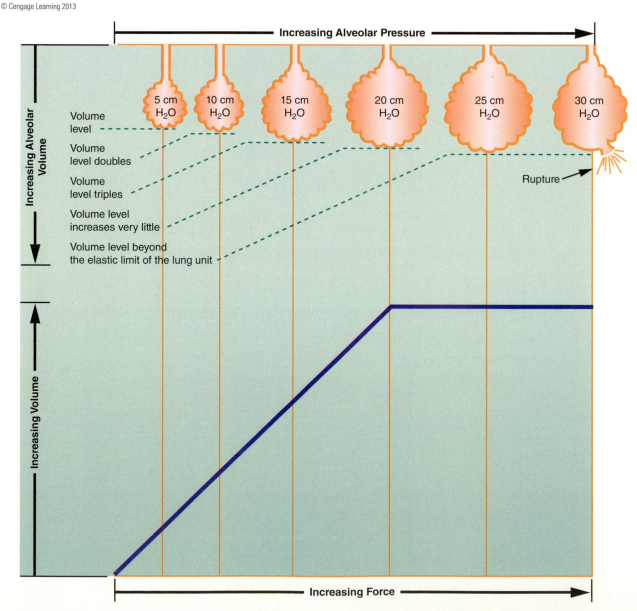

Clinical Connection—2-5

Positive-Pressure Ventilation

Clinically, when the patient is placed on a positive-pressure ventilator, the intrapleural pressures, intra-alveolar pressures, and the movement of the diaphragm will all be quite different than the normal mechanisms of pulmonary ventilation.

Inspiratory Phase of Positive-Pressure Ventilation

Figure 2–17 A shows that when the patient receives a positive-pressure breath from a mechanical ventilator, the intra-alveolar pressure progressively rises

above atmospheric pressure—similar to the positive pressure generated in an elastic balloon as it is being inflated. For example, if the mechanical ventilator delivered 30 cm H_2O pressure to the patient's lung during inspiration, the intra-alveolar pressure would increase to about 30 cm H_2O above the atmospheric pressure at the end of inspiration. As the pressure progressively increases in the alveoli during inspiration, the intrapleural pressure also increases.

As shown in Figure 2–17, the intrapleural pressure would gradually increase to about 30 cm H_2O above its

---

Figure 2–17

How a positive pressure breath from a mechanical ventilator affects the intra-alveolar pressure, intrapleural pressure, the excursion of the diaphragm, and gas flow during inspiration and expiration.

© Cengage Learning 2013

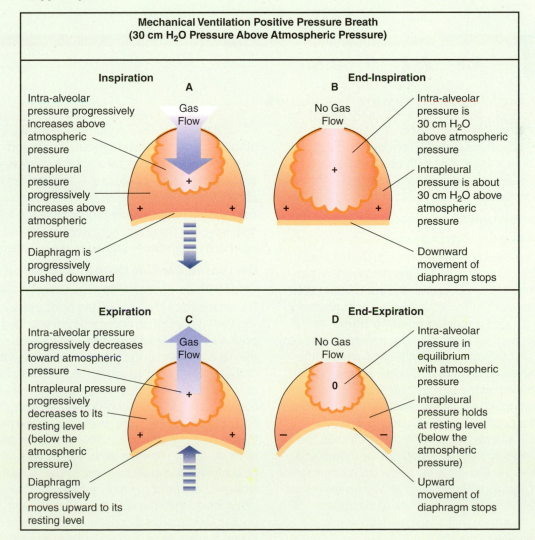

(continues)

Clinical Connection—2-5, continued

normal resting level, which, as illustrated in Figure 2–5, is normally below atmospheric pressure. Finally, as the intra-alveolar and intrapleural pressure increase during a positive-pressure breath, the lungs expand, pushing the diaphragm downward. This process continues until the positive-pressure breath stops (Figure 2-17 B).

Expiratory Phase of Positive-Pressure Ventilation

During exhalation, the intra-alveolar pressure decreases toward atmospheric pressure and allows the elastic properties of the lungs to return to their normal resting level—similar to the decreased positive pressure that occurs in an elastic balloon that is being allowed to return to the atmospheric pressure during deflation. This means that the high intra-alveolar pressure moves in the direction of the low atmospheric pressure until

the intra-alveolar pressure is in equilibrium with the atmospheric pressure. As the intra-alveolar pressure returns to normal, the intrapleural pressure decreases to its resting level (below the atmospheric pressure), and the diaphragm moves upward to its resting level (Figure 2-17 C).

At end-expiration, the intra-alveolar pressure is in equilibrium with atmospheric pressure. The intrapleural pressure is held at its resting level which, under normal circumstances, is below atmospheric pressure. The upward movement of the diaphragm stops at end-expiration (Figure 2-17 D). The administration of positive-pressure ventilation may also cause a number of adverse side effects, including lung rupture and gas accumulation between the lungs and chest wall (tension pneumothorax) and decreased cardiac output and blood pressure (see Clinical Connection 2–6: Hazards of Positive-Pressure Ventilation).

Clinical Connection—2-6

Hazards of Positive-Pressure Ventilation

The respiratory therapist must carefully monitor the patient on mechanical ventilation for a number of adverse affects associated with positive-pressure ventilation—including a sudden tension pneumothorax and decreased cardiac output and blood pressure.

Tension Pneumothorax

A patient receiving high positive pressures during mechanical ventilation is always at some degree of risk of a sudden lung rupture and resulting pneumothorax. A pneumothorax in which the intrapleural pressure is greater than the intra-alveolar (or atmospheric) pressure is called a **tension pneumothorax**. At the bedside, a number of clinical signs and symptoms can develop that indicate a sudden tension pneumothorax: (1) increased heart rate, (2) diminished or absent breath sounds on the affected side, (3) hyperresonant percussion note over the pneumothorax, (4) tracheal shift to the unaffected side, (5) displaced heart sounds, (6) an enlarged and immobile chest on the affected side, and (7) decreased cardiac output and blood pressure. A chest X-ray is used to confirm the extent of a pneumothorax and typically reveals (1) gas accumulation in the pleural cavity, (2) depressed diaphragm, and (3) shift of the mediastinum to the unaffected side of the chest.

The treatment for a pneumothorax is the insertion of a chest tube into the intrapleural space and the application of suction to draw out the air and re-expand the lung. Figure 2–18A illustrates a right-sided tension pneumothorax. Figure 2-18B shows a chest X-ray of a right-sided tension pneumothorax. Note the collapsed right lung, the depressed right diaphragm, and the heart and mediastinum pushed to the unaffected side.

Decreased Cardiac Output and Blood Pressure

The decreased cardiac output and blood pressure associated with a tension pneumothorax is caused by the **positive intrapleural pressure**—which is caused by the gas accumulation in the pleural cavity. As a result of the positive pleural pressure, the major intrathoracic veins—the inferior and superior vena cava—are compressed. This action impedes venous return to the heart. In general, the more severe the tension pneumothorax, (1) the greater the positive pressure in the pleural cavity, (2) the more the major intrathoracic veins will be compressed, and (3) the more cardiac output will be reduced. Because of the high resistance encountered by blood returning to the right atrium of the heart, blood pooling develops in the peripheral vascular system—mainly the legs, arms, and abdominal viscera.

Clinical Connection—2-6, continued

Figure 2–18

A. Illustrates a right-sided tension pneumothorax. **B.** Shows a chest X-ray of a right-sided tension pneumothorax caused by positive pressure ventilation. Note, in both A and B, the collapsed right lung (horizontal arrow in B), the depressed right diaphragm (vertical arrow in B), and the heart and mediastinum pushed to the unaffected side (i.e., pushed to the patient's left side).

Image A © Cengage Learning 2013

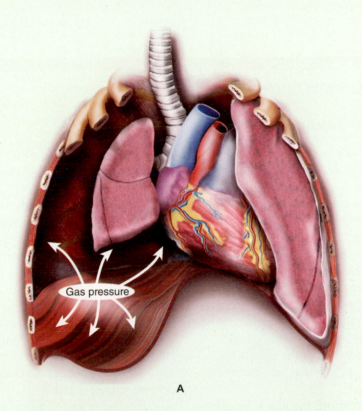

Gas pressure

A

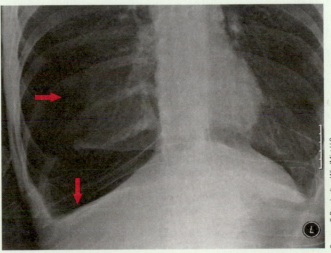

Courtesy T. Des Jardins, WindMist LLC

B

Surface Tension and Its Effect on Lung Expansion

In addition to the elastic properties of the lungs, the fluid (primarily H_2O) that lines the inner surface of the alveoli can profoundly resist lung expansion. To understand how the liquid coating the intra-alveolar surface can affect lung expansion, an understanding of the following is essential: (1) surface tension, (2) Laplace's law, and (3) how the substance called pulmonary surfactant off-sets alveolar surface tension.

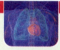

Clinical Connection—2-7

Negative-Pressure Ventilation

In 1928, Drinker and Shaw invented the first modern and practical negative-pressure ventilator—most commonly known as the "iron lung."[4] This early prototype negative-pressure ventilator consisted of an iron box and two vacuum cleaners. During the next few years, John H. Emerson developed a more cost-effective, commercial version of the iron lung. The iron lung was made famous for its important contributions during the poliomyelitis epidemics of the 1930s and 1950s. In general, the iron lung is a large elongated tank that encases the patient's body up to the neck. The neck is sealed with a rubber gasket so that only the patient's head is exposed to the atmosphere (i.e., barometric pressure).

To activate an **inspiration**, the iron lung uses a piston, pump-like mechanism that generates a negative pressure (vacuum) around the patient's chest, which, in turn, causes the thorax and lungs to expand (increased volume). This action causes the intra-alveolar pressure to decrease—remember, according to Boyle's law, as pressure deceases, the volume increases. Because the atmospheric pressure is higher than the intra-alveolar pressure—that is, a pressure gradient exists—gas from the atmosphere moves through the patient's nose or mouth to the alveoli (Figure 2–19A).

This gas flow continues until the intra-alveolar pressure and the atmospheric pressures are in equilibrium. Once the equilibrium point is reached, gas flow stops. This period of no gas flow is the **end-inspiration** phase of the negative-pressure ventilation cycle (Figure 2–19B).

To initiate **expiration**, the piston mechanism releases the negative pressure, which, in turn, allows the elastic recoil forces of the thorax and lungs to return to their normal—and smaller—size (decreased volume). This action causes the intra-alveolar pressure to increase—thus, creating a pressure gradient between the intra-alveolar pressure and atmospheric pressure. Because the intra-alveolar pressure is higher than the atmospheric pressure, gas from the alveoli moves through the tracheobronchial tree to the atmosphere (Figure 2–19C).

This gas flow will continue until the intra-alveolar pressure and the atmospheric pressure are in equilibrium. Once the equilibrium point is reached, gas flow stops. This period of no gas flow is the **end-expiration** phase of the negative-pressure ventilation cycle (Figure 2–19D).

There are several disadvantages associated with the full-body iron lung, including (1) patient access, (2) abdominal venous blood pooling, (3) decreased venous return, and (4) decreased cardiac output and blood pressure. Although the iron lung is still being utilized for long-term ventilation today, the prominent negative-pressure devices used are (1) the Porta-lung (offers the same level of efficiency as the iron lung, but in a lightweight portable unit), (2) the chest cuirass (an upper body only shell—named after the body armor worn by medieval soldiers), or (3) the body suit.

---

[4] Also called the Drinker tank or Shaw tank.

Clinical Connection—2-7, continued

Figure 2–19

How a negative pressure breath from a mechanical ventilator affects the intra-alveolar pressure, pleural pressure, and the excursion of the diaphragm, and gas flow during inspiration and expiration

© Cengage Learning 2013

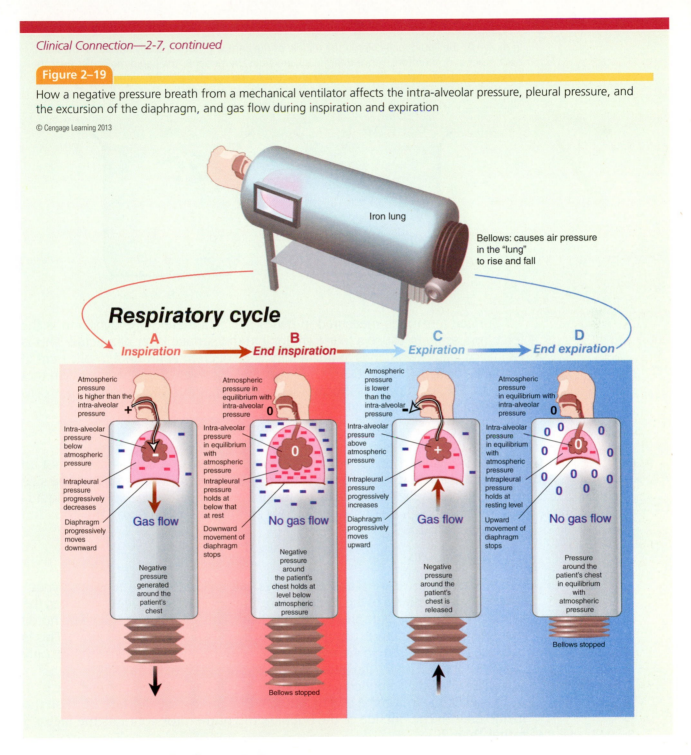

Surface Tension

When liquid molecules are completely surrounded by identical molecules, the molecules are mutually attracted toward one another and, therefore, move freely in all directions (Figure 2–20A on page 102). When a liquid–gas interface exists, however, the liquid molecules at the liquid–gas interface are strongly attracted to the liquid molecules within the liquid mass (Figure 2–20B). This molecular, cohesive force at the liquid–gas interface is called *surface tension*. It is the surface tension, for example, that maintains the shape of a water droplet, or makes it possible for an insect to move or stay afloat on the surface of a pond.

Figure 2–20

In model A, the liquid molecules in the middle of the container are mutually attracted toward each other and, therefore, move freely in all directions. In model B, the liquid molecules near the surface (liquid–gas interface) are strongly attracted to the liquid molecules within the liquid mass. This molecular force at the liquid–gas interface is called surface tension.

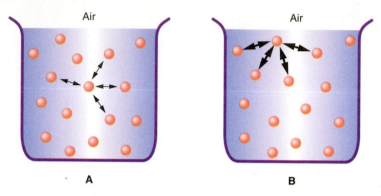

Surface tension is measured in dynes per centimeter. One dyne/cm is the force necessary to cause a tear 1 cm long in the surface layer of a liquid. This is similar to using two hands to pull a thin piece of cloth apart until a split 1 cm in length is formed (1 cm H_2O pressure equals 980 dynes/cm). The liquid film that lines the interior surface of the alveoli has the potential to exert a force in excess of 70 dynes/cm, a force that can easily cause complete alveolar collapse.

Laplace's Law

Laplace's law describes how the *distending pressure* of a liquid bubble (not an alveolus) is influenced by (1) the surface tension of the bubble and (2) the size of the bubble itself. When Laplace's law is applied to a sphere with one liquid–gas interface (e.g., a bubble completely submerged in a liquid), the equation is written as follows:

$$P = \frac{2\ ST}{r}$$

where P is the pressure difference (dynes/cm²), ST is surface tension (dynes/cm), and r is the radius of the liquid sphere (cm); the factor 2 is required when the law is applied to a liquid sphere with one liquid–gas interface. It should be noted that when Laplace's law is arranged as shown, it also applies to the lungs. This is because the alveoli are in constant contact with each other and, therefore, only have one surface area—the intra-alveolar surface area (refer to Figure 1–30).

When the law is applied to a bubble with two liquid–gas interfaces (e.g., a soap bubble blown on the end of a tube has a liquid–gas interface both on the inside and on the outside of the bubble), the numerator contains the factor 4 rather than 2:

$$P = \frac{4\ ST}{r}$$

Laplace's law shows that the *distending pressure* of a liquid sphere is (1) directly proportional to the surface tension of the liquid and (2) inversely proportional to the radius of the sphere.

In other words, the numerator of Laplace's law shows that (1) as the surface tension of a liquid bubble increases, the distending pressure necessary to hold the bubble open increases or (2) the opposite—when the surface tension of a liquid bubble decreases, the distending pressure of the bubble decreases (Figure 2–21). The denominator of Laplace's law shows that (1) when the

Figure 2–21

Bubbles A and B are the same size. The surface tension (ST) of bubble A is 10 dynes/cm and requires a distending pressure (P) of 5 cm H_2O to maintain its size. The surface tension of bubble B is 20 dynes/cm H_2O (twice that of bubble A) and requires a distending pressure of 10 cm H_2O (twice that of bubble A) to maintain its size (r = radius).

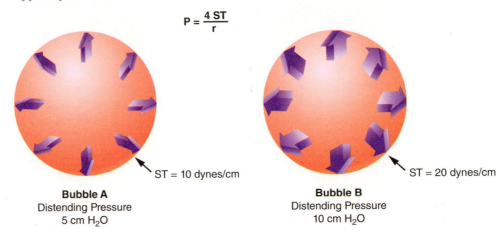

$$P = \frac{4\ ST}{r}$$

ST = 10 dynes/cm

ST = 20 dynes/cm

Bubble A
Distending Pressure
5 cm H_2O

Bubble B
Distending Pressure
10 cm H_2O

size of a liquid bubble increases, the distending pressure necessary to hold the bubble open decreases, or (2) the opposite—when the size of the bubble decreases, the distending pressure of the bubble increases (Figure 2–22). Because of this interesting physical phenomenon, when two different size bubbles—having the same surface tension—are in direct communication, the greater pressure in the smaller bubble will cause the smaller bubble to empty into the larger bubble (Figure 2–23 on page 104).

During the formation of a new bubble (e.g., a soap bubble blown on the end of a tube), the principles of Laplace's law do not come into effect until the distending pressure of the liquid sphere goes beyond what is called the *critical opening pressure*. As shown in Figure 2–24 on page 104, the critical opening pressure is the high pressure (with little volume change) that is initially required to overcome the liquid molecular force during the formation

Figure 2–22

The surface tension (ST) of bubbles A and B is identical. The radius (r) of bubble A is 2 cm, and it requires a distending pressure (P) of 5 cm H_2O to maintain its size. The radius of bubble B is 1 cm (one-half that of bubble A), and it requires a distending pressure of 10 cm H_2O (twice that of bubble A) to maintain its size.

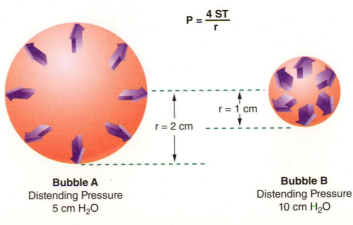

$$P = \frac{4\ ST}{r}$$

r = 1 cm

r = 2 cm

Bubble A
Distending Pressure
5 cm H_2O

Bubble B
Distending Pressure
10 cm H_2O

of a new bubble—similar to the high pressure first required to blow up a new balloon. Figure 2–24 also shows that, prior to the critical opening pressure, the distending pressure must progressively increase to enlarge the size of the bubble. In other words, the distending pressure is *directly proportional* to the radius of the bubble (the opposite of what Laplace's law states).

Figure 2–23

Bubbles A and B have the same surface tension. When the two bubbles are in direct communication, the higher pressure in the smaller bubble A causes it to empty into the large bubble B.

© Cengage Learning 2013

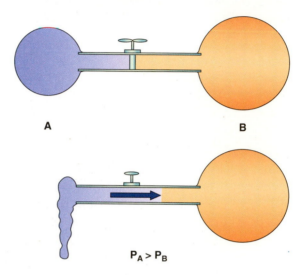

Figure 2–24

A. Model showing the formation of a new liquid bubble at the end of a tube. **B.** Graph showing the distending pressure required to maintain the bubble's size (volume) at various stages. Initially, a very high pressure, providing little volume change, is required to inflate the bubble. Once the critical opening pressure (same as critical closing pressure) is reached, however, the distending pressure progressively decreases as the size of the bubble increases. Thus, between the critical opening pressure and the point at which the bubble ruptures, the bubble behaves according to Laplace's law. Laplace's law applies to the normal functional size range of the bubble.

© Cengage Learning 2013

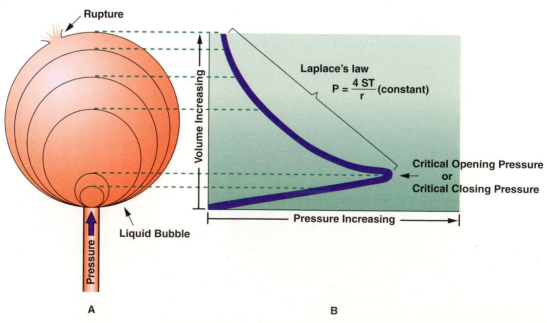

Once the critical opening pressure is reached, however, the distending pressure progressively decreases as the bubble increases in size—the distending pressure, as described by Laplace's law, is *inversely proportional* to the radius of the bubble. The distending pressure will continue to decrease until the bubble enlarges to its breaking point and ruptures. It is interesting to note that just before the bubble breaks, the distending pressure is at its lowest level (see Figure 2–24).

Conversely, Laplace's law shows that as an inflated bubble decreases in size, the distending pressure proportionally increases until the pressure reaches what is called the *critical closing pressure* (actually the same pressure as the critical opening pressure). When the size of the bubble decreases beyond this point, the liquid molecular force of the bubble becomes greater than the distending pressure and the bubble collapses (see Figure 2–24).

It should be emphasized that *Laplace's law does not state that the surface tension varies with the size of the bubble*. To the contrary, the law shows that as a liquid bubble changes in size, it is the *distending pressure—not* the *surface tension*—that varies inversely with the radius. In fact, as the radius of the sphere increases, the surface tension remains the same until the size of the bubble goes beyond its natural elastic limit and ruptures.

The fact that the surface tension remains the same while the radius of a liquid sphere changes can be illustrated mathematically by rearranging Laplace's law as follows:

1. Because surface tension is a property of the fluid and is constant for any specific fluid, Laplace's law can be restated as:

$$P = \frac{k}{r}$$

where k is a constant (in this case, the constant k equals surface tension) and P (pressure) is inversely proportional to r (radius).

2. The equation $P = k \div r$ can be rearranged as follows:

$$Pr = k$$

The formula now shows that the variable quantities (Pr) are inversely proportional and that their product is a constant (k). Thus, as one variable increases, the other must decrease to maintain a constant product (k).

To demonstrate this concept, consider taking a 400-mile automobile trip. With the formula distance = rate × time (d = rt), which represents product (d) and variable quantities (rt), we have:

$$400 = rt \quad (d = 400 \text{ miles})$$

or

$$\frac{400}{r} = t$$

On such a trip, assume that we travel at 50 miles per hour (mph) and that the trip takes 8 hours ($400 \div 50 = 8$). If we travel by train and increase the speed to 100 mph, the time of the trip decreases to 4 hours. If, however, we decrease the speed to 25 mph, the time increases to 16 hours ($400 \div 25 = 16$). In other words, as the speed increases the time decreases and vice versa, but the product (d) remains a constant 400 miles, which is determined by the length of the trip.

© Cengage Learning 2013

Figure 2–25

Rate and time are inversely proportional (as rate increases, time decreases; and as rate decreases, time increases).

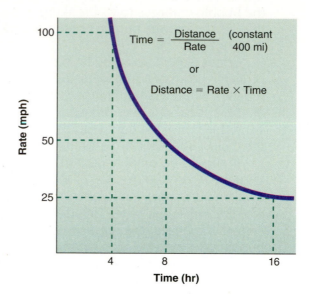

3. Thus, when two variables are inversely proportional, such as rt = 400 or t = 400 ÷ r, the time increases as the rate decreases, and time decreases as the rate increases (Figure 2–25). Note the similarity of the graph in Figure 2–25 to the portion of the graph that represents Laplace's law in Figure 2–24B.

Laplace's Law Applied to the Alveolar Fluid Lining

Because the liquid film that lines the alveolus resembles a bubble or sphere, according to Laplace's law, when the alveolar fluid is permitted to behave according to its natural tendency, a high transpulmonary pressure must be generated to keep the small alveoli open (see Figure 2–24). Fortunately, in the healthy lung, the natural tendency for the smaller alveoli to collapse is offset by a fascinating substance called pulmonary surfactant.

How Pulmonary Surfactant Regulates Alveolar Surface Tension

Pulmonary surfactant is an important and complex substance that is produced and stored in the alveolar type II cells (see Figure 1–30). It is composed of **phospholipids** (about 90 percent) and **protein** (about 10 percent). The primary surface tension-lowering chemical in pulmonary surfactant is the phospholipid **dipalmitoyl phosphatidylcholine (DPPC)**. The DPPC molecule has both a *hydrophobic* (water-insoluble) end and a *hydrophilic* (water-soluble) end. This unique hydrophobic/hydrophilic structure causes the DPPC molecule to position itself at the alveolar gas–liquid interface so that the hydrophilic end is toward the liquid phase and the hydrophobic end is toward the gas phase. Pulmonary surfactant at the alveolar liquid–gas interface can profoundly lower alveolar surface tension.

The DPPC molecule at the alveolar gas–liquid interface causes surface tension to decrease in proportion to its ratio to alveolar surface area. That is, when the alveolus decreases in size (exhalation), the proportion of DPPC to the alveolar surface area increases. This, in turn, increases the effect of the DPPC molecules and causes the alveolar surface tension to decrease (Figure 2–26A).

Figure 2–26

A. In the normal lung, the surface tension is low in the small alveolus because the ratio of surfactant to alveolar surface is high. **B.** As the alveolus enlarges, the surface tension steadily increases because the ratio of surfactant to alveolar surface decreases.

© Cengage Learning 2013

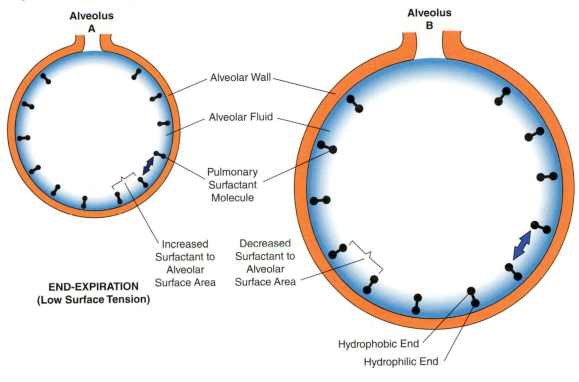

In contrast, when the alveolus increases in size (inhalation), the relative amount of DPPC to the alveolar surface area decreases (because the number of surfactant molecules does not change when the size of the alveolus changes), which decreases the effect of the DPPC molecules and causes the alveolar surface tension to increase (Figure 2–26B). In fact, as the alveolus enlarges, the surface tension will progressively increase to the value it would naturally have in the absence of pulmonary surfactant. Clinically, however, the fact that surface tension increases as the alveolus enlarges is not significant because according to Laplace's law, the distending pressure required to maintain the size of a bubble progressively decreases as the size of the bubble increases (see Figure 2–24).

It is estimated that the surface tension of the average alveolus varies from 5 to 15 dynes/cm (when the alveolus is very small) to about 50 dynes/cm (when the alveolus is fully distended) (Figure 2–27 on page 108). Because pulmonary surfactant has the ability to reduce the surface tension of the small alveoli, the high distending pressure that would otherwise be required to offset the critical closing pressure of the small alveoli is virtually eliminated.

In the absence of pulmonary surfactant, however, the alveolar surface tension increases to the level it would naturally have (50 dynes/cm), and the distending pressure necessary to overcome the recoil forces of the liquid film coating the small alveoli is very high. In short, the distending pressure required to offset the recoil force of the alveolar fluid behaves according to Laplace's law.

Figure 2–27

In the normal lung, the surface tension force progressively increases as the alveolar size increases. Similarly, as the alveolar size decreases, the surface tension force progressively decreases. Note that because of the alveolar surface tension, the actual physical change of the alveolus lags behind the pressure applied to it. When such a phenomenon occurs in the field of physics (i.e., a physical manifestation lagging behind a force), a hysteresis is said to exist. When this lung characteristic is plotted on a volume–pressure curve, the alveolus is shown to deflate along a different curve than that inscribed during inspiration and the curve has a looplike appearance. The hysteresis loop shows graphically that at any given pressure the alveolar volume is less during inspiration than it is during expiration. This alveolar hysteresis is virtually eliminated when the lungs are inflated experimentally with saline; such an experimental procedure removes the alveolar liquid–gas interface and, therefore, the alveolar surface tension. Inspiratory capacity is the volume of air that can be inhaled after a normal exhalation. Functional residual capacity is the volume of air remaining in the lungs after a normal exhalation.

© Cengage Learning 2013

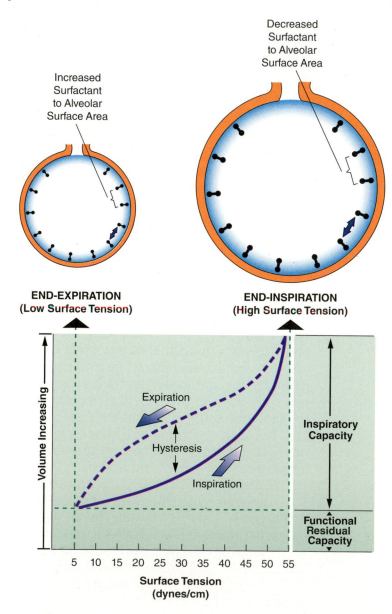

Table 2–1

Causes of Pulmonary Surfactant Deficiency

General Causes
Acidosis
Hypoxia
Hyperoxia
Atelectasis
Pulmonary vascular congestion
Specific Causes
Acute respiratory distress syndrome (ARDS)
Respiratory distress syndrome (RDS)
Pulmonary edema
Pulmonary embolism
Pneumonia
Excessive pulmonary lavage or hydration
Drowning
Extracorporeal oxygenation

© Cengage Learning 2013

As a result, when the distending pressure of the small alveoli falls below the critical closing pressure, the liquid molecular force pulls the alveolar walls together (see Figure 2–24). Once the liquid walls of the alveolus come into contact with one another, a liquid bond develops that strongly resists the re-expansion of the alveolus. Complete alveolar collapse is called **atelectasis**.

Table 2–1 lists some respiratory disorders that cause pulmonary surfactant deficiency.

Summary of the Elastic Properties of the Lungs

There are two major elastic forces in the lungs that cause an inflated lung to recoil inward: the elastic properties of the lungs and the surface tension of the liquid film that lines the alveoli.

Clinical Connection—2-8

Pulmonary Surfactant Deficiency

The respiratory therapist will encounter a number of pulmonary disorders that are associated with a pulmonary surfactant deficiency. For example, this problem is commonly seen in premature infants who are diagnosed with **respiratory distress syndrome (RDS)**. These babies are born before their type II alveolar cells are mature enough to produce a sufficient amount of pulmonary surfactant. Low levels of pulmonary surfactant increase the surface tension forces in the lungs and, in severe cases, cause the alveoli to collapse (atelectasis). Alveolar collapse shifts the baby's volume–pressure curve to the right, decreases lung compliance, decreases the baby's oxygenation level, and increases the work of breathing.

The treatment of choice during the early stages of RDS is **continuous positive airway pressure (CPAP)**. CPAP works to (1) re-inflate the lungs, (2) decrease the work of breathing, and (3) return the baby's oxygenation level to normal. Mechanical ventilation, in these cases, is avoided as long as possible. Because of the pulmonary surfactant deficiency associated with RDS, the administration of exogenous surfactant preparations such as **beractant** (Survanta®), **calfactant** (Infasurf®), and **poractant alfa** (Curosurf®) is often helpful.

Figure 2-28

In the normal lung, both the surface tension force (A) and the elastic force (B) progressively increase as the alveolus enlarges. The elastic force is the predominant force in both the small and the large alveoli. In the absence of pulmonary surfactant, the surface tension force (C) predominates in the small alveoli. The elastic force (B) still predominates in the large alveoli. Note that, as the alveolus enlarges, the pressure required to offset the "abnormal" surface tension force (C) ultimately decreases to the same pressure required to offset the "normal" surface tension force (B). Thus, it can be seen that when there is a deficiency of pulmonary surfactant, the surface tension of the small alveoli creates a high recoil force. If a high pressure is not generated to offset this surface tension force, the alveoli will collapse.

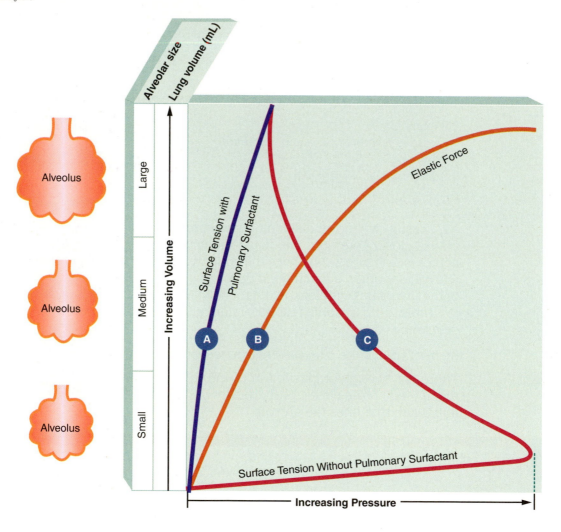

In the healthy lung, both the elastic tension and the degree of surface tension are low in the small alveoli. As the alveoli increase in size, both the elastic tension and the degree of surface tension progressively increase. The elastic tension, however, is the predominant force, particularly in the large alveoli (Figure 2–28).

In the absence of pulmonary surfactant, the alveolar fluid lining behaves according to Laplace's law—that is, a high pleural pressure must be generated to keep the small alveoli open. When such a condition exists, the surface tension force predominates in the small alveoli (see Figure 2–28).

Dynamic Characteristics of the Lungs

The term **dynamic** refers to the study of forces in action. In the lungs, dynamic refers to the movement of gas in and out of the lungs and the pressure changes required to move the gas. The dynamic features of the lung are best explained by Poiseuille's law for flow and pressure and the airway resistance equation.

Poiseuille's (Pwah-Sōy) Law for Flow and Pressure Applied to the Bronchial Airways

During a normal inspiration, pleural pressure decreases from its normal resting level (about −3 to −6 cm H_2O pressure), which causes the bronchial airways to lengthen and to increase in diameter *(passive dilation)*. During expiration, pleural pressure increases (or returns to its normal resting state), which causes the bronchial airways to decrease in length and in diameter *(passive constriction)* (Figure 2–29 on page 112). Under normal circumstances, these anatomic changes of the bronchial airways are not remarkable. In certain respiratory disorders (e.g., emphysema, chronic bronchitis), however, bronchial gas flow and pleural pressure may change significantly, particularly during expiration, when passive constriction of the tracheobronchial tree occurs. The reason for this is best explained in the relationship of factors described in Poiseuille's law. Poiseuille's law can be arranged for either flow or pressure.

Poiseuille's Law Arranged for Flow

When Poiseuille's law is arranged for flow, it is written as follows:

$$\dot{V} = \frac{\Delta P r^4 \pi}{8 l \eta}$$

where η = the viscosity of a gas (or fluid), ΔP = the change of pressure from one end of the tube to the other, r = the radius of the tube, l = the length of the tube, $\dot{V}$ = the gas (or fluid) flowing through the tube; and π and 8 = constants, which will be excluded from the discussion.

The equation states that flow is directly proportional to P and r^4 and inversely proportional to l and η. In other words, flow will decrease in response to decreased P and tube radius, and flow will increase in response to decreased tube length and fluid viscosity. Conversely, flow will increase in response to an increased P and tube radius and decrease in response to an increased tube length and fluid viscosity.

It should be emphasized that flow is profoundly affected by the radius of the tube. As Poiseuille's law illustrates, $\dot{V}$ is a function of the fourth power of the radius (r^4). In other words, assuming that pressure (P) remains constant, decreasing the radius of a tube by one-half reduces the gas flow to $\frac{1}{16}$ of its original flow.

For example, if the radius of a bronchial tube through which gas flows at a rate of 16 milliliters per second (mL/sec) is reduced to one-half its original size because of mucosal swelling, the flow rate through the bronchial tube would decrease to 1 mL/sec ($\frac{1}{16}$ the original flow rate) (Figure 2–30 on page 112).

Similarly, decreasing a tube radius by 16 percent decreases gas flow to one-half its original rate. For instance, if the radius of a bronchial tube through which gas flows at a rate of 16 mL/sec is decreased by 16 percent (e.g., because of mucosal swelling), the flow rate through the bronchial tube would decrease to 8 mL/sec (one-half the original flow rate) (Figure 2–31 on page 113).

Figure 2–29

During inspiration, the bronchial airways lengthen and increase in diameter. During expiration, the bronchial airways decrease in length and diameter.

© Cengage Learning 2013

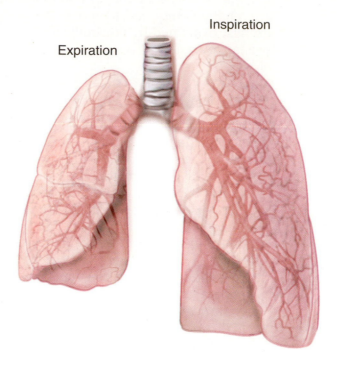

Inspiration

Expiration

Figure 2–30

Poiseuille's law for flow applied to a bronchial airway with its radius reduced 50 percent.

© Cengage Learning 2013

$$\dot{V} \simeq \Delta\, Pr^4$$

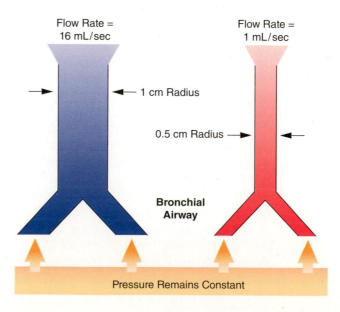

Flow Rate =
16 mL/sec

Flow Rate =
1 mL/sec

← 1 cm Radius

0.5 cm Radius →   ←

**Bronchial
Airway**

Pressure Remains Constant

© Cengage Learning 2013

Figure 2–31

Poiseuille's law for flow applied to a bronchial airway with its radius reduced 16 percent.

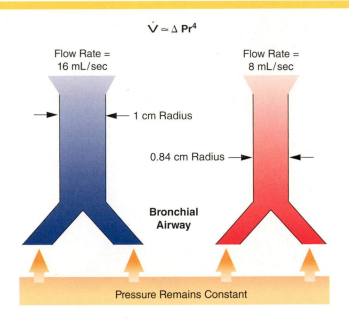

Poiseuille's Law Arranged for Pressure

When Poiseuille's law is arranged for pressure, it is written as follows:

$$P = \frac{\dot{V}8l\eta}{r^4\pi}$$

The equation now states that pressure is directly proportional to $\dot{V}$, l, and η and inversely proportional to r^4. In other words, pressure will increase in response to a decreased tube radius and decrease in response to a decreased flow rate, tube length, or viscosity. The opposite is also true: pressure will decrease in response to an increased tube radius and increase in response to an increased flow rate, tube length, or viscosity.

Pressure is a function of the radius to the fourth power (r^4) and therefore is profoundly affected by the radius of a tube. In other words, if flow ($\dot{V}$) remains constant, then decreasing a tube radius to one-half of its previous size requires an increase in pressure to 16 times its original level.

If the radius of a bronchial tube with a driving pressure of 1 cm H_2O is reduced to one-half its original size because of mucosal swelling, the driving pressure through the bronchial tube would have to increase to 16 cm H_2O ($16 \times 1 = 16$) to maintain the same flow rate (Figure 2–32 on page 114).

Similarly, decreasing the bronchial tube radius by 16 percent increases the pressure to twice its original level. For instance, if the radius of a bronchial tube with a driving pressure of 10 cm H_2O is decreased by 16 percent because of mucosal swelling, the driving pressure through the bronchial tube would have to increase to 20 cm H_2O (twice its original pressure) to maintain the same flow (Figure 2–33 on page 114).

Poiseuille's Law Rearranged to Simple Proportionalities

When Poiseuille's law is applied to the tracheobronchial tree during spontaneous breathing, the two equations can be rewritten as simple proportionalities:

$$\dot{V} \approx Pr^4$$

$$P \approx \frac{\dot{V}}{r^4}$$

Figure 2–32

Poiseuille's law for pressure applied to a bronchial airway with its radius reduced 50 percent.

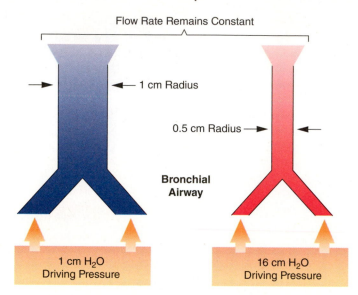

Figure 2–33

Poiseuille's law for pressure applied to a bronchial airway with its radius reduced 16 percent.

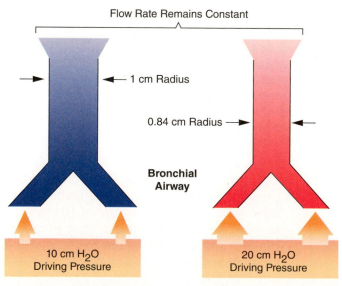

Based on the proportionality for flow, it can be stated that because gas flow varies directly with r^4 of the bronchial airway, flow must diminish during exhalation because the radius of the bronchial airways decreases. Stated differently, assuming that the pressure remains constant as the radius (r) of the bronchial airways decreases, gas flow ($\dot{V}$) also decreases. During normal spontaneous breathing, however, the reduction in gas flow during exhalation is negligible.

Clinical Connection—2-9

Respiratory Disorders That Decrease the Radius of the Airways

As described in more detail in the Clinical Application Section—Case 2 (page 139), any obstructive respiratory disorder—like asthma—that reduces the size of the bronchial airways can have a tremendous impact on gas flow and on the patient's work of breathing (Figure 2–34).

> **Figure 2–34**
>
> Asthma. Pathology includes (1) bronchial smooth muscle constriction, (2) inflammation and excessive production of thick, white bronchial secretions, and (3) alveolar hyperinflation.
>
> © Cengage Learning 2013

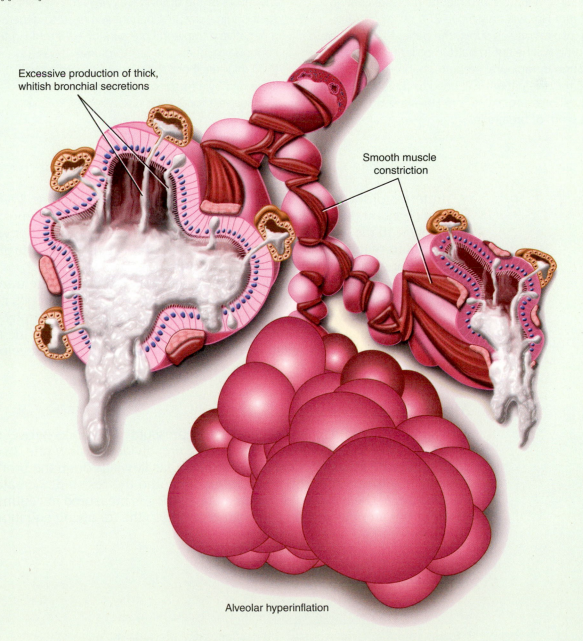

Excessive production of thick, whitish bronchial secretions

Smooth muscle constriction

Alveolar hyperinflation

(continues)

Clinical Connection—2-9, continued

According to Poiseuille's law for **flow**, airflow is directly proportional to the radius of the airway—raised to the fourth power (r^4). This means that the flow of gas drastically decreases in response to only a small decrease in the radius of the bronchial airway. For example, if a patient, who normally generates an intrapleural pressure of -3 mm Hg to inhale 500 mL of air, suddenly experiences an acute asthmatic episode that reduces the radius of the bronchial airways by only $\frac{1}{16}$ of their original size, the same negative intrapleural pressure change (-3 mm Hg) will only move 250 mL of gas during inspiration—in short, the patient's inspiration volume will be cut in half! In order to generate enough intrapleural pressure to inhale the original 500 mL, the patient will need to double the intrapleural pressure to -6 mm Hg—in short, double the work of breathing.

When applying Poiseuille's law for **pressure**, the intrapressure changes required to move gas are indirectly proportional to the radius of the airway—raised to the fourth power (r^4). Again, this means that the intrapleural pressure significantly increases in response to only a small decrease in the radius of the bronchial airway. For example, if a patient, who normally generates an intrapleural pressure of -3 mm Hg to inhale 500 mL of air, suddenly experiences an acute asthmatic episode that reduces the radius of the bronchial airways to one-half of their original size, the patient will need to generate a negative intrapleural pressure of -48 mm Hg to continue to inhale the same volume of gas (500 mL)—in short, the work of breathing will increased by a factor of 16 ($16 \times 3 = 48$).

See text for further discussion of Poiseuille's law.

In terms of the proportionality for pressure ($P \approx \dot{V} \div r^4$), if gas flow is to remain constant during exhalation, then the transthoracic pressure must vary inversely with the fourth power of the radius (r^4) of the airway. In other words, as the radius of the bronchial airways decreases during exhalation, the driving pressure must increase to maintain a constant gas flow.[5]

During normal spontaneous breathing, the need to increase the transrespiratory pressure during exhalation in order to maintain a certain gas flow is not significant. However, in certain respiratory disorders (e.g., emphysema, bronchitis, asthma), gas flow reductions and transthoracic pressure increases may be substantial as a result of the bronchial narrowing that develops in such disorders.

Airway Resistance

Airway resistance (R_{aw}) is defined as the pressure difference between the mouth and the alveoli (*transrespiratory pressure*) divided by flow rate. In other words, the rate at which a certain volume of gas flows through the bronchial airways is a function of the pressure gradient and the resistance created by the airways to the flow of gas. Mathematically, R_{aw} is measured in centimeters of water per liter per second (L/sec), according to the following equation:

$$R_{aw} = \frac{\Delta P (cm\ H_2O)}{\dot{V}(L/sec)}$$

---

[5] See mathematical discussion of Poiseuille's law in Appendix III.

For example, if an individual produces a flow rate of 4 L/sec during inspiration by generating a transrespiratory pressure of 4 cm H_2O, then R_{aw} would equal 1 cm H_2O/L/sec:

$$R_{aw} = \frac{\Delta P}{\dot{V}}$$

$$= \frac{4 \text{ cm } H_2O}{4 \text{ L/sec}}$$

$$= 1 \text{ cm } H_2O/\text{L/sec}$$

Normally, the R_{aw} in the tracheobronchial tree is about 0.5 to 1.5 cm H_2O/L/sec in adults. In patients with COPD (e.g., chronic bronchitis), however, R_{aw} may be very high. The value of R_{aw} is also much higher in newborn infants than in normal adults (refer to Chapter 11).

The movement of gas through a tube (or bronchial airway) can be classified as (1) laminar flow, (2) turbulent flow, or (3) a combination of laminar flow and turbulent flow—called tracheobronchial flow or transitional flow (Figure 2–35).

Laminar Flow

Laminar gas flow refers to a gas flow that is streamlined. The gas molecules move through the tube in a pattern parallel to the sides of the tube. This flow pattern occurs at low flow rates and at low-pressure gradients.

Turbulent Flow

Turbulent gas flow refers to gas molecules that move through a tube in a random manner. Gas flow encounters resistance from both the sides of the tube and from the collision with other gas molecules. This flow pattern occurs at high flow rates and at high-pressure gradients.

Figure 2–35

Types of gas flow.

© Cengage Learning 2013

Laminar

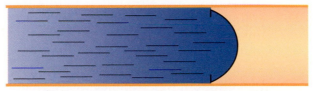

Turbulent

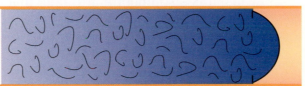

Tracheobronchial or Transitional Flow

Tracheobronchial gas flow occurs in the areas where the airways branch. Depending on the anatomic structure of the branching airways, and the velocity of gas flow, either laminar flow or turbulent flow may predominate.

Time Constants

A product of airway resistance (R_{aw}) and lung compliance (C_L) is a phenomenon called **time constant**, defined as the time (in seconds) necessary to inflate a particular lung region to about 60 percent[6] of its potential filling capacity. Lung regions that have either an increased R_{aw} or an increased C_L require more time to inflate. These alveoli are said to have a *long time constant.* In contrast, lung regions that have either a decreased R_{aw} or a decreased C_L require less time to inflate. These alveoli are said to have a *short time constant.*

Mathematically, the time constant (T_c) is expressed as follows:

$$T_c \text{ (sec)} = \underbrace{\frac{\Delta P(\text{cm H}_2\text{O})}{\dot{V}(\text{L/sec})}}_{(R_{aw})} \times \underbrace{\frac{\Delta V(\text{L})}{\Delta P(\text{cm H}_2\text{O})}}_{(C_L)}$$

$$= \frac{\text{cm H}_2\text{O} \times \text{L}}{\text{L/sec} \times \text{cm H}_2\text{O}}$$

This equation shows that as R_{aw} increases, the value for pressure (P, in cm H_2O) in the numerator increases. Or, when C_L decreases, the value for volume (V) in liters (L) in the numerator decreases.

Thus, assuming that all other variables remain constant, if the R_{aw} of a specific lung region doubles, then the time constant will also double (i.e., the lung unit will take twice as long to inflate). In contrast, if the C_L is reduced by half, then the time constant will also be reduced by half—and, importantly, the potential filling capacity of the lung region is also reduced by half. To help illustrate this concept, consider the time constants illustrated in Figure 2–36.

In Figure 2–36A, two alveolar units have identical R_{aw} and C_L. Thus, the two alveoli require the same amount of time to inflate—they have the same time constants.

Figure 2–36B shows two alveolar units with the same R_{aw} but with two different C_L. Because the C_L in unit B is one-half the C_L of unit A, unit B (low compliance) receives one-half the volume of unit A (high compliance). It is important to realize that unit B has a shorter time constant than unit A and unit B receives only one-half the volume received by unit A.

In Figure 2–36C, the two alveolar units have the same compliance, but two different R_{aw}. Because the R_{aw} leading to unit B is twice the R_{aw} leading to unit A, unit B (high R_{aw}) requires twice the time to fill to the same volume as unit A (low R_{aw}). It is important to note that the two alveolar units do not have the same time constant—the time constant for unit B is twice that of unit A. Thus, it is also important to note that as the breathing frequency increases, the time necessary to fill unit B may not be adequate. Clinically, how readily a lung region fills with gas during a specific time period is called **dynamic compliance**.

---

[6] Technically, 63 percent.

Figure 2–36

Time constants for hypothetical alveoli with differing lung compliances (C_L), supplied by airways with differing resistances (R_{aw}).

© Cengage Learning 2013

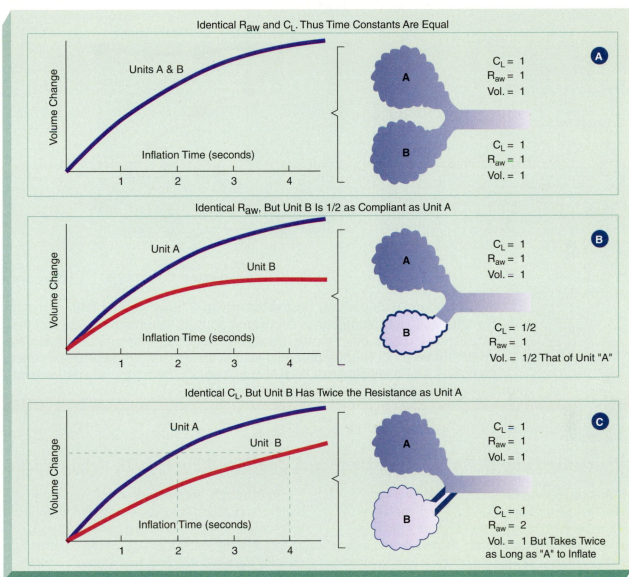

Dynamic Compliance

The measurement called dynamic compliance is a product of the time constants. Dynamic compliance is defined as the change in the volume of the lungs divided by the change in the transpulmonary pressure (obtained via a partially swallowed esophageal pressure balloon) during the time required for one breath. Dynamic compliance is distinctively different from the lung compliance (C_L) defined earlier in this chapter as the change in lung volume (ΔV) per unit pressure change (ΔP) (see Figure 2–13). In short, lung compliance is determined during a period of no gas flow, whereas dynamic compliance is measured during a period of gas flow.

In the healthy lung, the dynamic compliance is about equal to lung compliance at all breathing frequencies (the ratio of dynamic compliance to lung compliance is 1:1) (Figure 2–37 on page 120).

Figure 2–37

Dynamic compliance/lung compliance ratio at different breathing frequencies. In normal individuals there is essentially no ratio change. In individuals with obstructive disorders, however, the ratio decreases dramatically as the respiratory rate increases.

© Cengage Learning 2013

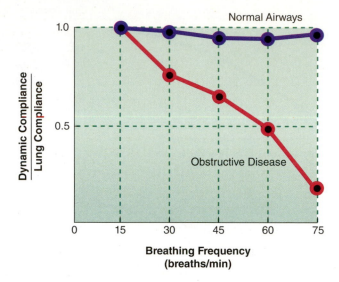

In patients with partially obstructed airways, however, the ratio of dynamic compliance to lung compliance falls significantly as the breathing frequency rises (see Figure 2–37). In other words, the alveoli distal to the obstruction do not have enough time to fill to their potential filling capacity as the breathing frequency increases. The compliance of such alveoli is said to be **frequency dependent**.

Clinical Connection—2-10

Restrictive Lung Disorders, Time Constants, and Breathing Pattern Relationships

Common restrictive respiratory disorders that decrease lung compliance (C_L)—and, therefore, decrease the time constant—include atelectasis, pneumonia, pneumothorax, pleural effusion, pulmonary edema, acute respiratory distress syndrome, and interstitial lung diseases. A decreased time constant simply means that the actual time it takes to inflate stiff—noncompliant—alveoli is shorter, but at the undesirable cost of less alveolar volume.

To offset the decreased C_L—and, therefore, the decreased lung volume—associated with these respiratory disorders, the patient typically adopts a faster ventilatory rate. In other words, because the patient is only able to inhale smaller tidal volumes, they simply breathe more times per minute. This breathing pattern works to maintain the overall minute volume at, or beyond, the patient's normal minute volume.

Clinical Connection—2-11

Obstructive Lung Disorders, Time Constants, and Breathing Pattern Relationships

Common obstructive respiratory disorders that increase airway resistance (R_{aw})—and, therefore, increase the time constant—include asthma, chronic bronchitis, emphysema, and cystic fibrosis.

Figure 2–38 shows the major bronchial airway changes associated with chronic bronchitis. A longer time constant simply means that the actual time it takes to inflate the alveoli is longer. This is because

Clinical Connection—2-11, continued

it takes more time for gas to move through partially obstructed ($\uparrow R_{aw}$) bronchial airways—similar to trying to inhale normally through a straw.

An interesting irony in these cases is this: the faster the patient's ventilatory rate, the smaller the volume of air they inhale during each breath—the patient's lung compliance (C_L) is then said to be **frequency dependent.**

To offset the increased R_{aw}—and, therefore, the decreased lung volume—associated with obstructive respiratory disorders, the patient typically adopts a slower ventilatory rate and a larger tidal volume per breath. By slowing the ventilatory rate down and taking deeper breaths, the overall minute volume will remain at, or near, the patient's normal.

Figure 2–38

Chronic bronchitis. Pathology includes (1) inflammation and swelling of the peripheral airways, (2) excessive mucus production and accumulation, and (3) alveolar hyperinflation. Because of the abnormal airway changes associated with chronic bronchitis, there is an increased resistance (R_{aw}) and an increased time constant. The patient's lung compliance is said to be **frequency dependent**—the faster the ventilator rate, the smaller the volume of air moved.

© Cengage Learning 2013

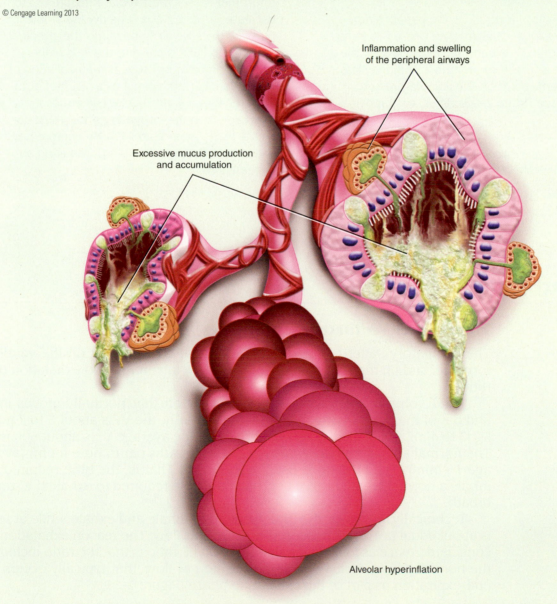

Inflammation and swelling of the peripheral airways

Excessive mucus production and accumulation

Alveolar hyperinflation

Clinical Connection—2-12

Auto-PEEP and Its Relationship to Airway Resistance during Rapid Ventilatory Rates

During rapid ventilatory rates, small airways with high R_{aw} may not have sufficient time to fully deflate during exhalation. The pressure in the alveoli distal to these airways may still be positive (greater than the atmospheric pressure) when the next inspiration begins. Clinically, the **positive end-expiratory pressure (PEEP)** caused by inadequate expiratory time is called **auto-PEEP**.[7] Auto-PEEP increases a patient's *work of breathing* (WOB) in two ways:

1. As a result of auto-PEEP, the patient's *functional residual capacity* (FRC) increases (refer to Chapter 3). When the FRC increases, the patient is forced to breathe at a higher, less compliant, point on the *volume-pressure curve* (see Figure 2–13). Thus, air trapping

and alveolar hyperinflation (auto-PEEP) decrease lung compliance, causing the WOB to increase.

2. When auto-PEEP produces air trapping and alveolar hyperinflation, the patient's diaphragm is pushed downward; this causes the patient's inspiratory efforts to become less efficient, causing the WOB to increase. Normally, an individual needs to create an inspiratory effort that causes the alveolar pressure (P_A) to decrease −1 or 2 cm H_2O below the ambient pressure to cause air to flow into the alveoli. When auto-PEEP is present, the P_A is higher than the ambient pressure at the beginning of inspiration. For example, if as a result of auto-PEEP the P_A is +4 cm H_2O (above atmospheric pressure), then the inspiratory effort must decrease the P_A more than 4 cm H_2O before gas can start to flow into the lungs, requiring an increased WOB.

---

[7] Auto-PEEP is also called air trapping, intrinsic PEEP, occult PEEP, inadvertent PEEP, and covert PEEP.

Ventilatory Patterns

The Normal Ventilatory Pattern

The ventilatory pattern consists of (1) the tidal volume (V_T), (2) the ventilatory rate, and (3) the time relationship between inhalation and exhalation (I:E ratio).

Tidal volume is defined as the volume of air that normally moves into and out of the lungs in one quiet breath. Normally, the V_T is about 5 to 7 mL/ kg (3 to 4 mL/lb) of ideal body weight (IBW). The average V_T is about 500 mL. The normal adult ventilatory rate is 12 to 18 breaths per minute (bpm) (average 15 bpm). The I:E ratio is usually about 1:2. That is, the time required to inhale a normal breath is about one-half the time required to exhale the same breath.

Technically, however, the time required to inhale and exhale while at rest is about equal (a 1:1 ratio) in terms of "true" gas flow. The reason exhalation is considered twice as long as inhalation in the I:E ratio is that the ratio includes the normal pause, during which there is no gas flow, that typically occurs at end-expiration as part of the exhalation phase (Figure 2–39).

Figure 2–39

Normal, spontaneous breathing (eupnea). The I:E ratio typically is 1:2.

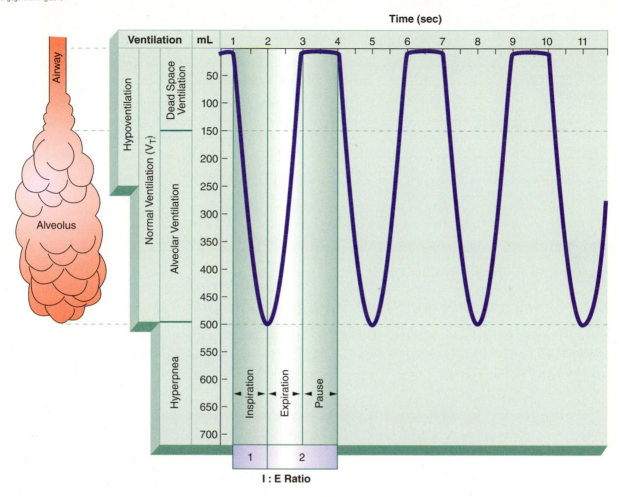

This normal pause that occurs at end-exhalation is usually about equal, in terms of time, to either the inspiratory or expiratory phase. Thus, when an individual is at rest, the time required for a normal ventilatory cycle consists of approximately three equal phases: (1) the inspiratory phase, (2) the expiratory phase, and (3) the pause phase at end-expiration (see Figure 2–39).

Clinical Connection—2-13

Normal Respiratory Rates for Different Age Groups

In the clinical setting, there are wide ranges of patient ages that are receiving respiratory care. Because the normal breathing rate varies between the different age groups, the respiratory care practitioner must have working knowledge of what is a normal respiratory rate among the different age groups—even when the rate is very fast (e.g., newborn infants and toddlers). The average, normal breathing rate range according to different age groups is as follows:

(continues)

Clinical Connection—2-13, continued

Age Group	Age	Breathing Rate
Newborn infant	1 month–1 year	30–60
Toddler	1–3 years	25–40
Preschooler	3–6 years	20–35
Child	6–12 years	20–30
Adolescent	12–18 years	12–20
Adult	19+ years	12–20

Normal Respiratory Rates for Different Age Groups

The reader is challenged to quietly observe the breathing rates of people in different age groups.

Clinical Connection—2-14

Tidal Volume and Breathing Rate Strategies for Mechanical Ventilation

Although the precise tidal volume and breathing rate selected for a patient on a mechanical ventilator is always based on the patient's specific needs—for example, patient history, arterial blood gas values, chest X-rays, and cardiac status—a generally accepted starting point for some specific pulmonary disorders are as follows:

Common Assist-Control Mechanical Ventilatory Management Strategies Good Starting Points

Pulmonary Status	Disease Characteristic	Tidal Volume	Ventilatory Set Rate—Breaths per Minute (bpm)
Normal lung mechanics	Normal compliance and airway resistance	10–12 mL/kg of IBW	10–12 bpm
Asthma, bronchitis or emphysema (COPD)	High airway resistance, high lung compliance with COPD	8–10 mL/kg When air-trapping is extensive, a lower V_T (5–6 mL/kg) may be helpful.	10–12 bpm When air-trapping is extensive, a slower rate may be required.
Acute respiratory distress syndrome	Low lung compliance due to diffuse, uneven alveolar injury	6–8 mL/kg	As high as 35 bpm
Postoperative ventilatory support (e.g., coronary artery bypass surgery)	Often normal compliance and airway resistance	10–12 mL/kg	12 bpm
Neuromuscular disorder (e.g., myasthenia gravis or Guillain-Barré syndrome)	Normal compliance and airway resistance	10–15 mL/kg	10–12 bpm

Alveolar Ventilation versus Dead Space Ventilation

Only the inspired air that reaches the alveoli is effective in terms of gas exchange. This portion of the inspired gas is referred to as alveolar ventilation. The volume of inspired air that does not reach the alveoli is not effective. This portion of gas is referred to as dead space ventilation (Figure 2–40). There are three types of dead space: (1) anatomic, (2) alveolar, and (3) physiologic.

Anatomic Dead Space

Anatomic dead space is the volume of gas in the conducting airways: the nose, mouth, pharynx, larynx, and lower airways down to, but not including, the respiratory bronchioles. The volume of anatomic dead space is approximately equal to 1 mL/lb (2.2 mL/kg) of "ideal" body weight. Thus, if an individual weighs 150 pounds, approximately 150 mL of inspired gas would be anatomic dead space gas (or physiologically ineffective).

Moreover, because of the anatomic dead space, the gas that does enter the alveoli during each inspiration (alveolar ventilation) is actually a combination of anatomic dead space gas (non-fresh gas) and gas from the atmosphere (fresh gas). To visualize this, consider the inspiration and expiration of 450 mL (V_T) in an individual with an anatomic dead space of 150 mL (Figure 2–41 on page 126).

Inspiration. As shown in Figure 2–41A, 150 mL of gas fill the anatomic dead space at pre-inspiration. This gas was the last 150 mL of gas to leave the

---

Figure 2–40

Dead space ventilation (V_D).

© Cengage Learning 2013

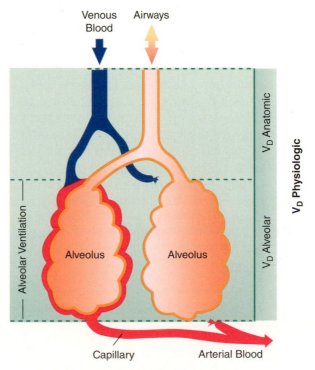

Dead Space Ventilation (V_D)

Figure 2–41

Alveolar ventilation versus dead space ventilation during one ventilatory cycle.

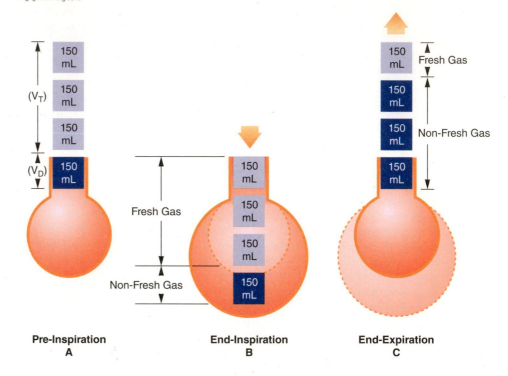

Pre-Inspiration
A

End-Inspiration
B

End-Expiration
C

alveoli during the previous exhalation. Thus, as shown in Figure 2–41B, the first 150 mL of gas to enter the alveoli during inspiration are from the anatomic dead space (non-fresh gas). The next 300 mL of gas to enter the alveoli are from the atmosphere (fresh gas). The last 150 mL of fresh gas inhaled fill the anatomic dead space (see Figure 2–41B). Thus, of the 450 mL of gas that enter the alveoli, 150 mL come from the conducting airways (non-fresh gas) and 300 mL come from the atmosphere (fresh gas).

Expiration. As shown in Figure 2–41C, 450 mL of gas are forced out of the alveoli during expiration. The first 150 mL of gas exhaled are from the anatomic dead space. This gas was the last 150 mL that entered the conducting airways during the previous inspiration (see Figure 2–41B). The next 300 mL of gas exhaled come from the alveoli. The last 150 mL of gas to leave the alveoli fill the anatomic dead space. During the next inspiration, the last 150 mL of gas exhaled from the alveoli will, again, reenter the alveoli, thus diluting the oxygen concentration of any atmospheric gas that enters the alveoli (see Figure 2–41A).

Therefore, minute alveolar ventilation (V_A) is equal to the tidal volume (V_T) minus the dead space ventilation (V_D) multiplied by the breaths per minute (frequency):

$$\dot{V}_A = (V_T - V_D) \times \text{breaths/min}$$

For example, if:

$$V_T = 450 \text{ mL}$$
$$V_D = 150 \text{ mL}$$

breaths/min = 12

then minute alveolar ventilation would be computed as follows:

$$\dot{V}_A = V_T - V_D \times \text{breaths/min}$$
$$= 450 \text{ mL} - 150 \text{ mL} \times 12$$
$$= 300 \text{ mL} \times 12$$
$$= 3600 \text{ mL}$$

Finally, an individual's breathing pattern (depth and rate of breathing) can profoundly alter the total alveolar ventilation. For example, Table 2–2 shows three different subjects, each having a total minute ventilation (MV) of 6000 mL and each having an anatomic dead space volume of 150 mL. Each subject, however, has a different tidal volume and breathing frequency. Subject A has a tidal volume of 150 mL and a breathing frequency of 40 breaths/min. Even though gas rapidly moves in and out of the lungs, the actual alveolar ventilation is zero. Subject A is merely moving 150 mL of gas in and out of the anatomic dead space at a rate of 40 times per minute. Clinically, this subject would become unconscious in a few minutes.

Subject B has a tidal volume of 500 mL and a breathing frequency of 12 breaths/min. This subject has an alveolar ventilation of 4200 mL. Subject C has a tidal volume of 1000 mL and a frequency of 6 breaths/min. This subject has an alveolar ventilation of 5100 mL.

The important deduction to be drawn from Table 2–2 is this: **an increased depth of breathing is far more effective than an equivalent increase in breathing rate in terms of increasing an individual's total alveolar ventilation.** Or, conversely, a decreased depth of breathing (decreased tidal volume) can lead to a significant and, perhaps, a critical reduction of alveolar ventilation. This is because the anatomic dead space volume represents a fixed volume (normally about one-third), and the fixed volume will make up a larger portion of a decreasing tidal volume. This fraction increases as the tidal volume decreases until, as demonstrated by subject A, it represents the entire tidal volume. On the other hand, any increase in the tidal volume beyond the anatomic dead space goes entirely toward increasing alveolar ventilation.

Table 2–2

Effect of Breathing Depth and Frequency on Alveolar Ventilation

Subject	Breathing Depth (V_T) (mL)		Breathing Frequency (breaths/min)		Total MV* (mL/min)	$V_D^\dagger$ (mL/min)	$V_A^\ddagger$ (mL/min)
A	150	×	40	=	6000	150 × 40 = 6000	0
B	500	×	12	=	6000	150 × 12 = 1800	4200
C	1000	×	6	=	6000	150 × 6 = 900	5100

© Cengage Learning 2013

* Total alveolar ventilation, or minute ventilation (MV), is the product of breathing depth, or tidal volume (V_T), times breathing frequency, or breaths per minute.
† Total dead space ventilation (V_D) is the product of anatomic dead space volume (150 mL in each subject) times breathing frequency.
‡ V_A = alveolar ventilation.

Alveolar Dead Space

Alveolar dead space occurs when an alveolus is ventilated but not perfused with pulmonary blood. Thus, the air that enters the alveolus is not effective in terms of gas exchange, because there is no pulmonary capillary blood flow. The amount of alveolar dead space is unpredictable.

Clinical Connection—2-15

A Giraffe's Neck: Alveolar Ventilation versus Dead Space Ventilation

It is interesting to note that a giraffe's neck (anatomic dead space) can be up to 12 feet long (Figure 2–42). Although the giraffe's trachea has a small diameter relative to the length, it is estimated that the trachea dead space ventilation is about 3 L of gas per breath. Fortunately, the giraffe's lungs are capable of accommodating between 4 and 15 L of air per breath. This large volume of gas is more than enough to offset the 3 L of dead space ventilation. The giraffe's normal respiratory rate is about ⅓ of a human—or about 6 breaths per minute.

The reader is challenged to cut a yard of large bore corrugated tubing, and then attempt to breathe in and out through the tube as long as possible—similar to breathing through a snorkel. How long do you think you can breathe through the tubing before you feel very short of breath? How much more air would you need to inhale in order to move fresh gas into your lungs? Consider how the tubing—between the tubing circuitry on a mechanical ventilator and the endotracheal tube—might affect the patient's dead space ventilation.

Figure 2–42

A giraffe's anatomic dead space is about 3 liters.

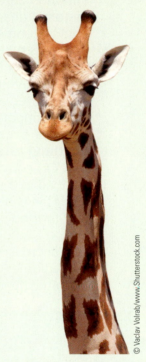

© Vaclav Volrab/www.Shutterstock.com

Clinical Connection—2-16

Pulmonary Embolus and Dead Space Ventilation

A blood clot that travels through the venous system and lodges in the pulmonary arteries or arterioles is called a **pulmonary embolus**. A pulmonary embolus reduces or completely blocks the pulmonary blood flow from traveling further down stream to the alveoli. As a result, the alveolar ventilation beyond the obstruction is wasted, or dead space, ventilation. In other words, no carbon dioxide or oxygen exchanges can occur in these alveoli. Pulmonary embolisms are extremely dangerous. The respiratory therapist should always be on alert for this respiratory disorder—particularly in patients with a recent history of bone fractures (especially the pelvis and long bones of the lower extremities), prolonged inactivity, hypercoagulation disorders, pregnancy and childbirth, and obesity.

Physiologic Dead Space

Physiologic dead space is the sum of the anatomic dead space and alveolar dead space. Because neither of these two forms of dead space is effective in terms of gas exchange, the two forms are combined and are referred to as physiologic dead space.

How Normal Pleural Pressure Differences Cause Regional Differences in Normal Lung Ventilation

As discussed earlier, the diaphragm moves air in and out of the lungs by changing the pleural and intra-alveolar pressures. Ordinarily, the pleural pressure is always below atmospheric pressure during both inspiration and expiration (see Figure 2–5).

The pleural pressure, however, is not evenly distributed within the thorax. In the normal individual in the upright position, there is a natural pleural pressure gradient from the upper lung region to the lower. The negative pleural pressure at the apex of the lung is normally greater (from -7 to -10 cm H_2O pressure) than at the base (from -2 to -3 cm H_2O pressure). This gradient is gravity dependent and is thought to be due to the normal weight distribution of the lungs above and below the hilum. In other words, because the lung is suspended from the hilum, and because the lung base weighs more than the apex (primarily due to the increased blood flow in the lung base), the lung base requires more pressure for support than does the lung apex. This causes the negative pleural pressure around the lung base to be less.

Because of the greater negative pleural pressure in the upper lung regions, the alveoli in those regions are expanded more than the alveoli in the lower regions. In fact, many of the alveoli in the upper lung regions may be close to, or at, their total filling capacity. This means, therefore, that the compliance of the alveoli in the upper lung regions is normally less than the compliance of the alveoli in the lower lung regions in the normal person in the upright position. As a result, during inspiration the alveoli in the upper lung regions are unable to accommodate as much gas as the alveoli in the lower lung regions. Thus, in the normal individual in the upright position, ventilation is usually much greater and more effective in the lower lung regions (Figure 2–43 on page 130).

The Effect of Airway Resistance and Lung Compliance on Ventilatory Patterns

As already mentioned, the respiratory rate and tidal volume presented by an individual are known as the *ventilatory pattern*. The average normal ventilatory pattern is a respiratory rate of 15 breaths per minute and a tidal volume of about 500 mL. Although the precise mechanism is not clear, it is well documented that these ventilatory patterns frequently develop in response to changes in lung compliance and airway resistance.

Figure 2–43

Intrapleural pressure gradient in the upright position. The negative intrapleural pressure normally is greater in the upper lung regions compared with the lower lung regions. Because of this, the alveoli in the upper lung regions expand more than those in the lower lung regions. This condition causes alveolar compliance to be lower in the upper lung regions and ventilation to be greater in the lower lung regions.

© Cengage Learning 2013

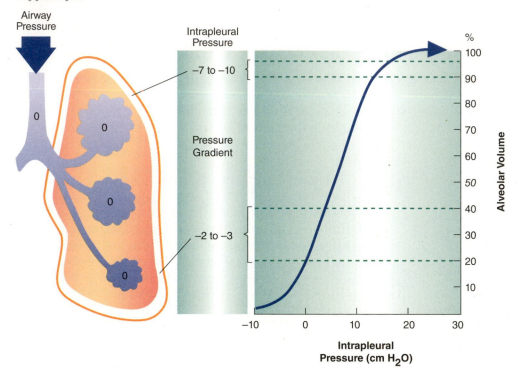

Clinical Connection—2-17

How the Adopted Breathing Pattern Changes in Chronic Obstructive Lung Disorders When Compromised by a Restrictive Lung Disorder

The patient's adopted ventilatory pattern is frequently modified in the clinical setting because of secondary complications. For example, a patient with emphysema (chronic obstructive lung disorder), who has adopted a decreased ventilatory rate and an increased tidal volume because of the increased R_{aw} and increased time constant associated with the disorder, may in fact demonstrate an increased ventilatory rate and decreased tidal volume in response to a lung infection (pneumonia) that causes lung compliance to decrease.

As will be discussed later in Chapter 7, because acute ventilatory changes (i.e., hyperventilation or hypoventilation) are commonly seen in patients who have chronic obstructive pulmonary disorders, the respiratory therapist must be familiar with—and on the alert for—clinical signs and symptoms that indicate the patient's ventilatory status is

changing from their normal. For example, an arterial blood gas on the patient with chronic obstructive pulmonary disease often confirms the patient is hyperventilating—that is, breathing faster than his or her normal—because of a secondary pneumonia. Clinically, this arterial blood gas is classified as "acute alveolar hyperventilation superimposed on chronic ventilatory failure"[8] and, importantly, the patient is in "impending ventilatory failure." The reader will learn more about these interesting arterial blood gas measurements later in the textbook.

---

[8] Clinically, this arterial blood gas (ABG) is also called acute hyperventilation superimposed on compensated respiratory acidosis. The importance of arterial blood gas interpretations will be discussed in greater detail in Chapter 7—Acid–Base Balance and Regulation.

Figure 2–44

The effects of increased airway resistance and decreased lung compliance on ventilatory frequency and tidal volume.

© Cengage Learning 2013

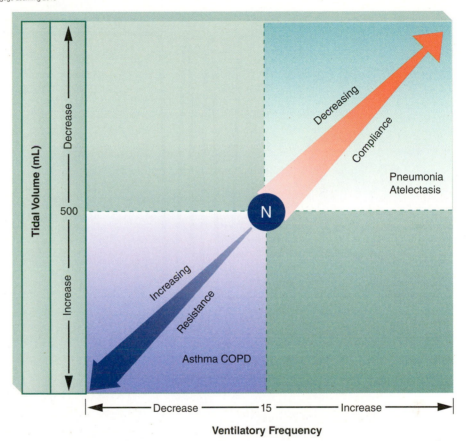

Ventilatory Frequency

When lung compliance decreases, the patient's ventilatory rate generally increases while, at the same time, the tidal volume decreases. When airway resistance increases, the patient's ventilatory frequency usually decreases while, at the same time, the tidal volume increases (Figure 2–44).

The ventilatory pattern is determined by both **ventilatory efficiency** (to minimize dead space ventilation) and **metabolic efficiency** (to minimize the work or oxygen cost of breathing). The body is assumed to adjust both rate and depth of breathing to give the best trade-off between the two. In severe cases, an increase in ventilation will ultimately reach a point in which the increase in oxygen delivery is exceeded by the increase in oxygen demanded by the respiratory muscles. In short, the ventilatory pattern adopted by a patient is based on minimum work requirements, rather than ventilatory efficiency.

In physics, work is defined as the force applied multiplied by the distance moved (work = force × distance). In respiratory physiology, the changes in transpulmonary pressure (force) multiplied by the change in lung volume (distance) may be used to quantitate the amount of work required to breathe (work = pressure × volume). Normally, about 5 percent of an individual's total energy output goes to the work of breathing.

Thus, because the patient may adopt a ventilatory pattern based on the **expenditure of energy** rather than the efficiency of ventilation, it cannot be assumed that the ventilatory pattern acquired by the patient in response to a

Figure 2–45

Biot's breathing: Short episodes of rapid, uniformly deep inspirations, followed by 10 to 30 seconds of apnea.

© Cengage Learning 2013

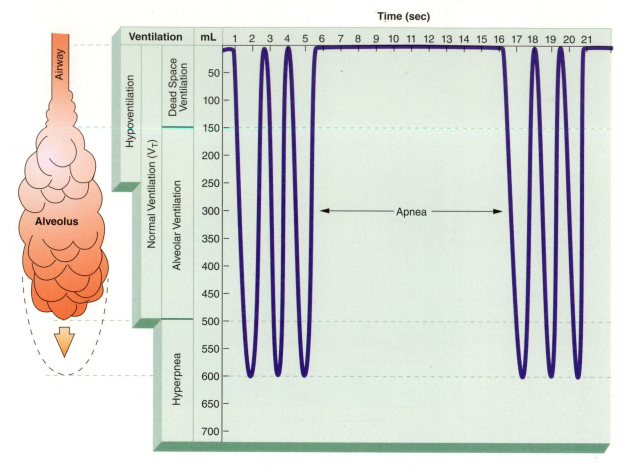

certain respiratory disorder is the most efficient one in terms of physiologic gas exchange. Such ventilatory patterns are usually seen in the more severe pulmonary disorders that cause lung compliance to decrease or airway resistance to increase.

Overview of Specific Breathing Conditions

The following are types of breathing conditions frequently seen by the respiratory care practitioner in the clinical setting.

Apnea: Complete absence of spontaneous ventilation. This causes the $P_{A_{O_2}}$[9] and Pa_{O_2}[10] to rapidly decrease and the $P_{A_{CO_2}}$[11] and Pa_{CO_2}[12] to increase. Death will ensue in minutes.

Eupnea: Normal, spontaneous breathing (see Figure 2–39).

Biot's breathing: Short episodes of rapid, uniformly deep inspirations, followed by 10 to 30 seconds of apnea (Figure 2–45). This pattern was first described in patients suffering from meningitis.

---

[9]$P_{A_{O_2}}$ = *alveolar oxygen tension.*

[10]Pa_{O_2} = *arterial oxygen tension.*

[11]$P_{A_{CO_2}}$ = *alveolar carbon dioxide tension.*

[12]Pa_{CO_2} = *arterial carbon dioxide tension.*

Figure 2–46

Hyperpnea: Increased depth of breathing.

© Cengage Learning 2013

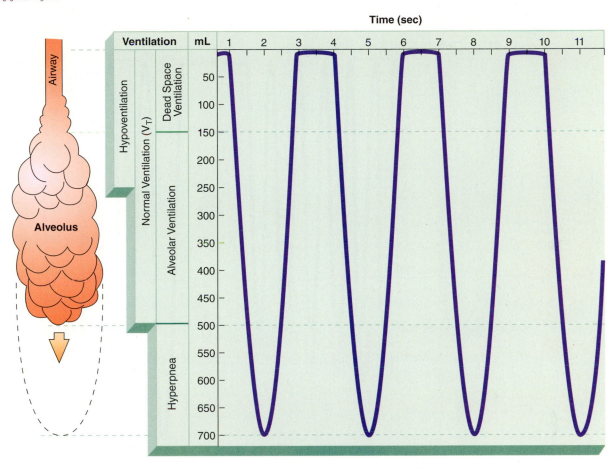

Hyperpnea: Increased depth (volume) of breathing with or without an increased frequency (Figure 2–46).

Hyperventilation: Increased alveolar ventilation (produced by any ventilatory pattern that causes an increase in either the ventilatory rate or the depth of breathing) that causes the $P_{A_{CO_2}}$ and, therefore, the Pa_{CO_2} to decrease (Figure 2–47 on page 134).

Hypoventilation: Decreased alveolar ventilation (produced by any ventilatory pattern that causes a decrease in either the ventilatory rate or the depth of breathing) that causes the $P_{A_{CO_2}}$ and, therefore, the Pa_{CO_2} to increase (Figure 2–48 on page 135).

Tachypnea: A rapid rate of breathing.

Cheyne-Stokes breathing: Ten to 30 seconds of apnea, followed by a gradual increase in the volume and frequency of breathing, followed by a gradual decrease in the volume of breathing until another period of apnea

Hyperventilation: Increased rate (A) or depth (B), or some combination of these, of breathing that causes the $P_{A_{CO_2}}$ and, therefore, the Pa_{CO_2} to decrease.

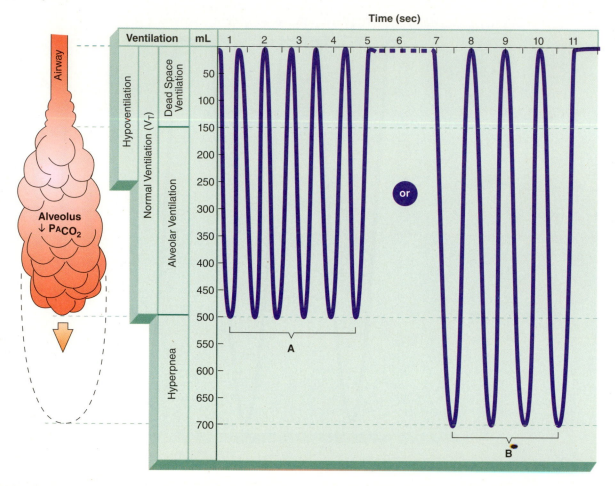

Clinical Connection—2-18

The Arterial Carbon Dioxide Level and Its Relationship to the Clinical Verification of Hyperventilation and Hypoventilation

A patient's breathing rate can often be very misleading. For example, even though a fast respiratory rate is often associated with hyperventilation, the patient's rapid breathing rate alone is not enough to make the assessment of hyperventilation. The absolute confirmation of hyperventilation can only be made by evaluating the patient's arterial carbon dioxide partial pressure—(Pa_{CO_2}). Hyperventilation is verified when the patient's arterial blood gas values reveal an acute respiratory alkalosis (increased pH) as a result of a sudden decrease in the Pa_{CO_2} level. On the other hand, hypoventilation is established when the arterial

blood gas values show an acute respiratory acidosis (decreased pH) as a result of an elevated Pa_{CO_2} level.

In the clinical setting, the respiratory therapist frequently evaluates the patient's arterial blood gas values—pH, Pa_{CO_2}, HCO_3^-, and Pa_{O_2}—to determine the patient's ventilatory status. Oftentimes, the therapist must adjust the rate and tidal volume on the mechanical ventilator to correct the patient's Pa_{CO_2} level. The importance of the Pa_{CO_2} and its relationship to arterial blood gas interpretations will be discussed in greater detail in Chapter 7—Acid–Base Balance and Regulation.

Figure 2–48

Hypoventilation: Decreased rate (A) or depth (B), or some combination of both, of breathing that causes the $P_{A_{CO_2}}$ and, therefore, the Pa_{CO_2} to increase.

© Cengage Learning 2013

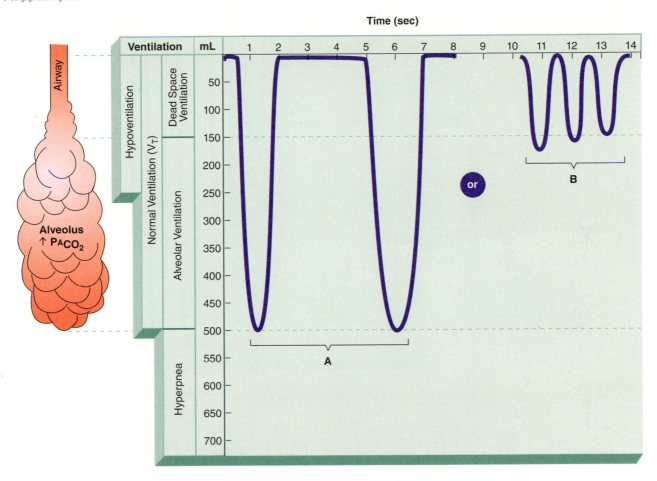

occurs (Figure 2–49 on page 136). As the depth of breathing increases, the $P_{A_{CO_2}}$ and Pa_{CO_2} fall and the $P_{A_{O_2}}$ and Pa_{O_2} rise. Cheyne-Stokes breathing is associated with cerebral disorders and congestive heart failure (CHF).

Kussmaul's breathing: Both an increased depth (hyperpnea) and rate of breathing (Figure 2–50 on page 136). This ventilatory pattern causes the $P_{A_{CO_2}}$ and Pa_{CO_2} to decline and the $P_{A_{O_2}}$ and Pa_{O_2} to increase. Kussmaul's breathing is commonly associated with diabetic acidosis (ketoacidosis).

Orthopnea: A condition in which an individual is able to breathe most comfortably only in the upright position.

Dyspnea: Difficulty in breathing, of which the individual is aware.

Figure 2–49

Cheyne-Stokes
breathing: A
gradual increase
and decrease in
the volume and
rate of breathing,
followed by 10
to 30 seconds of
apnea.

© Cengage Learning 2013

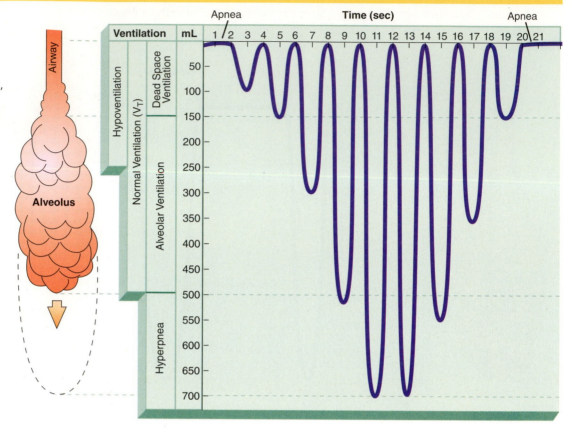

Figure 2–50

Kussmaul's
breathing:
Increased rate and
depth of breathing.
This breathing
pattern causes
the PA_{CO_2} and Pa_{CO_2}
to decrease and
PA_{O_2} and Pa_{O_2} to
increase.

© Cengage Learning 2013

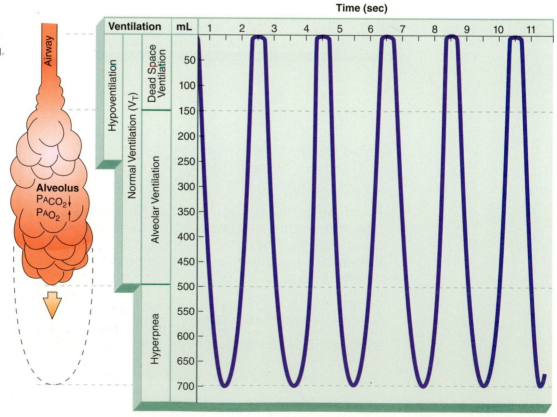

Chapter Summary

The essential knowledge base for ventilation consists of four major areas. *First,* the respiratory therapist must understand the primary mechanisms of pulmonary ventilation. Important to this subject includes how the atmosphere pressure, Boyle's law, and pressure gradients are connected to (1) the excursion of the diaphragm; (2) pleural pressure; (3) intra-alveolar pressure; and (4) gas flow during inspiration, end-inspiration, expiration, and end-expiration. In addition, key pressure gradients related to the mechanisms of ventilation are the driving pressure, transrespiratory pressure, transmural pressure, transpulmonary pressure, and transthoracic pressure. Clinical connections associated with the mechanisms of ventilation include inspiratory intercostal retractions and the harmful effects of pressure gradients when the thorax is unstable.

Second, the respiratory therapist must understand the elastic properties of the lungs. Major components of this subject are (1) lung compliance, including the calculation of lung compliance; (2) elastance, including Hooke's law; and (3) surface tension and its relationship to Laplace's law, pulmonary surfactant, and the deficiency of pulmonary surfactant. Clinical connections associated with all the above topics include (1) pulmonary disorders that force the patient to breathe at the top—flat portion—of the volume-pressure curve; (2) pulmonary disorders that shift the volume-pressure curve to the right—decreased lung compliance; (3) positive-pressure ventilation and related hazards; (4) negative-pressure ventilation; and (5) pulmonary surfactant deficiency.

Third, the therapist must have a good understanding of the dynamic characteristics of the lungs. This important subject includes (1) how Poiseuille's law arranged for either flow or pressure relates to the radius of the bronchial airways; (2) airway resistance, including its calculation, and its relationship to laminar and turbulent flow; and (3) dynamic compliance and its relationship to increased airway resistance and frequency dependence. Clinical connections associated with these topics include (1) respiratory disorders that decrease the radius of the airways; (2) restrictive lung disorders, time constants, and breathing pattern relationships; (3) obstructive lung disorders, time constants, and breathing pattern relationships; and (4) auto-PEEP and its relationship to airway resistance during rapid ventilatory rates.

Finally, the respiratory therapist needs a good knowledge base of the characteristics of normal and abnormal ventilatory patterns. This subject consists of (1) knowing the meaning of the normal ventilatory pattern, including the tidal volume, ventilatory rate, and IE ratio; (2) differentiating between alveolar ventilation and dead space ventilation; (3) knowing how the depth and rate of breathing affects alveolar ventilation; (4) being able to calculate an individual's alveolar ventilation; (5) understanding how the normal pleural pressure differences cause regional differences in normal lung ventilation; (6) knowing how the respiratory rate and tidal volume change in response to a decreased lung compliance or an increased airway resistance; and (7) the ability to recognize specific breathing conditions, such as Biot's breathing, hypoventilation, tachypnea, Cheyne-Stokes breathing, Kussmaul's breathing, orthopnea, and dyspnea.

Clinical connections associated with these topics include (1) the normal respiratory rates for different age groups; (2) the tidal volume and respiratory rate strategies for mechanical ventilation; (3) how dead space ventilation relates to an endotracheal tube, or the tubing circuitry on a mechanical ventilator, or a pulmonary embolus; (4) how the adopted breathing pattern changes in chronic obstructive lung disorders when compromised by a restrictive lung disorder; and (5) the arterial carbon dioxide level and its relationship to the clinical verification of hyperventilation and hypoventilation.

1 Clinical Application Case

A 22-year-old male who had been in a motorcycle crash was brought to the emergency department with several facial, neck, and shoulder abrasions and lacerations, and multiple broken ribs. During each breath, the patient's right anterior chest moved inward during inspiration and outward during exhalation (clinically this is called a *flail chest*). The patient was alert, in pain, and stated, "I can't breathe. Am I going to die?"

The patient's skin was pale and blue. His vital signs were blood pressure—166/93 mm Hg, heart rate—135 beats/min, and respiratory rate—26 breaths/min and shallow. While on a simple oxygen mask, the patient's peripheral oxygen saturation level (Sp_{O_2}), measured over the skin of his index finger, was 79 percent (normal, 97 percent). Chest X-ray showed that the third, fourth, fifth, sixth, and seventh ribs were each broken in two or three places on the right anterior chest. The chest X-ray also revealed that his right lung was partially collapsed.

A chest tube was inserted and the patient was immediately transferred to the intensive care unit (ICU), sedated, intubated, and placed on a mechanical ventilator. The mechanical ventilator was set at a ventilatory rate of 12 breaths/minute, an oxygen concentration of 0.5, and a positive end-expiratory pressure (PEEP) of +5 cm H_2O.[13] No spontaneous breaths were present between the mandatory mechanical breaths.

Four hours later, the patient appeared comfortable and his skin color was normal. The ventilator was set at a rate of 12 breaths/min, an inspired oxygen concentration ($F_{I_{O_2}}$) of 0.3, and a PEEP of +5 cm H_2O. No spontaneous breaths were generated between each mechanical ventilation. During each mechanical breath, both the right and left side of the patient's chest expanded symmetrically. His blood pressure was 127/83 mm Hg and heart rate was 76 beats/min. A second chest X-ray revealed that his right lung had re-expanded. His peripheral oxygen saturation level was 97 percent.

Discussion

This case illustrates (1) the effects on *transthoracic pressure and transpulmonary pressure* when the thorax is unstable, (2) how the excursions of the diaphragm affect the pleural pressure, (3) acute decreased lung compliance, and (4) the therapeutic effects of positive-pressure ventilation in flail chest cases.

Under normal conditions, on each inhalation, the diaphragm moves downward and causes the pleural pressure and alveolar pressure to decrease (see Figure 2–5). In this case, however, the patient's ribs were broken on the right side and caved in during each inspiration when the pleural and alveolar pressure decreased. This caused the right lung to partially collapse—an acute decreased lung compliance condition (see Figure 2–13).

This process was corrected when the patient was ventilated with positive pressure. The patient no longer had to generate negative pressure to inhale. During each positive-pressure breath, the chest wall expanded evenly and returned to normal resting level at the end of each expiration. This process allowed the ribs to heal. After 10 days, the patient was weaned from the ventilator. He was discharged 3 days later.

---

[13] At the end of a normal spontaneous expiration, the pressure in the alveoli is equal to the barometric pressure. A +5 cm H_2O of PEEP means that at the end of each exhalation, the patient's alveoli still had a positive pressure of 5 cm H_2O above atmospheric pressure. Therapeutically, this helps to re-expand collapsed alveoli or prevent the collapse of alveoli.

2 Clinical Application Case

This 14-year-old girl with a long history of asthma presented in the emergency department in moderate to severe respiratory distress. She appeared very frightened and tears were running down her face. She was sitting perched forward with her arms braced in a tripod-like position on the side of a gurney, hands clutching the edge of the gurney. She was using her accessory muscles of inspiration. When asked about her condition, she stated, "I can't get enough air." She could only speak two or three words at a time, between each breath.

The patient's skin appeared pale and bluish. She had a frequent and strong cough, productive of large amounts of thick, white secretions. Her vital signs were blood pressure—151/93 mm Hg, heart rate—106 beats/min and strong, and respiratory rate—32 breaths/min. Wheezes were heard over both lung fields. Chest X-ray showed that her lungs were hyperinflated and that her diaphragm was depressed. Her peripheral oxygen saturation level (Sp_{O_2}), measured by pulse oximetry over the skin of her index finger was 89 percent (normal, 97 percent).

The respiratory therapist working in the emergency department started the patient on oxygen via a 6-liter (6 L/min) nasal cannula, and on a bronchodilator continuously, via a handheld aerosol. The therapist also remained at the patient's bedside to monitor the patient's response to treatment, and to encourage the patient to take slow, deep inspirations.

Forty-five minutes later, the patient had substantially improved. She was sitting up in bed and no longer appeared to be in respiratory distress. She could speak in longer sentences without getting short of breath. Her skin color was normal. Her vital signs were blood pressure—126/83 mm Hg, heart rate—87 beats/min, and respiratory rate—14 breaths/min.

When instructed to cough, she generated a strong, nonproductive cough. Although wheezes could still be heard over the patient's lungs, they were not as severe as they were on admission. A second chest X-ray showed that her lungs were normal and her diaphragm was no longer depressed. Her Sp_{O_2} was 94 percent.

Discussion

This case illustrates (1) an acute decreased lung compliance condition, (2) how *Poiseuille's law* can be used to demonstrate the effects of bronchial constriction and excessive airway secretions on bronchial gas flow and the work of breathing, (3) the effects of an increased *airway resistance* (R_{aw}) on *time constants*, and (4) the *frequency-dependent* effects of a decreased ventilatory rate on the ventilation of alveoli.

As the severity of the tracheobronchial tree constriction progressively increased, the patient's ability to exhale fully declined. This process caused the patient's lungs to hyperinflate (but not with fresh air). As a result of the hyperinflation, the patient's work of breathing increased, because her lungs were functioning at the very top of their volume–pressure curve—the flat portion of the curve (see Figure 2–13). As the volume–pressure curve shows, lung compliance is very low on the upper, flat portion of the volume–pressure curve. Because of this, the patient was working extremely hard to breathe (i.e., generating large pleural pressure changes), with little or no change in her alveolar ventilation (volume), as shown in Figure 2–13.

In addition, as Poiseuille's law demonstrates, the tracheobronchial tree constriction and excessive airway secretions, both caused by the asthma attack, can have a tremendous impact on gas flow and on the patient's work of breathing. Poiseuille's law shows that gas flow is *directly* related to the fourth power of the radius (r^4) of the tracheobronchial tree, and pressure (e.g., pleural pressure changes) is *indirectly* related to the fourth power of the radius of the airways. Thus, if the patient's bronchial constriction and bronchial secretions decreased the radius of the airways by one-half, the flow of gas would decrease to $1/16$ of the original flow (see Figure 2–29). Similarly, in order for the patient to maintain the same flow rate, she would have to increase her work of breathing to 16 times her original level (see Figure 2–31).

Airway resistance (R_{aw}) can be defined as the pleural pressure difference (ΔP) generated by the patient to move a volume of gas divided by the flow rate ($\dot{V}$). Again, according to Poiseuille's law, it can be seen that

(continues)

as the airways narrow, pleural pressure will increase significantly while, at the same time, gas flow through the airways will decrease. Because $R_{aw} = \Delta P \div \dot{V}$, it is easy to see mathematically how quickly airway resistance can increase during an asthmatic episode.

Finally, as the airway resistance (R_{aw}) increased, the alveoli distal to the bronchial constriction required a longer time to inflate. These alveoli are said to have a long *time constant* (see Figure 2–30). A product of the time constants is the measurement called *dynamic compliance*, which is the change in volume of the lungs divided by the change in the transpulmonary pressure during the time required for one breath (i.e., during a period of gas flow).

In the healthy lung, the dynamic compliance is approximately equal to lung compliance at all breathing frequencies. In the patient with partially obstructed airways, however, the ratio of dynamic compliance to lung compliance decreases as the respiratory rate increases. The alveoli distal to the airway obstruction do not have enough time to fully inflate as the breathing frequency rises. The compliance of these alveoli is said to be *frequency dependent*. This is why it was important for the respiratory therapist to remain at the bedside and encourage the patient to take slow, deep breaths.

Because the patient was having trouble inhaling a normal volume of gas and because her oxygen saturation level (Sp_{O_2}) was below normal, oxygen therapy was clearly indicated. The continuous bronchodilator therapy was also indicated and worked to offset the effects of airway constriction (as described by Poiseuille's law), increased airway resistance, air trapping, and hyperinflation. As the lung hyperinflation progressively declined, lung compliance steadily increased, or returned to normal (i.e., returned back to the steep portion of the volume-pressure curve). The patient continued to improve and was discharged from the hospital by the next afternoon.

Review Questions

1. The average compliance of the lungs and chest wall combined is
  A. 0.1 L/cm H_2O
  B. 0.2 L/cm H_2O
  C. 0.3 L/cm H_2O
  D. 0.4 L/cm H_2O

2. Normally, the airway resistance in the tracheobronchial tree is about
  A. 0.5–1.5 cm H_2O/L/sec
  B. 1.0–2.0 cm H_2O/L/sec
  C. 2.0–3.0 cm H_2O/L/sec
  D. 3.0–4.0 cm H_2O/L/sec

3. In the normal individual in the upright position
  1. the negative pleural pressure is greater (i.e., more negative) in the upper lung regions
  2. the alveoli in the lower lung regions are larger than the alveoli in the upper lung regions
  3. ventilation is more effective in the lower lung regions
  4. the pleural pressure is always below atmospheric pressure during a normal ventilatory cycle
    A. 1 and 2 only
    B. 2 and 3 only
    C. 2, 3, and 4 only
    D. 1, 3, and 4 only

4. When lung compliance decreases, the patient commonly has
   1. an increased ventilatory rate
   2. a decreased tidal volume
   3. an increased tidal volume
   4. a decreased ventilatory rate
      A. 1 only
      B. 2 only
      C. 3 and 4 only
      D. 1 and 2 only

5. When arranged for flow Poiseuille's law states that flow is
   1. inversely proportional to r^4
   2. directly proportional to P
   3. inversely proportional to η
   4. directly proportional to l
      A. 1 only
      B. 2 only
      C. 2 and 3 only
      D. 3 and 4 only

6. During a normal exhalation, the
   1. intra-alveolar pressure is greater than the atmospheric pressure
   2. pleural pressure is less than the atmospheric pressure
   3. intra-alveolar pressure is in equilibrium with the atmospheric pressure
   4. pleural pressure progressively decreases
      A. 1 only
      B. 4 only
      C. 1 and 2 only
      D. 3 and 4 only

7. At rest, the normal pleural pressure change during quiet breathing is about
      A. 0–2 mm Hg
      B. 2–4 mm Hg
      C. 4–6 mm Hg
      D. 6–8 mm Hg

8. Normally, an individual's tidal volume is about
      A. 1–2 mL/lb
      B. 3–4 mL/lb
      C. 5–6 mL/lb
      D. 7–8 mL/lb

9. A rapid and shallow ventilatory pattern is called
      A. hyperpnea
      B. apnea
      C. alveolar hyperventilation
      D. tachypnea

10. Assuming that pressure remains constant, if the radius of a bronchial airway through which gas flows at a rate of 400 L/min is reduced to one-half of its original size, the flow through the bronchial airway would change to
      A. 10 L/min
      B. 25 L/min
      C. 100 L/min
      D. 200 L/min

11. The difference between the alveolar pressure and the pleural pressure is called the
   A. transpulmonary pressure
   B. transthoracic pressure
   C. driving pressure
   D. transrespiratory pressure

12. According to Laplace's law, if a bubble with a radius of 4 cm and a distending pressure of 10 cm H_2O is reduced to a radius of 2 cm, the new distending pressure of the bubble will be
   A. 5 cm H_2O
   B. 10 cm H_2O
   C. 15 cm H_2O
   D. 20 cm H_2O

13. If alveolar unit A has one-half the compliance of alveolar unit B, then the
   1. time constant of unit A is essentially the same as that of unit B
   2. volume in unit B is two times greater than volume in unit A
   3. time constant of unit B is twice as long as that of unit A
   4. volume in unit B is essentially the same as the volume of unit A
      A. 1 only
      B. 3 only
      C. 4 only
      D. 2 and 3 only

14. If a patient weighs 175 pounds and has a tidal volume of 550 mL and a respiratory rate of 17 breaths/min, what is the patient's minute alveolar ventilation?

_____

15. Lung compliance study

   Part I: If a patient generates a negative pleural pressure change of −8 cm H_2O during inspiration, and the lungs accept a new volume of 630 mL, what is the compliance of the lungs?

_____

   Part II: If the same patient, 6 hours later, generates an pleural pressure of −12 cm H_2O during inspiration, and the lungs accept a new volume of 850 mL, what is the compliance of the lungs?

_____

   Part III: In comparing Part II to Part I, the patient's lung compliance is
   A. increasing
   B. decreasing

16. If a patient produces a flow rate of 5 L/sec during a forced exhalation by generating a transrespiratory pressure of 20 cm H_2O, what is the patient's R_{aw}?
   A. 1 cm H_2O/L/sec
   B. 2 cm H_2O/L/sec
   C. 3 cm H_2O/L/sec
   D. 4 cm H_2O/L/sec

17. As R_{aw} increases, the patient commonly manifests
    1. a decreased ventilatory rate
    2. an increased tidal volume
    3. a decreased tidal volume
    4. an increased ventilatory rate
        A. 1 only
        B. 2 only
        C. 1 and 2 only
        D. 3 and 4 only

18. If the radius of a bronchial airway, which has a driving pressure of 2 mm Hg, is reduced by 16 percent of its original size, what will be the new driving pressure required to maintain the same gas flow through the bronchial airway?
    A. 4 mm Hg
    B. 8 mm Hg
    C. 12 mm Hg
    D. 16 mm Hg

19. In the healthy lung, when the alveolus decreases in size during a normal exhalation, the
    1. surface tension decreases
    2. surfactant to alveolar surface area increases
    3. surface tension increases
    4. surfactant to alveolar surface area decreases
        A. 1 only
        B. 3 only
        C. 4 only
        D. 1 and 2 only

20. At end-expiration, P_{ta} is
    A. 0 mm Hg
    B. 2 mm Hg
    C. 4 mm Hg
    D. 6 mm Hg

Clinical Application Questions

Case 1

1. Because this patient's ribs were broken on the right side, his right chest (bulged outward _____; caved inward _____) during each inspiration.

2. As a result of the previously described condition described, the patient's right lung _____, which in turn caused an acute (decreased _____; increased _____) lung compliance condition.

3. The pathophysiologic process that developed in this case was corrected with _____. During each breath, the patient's chest wall (caved inward _____; moved outward _____) and then returned to normal _____ at the end of each expiration.

Case 2

1. As a result of the hyperinflation, the patient's work of breathing increased because her lungs were inflated to the very top of their volume–pressure curve. As the volume-pressure curve illustrates, lung compliance is very (high _____; low _____) on the upper, flat portion of the volume–pressure curve.

2. Because of the lung hyperinflation described in question 1, the patient was generating (small _____; large _____) pleural pressure changes with (little or no _____; moderate to large _____) volume changes.

3. What two major tracheobronchial tree changes occurred during the asthma attack that caused gas flow to significantly decrease, as described by Poiseuille's law?

   _____

   _____

4. As the airway resistance increased in this case, the alveoli distal to the bronchial constriction required (shorter _____; longer _____) time to inflate. These alveoli are said to have a (short _____; long _____) time constant.

5. A product of the time constants is the measurement called dynamic compliance, which is the change in volume of the lungs divided by the change in the transpulmonary pressure during the time for one breath. During an asthmatic episode, the patient's dynamic compliance (increases _____; decreases _____; remains the same _____).

Chapter 3

Pulmonary Function Measurements

Objectives

By the end of this chapter, the student should be able to:

1. Define the following *lung volumes:*
   - Tidal volume
   - Inspiratory reserve volume
   - Expiratory reserve volume
   - Residual volume
2. Define the following *lung capacities:*
   - Vital capacity
   - Inspiratory capacity
   - Functional residual capacity
   - Total lung capacity
3. Identify the approximate lung volumes and capacities in milliliters in the average healthy man and woman between 20 and 30 years of age.
4. Identify the lung volumes and lung capacities changes that occur in obstruction and restrictive lung disorders.
5. Discuss the clinical connection associated with obstructive lung disorders.
6. Discuss the clinical connections associated with restrictive lung disorders.
7. Compare and contrast how the following methods indirectly measure the residual volume and the capacities containing the residual volume:
   - Closed circuit helium dilution
   - Open circuit nitrogen washout
   - Body plethysmography
8. Compare and contrast the following *expiratory flow rate measurements:*
   - Forced vital capacity
   - Forced expiratory volume timed
   - Forced expiratory volume$_{1\,sec}$/forced vital capacity ratio
   - Forced expiratory flow$_{25\%-75\%}$
   - Forced expiratory flow$_{200-1200}$
   - Peak expiratory flow rate

   - Maximum voluntary ventilation
   - Flow-volume curves
9. Identify the following average dynamic flow rate measurements for the healthy man and woman between 20 and 30 years of age:
   - Forced expiratory volume timed for periods of 0.5, 1.0, 2.0, and 3.0 seconds
   - Forced expiratory flow$_{200-1200}$
   - Forced expiratory flow$_{25\%-75\%}$
   - Peak expiratory flow rate
   - Maximum voluntary ventilation
10. Describe the clinical connection associated with FEV$_1$/FVC ratio and FEV$_1$ in the assessment and management of chronic obstructive pulmonary disease (COPD).
11. Describe the clinical connection associated with differentiating between an obstructive and restrictive lung disorder.
12. Describe the clinical connection associated with an asthma action plan—the green, yellow, and red zones.
13. Describe the clinical connection associated with both an obstructive and restrictive lung disorder.
14. Describe the *effort-dependent portion* of a forced expiratory maneuver.
15. Describe the *effort-independent portion* of a forced expiratory maneuver.
16. Explain how the *dynamic compression mechanism* limits the flow rate during the last 70 percent of a forced vital capacity, and define the equal pressure point.
17. Describe the clinical connection associated with how spirometry can confirm dynamic compression.
18. Describe the clinical connection associated with pursed-lip breathing.

(continues)

19. Describe the diffusion capacity of carbon monoxide study.
20. Describe how the following are used to evaluate the patient's ability to maintain spontaneous, unassisted ventilation:
—Maximum inspiratory pressure (MIP)
—Maximum expiratory pressure (MEP)
—Rapid shallow breathing index (RSBI) ratio

21. Describe the clinical connection associated with the ventilatory mechanics used to predict mechanical ventilation weaning success.
22. Describe the clinical connection associated with broadening one's career by pursuing a certified pulmonary function technologist or registered pulmonary function technologist credential.
23. Complete the review questions at the end of this chapter.

Lung Volumes and Capacities

The volume of air that moves in and out of the lungs—and remains in the lungs—is a matter of great importance to the study of cardiopulmonary physiology. The total amount of air that the lungs can accommodate is divided into these two major categories—the lung volumes and lung capacities. There are four different lung volumes, and four different lung capacities—which are composed of two or more lung volumes (Figure 3-1).

Lung Volumes

The four lung volumes are the tidal volume, inspiratory reserve volume, expiratory reserve volume, and residual volume. During normal quiet breathing, about 500 mL of air moves in and out of the lungs with each breath. This volume is tidal volume (V_T). The amount of air that can be forcibly inhaled beyond the V_T is the inspiratory reserve volume (IRV). The amount of air that can be forcibly exhaled after a normal V_T is the expiratory reserve volume (ERV). The amount of air still in the lungs after a forced ERV is the residual volume (RV). The RV is important for keeping the alveoli open

---

Figure 3–1

Normal lung volumes and capacities. IRV = inspiratory reserve volume; V_T = tidal volume; ERV = expiratory reserve volume; RV = residual volume; VC = vital capacity; TLC = total lung capacity; IC = inspiratory capacity; FRC = functional residual capacity.

© Cengage Learning 2013

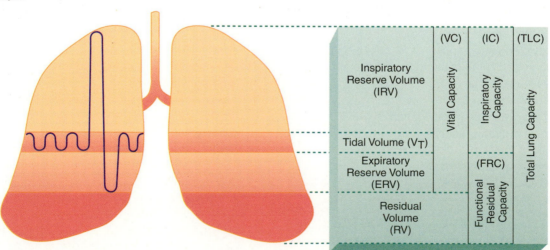

© Cengage Learning 2013

Table 3–1

Approximate Lung Volumes and Capacities in Healthy Men and Women 20 to 30 Years of Age

	Measurement	Description	Adult Male Average Value	Adult Female Average Value
Lung Volumes	**Tidal volume (V$_T$)**	The amount of air inhaled and exhaled with each breath during quiet breathing	500 mL	400–500 mL
	Inspiratory reserve volume (IRV)	The amount of air that can be forcibly inhaled beyond the V$_T$	3100 mL	1900 mL
	Expiratory reserve volume (ERV)	The amount of air that can be forcibly exhaled after a normal V$_T$	1200 mL	800 mL
	Residual volume (RV)	The amount of air still in the lungs after a forced ERV	1200 mL	1000 mL
Lung Capacities	**Vital capacity (VC)**	The maximum volume of air that can be exhaled after a maximal inspiration (VC = IRV + V$_T$ + ERV).	4800 mL	3200 mL
	Inspiratory capacity (IC)	The volume air that can be inhaled after a normal exhalation (IC = V$_T$ + IRV).	3600 mL	2400 mL
	Functional residual capacity (FRC)	The volume of air remaining in the lungs after a normal exhalation (FRC = ERV + RV).	2400 mL	1800 mL
	Total lung capacity (TLC)	The maximum amount of air that the lungs can accommodate (TLC = V$_T$ + IRV + ERV + RV).	6000 mL	4200 mL

and overall gas exchange. Table 3–1 provides a description of the lung volumes and the average normal values for males and females between 20 and 30 years of age.

Lung Capacities

The four lung capacities are the vital capacity, inspiratory capacity, functional residual capacity, and total lung capacity. The **vital capacity (VC)** is the maximum volume of air that can be exhaled after a maximal inspiration. The VC is the sum of the IRV + V$_T$ + ERV. There are two major VC measurements: the **slow vital capacity (SVC)**, in which exhalation is performed slowly; and the **forced vital capacity (FVC)**, in which maximal effort is made to exhale as rapidly as possible. The FVC will be discussed in more detail later in this chapter.

The **inspiratory capacity (IC)** is the volume air that can be inhaled after a normal exhalation. The IC is the sum of the V_T + IRV. The **functional residual capacity (FRC)** is the volume of air remaining in the lungs after a normal exhalation. The FRC is the sum of the ERV + RV. The total lung capacity (TLC) is the maximum amount of air that the lungs can accommodate. The TLC is the sum of the V_T + IRV + ERV + RV. Table 3–1 provides a description of the lung capacities and the average normal values for males and females between 20 and 30 years of age.

Lung Volumes and Capacities in Obstructive and Restrictive Lung Disorders

The lung volumes and lung capacities are abnormally altered in any respiratory disorder to some degree. Pulmonary function studies are routinely administered to these patients to (1) determine if the lung problem is an obstructive or restrictive lung disorder, (2) evaluate the severity of the pulmonary disorder, (3) determine if the lung problem is an obstructive or restrictive lung disorder, and (4) monitor the progress of chronic pulmonary disorders.

In an **obstructive lung disorder**, the RV, V_T, and FRC, are increased; and the VC, IC, IRV, and ERV are decreased (Figure 3–2). In a **restrictive lung disorder**, the VC, IC, RV, FRC, V_T, and TLC are all decreased (Figure 3–3). Relative to the degree of severity, both an obstructive or a restrictive lung disorder disrupt the exchange of oxygen and carbon dioxide between the alveoli and pulmonary capillary blood.

Figure 3–2

How obstructive lung disorders alter lung volumes and capacities. IRV = inspiratory reserve volume; V_T = tidal volume; ERV = expiratory reserve volume; RV = residual volume; VC = tidal capacity; IC = inspiratory capacity; FRC = functional residual capacity; TLC = total lung capacity.

© Cengage Learning 2013

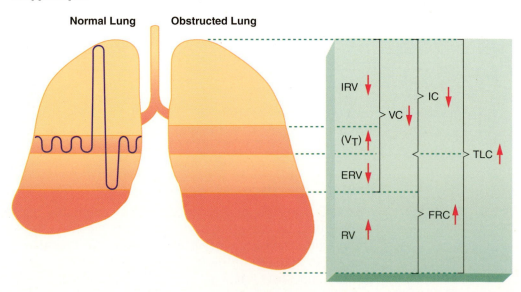

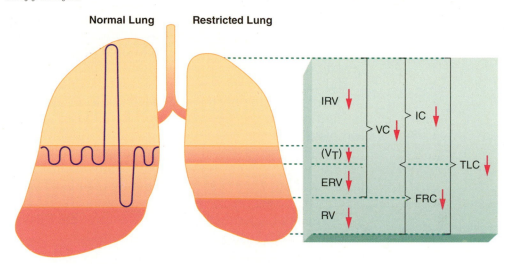

Figure 3–3

How restrictive lung disorders alter lung volumes and capacities. IRV = inspiratory reserve volume; V_T = tidal volume; ERV = expiratory reserve volume; RV = residual volume; VC = vital capacity; IC = inspiratory capacity; FRC = functional residual capacity; TLC = total lung capacity.

© Cengage Learning 2013

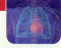

Clinical Connection—3-1

Obstructive Lung Disorders

An obstructive lung disorder is characterized by a variety of abnormal conditions of the tracheobronchial tree—such as bronchial secretions, mucus plugging, bronchospasm, and distal airway weakening—that cause a reduction of gas flow out of the lungs and air trapping. The flow of gas is especially reduced during a forced exhalation. The FEV_1/FVC ratio is the best indicator of an obstructive lung disorder. There are only a few obstructive lung disorders—**cystic fibrosis, bronchitis, asthma, bronchiectasis,** and **emphysema**. These can be remembered by the acronym CBABE, which is the first letter of each condition. The respiratory therapist will often treat patients with these diseases. When chronic bronchitis and emphysema appear together as one disease complex, the patient is said to have **chronic obstructive pulmonary disease (COPD)**.

Clinical Connection—3-2

Restrictive Lung Disorders

A restrictive lung disorder is characterized by any pathologic condition that causes a restriction of the lungs or chest wall—which, in turn, causes a decrease in lung volumes and capacities. Common restrictive lung disorders treated by the respiratory therapist include pneumonia, pulmonary edema, flail chest, pneumothorax, pleural effusion, chronic interstitial lung disease, lung cancer, acute respiratory distress syndrome, and postoperative alveolar collapse (altelectasis).

Indirect Measurements of the Residual Volume and Capacities Containing the Residual Volume

Because the *residual volume* (RV) cannot be exhaled, the RV, and lung capacities that contain the RV, is measured indirectly by one of the following methods: *closed-circuit helium dilution, open-circuit nitrogen washout,* or *body plethysmography.* A brief description of each of these methods follows.

The **closed-circuit helium dilution** test requires the patient to rebreathe from a spirometer that contains a known volume of gas (V_1) and a known concentration (C_1) of helium (He), usually 10 percent. The patient is "switched-in" to the closed-circuit system at the end of a normal tidal volume breath (i.e., the level at which only the FRC is left in the lungs). A helium analyzer continuously monitors the He concentration. Exhaled carbon dioxide is chemically removed from the system. The gas in the patient's FRC, which initially contains no He, mixes with the gas in the spirometer. This dilutes the He throughout the entire system (i.e., patient's lungs, spirometer, and circuit). The test lasts for about 7 minutes. When the He changes by less than 0.2 percent over a period of 1 second, the test is terminated. The He concentration at this point is C_2. The final volume of the entire system—the He circuit and lungs (V_2)—can be calculated by using the following formula:

$$V_1 C_1 = V_2 C_2$$

which is rearranged to solve for V_2 as follows

$$V_2 = \frac{V_1 C_1}{C_2}$$

The FRC can then be calculated by subtracting the initial spirometer volume (V_1) from the equilibrium volume (V_2). (FRC = $V_2 - V_1$). The RV is determined by FRC − ERV. The TLC can be calculated by RV + VC.

In the **open-circuit nitrogen washout** test, the patient breathes 100 percent oxygen through a one-way valve for up to 7 minutes. The patient is "switched-in" to the system at the end of a normal tidal volume (i.e., the level at which only the FRC is left in the lungs). At the beginning of the test, the nitrogen (N_2) concentration in the alveoli is 79 percent (C_1). During each breath, oxygen is inhaled and N_2-rich gas from the FRC is exhaled. Over several minutes, the N_2 in the patient's FRC is effectively washed out. In patients with normal lungs this occurs in 3 minutes or less. Patients with obstructive lung disease may not wash out completely even after 7 minutes.

During the washout period, the exhaled gas volume is measured and the average concentration of N_2 is determined with a nitrogen analyzer. The test is complete when the N_2 concentration drops from 79 to 1.5 percent or less. The FRC (V_1) can then be determined by taking the initial concentration of N_2 in the FRC gas (C_1), the total volume of gas exhaled during the washout period (V_2), and the average concentration of N_2 in the exhaled gas (C_2) and inserting the findings into the following equation:

$$V_1 = \frac{C_2 V_2}{C_1}$$

The FRC can then be calculated by subtracting the known volume of the breathing circuit (V_{bc}) and correcting for the volume of N_2 excreted into the lungs from the plasma and body tissues during the test (V_{tis}):

$$FRC = V_1 - V_{bc} + V_{tis}$$

Body plethysmography measures the gas volume within the lungs (thoracic gas volume [V_{TG}]) indirectly by using a modification of Boyle's law. During the test, the patient sits in an airtight chamber called a *body box*. Initially, the patient is permitted to breathe quietly through an open valve (shutter). Once the patient is relaxed, the test begins at the precise moment the patient exhales to the end tidal volume level (FRC). At this point, the shutter is closed and the patient is instructed to pant against the closed shutter. Pressure and volume changes are monitored during this period. The alveolar pressure changes caused by the compression and decompression of the lungs are estimated at the mouth. Because there is no airflow during this period, and because the temperature is kept constant, the pressure and volume changes can be used to determine the trapped volume (FRC) by applying Boyle's law. This method is generally considered to be the most accurate of the three methods for measuring RV.

Pulmonary Mechanics

In addition to measuring volumes and capacities, the rate at which gas flows in and out of the lungs can also be measured. Expiratory flow rate measurements provide data on the integrity of the airways and the severity of airway impairment, as well as indicating whether the patient has a large airway or a small airway problem. Collectively, the tests for measuring expiratory flow rates are referred to as the pulmonary mechanic measurements.

Pulmonary Mechanic Measurements
Forced Vital Capacity (FVC)

The FVC is the maximum volume of gas that can be exhaled as forcefully and rapidly as possible after a maximal inspiration (Figure 3–4). The FVC is the

Figure 3–4

Forced vital capacity (FVC). A = point of maximal inspiration and the starting point of an FVC.

© Cengage Learning 2013

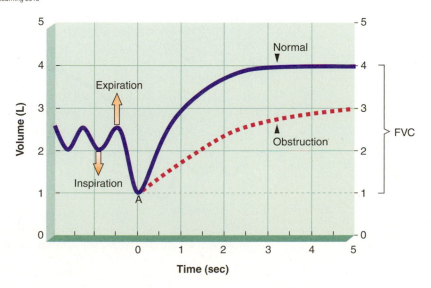

most commonly performed pulmonary function measurement. In the normal individual, the *total expiratory time* (TET) required to completely exhale the FVC is 4 to 6 seconds. In obstructive lung disease (e.g., chronic bronchitis), the TET increases. TETs greater than 10 seconds have been reported in these patients.

In the normal individual, the FVC and the slow vital capacity (SVC) are usually equal. In the patient with obstructive lung disease, the SVC is often normal and the FVC is usually decreased because of air trapping. The FVC is also decreased in restrictive lung disorders (e.g., pulmonary fibrosis, adult respiratory distress syndrome, pulmonary edema). This is primarily due to the low vital capacity associated with restrictive disorders. The TET needed to exhale the FVC in a restrictive disorder, however, is usually normal or even lower than normal, because the elasticity of the lung is high (low compliance) in restrictive disorders.

Forced Expiratory Volume Timed (FEV$_T$)

The FEV$_T$ is the maximum volume of gas that can be exhaled within a specific time period. This measurement is obtained from an FVC. The most frequently used time period is 1 second. Other commonly used periods are 0.5, 2, and 3 seconds (Figure 3–5). Normally, the percentage of the total FVC exhaled during these time periods is as follows: FEV$_{0.5}$, 60 percent; FEV$_1$, 83 percent; FEV$_2$, 94 percent; and FEV$_3$, 97 percent. Patients with *obstructive pulmonary disease* have a decreased FEV$_T$. Patients with *restrictive lung disease* also have a decreased FEV$_T$, primarily due to the low vital capacity associated with such disease. The FEV$_T$ decreases with age.

Forced Expiratory Volume$_{1\ Sec}$/Forced Vital Capacity Ratio (FEV$_1$/FVC Ratio)

The *FEV$_1$/FVC ratio* is the comparison of the amount of air exhaled in 1 second to the total amount exhaled during an FVC maneuver. Because the

---

Figure 3–5

Forced expiratory volume timed (FEV$_T$).

© Cengage Learning 2013

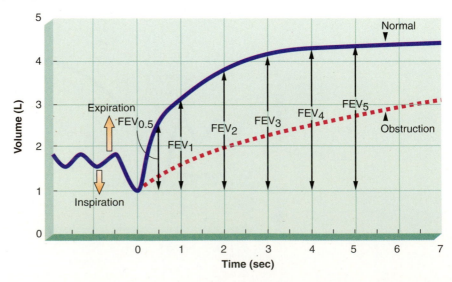

FEV_1/FVC ratio is expressed as a percentage, it is commonly referred as a *forced expiratory volume in 1 second percentage* ($FEV_{1\%}$). As mentioned previously, the normal adult exhales 83 percent or more of the FVC in 1 second (FEV_1). Thus, under normal conditions the patient's $FEV_{1\%}$ should also be 83 percent or greater. Clinically, however, an $FEV_{1\%}$ of 65 percent or more is often used as an acceptable value in older patients.

Key Pulmonary Function Measurements Used to Differentiate between an Obstructive or Restrictive Pulmonary Disorder

Collectively, the **FVC**, **FEV_1**, and the **FEV_1/FEV ratio**—(commonly called the **$FEV_{1\%}$**) are the three most commonly used pulmonary function measurements to (1) differentiate between an obstructive and restrictive lung disorder and (2) determine the severity of a patient's pulmonary disorder. For different reasons, the FVC and FEV_1 are both reduced in obstructive and restrictive lung disorders:

In a restrictive lung disorder, the patient can only inhale smaller volumes of air. As a result, only smaller volumes of air can be exhaled—a smaller FVC and FEV_1. In an obstructive lung disorder, the FEV_1 is reduced because of the increased airway resistance. The FVC is reduced because of early airway closure and air trapping. In other words, the trapped air is blocked from being available for the FVC measurement.

The $FEV_{1\%}$ serves as the key pulmonary function measurement to differentiate between an obstructive and restrictive lung disorder. In other words, the comparison of the FEV_1 with the FVC—the FEV_1/FEV ratio—provides a clear distinction between these two pulmonary disorders as follows:

- In an **obstructive lung disorder**, the $FEV_{1\%}$ is *decreased.* As discussed earlier, a normal $FEV_{1\%}$ is 83 percent or greater. Only a patient with an obstructive disorder will exhale less than 70 percent of their FVC in the first second.
- In a **restrictive lung disorder**, the $FEV_{1\%}$ is normal or *increased.*

 Clinical Connection—3-3

The FEV_1/FVC Ratio and FEV_1 in the Assessment and Management of Chronic Obstructive Pulmonary Disease (COPD)

The **Global Initiative for Chronic Obstructive Lung Disease (GOLD)** provides an excellent framework using the FEV_1/FVC ratio (commonly written as: $FEV_{1\%}$) and FEV_1 values to categorize a patient's COPD as **stage I** (mild), **stage II** (moderate), **stage III** (severe), or **stage IV** (very severe). Based on the patient's COPD stage category, an appropriate treatment program can easily be developed (Figure 3–6). For example, if a COPD patient demonstrated an FEV_1/FVC of 65 percent of predicted and an FEV_1 of 45 percent of predicted, the severity of the patient's COPD would be classified as stage III. Thus, in addition to any of treatment modalities the patient is presently receiving—for example, work to reduce all risk factors, the administration of short-long and long-term bronchodilators, and any pulmonary rehabilitation—glucocorticosteroids would now be indicated because of the stage III assessment (see Figure 3–6 on page 154).

(continues)

Clinical Connection—3-3, continued

Figure 3–6

The Global Initiative for Chronic Obstructive Lung Disease (GOLD) provides an excellent framework to evaluate the severity of COPD and management guidelines.

© Cengage Learning 2013

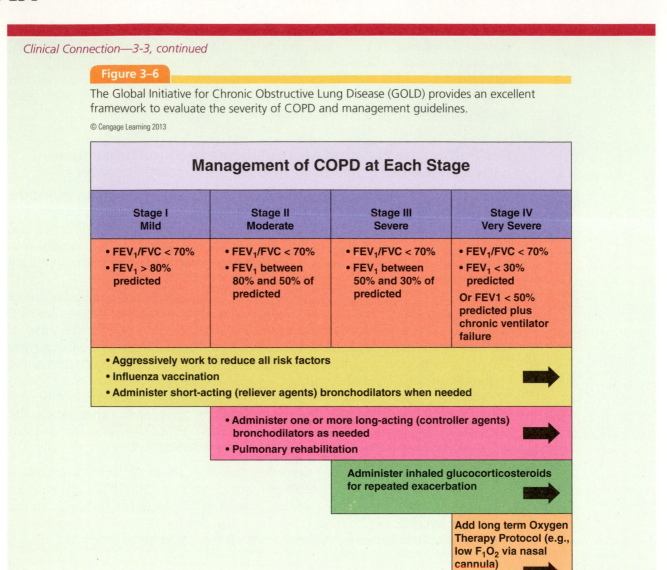

Management of COPD at Each Stage

Stage I Mild	Stage II Moderate	Stage III Severe	Stage IV Very Severe
• $FEV_1/FVC < 70\%$ • $FEV_1 > 80\%$ predicted	• $FEV_1/FVC < 70\%$ • FEV_1 between 80% and 50% of predicted	• $FEV_1/FVC < 70\%$ • FEV_1 between 50% and 30% of predicted	• $FEV_1/FVC < 70\%$ • $FEV_1 < 30\%$ predicted Or $FEV1 < 50\%$ predicted plus chronic ventilator failure

• **Aggressively work to reduce all risk factors**
• **Influenza vaccination**
• **Administer short-acting (reliever agents) bronchodilators when needed** →

• **Administer one or more long-acting (controller agents) bronchodilators as needed**
• **Pulmonary rehabilitation** →

Administer inhaled glucocorticosteroids for repeated exacerbation →

Add long term Oxygen Therapy Protocol (e.g., low F_1O_2 via nasal cannula) →

Forced Expiratory Flow$_{25\%-75\%}$ (FEF$_{25\%-75\%}$)

The FEF$_{25\%-75\%}$ is the average flow rate that occurs during the middle 50 percent of an FVC measurement (Figure 3–7). This average measurement reflects the condition of *medium- to small-sized airways.* The average FEF$_{25\%-75\%}$ for normal healthy men aged 20 to 30 years is about 4.5 L/sec (270 L/min), and for women of the same age, about 3.5 L/sec (210 L/min). The FEF$_{25\%-75\%}$ decreases with age and in obstructive lung disease. In obstructive lung disease, flow rates as low as 0.3 L/sec (18 L/min) have been reported.

The FEF$_{25\%-75\%}$ is also decreased in patients with restrictive lung disorders, primarily because of the low vital capacity associated with restrictive lung disorders. Although the FEF$_{25\%-75\%}$ has no value in distinguishing between obstructive and restrictive disease, it is helpful in further confirming—or ruling out—an obstructive pulmonary disease in patients with borderline low FEV$_{1\%}$. Conceptually, the FEF$_{25\%-75\%}$ is similar to measuring, and then averaging, the flow rate from a water faucet when 25 and 75 percent of a specific volume of water have accumulated in a measuring container (Figure 3–8 on page 156).

Clinical Connection—3-4

Differentiating between Obstructive and Restrictive Lung Disorders

Clinically, the FVC, FEV_1, and $FEV_{1\%}$ are commonly used to determine if a patient is suffering from either an obstructive lung disorder or a restrictive lung disorder. For example, a respiratory therapist is called to help care for a 71-year-old male patient who presents in the emergency room short of breath. The patient is using his accessory muscles of inspiration and is pursed-lip breathing. His face appears blue and his blood pressure is 155/95. The patient states that he might have the flu and has been short of breath for the past two days. The patient also states that he had been diagnosed with pneumonia a few years earlier. The doctor asks that the respiratory therapist have the patient perform a bedside spirometry test to help determine if the patient might have a restrictive or obstructive lung problem. The patient demonstrates the following pulmonary function values.

PFT Measurement	Predicted	Actual	Percent of Predicted
FVC	4.5 L	3.4 L	75%
FEV_1	3.6 L	2.1 L	58%
$FEV_{1\%}$ (FEV_1/FVC ratio)	>83%	62%	—

Based on the data provided by this relatively simple bedside spirometry test, an $FEV_{1\%}$ lower than predicted means the patient is demonstrating an obstructive lung problem. Only a patient with an obstructive lung disorder has a reduced $FEV_{1\%}$. When a patient has a restrictive lung problem, the $FEV_{1\%}$ is either normal or increased. To develop a complete therapeutic plan for this patient, a number of clinical procedures will need to be performed, including (1) obtaining a complete patient history, (2) a more comprehensive pulmonary function study, (3) arterial blood gas measurements, and (4) chest X-rays.

Figure 3–7

Forced expiratory flow$_{25\%-75\%}$ ($FEF_{25\%-75\%}$).

© Cengage Learning 2013

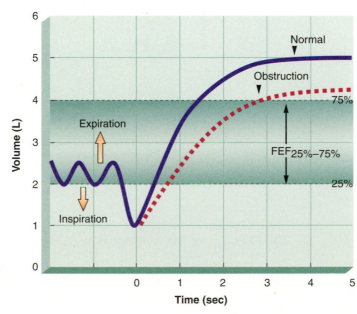

Figure 3–8

The $FEF_{25\%-75\%}$ is similar to measuring and then averaging the flow rate from a faucet when 1 and 3 liters of water have accumulated in a 4-liter container. **A.** Picture the flow rate from the faucet being measured when 1 liter (25%) of water has entered a 4-liter container **B.** Again, picture the flow rate from the faucet being measured when 3 liters (75 percent) of water have entered the 4-liter container. Taking the average of the two flow rates would be similar to the $FEF_{25\%-75\%}$, which measures and then averages the flow rate when an individual exhales 25 and 75 percent of the FVC.

© Cengage Learning 2013

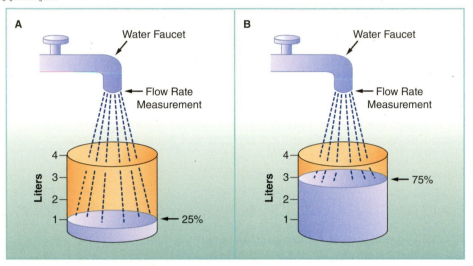

Figure 3–9

Forced expiratory flow$_{200-1200}$ ($FEF_{200-1200}$).

© Cengage Learning 2013

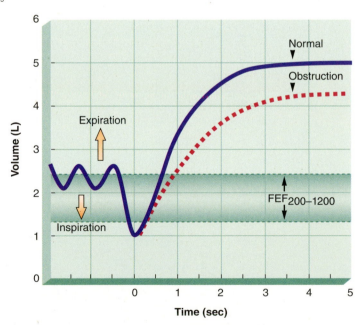

Forced Expiratory Flow$_{200-1200}$ ($FEF_{200-1200}$)

The $FEF_{200-1200}$ is the average flow rate that occurs between 200 and 1200 mL of the FVC (Figure 3–9). The first 200 mL of the FVC is usually exhaled more slowly than the average flow rate because of the inertia involved in the respiratory maneuver and the unreliability of response time of the equipment. Because the

$FEF_{200-1200}$ measures expiratory flows at high lung volumes, it is a good index of the integrity of *large airway function* (above the bronchioles). Flow rates that originate from the large airways are referred to as the effort-dependent portion of the FVC.[1] Thus, the greater the patient effort, the higher the $FEF_{200-1200}$ value. The average $FEF_{200-1200}$ for healthy men ages 20 to 30 years is about 8 L/sec (480 L/min), and for women of the same age, about 5.5 L/sec (330 L/min).

The $FEF_{200-1200}$ decreases with age and in obstructive lung disease. Flow rates as low as 1 L/sec (60 L/min) have been reported in some patients with obstructive lung disease. The $FEF_{200-1200}$ is also decreased in patients with restrictive lung disorders. This is primarily because of the low vital capacity associated with restrictive lung disorders. Conceptually, the $FEF_{200-1200}$ is similar to measuring, and then averaging, the flow rate from a water faucet when 200 and 1200 mL have accumulated in a measuring container (Figure 3–10).

Peak Expiratory Flow Rate (PEFR)

The peak expiratory flow rate (PEFR) (also known as the *peak flow rate*) is the maximum flow rate that can be achieved during an FVC maneuver (Figure 3–11 on page 158). The PEFR is most commonly measured at the bedside using a small, handheld flow-sensing device called a **peak flow meter**. Similar to the $FEF_{200-1200}$ measurement, the PEFR reflects initial flows originating from the large airways during the first part of an FVC maneuver (the effort-dependent portion of the FVC).[2] Thus, the greater the patient effort, the higher the PEFR value.

Figure 3–10

The $FEF_{200-1200}$ is similar to measuring and then averaging the flow rate of water from a faucet at the precise moment when 200 and 1200 mL of water have accumulated in a container **A.** Picture the flow rate from the faucet being measured when 200 mL of water have entered the container **B.** Then picture the flow rate from the faucet being measured when 1200 mL of water have entered container. Taking the average of the two flow rates would be similar to the $FEF_{200-1200}$, which measures and then averages the flow rate at the precise point when 200 and 1200 mL of gas have been exhaled during an FVC maneuver.

© Cengage Learning 2013

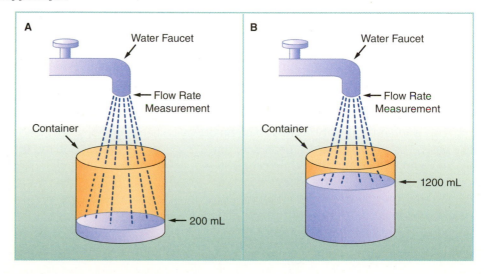

[1,2] See "The Effort-Dependent Portion of a Forced Expiratory Maneuver" later in this chapter.

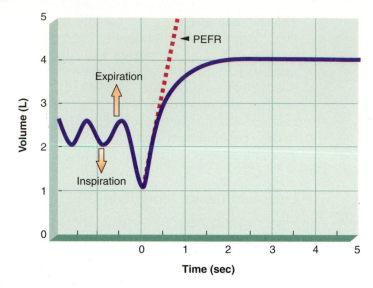

Figure 3–11

Peak expiratory flow rate (PEFR).

Clinical Connection—3-5

Asthma Action Plan—The Green, Yellow, and Red Zones

It is often recommended in children who have asthma that an **asthma action plan** be developed between the parents and the child's doctor. A patient is given a peak flow meter and taught to perform the measurement. Over the course of days and weeks, the patient records his or her personal best peak flow. An asthma action plan is a guide to help monitor the asthma and determine what to do in response to specific symptoms. A common asthma action plan is divided into three zones—green, yellow, and red—similar to the colors on a traffic light. The green zone is 80 percent or better of the personal best peak flow. This is where you want a child to be on a daily basis. The yellow zone is a peak flow that falls between 80 percent and 50 percent of the personal best peak flow. The yellow zone is a warning that the asthma is getting worse and action is needed to prevent an asthmatic attack. The red zone—or less than 50 percent of the patient's personal best peak flow—means the patient is in immediate danger and emergency action must be taken right away! Figure 3–12 provides an overview of the green, yellow, and red asthma action plan.

Note that the peak flow meter used in the asthma action plan is a very important—and very easy to use—diagnostic tool to help monitor a patient with moderate or severe asthma. When patients know their personal best peak flow number,[3] they can actually identify when an asthmatic episode is getting worse—oftentimes, even before they feel any symptoms. The doctor uses the personal best peak flow rate to help determine the patient's green, yellow, and red zones. Although the green, yellow, and red action plan zones are most commonly used with children, the monitoring of peak flow rates can be very beneficial for all asthma patients in all age groups.

---

[3] *Peak flow personal best* means the highest peak flow number that can be achieved over a 2- to 3-week period.

Clinical Connection—3-5, continued

Figure 3-12

Asthma action plan: green, yellow, and red zones.

Source: National Heart, Lung, and Blood Institute, National Institute of Health, U.S. Department of Health and Human Services. NIH Publication No 07-5251, April 2007. For more information, go to: www.nhlbi.nih.gov

Asthma Action Plan

For: _____ Doctor: _____ Date: _____

Doctor's Phone Number _____ Hospital/Emergency Department Phone Number _____

GREEN ZONE

Doing Well

- No cough, wheeze, chest tightness, or shortness of breath during the day or night
- Can do usual activities

And, if a peak flow meter is used,

Peak flow: more than _____
(80 percent or more of my best peak flow)

My best peak flow is: _____

Take these long-term control medicines each day (include an anti-inflammatory).

Medicine	How much to take	When to take it

☐ Before exercise ☐ 2 or ☐ 4 puffs 5 to 60 minutes before exercise

YELLOW ZONE

Asthma Is Getting Worse

- Cough, wheeze, chest tightness, or shortness of breath, or
- Waking at night due to asthma, or
- Can do some, but not all, usual activities

-Or-

Peak flow: _____ to _____
(50 to 79 percent of my best peak flow)

First **Add: quick-relief medicine—and keep taking your GREEN ZONE medicine.**

_____ ☐ 2 or ☐ 4 puffs, every 20 minutes for up to 1 hour
(short-acting beta₂-agonist) ☐ Nebulizer, once

Second **If your symptoms (and peak flow, if used) return to GREEN ZONE after 1 hour of above treatment:**

☐ Continue monitoring to be sure you stay in the green zone.

-Or-

If your symptoms (and peak flow, if used) do not return to GREEN ZONE after 1 hour of above treatment:

☐ Take: _____ ☐ 2 or ☐ 4 puffs or ☐ Nebulizer
(short-acting beta₂-agonist)

☐ Add: _____ _____ mg per day For _____ (3–10) days
(oral steroid)

☐ Call the doctor ☐ before/ ☐ within _____ hours after taking the oral steroid.

RED ZONE

Medical Alert!

- Very short of breath, or
- Quick-relief medicines have not helped, or
- Cannot do usual activities, or
- Symptoms are same or get worse after 24 hours in Yellow Zone

-Or-

Peak flow: less than _____
(50 percent of my best peak flow)

Take this medicine:

☐ _____ ☐ 4 or ☐ 6 puffs or ☐ Nebulizer
(short-acting beta₂-agonist)

☐ _____ _____ mg
(oral steroid)

Then call your doctor NOW. Go to the hospital or call an ambulance if:
- You are still in the red zone after 15 minutes AND
- You have not reached your doctor.

DANGER SIGNS
- Trouble walking and talking due to shortness of breath
- Lips or fingernails are blue

- Take ☐ 4 or ☐ 6 puffs of your quick-relief medicine AND
- Go to the hospital or call for an ambulance _____ NOW!
  (phone)

Figure 3–13

Maximum voluntary ventilation (MVV).

© Cengage Learning 2013

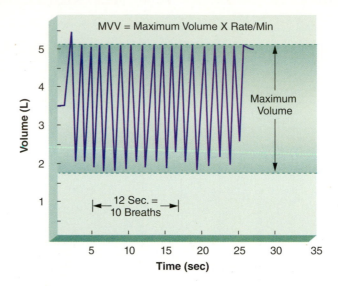

The average PEFR for normal healthy men ages 20 to 30 years is about 10 L/sec (600 L/min), and for women of the same age, about 7.5 L/sec (450 L/min). The PEFR decreases with age and in obstructive lung disease. The PEFR is an inexpensive and effective bedside measurement that is used both in the hospital and home care setting to evaluate gross changes in airway function and to assess the patient's response to bronchodilator therapy.

Maximum Voluntary Ventilation (MVV)

The MVV is the largest volume of gas that can be breathed voluntarily in and out of the lungs in 1 minute (the patient actually performs the test for only 12 seconds—or a minimum of 6 seconds); it is also known as *maximum breathing capacity* (MBC) (Figure 3–13). The MVV is a general test that evaluates the performance of the respiratory muscles' strength, the compliance of the lung and thorax, airway resistance, and neural control mechanisms. The MVV is a broad test and only large reductions are significant. The average MVV for healthy men ages 20 to 30 years is about 170 L/min, and for women of the same age it is about 110 L/min. The MVV decreases with age and chronic obstructive pulmonary disease. The MVV is relatively normal in restrictive pulmonary disease. The MVV decreases with age.

Table 3–2 provides a summary of the normal forced expiratory flow measurements in the healthy male and female 20 years of age.

Flow-Volume Loop

The flow-volume loop is a graphic presentation of a forced vital capacity (FVC) maneuver followed by a forced inspiratory volume (FIV) maneuver. When the FVC and FIV are plotted together, the illustration produced by the two curves is called a **flow-volume loop** (Figure 3–14 on page 164). The flow-volume loop compares both the *flow rates* and *volume changes* produced at different points of an FVC and FIV maneuver. Although the flow-volume loop does not measure the $FEF_{200-1200}$ and $FEF_{25\%-75\%}$, it does show the *maximum flows* ($\dot{V}_{max}$) at

Table 3–2

Overview of Normal Forced Expiratory Flow Rate Measurements in the Healthy Male and Female 20 to 30 Years of Age

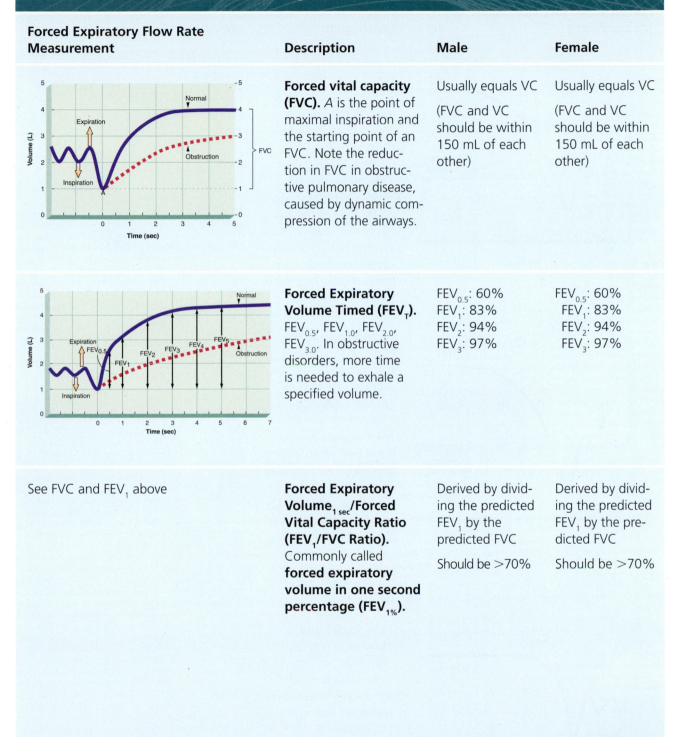

Forced Expiratory Flow Rate Measurement	Description	Male	Female
	Forced vital capacity (FVC). *A* is the point of maximal inspiration and the starting point of an FVC. Note the reduction in FVC in obstructive pulmonary disease, caused by dynamic compression of the airways.	Usually equals VC (FVC and VC should be within 150 mL of each other)	Usually equals VC (FVC and VC should be within 150 mL of each other)
	Forced Expiratory Volume Timed (FEV$_T$). FEV$_{0.5}$, FEV$_{1.0}$, FEV$_{2.0}$, FEV$_{3.0}$. In obstructive disorders, more time is needed to exhale a specified volume.	FEV$_{0.5}$: 60% FEV$_1$: 83% FEV$_2$: 94% FEV$_3$: 97%	FEV$_{0.5}$: 60% FEV$_1$: 83% FEV$_2$: 94% FEV$_3$: 97%
See FVC and FEV$_1$ above	**Forced Expiratory Volume$_{1 sec}$/Forced Vital Capacity Ratio (FEV$_1$/FVC Ratio).** Commonly called **forced expiratory volume in one second percentage (FEV$_{1\%}$).**	Derived by dividing the predicted FEV$_1$ by the predicted FVC Should be >70%	Derived by dividing the predicted FEV$_1$ by the predicted FVC Should be >70%

(continues)

Table 3–2

(Continued)

Forced Expiratory Flow Rate Measurement	Description	Male	Female
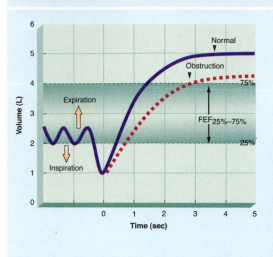	**Forced Expiratory Flow$_{25\%-75\%}$ (FEF$_{25\%-75\%}$).** This test measures the average rate of flow between 25 and 75% of an FVC. The flow rate is measured when 25% of the FVC has been exhaled and again when 75% of the FVC has been exhaled. The average rate of flow is derived by dividing the combined flow rates by 2.	4.5 L/sec (270 L/min)	3.5 L/sec (210 L/min)
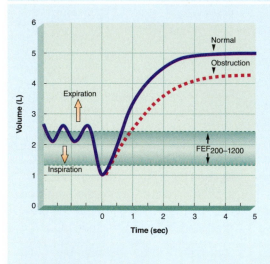	**Forced Expiratory Flow$_{200-1200}$ (FEF$_{200-1200}$).** This test measures the average rate of flow between 200 and 1200 mL of an FVC. The flow rate is measured when 200 mL have been exhaled and again when 1200 mL have been exhaled. The average rate of flow Is derived by dividing the combined flow rates by 2.	8 L/sec (480 L/min)	5.5 L/sec (330 L/min)
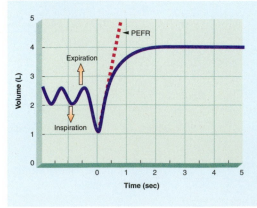	**Peak Expiratory Flow Rate (PEFR).** The maximum flow rate (steepest slope of the volume/time trace) generated during an FVC maneuver.	8–10 L/sec (500–600 L/min)	7.5 L/sec (450 L/min)

Forced Expiratory Flow Rate Measurement	Description	Male	Female
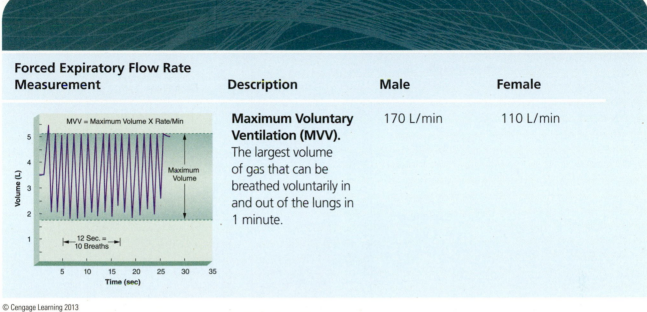	**Maximum Voluntary Ventilation (MVV).** The largest volume of gas that can be breathed voluntarily in and out of the lungs in 1 minute.	170 L/min	110 L/min

© Cengage Learning 2013

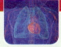

Clinical Connection—3-6

Both an Obstructive and a Restrictive Lung Disorder

In the Clinical Application Section—Case 2 (page 176), the respiratory therapist is called to help care for a 29-year-old with no previous history of pulmonary disease who enters the hospital system complaining of a frequent cough and shortness of breath. The patient reports that his respiratory distress developed shortly after breathing paint fumes while working in a small and confined area. This case illustrates a patient with both an acute obstructive and a restrictive lung disorder. Because of the excessive secretions caused by the paint fumes and subsequent airway infection, the patient's pulmonary mechanic measurements (e.g., FVC, FEV_T,

and PEFR) all were decreased. In addition, because of the mucus plugging and subsequent alveolar collapse, the patient's lung volumes and capacities (e.g., RV, FRC, and VC) all decrease. This case further demonstrates how a variety of pulmonary function measurements are used to evaluate and verify the patient's pulmonary status. Note: This clinical case example is of a patient with an acute obstructive and acute restrictive lung disorder. With appropriate treatment, acute pulmonary problems often resolve without long-term lung injury. Chronic obstructive and chronic restrictive lung conditions will not resolve.

any point of the FVC. The most commonly reported maximum flows are $FEF_{25\%}$, $FEF_{50\%}$, and $FEF_{75\%}$. In healthy individuals, the $FEF_{50\%}$ (also called the $\dot{V}_{max_{50}}$) is a straight line because the expiratory flow decreases linearly with volume throughout most of the FVC range. In subjects with obstructive lung disease, however, the flow rate decreases at low lung volumes, causing the $FEF_{50\%}$ to decrease. This causes a cuplike or scooped out effect on the flow-volume loop.

To summarize, depending on the sophistication of the equipment, several important measurements can be obtained from the flow-volume loop, including the following:

- PEFR
- PIFR
- FVC
- FEV_T

- FEV_1/FVC ratio ($FEV_{1\%}$)
- $FEF_{25\%}$
- $FEF_{50\%}$ ($\dot{V}_{max_{50}}$)
- $FEF_{75\%}$

© Cengage Learning 2013

Figure 3–14

Normal flow-volume loop. PEFR = peak expiration flow rate; PIFR = peak inspiratory flow rate; FVC = forced vital capacity; FEF$_{25\%-75\%}$ = forced expiratory flow$_{25\%-75\%}$; FEF$_{50\%}$ = forced expiratory flow$_{50\%}$ (also called $\dot{V}_{max_{50}}$).

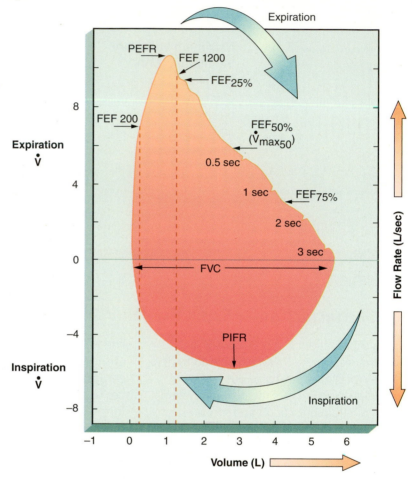

Flow-volume loop measurements graphically illustrate both obstructive (Figure 3–15) and restrictive lung problems (Figure 3–16 on page 166). Table 3–3 on page 166 summarizes the average dynamic flow rate values found in healthy men and women ages 20 to 30 years.

Factors Affecting Predicted Normal Values

A number of factors affect the normal predicted lung volumes and capacities, including height, weight, age, gender, and race. Among individuals of the same gender, **height** is the most important factor that affects pulmonary function. Taller subjects have greater pulmonary function values—especially in terms of lung volumes, lung capacities, and diffusion capacity values. An individual's height is not as significant in expiratory flow rate measurements (e.g., FVC, FEV$_1$, or PEFR). In children, normal pulmonary function values are more directly related to height than age, up until the child is about 60 inches (152 cm) tall. After a child reaches this height, the age of the patient begins to be a factor in predicting normal values.

A patient's **weight** is sometimes taken into account along with height. The effect of weight on a patient's lung volumes can be seen when comparing

Figure 3–15

Flow-volume loop, obstructive pattern. FVC = forced vital capacity.

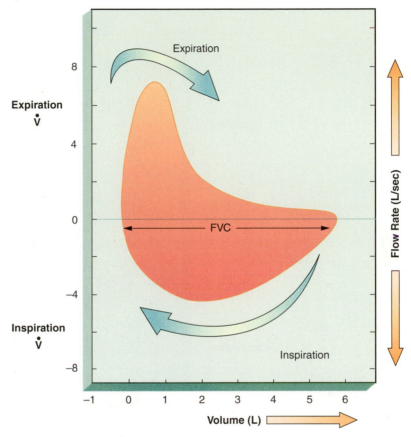

adult subjects of the same height—especially in the obese patient. In general, as weight increases beyond a patient's normal, lung volumes decrease. A patient's **age** can affect a patient's normal lung volumes and capacity values. After the age of 25, lung volumes, expiratory flow rates, and diffusing capacity values tend to decrease.

The **gender** of the patient affects the predicted normal pulmonary function values. Male subjects typically generate greater predicted lung volumes, expiratory flow rates, and diffusing capacities than female subjects of the same age and height. Finally, a patient's race or ethnic origin has been shown to have some effect on normal predicted values. Black, Hispanic, and Asian patients typically have smaller predicted pulmonary function values than subjects of European-descent origin.

How the Effects of Dynamic Compression Decrease Expiratory Flow Rates

The Effort-Dependent Portion of a Forced Expiratory Maneuver

During approximately the first 30 percent of an FVC maneuver, the maximum peak flow rate is dependent on the amount of muscular effort exerted by the individual. This portion of the FVC maneuver originates from the large airways and is referred to as **effort dependent**. As discussed earlier, the $FEF_{200-1200}$ and PEFR measurements reflect flow rates from the large airways. Thus, the greater the patient effort, the higher the $FEF_{200-1200}$ and PEFR values.

Figure 3–16

Flow-volume loop, restrictive pattern. FVC = forced vital capacity.

© Cengage Learning 2013

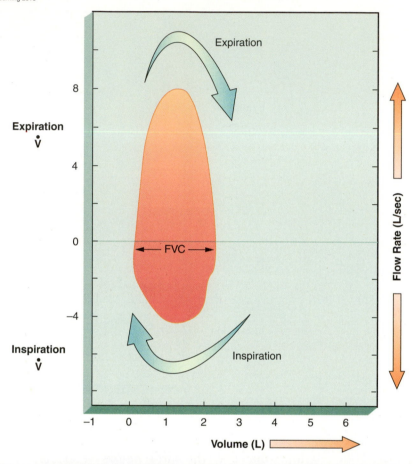

Table 3–3

Average Dynamic Flow Rate Measurements in Healthy Men and Women 20 to 30 Years of Age

Measurement*	Men	Women
FEV_T		
$FEV_{0.5}$	60%	60%
$FEV_{1.0}$	83%	83%
$FEV_{2.0}$	94%	94%
$FEV_{3.0}$	97%	97%
$FEF_{200-1200}$	8 L/sec (480 L/min)	5.5 L/sec (330 L/min)
$FEF_{25\%-75\%}$	4.5 L/sec (270 L/min)	3.5 L/sec (210 L/min)
PEFR	10 L/sec (600 L/min)	7.5 L/sec (450 L/min)
MVV	170 L/min	110 L/min

© Cengage Learning 2013

* See text for explanation of abbreviations.

Figure 3–17

The effort-dependent and effort-independent portions of a forced expiratory maneuver in a flow-volume loop measurement. FVC = forced vital capacity.

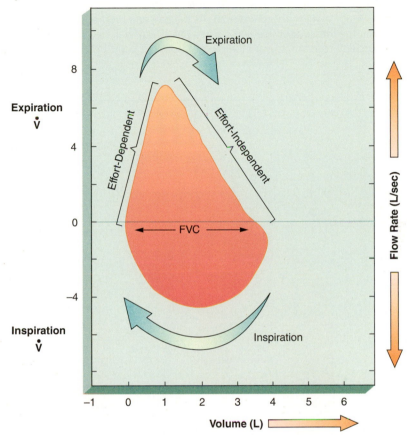

The Effort-Independent Portion of a Forced Expiratory Maneuver

The flow rate during approximately the last 70 percent of an FVC maneuver is **effort independent**. That is, once a maximum flow rate has been attained, the flow rate cannot be increased by further muscular effort.

The lung volume at which the patient initiates a forced expiratory maneuver also influences the maximum flow rate. As lung volumes decline, flow also declines. The reduced flow, however, is the maximum flow for that particular volume.

Figure 3–17 illustrates where the effort-dependent and effort-independent portions of a forced expiratory maneuver appear on a flow-volume loop.

Dynamic Compression of the Bronchial Airways

The limitation of the flow rate that occurs during the last 70 percent of an FVC maneuver is due to the **dynamic compression** of the walls of the airways. As gas flows through the airways from the alveoli to the atmosphere during passive expiration, the pressure within the airways diminishes to zero (Figure 3–18A).

During a forced expiratory maneuver, however, as the airway pressure decreases from the alveoli to the atmosphere, there is a point at which the pressure within the lumen of the airways equals the pleural pressure surrounding the airways. This point is called the **equal pressure point**.

Figure 3–18

The dynamic compression mechanism. **A.** During passive expiration, static elastic recoil pressure of the lungs (P_{stL}) is 10, pleural pressure (P_{pl}) at the beginning of expiration is −5, and alveolar pressure (P_{alv}) is +5. In order for gas to move from the alveolus to the atmosphere during expiration, the pressure must decrease progressively in the airways from +5 to 0. As A shows, P_{pl} is always less than the airway pressure. **B.** During forced expiration, P_{pl} becomes positive (+10 in this illustration). When this P_{pl} is added to the P_{stL} of +10, P_{alv} becomes +20. As the pressure progressively decreases during forced expiration, there must be a point at which the pressures inside and outside the airway wall are equal. This point is the equal pressure point. Airway compression occurs downstream (toward the mouth) from this point because the lateral pressure is less than the surrounding wall pressure.

© Cengage Learning 2013

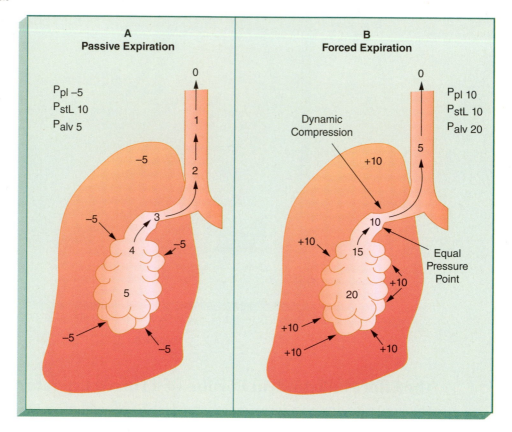

Downstream (i.e., toward the mouth) from the equal pressure point, the lateral pressure within the airway becomes less than the surrounding pleural pressure. Consequently, the airways are compressed. As muscular effort and pleural pressure increase during a forced expiratory maneuver, the equal pressure point moves upstream (i.e., toward the alveolus). Ultimately, the equal pressure point becomes fixed where the individual's flow rate has achieved maximum (Figure 3–18B). In essence, once dynamic compression occurs during a forced expiratory maneuver, increased muscular effort merely augments airway compression, which, in turn, increases airway resistance.

As the structural changes associated with certain respiratory diseases (e.g., COPD) intensify, the patient commonly responds by increasing intrapleural pressure during expiration to overcome the increased airway resistance produced by the disease. By increasing intrapleural pressure during expiration, however, the patient activates the dynamic compression mechanism, which in turn further reduces the diameter of the bronchial airways. This results in an even greater increase in airway resistance.

Clinical Connection—3-7

Spirometry Confirmation of Dynamic Compression

In the Clinical Application Section—Case 1 (see page 174), the respiratory therapist is called to help care for a 16-year-old girl with a long history of asthma who became short of breath while playing volleyball during her high school gym class. The case demonstrates how the measurement of a patient's pulmonary mechanics can serve as an important clinical monitor (e.g., FVC, FEV$_1$, and PEFR) and the effects of the effort-independent portion of an FVC, dynamic compression, and the equal pressure point. This case further shows that even when the patient makes a strong muscular effort on a FVC test, the closure of her airways—caused by equal pressure point changes and dynamic compression—moves closer to her alveoli. This action, in turn, further increases airway resistance and offsets any improvement in the FVC.

Clinical Connection—3-8

Pursed-Lip Breathing

Pursed-lip breathing is commonly seen in patients suffering from chronic obstructive pulmonary disease (COPD). It is a relatively simple—but effective—technique that many patients learn without formal training. Pursed-lip breathing is characterized by a deep inhalation followed by prolonged expiration through pursed lips—similar to that used for whistling, kissing, or blowing through a flute. Pursed-lip breathing increases the airway pressure during exhalation and, thereby, works to offset the adverse effects of dynamic compression—which, in turn, causes early airway collapse, air trapping, and alveolar overinflation. Pursed-lip breathing creates a natural **continuous positive airway pressure (CPAP)** to hold the airways open from the inside. In addition, pursed-lip breathing has been shown to decrease the patient's breathing rate and yield a ventilatory pattern that is more effective in alveolar gas mixing (Figure 3–19).

Figure 3–19

A. Schematic illustration of alveoli compression of weakened bronchiole airways during normal expiration in patients with COPD. **B.** The effects of pursed-lip breathing in patients with COPD. The weakened bronchiole airways are kept open by the effects of positive pressure created by pursed lips during expiration.

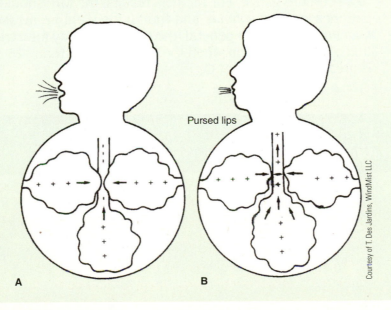

Pursed lips

A   B

Courtesy of T. Des Jardins, WindMist LLC

Flow normally is not limited to effort during inspiration. This is because the airways widen as greater inspiratory efforts are generated, thus enhancing gas flow (refer to Figure 2-29).

Diffusion Capacity of Carbon Monoxide ($D_{L_{CO}}$)

The $D_{L_{CO}}$ study measures the amount of carbon monoxide (CO) that moves across the alveolar-capillary membrane. CO has an affinity for hemoglobin that is about 210 times greater than that of oxygen. Thus, in individuals who have normal amounts of hemoglobin and normal ventilatory function, the only limiting factor to the diffusion of CO is the thickness of the alveolar-capillary membrane. In essence, the $D_{L_{CO}}$ study measures the physiologic status of the various anatomic structures that compose the alveolar-capillary membrane.

The CO single-breath technique is commonly used for this measurement. Under normal conditions, the average $D_{L_{CO}}$ value for the resting male is 25 mL/min/mm Hg (standard temperature and pressure, dry [STPD]). This value is slightly lower in females, presumably because of their smaller normal lung volumes. The $D_{L_{CO}}$ may increase threefold in healthy subjects during exercise. The $D_{L_{CO}}$ generally decreases in response to lung disorders that affect the alveolar-capillary membrane. For example, the $D_{L_{CO}}$ is decreased in emphysema because of the alveolar-capillary destruction associated with this lung disease. Other respiratory disorders that decrease a patient's $D_{L_{CO}}$ include chronic interstitial lung disease, pneumonia (alveolar consolidation), pulmonary edema, and acute respiratory distress syndrome.

Maximum Inspiratory and Expiratory Pressure

An individual's **maximum inspiratory pressure** (MIP) and **maximum expiratory pressure** (MEP) are directly related to muscle strength. Table 3–4 shows the average MIP and MEP for the normal, healthy adult. Clinically, the MIP and MEP are used to evaluate the patient's ability to maintain spontaneous, unassisted ventilation. Both the MIP and MEP are commonly measured while the patient inhales and exhales through an endotracheal tube that is attached to a pressure gauge. For the best results, the MIP should be measured at the patient's *residual volume,* and the MEP should be measured at the patient's *total lung capacity.* In general, the patient is ready for a trial of spontaneous or unassisted ventilation when the MIP is greater than –25 cm H_2O and the MEP is greater than 50 cm H_2O.

Table 3–4		
Maximum Inspiratory and Expiratory Pressures		
	MIP	**MEP**
Male	−125 cm H_2O	230 cm H_2O
Female	−90 cm H_2O	150 cm H_2O

Rapid Shallow Breathing Index (RSBI) Ratio

The rapid shallow breathing index (RSBI) ratio is commonly used to help determine if a mechanically ventilated patient can be successfully weaned of the ventilator. The RSBI is the ratio of the patient's spontaneous breathing rate (breaths/min) to the tidal volume (liters)—also referred to as the frequency to tidal volume (f/V_T) ratio. The RSBI is considered an excellent clinical predictor of weaning success in mechanically ventilated patients. The RSBI is an easy test to perform and, importantly, is independent of the patient's effort and cooperation.

The RSBI measurement is taken 1 minute after disconnecting the spontaneously breathing patient form the ventilator. The discontinuation of ventilator support is likely to be successful when the RSBI is below 105 (normal range, 60 to 105). An RSBI value greater than 105 indicates that the patient will likely fail a weaning trial. For example, if a patient, who is being considered for weaning from mechanical ventilation, demonstrates a spontaneous ventilatory rate of 28 breaths/minute and an average tidal volume of 0.35 liter, the patient's RSBI would easily be calculated as follows:

$$RSBI = 28 \text{ bpm} \div 0.35 \text{ L} = 80$$

Because the patient is clearly below the threshold criteria of 105, and assuming all other weaning criteria are acceptable (e.g., acid-base status, oxygenation status, lung compliance, airway resistance, V_D/V_T, and maximum inspiratory pressure), the patient will likely be successfully weaned off the ventilator.

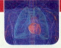

Clinical Connection—3-9

Ventilator Mechanics Used to Predict Mechanical Ventilation Weaning Success

The respiratory therapist uses a number of the pulmonary function measurements to evaluate the patient's readiness to be successfully weaned off a mechanical ventilator. Common bedside pulmonary function measurements used, and the desired criteria are shown in the table below.

Additional pulmonary measurements used to help determine the possible success of weaning a patient off of a mechanical ventilator include (1) acid–base evaluations, (2) oxygenation assessments, and (3) work of breathing measurements (e.g., dynamic and static compliance).

Common Pulmonary Function Measurements Used to Determine Readiness for Weaning and Ventilator Discontinuation

Measurement	Criteria
Spontaneous breathing trial	Tolerates 12–30 min
Respiratory rate (f)	<30 breaths/min
Tidal volume (V_T)	>5–8 mL/kg
Vital capacity (VC)	>10–15 mL/kg
Minute ventilation (V_E)	<10–15 L/min
Maximum inspiratory pressure (MIP)	>−20 to −30 cm H_2O in 20 sec
Dead space to tidal volume ratio (VD/V_T)	<0.6
Static lung compliance (C_L)	>25 mL/cm H_2O
Rapid shallow breathing index (RSBI) ratio or (f/V_T)	<100 (spontaneous breathing pattern)

Clinical Connection—3-10

Certified Pulmonary Function Technologist and Registered Pulmonary Function Technologist

The respiratory care practitioner can further broaden his or her career by pursuing additional education and training as a Certified Pulmonary Function Technologist (CPFT) or a Registered Pulmonary Function Technologist (RPFT). The **National Board for Respiratory Care Inc. (NBRC)** administers the CPFT and RPFT credentialing examinations (www.nbrc.org). Applicants must be 18 years of age or older and satisfy one of the following criteria:

- Have a minimum of an associate degree from a respiratory therapy educational program supported or accredited by the Commission on Accreditation for Respiratory Care (CoARC), or accredited by the Commission on Accreditation of Allied Health Education Programs (CAAHEP).

- Be a Certified Respiratory Therapist (CRT) credentialed by the NBRC.

- Be a Registered Respiratory Therapist (RRT) credentialed by the NBRC.

- Complete 62 semester hours of college credit from a college or university accredited by its regional association or its equivalent, including college credit level courses in biology, chemistry, and mathematics. A minimum of 6 months of clinical experience[4] in the field of pulmonary function technology under the direction of a Medical Director of a pulmonary function laboratory or a special care area is also required prior to applying for the examination.

- Be a high school graduate (or the equivalent) and complete two years of clinical experience in the field of pulmonary function technology under the direction of a Medical Director or a pulmonary function laboratory or a special care area prior to applying for the examination.

---

[4] Clinical experience is defined as a minimum of eight hours per week for a calendar year in pulmonary technology under the supervision of a medical director of a pulmonary function laboratory or a special care area acceptable to the Board. Clinical experience must be completed before the candidate applies for this examination.

Chapter Summary

The total amount of air that the lungs can accommodate is divided into four separate volumes and four capacities. The lung volumes are the tidal volume (V_T), inspiratory reserve volume (IRV), expiratory reserve volume (ERV), and residual volume (RV). The capacities consist of the vital capacity (VC), inspiratory capacity (IC), functional residual capacity (FRC), and total lung capacity (TLC).

In obstructive lung disorders, the RV, V_T, FRC, and TLC are increased; the VC, IC, IRV, and ERV are decreased. In restrictive lung disorders, the VC, IC, RV, FRC, V_T, and TLC are all decreased. Obstructive lung disorders include chronic bronchitis, emphysema, asthma, cystic fibrosis, and bronchiectasis. Restrictive lung disorders include pneumonia, pulmonary edema, flail chest, pneumothorax, pleural effusion, chronic interstitial lung disease, lung cancer, acute respiratory distress syndrome, and postoperative alveolar collapse.

Because the RV cannot be exhaled, the RV, and lung capacities that contain the RV, is measured indirectly by the closed-circuit helium dilution method, the open-circuit nitrogen washout method, or body plethymosgraphy.

In addition to measuring volumes and capacities, the rate at which gas flows into and out of the lungs can be measured. Collectively, the tests used to measure expiratory flow rates are referred to as pulmonary mechanic measurements. These tests include the forced vital capacity (FVC), forced expiratory volume time (FEV_T), forced expiratory volume 1 sec/forced vital capacity ratio (FEV_1/FVC)—commonly written as $FEV_{1\%}$—forced expiratory flow 25%–75% ($FEF_{25\%-75\%}$), forced expiratory flow$_{200-1200}$ ($FEF_{200-1200}$), peak expiratory flow rate (PEFR), and the maximum voluntary ventilation (MVV).

The flow-volume loop is a graphic presentation of an FVC followed by a forced inspiratory volume (FIV) maneuver. The flow-volume loop compares both the flow rates and volume changes produced at different points of the FVC and FIV maneuver. A number of measurements can be obtained from the flow-volume loop, including the PEFR, PIFR, FVC, FEV_T, FEV_1/FVC ratio, $FEF_{25\%}$, $FEF_{50\%}$ ($\dot{V}_{max50}$), and $FEF_{75\%}$. The FVC, FEV_1, and the FEV_1/FVC ratio are the most commonly used pulmonary function measurements to (1) evaluate the severity of COPD, (2) help develop a treatment plan, and (3) differentiate between an obstructive and restrictive lung disorder.

To fully understand the pulmonary mechanic measurements, the respiratory therapist must have a basic knowledge of how the effects of dynamic compression decrease expiratory flow rates, including the influences of (1) the effort-dependent portion of a forced expiratory maneuver, (2) the effort-independent portion of a forced expiratory maneuver, and (3) the dynamic compression of the bronchial airways. A clinical connection associated with offsetting the adverse affects of dynamic airway compression is pursed-lip breathing.

Finally, the diffusion capacity of carbon monoxide ($D_{L_{CO}}$) is routinely used to evaluate the physiologic status of the various anatomic structures of the alveolar-capillary membrane. The maximum inspiratory pressure (MIP) and maximum expiratory pressure (MEP) are used to directly measure muscle strength to help in predicting mechanical ventilator weaning success. The rapid shallow breathing index ratio (RSBI) is an excellent tool to help in assessing a patient's readiness to be successfully weaned off a ventilator.

Clinical connections associated with the preceding topics include (1) obstructive lung disorders; (2) restrictive lung disorders; (3) the FEV_1/FVC ratio and the FEV_1 in the assessment and management of chronic obstructive pulmonary disease (COPD); (4) differentiating between obstructive and restrictive lung disorders; (5) the asthma action plan—the green, yellow, and red zone; (6) both an obstructive and restrictive lung disorder; (7) spirometry confirmation of dynamic compression; (8) pursed-lip breathing; (9) ventilator mechanics used to predict mechanical ventilation weaning success; and (10) broadening one's career by pursuing a certified pulmonary function technologist or registered pulmonary function technologist credential.

Clinical Application Case

A 16-year-old girl with a long history of asthma became short of breath while playing volleyball during her high school gym class. The head coach took her out of the game and had an assistant coach watch her closely. Even though the patient inhaled a total of four puffs of the bronchodilator albuterol from a metered-dose inhaler over the next 30 minutes, her condition progressively worsened. Concerned, the coach called the patient's mother. Because the patient had had to be given mechanical ventilation on two different occasions, the patient's mother asked the coach to take her daughter directly to the emergency department of the local hospital.

In the emergency department, the patient was observed to be in severe respiratory distress. Her skin was blue and she was using her accessory muscles of inspiration. The patient stated, "My asthma is really getting bad." Her vital signs were blood pressure—180/110 mm Hg, heart rate—130 beats/min, respiratory rate—36 breaths/min, and oral temperature 37°C. While on 4 L/min oxygen via nasal cannula, her hemoglobin oxygen saturation measured by pulse oximetry over the skin of her index finger, was 83 percent.

A portable chest X-ray showed that her lungs were hyperinflated and that her diaphragm was depressed (Figure 3–20). Measurement of the patient's forced vital capacity provided the data shown in the table on top of next page.

Figure 3–20

X-ray showing presence of asthma.

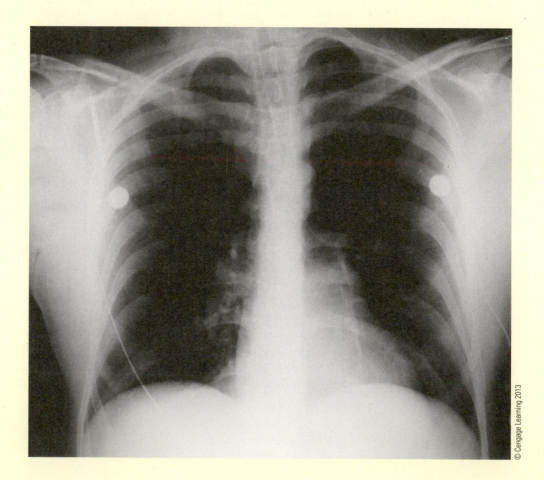

Bedside Spirometry		
Parameter*	Predicted	Actual
FVC	2800 mL	1220 mL
FEV$_1$	>83%	44%
PEFR	400 L/min	160 L/min

*FVC = forced vital capacity; FEV$_1$ = forced expiratory volume in 1 second (see text); PEFR = peak expiratory flow rate.

Because the respiratory therapist felt that the patient did not produce a good effort on her first FVC test, a second test was done. Even though the patient appeared to exhale much more forcefully during the second FVC test, the spirometry results were identical to the previous ones. The patient's mother stated that her daughter's "personal best" peak expiratory flow rate (PEFR) at home was 360 L/min. While the patient was in the emergency department, the nurse started an intravenous infusion. The respiratory therapist increased the patient's oxygen via nasal cannula to 6 L/min. The patient was then given a continuous bronchodilator therapy via a handheld nebulizer per the respiratory care protocol. The medical director of the respiratory care department was notified, and a mechanical ventilator was placed on standby.

One hour later, the patient stated that she was breathing easier. Her skin appeared pink, and she was no longer using her accessory muscles of inspiration. Her vital signs were blood pressure—122/76 mm Hg, heart rate—82 beats/min, and respiratory rate—14 breaths/min. On 2 L/min oxygen via nasal cannula, her Sp$_{O_2}$ was 97 percent. Her bedside spirometry results at this time were as follows:

Bedside Spirometry		
Parameter*	Predicted	Actual
FVC	2800 mL	2375 mL
FEV$_1$	>83%	84%
PEFR	400 L/min	345 L/min

*FVC = forced vital capacity; FEV$_1$ = forced expiratory volume in 1 second; PEFR = peak expiratory flow rate.

The patient continued to improve, and her oxygen therapy, bronchodilator therapy, and IV were all discontinued the next morning. Her bedside spirometry results were FVC, 2810 mL; FEV$_1$, 87 percent; and PEFR, 355 L/min. She was discharged on the afternoon of the second day. During her exit interview, she was instructed to use her metered-dose inhaler about 15 minutes before each gym class.

Discussion

This case illustrates how the measurement of a patient's pulmonary mechanics can serve as an important clinical monitor and the effects and interrelationships of the following on the bronchial airways during a forced expiratory maneuver: the *effort-independent* portion of a forced expiratory maneuver, *dynamic compression,* and the *equal pressure point.*

When the patient was in the emergency department, the fact that her mother knew her daughter's "personal best" PEFR served as an important clinical indicator of the severity of the patient's asthma attack. Today, asthma patients commonly monitor their own PEFR at home to evaluate the severity of an asthmatic episode. Some physicians instruct their patients to call them or to go directly to the hospital when their PEFR decreases to a specific level.

The fact that the respiratory therapist obtained the same bedside spirometry results on the second test demonstrated the effects of *effort-independent flow rate, dynamic compression,* and the *equal pressure point* on the bronchial airways during an FVC maneuver. Remember, approximately the last 70 percent of an FVC maneuver is effort independent because of the dynamic compression of the bronchial airways. When the patient made a stronger muscular effort on the second FVC test, she only moved the equal pressure point (and dynamic compression) of her airways closer to the alveoli—which, in turn, further increased airway resistance and offset any increase in her FVC (see Figure 3–16).

2 Clinical Application Case

A 29-year-old man with no previous history of pulmonary disease presented at his family physician's office complaining of a frequent cough and shortness of breath. He stated that his cough had started about 2 weeks prior to this visit as a result of breathing paint fumes while working in a small and confined area. Even though the patient stated that he had stopped painting in the enclosed area immediately, his cough and his ability to breathe progressively worsened. At the time of this office visit, he had been too ill to work for 2 days. The physician admitted the patient to the hospital and requested a pulmonary consultation.

In the hospital, the patient appeared healthy but in severe respiratory distress. His skin was blue, and his hospital gown was damp from perspiration. He had a frequent and weak cough. During each coughing episode, he produced a moderate amount of thick, white and yellow sputum. His vital signs were blood pressure—155/96 mm Hg, heart rate—90 beats/min, respiratory rate—26 breaths/min, and oral temperature of 37°C. Dull percussion notes were elicited over the lower lobe of the patient's left lung. Rhonchi were heard over both lungs during exhalation, and loud bronchial rales were heard over the left lower lobe.

On administration of 4 L/min oxygen via nasal cannula, the patient's arterial oxygen pressure was Pa_{O_2} 63 mm Hg (normal, 80–100 mm Hg). A chest X-ray showed several areas of alveolar collapse (*atelectasis*) throughout the left lower lobe. A pulmonary function study revealed the following results:

Pulmonary Function Study No. 1		
Parameter*	**Predicted**	**Actual**
FVC	4600 mL	2990 mL
FEV_1	>83%	67%
$FEF_{200-1200}$	470 L/min	306 L/min
PEFR	>400 L/min	345 L/min
VC	4600 mL	2900 mL
RV	1175 mL	764 mL
FRC	2350 mL	1528 mL

*FVC = forced vital capacity; FEV_1 = forced expiratory volume in first second of an FVC maneuver; $FEF_{200-1200}$ = forced expiratory flow$_{200-1200}$; see text; PEFR = peak expiratory flow rate; VC = vital capacity; RV = residual volume; FRC = functional residual capacity.

In the patient's chart, the physician noted that the excessive bronchial secretions were a result of an acute tracheobronchial tree inflammation (acute bronchitis) caused by the inhalation of noxious paint fumes. The physician also noted that the patches of atelectasis (see Figure 3–10) identified in the patient's left lower lung lobe were most likely caused by excessive airway secretions and mucous plugging.

The respiratory therapist working with the patient obtained a sputum sample and sent it to the laboratory for culture. To help mobilize and clear the excessive bronchial secretions and to offset the mucous plugging, the patient was started on aggressive bronchial hygiene therapy, which consisted of coughing and deep breathing, chest physical therapy, and postural drainage. To treat the atelectasis in the left lower lobe, the patient received lung expansion therapy (hyperinflation therapy), which consisted of incentive spirometry, coughing and deep breathing, and continuous positive airway pressure (CPAP) via a face mask.

Three days later, the patient's general appearance had improved significantly, and he no longer appeared to be in respiratory distress. His skin was pink. He no longer had a cough. When the patient was asked to cough, the cough was strong and nonproductive. At this time, he was receiving antibiotic therapy for a streptococcal infection that had been identified from a sputum culture. His vital signs were blood pressure—116/66 mm Hg, heart rate—64 beats/min, respiratory rate—12 breaths/min, and oral temperature of 37°C. Normal percussion notes were elicited over both lungs. Normal bronchial vesicular breath sounds were heard over both lungs.

On room air, the patient's Pa_{O_2} was 96 mm Hg. A chest X-ray showed no problems. A second pulmonary function study revealed the results shown in the following table. The patient was discharged the next day.

Pulmonary Function Study No. 2		
Parameter*	**Predicted**	**Actual**
FVC	4600 mL	4585 mL
FEV_1	>83%	83%
$FEF_{200-1200}$	470 L/min	458 L/min
PEFR	>400 L/min	455 L/min
VC	4600 mL	4585 mL
RV	1175 mL	1165 mL
FRC	2350 mL	2329 mL

*FVC = forced vital capacity; FEV_1 = forced expiratory volume in first second of an FVC maneuver; $FEF_{200-1200}$ = forced expiratory flow$_{200-1200}$; see text; PEFR = peak expiratory flow rate; VC = vital capacity; RV = residual volume; FRC = functional residual capacity.

Discussion

This case illustrates both an obstructive and restrictive lung disorder. Because of the excessive bronchial secretions produced by the inhalation of paint fumes and the subsequent streptococcal infection, the patient's FVC, FEV_1, $FEF_{200-1200}$, and PEFR were all decreased at the time of admission.

In addition, the excessive bronchial secretions (and the patient's weak cough effort) caused mucous pooling, and mucous plugging, of the bronchial airways in the left lower lobe. As a result of the mucous plugging, the alveoli distal to the bronchial obstructions could not be ventilated and eventually collapsed. This condition was verified by the chest X-ray and by the decreased VC, RV, and FRC.

Fortunately, his respiratory problems were reversible with aggressive bronchial hygiene therapy and lung expansion therapy. Once the bronchial secretions were cleared, the obstructive problem was no longer present. This was verified by the increased values shown of the FVC, FEV_1, $FEF_{200-1200}$, and PEFR. When the mucous plugs were cleared and the lungs were re-expanded, the restrictive problem was no longer present. This was verified by the increased values of the VC, FRC, and RV.

Review Questions

1. The volume of air that can be exhaled after a normal tidal volume exhalation is the
   A. IRV
   B. FRC
   C. FVC
   D. ERV

2. In an obstructive lung disorder, the
   1. FRC is decreased
   2. RV is increased
   3. VC is decreased
   4. IRV is increased
      A. 1 and 3 only
      B. 2 and 3 only
      C. 2 and 4 only
      D. 2, 3, and 4 only

3. The PEFR in normal healthy men ages 20 to 30 years may exceed
   A. 300 L/min
   B. 400 L/min
   C. 500 L/min
   D. 600 L/min

4. Which of the following can be obtained from a flow-volume loop study?
   1. FVC
   2. PEFR
   3. FEV_T
   4. $FEF_{25\%-75\%}$
      A. 1 and 2 only
      B. 2 and 3 only
      C. 1, 3, and 4 only
      D. 1, 2, 3, and 4

5. The MVV in normal healthy men ages 20 to 30 years is
   A. 60 L/min
   B. 100 L/min
   C. 170 L/min
   D. 240 L/min

6. Approximately how much of a forced expiratory maneuver is effort dependent?
   A. 20%
   B. 30%
   C. 40%
   D. 50%

7. Which of the following forced expiratory measurements reflects the status of medium-sized to small-sized airways?
   A. $FEF_{200-1200}$
   B. PEFR
   C. MVV
   D. $FEF_{25\%-75\%}$

8. Normally, the percentage of the total volume exhaled during an FEV_1 by a 20-year-old individual is
   A. 60%
   B. 83%
   C. 94%
   D. 97%

9. Which of the following forced expiratory measurements is a good index of the integrity of large airway function?
   A. FEV_T
   B. $FEF_{200-1200}$
   C. $FEF_{25\%-75\%}$
   D. MVV

10. The residual volume/total lung capacity ratio in healthy men ages 20 to 30 years is
    A. 15%   C. 25%
    B. 20%   D. 30%

11. A 73-year-old man with a long history of smoking demonstrates the following clinical data on a pulmonary function test (PFT):

Pulmonary Function Test			
PFT	**Below Normal**	**Normal**	**Above Normal**
VC	X		
RV			X
FRC			X
ERV	X		
FEV_T	X		
$FEV_{1\%}$	X		
$FEF_{25\%-75\%}$	X		
PEFR	X		
MVV	X		

Based on the information shown, the patient appears to have
- A. An obstructive lung disorder
- B. A restrictive lung disorder
- C. Both obstructive and restrictive lung disorders
- D. Neither an obstructive or restrictive lung disorder

Clinical Application Questions

Case 1

1. When the patient was in the emergency department, what pulmonary function measurement served as an important clinical indicator of the severity of the patient's asthma attack?

2. The fact that the respiratory therapist obtained the same bedside spirometry results on the second test demonstrated the presence of what three physiologic effects?

3. When the patient made a stronger muscular effort on the second FVC test, she only moved the equal pressure point of her airways

Case 2

1. This patient demonstrated both obstructive and restrictive lung disorders. During the first part of the case, which pulmonary function studies verified that the patient had an obstructive pulmonary disorder?

2. Which pulmonary function studies verified that the patient had a restrictive pulmonary disorder?

3. After aggressive bronchial hygiene therapy and lung expansion therapy, the patient's FEV_1 (increased _____; decreased _____; remained the same _____), and the RV (increased _____; decreased _____; remained the same _____).

Chapter 4

The Diffusion of Pulmonary Gases

Objectives

By the end of this chapter, the student should be able to:

1. Describe Dalton's law—the law of partial pressures
2. Explain how Dalton's law relates to the partial pressure of atmospheric gases
3. Identify the percentage and partial pressure of the gases that compose the barometric pressure:
   —Nitrogen
   —Oxygen
   —Argon
   —Carbon dioxide
4. Differentiate between pressure gradients and diffusion gradients
5. Identify the partial pressure of the gases in the air, alveoli, and blood:
   —Oxygen (P_{O_2})
   —Carbon dioxide (P_{CO_2})
   —Water (P_{H_2O})
   —Nitrogen (P_{N_2})
6. Calculate the *ideal alveolar gas equation*.
7. Name the nine major structures of the *alveolar-capillary membrane* through which a gas molecule must diffuse.
8. Describe how oxygen and carbon dioxide normally diffuse across the alveolar-capillary membrane.
9. Describe the clinical connection associated with pulmonary disorders that increase the alveolar-capillary thickness.
10. Explain how *Fick's law* relates to gas diffusion.

11. Describe how the following relate to the *diffusion constants* in Fick's law:
    —Henry's law
    —Graham's law
12. Describe the clinical connection associated with hyperbaric oxygen therapy and the clinical application of Henry's law.
13. Describe the clinical connection associated with oxygen toxicity.
14. Describe the clinical connection associated with Fick's law, including Case 1 and Case 2 at the end of the chapter.
15. Describe the clinical connection associated with respiratory disorders that decrease the alveolar surface area.
16. Define *perfusion limited,* and explain how it relates to a gas such as nitrous oxide.
17. Define *diffusion limited,* and explain how it relates to a gas such as carbon monoxide.
18. Describe how oxygen can be classified as perfusion or diffusion limited.
19. Describe the clinical connection associated with why a decreased $D_{L_{CO}}$ is a classic diagnostic sign of emphysema.
20. Complete the review questions at the end of this chapter.

Introduction

As described in Chapter 2, the flow of air between the atmosphere and the alveoli occurs as a result of pressure gradients created by the diaphragm during inspiration and expiration. This mechanism of ventilation moves oxygenated air from the atmosphere to the alveoli during inspiration and carbon dioxide from the alveoli to the external environment during expiration.

Gas A	Gas B	Gas A + B
Pressure = 10	Pressure = 5	Pressure = 15

The mechanics of ventilation, however, only moves bulk amounts of air in and out of the lungs. The next step in the process of respiration is the movement of gases across the alveolar-capillary membrane (AC-membrane). This process occurs by what is called **gas diffusion**.

To fully appreciate *gas diffusion*, the reader must understand (1) **Dalton's law**; (2) the **partial pressures of atmospheric gases**; and (3) the fundamental differences between (a) **pressure gradients**, which move gas in and out of the lungs, and (b) **diffusion gradients**, which move gas across the alveolar-capillary membrane.

Dalton's Law

According to **Dalton's law**—the **law of partial pressures**,[1,2] the total pressure exerted by a mixture of gases is equal to the sum of the pressures exerted independently by each gas in the mixture. In addition, the pressure exerted by each gas—its partial pressure—is directly proportional to the percentage of that gas in the gas mixture. For example, if 10 molecules of gas are enclosed in a container, the total pressure may be expressed as 10; if 5 molecules of a different gas are enclosed in another container of equal volume, the total pressure may be expressed as 5; if both these gases are enclosed in a container of equal volume, the total pressure may be expressed as 15 (Figure 4–1).

It should be emphasized that the pressure produced by a particular gas is completely unaffected by the presence of another gas. Each gas in a mixture will individually contribute to the total pressure created by the mixture of gases.

---

[1] The term **partial pressure** refers to the force exerted by one gas in a mixture of gases—or in a liquid.

[2] It should be noted that it is common to use either **mm Hg** or **torr** gas pressure values (e.g., P_{O_2}, P_{CO_2}, N_2). The *torr* was named after Evangelista Torricelli, an Italian physicist and mathematician, who discovered the principle of the mercury barometer in 1644. In honor of Torricelli, the torr was defined as a unit of pressure equal to 1 mm Hg—i.e., 1 torr = 1 mm Hg.

The **National Board for Respiratory Care (NBRC)** uses the following on national board exams:

- **torr** is used for blood gases values (e.g., Pa_{O_2} or Pa_{CO_2}).

- **mm Hg** is used for blood pressure and barometric values.

Partial Pressures of Atmospheric Gases

The earth's atmospheric gases consist of nitrogen (N_2), oxygen (O_2), carbon dioxide (CO_2), and other trace gases (e.g., argon). Because the partial pressure of each gas that surrounds the earth is directly related to its concentration—relative to the barometric pressure (P_B)—the partial pressure of each gas can easily be determined by multiplying the P_B by the percentage of the gas in the atmosphere. For example, because the percentage of oxygen in the atmosphere is about 21 percent—and assuming a normal P_B of 760 mm Hg at sea level—the partial pressure of oxygen is calculated as follows:

Atmospheric $P_{O_2} = 0.21 \times 760 = 159.6$ mm Hg

The partial pressure of each of the atmospheric gases—P_{N_2}, P_{O_2}, P_{CO_2}, and some trace gases—collectively make a total atmospheric pressure of 760 mm Hg. Figure 4–2 shows the atmospheric gases, their respective percentages, and the partial pressure of each gas at sea level.

Figure 4–2

Atmospheric gases, their respective percentages, and partial pressure of each gas at sea level.

© Cengage Learning 2013

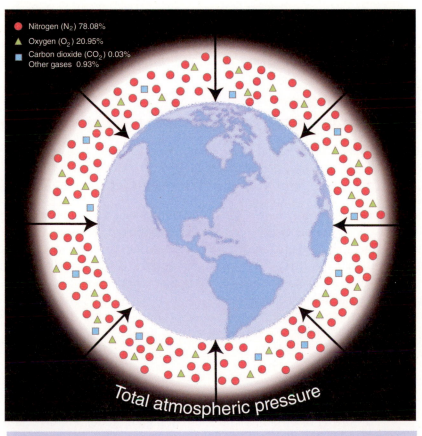

Total atmospheric pressure		P_{N_2}	P_{O_2}	P_{CO_2}	P_{other}
760 mm Hg	=	592.8 mm Hg +	159.6 mm Hg +	0.2 mm Hg +	7 mm Hg
(100%)		(78.08%)	(20.95%)	(0.03%)	(0.93%)

1 mm Hg = 1 torr (see footnote 2, page 182)

The atmospheric pressure decreases with an increase in altitude. This is because the density of the different gases surrounding the earth decreases with increased altitude. As the density of the atmospheric gases decrease, the partial pressure exerted by each gas—e.g., the P_{O_2}—also decreases. However, it is important to remember that even though the barometric pressure decreases with the altitude, the concentration of all the atmospheric gases remains the same at both high and low elevations. In other words, the percentage of oxygen is always about 21 percent—both at sea level and at the top of Mt. Everest (29,035 above sea level). What changes at different altitudes are the partial pressures of the atmospheric gases.

Finally, it should be noted that moving in the opposite direction has the reverse effect. That is, the atmospheric pressure increases by 1 atmosphere (760 mm Hg) for each 33 feet of descent (in water) below sea level. For example, at 99 feet below sea level, the total pressure exerted on the body is equal to 4 atmospheres—or 3030 mm Hg. Thus, the partial pressure exerted by each gas in the atmosphere is increased four times. This means the partial pressure of oxygen increases from about 159 mm Hg to 636 mm Hg.[3]

Gas Diffusion—Pressure Gradients versus Diffusion Gradients

As described in Chapter 2, a **pressure gradient** is defined as the movement of gas from an area of high pressure (high concentration) to an area of low pressure (low concentration). A pressure gradient is the primary mechanism responsible for moving air in and out of the lungs during ventilation.

Clinical Connection—4-1

Pulmonary Disorders That Increase the Alveolar-Capillary Thickness

In the clinical setting, the respiratory therapist will treat countless patients with respiratory disorders that cause the alveolar-capillary membrane thickness to increase. Such pulmonary disorders include pulmonary edema, pneumonia, interstitial lung diseases (e.g., scleroderma, sarcoidosis, or Goodpasture's syndrome), acute respiratory distress syndrome (ARDS), and respiratory distress syndrome (RDS) in newborn infants. In patients who have these conditions, even the total transit time (0.75 second) it takes venous blood to move through the alveolar-capillary system may not be enough for adequate gas exchange. In these cases, the treatment efforts are usually directed at increasing the patient's inspired oxygen concentration.

---

[3] For further discussion of pressure at high altitude, refer to Chapter 19, High Altitudes and Its Effects on the Cardiopulmonary System. For further discussion of pressure at high-pressure environments, refer to Chapter 20, High-Pressure Environments and Their Effects on the Cardiopulmonary System.

Clinical Connection—4-2

Hyperbaric Oxygen Therapy—A Clinical Application of Henry's Law

Hyperbaric oxygen therapy (HBOT) (also known as hyperbaric medicine) is the therapeutic application of oxygen at pressures greater than 1 atm. A patient receiving HBOT is placed in a sealed hyperbaric chamber and exposed to selected oxygen concentrations at 1.5 to 3 times above the normal atmospheric pressure (760 mm Hg). Thus, if a patient receives 100 percent oxygen at 3 atm, the partial pressure of oxygen (P_{O_2}) in the chamber would be 2280 mm Hg ($3 \times 760 = 2280$).

Remember, according to Henry's law, the amount of gas that dissolves in a liquid is directly related to the partial pressure of the gas. In other words, the higher the partial pressure of oxygen (P_{O_2}) in the hyperbaric chamber, the greater the amount of oxygen that will be forced into the patient's pulmonary capillary blood. Although the application of hyperbaric medicine was originally developed to treat underwater divers who were suffering from decompression sickness (the bends), it is now commonly used to treat the following conditions:

Indications for Hyperbaric Oxygenation

Gas disorders
- Gas embolism
- Decompression sickness

Vascular disorders
- Radiation necrosis
- Diabetic wounds of the lower extremities
- Nonhealing skin grafts
- Crush injuries
- Acute traumatic ischemias
- Thermal burns

Infections
- Clostridial gangrene
- Necrotizing soft-tissue infections (flesh-eating bacteria)
- Refactory osteomyelitis

Oxygen transport disorders
- Carbon monoxide (CO) poisoning
- Cyanide poisoning
- Severe blood loss or anemia

It is important to point out that the pressure gradients generated during ventilation always move a bulk volume of gas in the same direction—either in or out of the lungs. This also means that each individual gas (e.g., N_2, O_2, CO_2, trace gases) moves in the same direction—either in or out of the lungs. As will be described next, individual gases molecules can move in opposite directions during gas diffusion.

Gas diffusion is defined as the movement of "individual gas molecules" from an area of high pressure (high concentration) to an area of low pressure (low concentration). In other words, each individual gas (e.g., N_2, O_2, CO_2) can continue to move independently from the other gases from a high-pressure area to a low-pressure. Individual gas partial pressure differences are known as **diffusion gradients**. Kinetic energy is the driving force responsible for diffusion.

This means that when a volume of gas reaches its destination—for example, the alveoli by means of a pressure gradient, or the alveoli by way of the pulmonary capillary blood flow—each individual gas can move according to its own diffusion gradient. In other words, two different gases can move (diffuse) in opposite directions based on their individual diffusion gradients. For example, under normal circumstances, O_2 diffuses from the alveoli into the pulmonary capillaries; while, at the same time, CO_2 diffuses from the pulmonary capillaries into the alveoli. The diffusion of O_2 and CO_2 continues until the partial pressures of O_2 and CO_2 are in equilibrium.

The Partial Pressures of Gases in the Air, Alveoli, and Blood

Table 4–1 shows the partial pressure of gases in dry air, alveolar gas, arterial blood, and venous blood. Note that even though the total barometric pressure is the same in the atmosphere and in the alveoli, the partial pressure of oxygen in the atmosphere (159 torr) is significantly higher than the partial pressure of oxygen in the alveoli (100 torr). This is because alveolar oxygen must mix—or compete, in terms of partial pressures—with alveolar CO_2 pressure (PA_{CO_2} = 40 torr) and alveolar water vapor pressure (P_{H_2O} = 47 torr), which are not nearly as high in the atmosphere. In short, by the time the oxygen molecules reach the alveoli, they are diluted by the addition of CO_2 and H_2O molecules. This leads to a decrease in the partial pressure of oxygen in the alveoli (PA_{O_2}).

Depending on the surrounding temperature and pressure, water can exist as a liquid, gas, or solid. Water in the gaseous form is called *water vapor,* or *molecular water.* When water vapor is present in a volume of gas, it behaves according to the gas laws and exerts a partial pressure. Because alveolar gas is 100 percent humidified (saturated) at body temperature, the alveolar gas is assumed to have an *absolute humidity* of 44 mg/L, and a *water vapor pressure* (P_{H_2O}) of 47 torr—regardless of the humidity of the inspired air (Table 4–2).

Table 4–1				
Partial Pressure (torr)* of Gases in the Air, Alveoli, and Blood**				
Gases	**Dry Air**	**Alveolar Gas**	**Arterial Blood**	**Venous Blood**
P_{O_2}	159.0	100.0	95.0	40.0
P_{CO_2}	0.2	40.0	40.0	46.0
P_{H_2O} (water vapor)	0.0	47.0	47.0	47.0
P_{N_2} (and other gases in minute quantities)	600.8	573.0	573.0	573.0
Total	760.0	760.0	755.0	706.0

© Cengage Learning 2013

* 1 torr = 1 mm Hg
** The values shown are based on standard pressure and temperature.

Table 4–2

Relationship Between Temperature, Absolute Humidity, and Water Vapor Pressure*

Temperature (Celsius)	Absolute (Maximum) Humidity (mg/L)	Water Vapor Pressure (torr)
37°	44.0	47.0
35°	39.6	42.2
30°	30.4	31.8
27°	25.8	26.7
25°	23.0	23.8
20°	17.3	17.5

© Cengage Learning 2013

* At sea level (760 torr).
1 torr = 1 mm Hg

The Ideal Alveolar Gas Equation

Clinically, the alveolar oxygen tension ($P_{A_{O_2}}$) can be computed from the **ideal alveolar gas equation**. A useful clinical approximation of the ideal alveolar gas equation is as follows:

$$P_{A_{O_2}} = [P_B - P_{H_2O}]F_{I_{O_2}} - P_{a_{CO_2}} (1.25)$$

or

$$P_{A_{O_2}} = [P_B - P_{H_2O}] F_{I_{O_2}} - \frac{P_{a_{CO_2}}}{0.8}$$

where $P_{A_{O_2}}$ is the partial pressure of oxygen in the alveoli, P_B is the barometric pressure, P_{H_2O} is the partial pressure of water vapor in the alveoli (P_{H_2O} = 47 torr), $F_{I_{O_2}}$ is the fractional concentration of inspired oxygen, and $P_{a_{CO_2}}$ is the partial pressure of arterial carbon dioxide. The number 1.25 is a factor that adjusts for alterations in oxygen tension due to variations in the *respiratory exchange ratio* (RR), which is the ratio of the amount of oxygen that moves into the pulmonary capillary blood to the amount of carbon dioxide that moves out of the pulmonary blood and into the alveoli. Normally, about 200 mL/minute of carbon dioxide move into the alveoli while about 250 mL/minute of oxygen move into the pulmonary capillary blood, making the respiratory exchange ratio about 0.8.

Thus, if a patient is receiving an $F_{I_{O_2}}$ of 0.40 on a day when the barometric pressure is 755 torr, and if the $P_{a_{CO_2}}$ is 55 torr, then the patient's alveolar oxygen tension ($P_{A_{O_2}}$) can be calculated as follows:

$$P_{A_{O_2}} = [P_B - P_{H_2O}]F_{I_{O_2}} - P_{a_{CO_2}}(1.25)$$
$$= [755 - 47]0.40 - 55(1.25)$$
$$= [708]0.40 - 68.75$$
$$= [283.2] - 68.75$$
$$= 214.45$$

Clinically, when the Pa_{CO_2} is less than 60 torr, and when the patient is receiving oxygen therapy greater than 0.6, the following simplified version of the alveolar gas equation may be used:

$$PA_{O_2} = [P_B - P_{H_2O}]FI_{O_2} - Pa_{CO_2}$$

The Diffusion of Pulmonary Gases

The process of diffusion is the passive movement of gas molecules from an area of high partial pressure to an area of low partial pressure until both areas are equal in pressure. Once equilibrium occurs, diffusion ceases.

In the lungs, a gas molecule must diffuse through the alveolar-capillary membrane (Figure 4–3), which is composed of (1) the liquid lining the intra-alveolar membrane, (2) the alveolar epithelial cell, (3) the basement membrane of the alveolar epithelial cell, (4) loose connective tissue (the interstitial space), (5) the basement membrane of the capillary endothelium, (6) the capillary endothelium, (7) the plasma in the capillary blood, (8) the erythrocyte membrane, and (9) the intracellular fluid in the erythrocyte until a hemoglobin molecule is encountered. The thickness of these physical barriers is between 0.36 and 2.5 mm. Under normal circumstances, this is a negligible barrier to the diffusion of oxygen and carbon dioxide.

Figure 4–3

The major barriers of the alveolar-capillary membrane through which a gas molecule must diffuse.

© Cengage Learning 2013

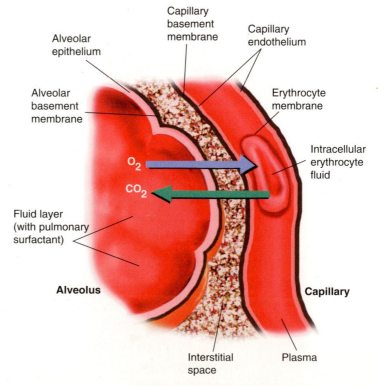

ALVEOLAR-CAPILLARY MEMBRANE

Oxygen and Carbon Dioxide Diffusion Across the Alveolar-Capillary Membrane

In the healthy resting individual, venous blood entering the alveolar-capillary system has an average oxygen tension ($P\bar{v}_{O_2}$) of 40 torr and an average carbon dioxide tension ($P\bar{v}_{CO_2}$) of 46 torr. As blood passes through the capillary, the average alveolar oxygen tension ($P_{A_{O_2}}$) is about 100 torr, and the average alveolar carbon dioxide tension ($P_{A_{CO_2}}$) is about 40 torr (see Table 4–1).

Thus, when venous blood enters the alveolar-capillary system, there is an oxygen pressure gradient of about 60 torr and a carbon dioxide pressure gradient of about 6 torr. As a result, oxygen molecules diffuse across the alveolar-capillary membrane into the blood while, at the same time, carbon dioxide molecules diffuse out of the capillary blood and into the alveoli (Figure 4–4).[4]

The diffusion of oxygen and carbon dioxide will continue until equilibrium is reached; this is usually accomplished in about 0.25 second. Under normal resting conditions, the total transit time for blood to move through the alveolar-capillary system is about 0.75 second. Thus, the diffusion of oxygen and carbon dioxide is completed in about one-third of the time available (Figure 4–5 on page 190).

Figure 4–4

Normal gas pressures for oxygen (O_2) and carbon dioxide (CO_2) as blood moves through the alveolar-capillary membrane. $P\bar{v}_{O_2}$ = partial pressure of oxygen in mixed venous blood; $P\bar{v}_{CO_2}$ = partial pressure of carbon dioxide in mixed venous blood; $P_{A_{O_2}}$ = partial pressure of oxygen in alveolar gas; $P_{A_{CO_2}}$ = partial pressure of carbon dioxide in alveolar gas; Pa_{O_2} = partial pressure of oxygen in arterial blood; Pa_{CO_2} = partial pressure of carbon dioxide in arterial blood.

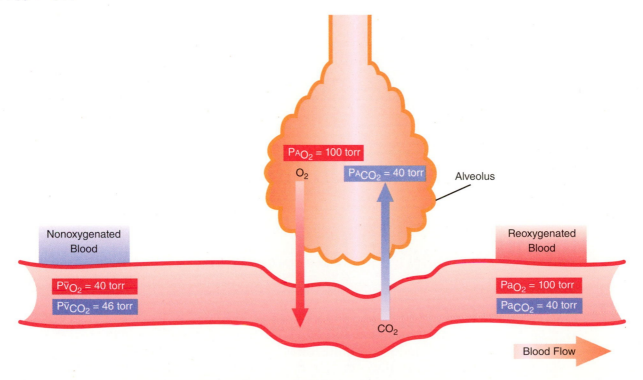

---

[4] The exhaled P_{CO_2} leaving at the level of the mouth is about 35 torr because of different alveolar emptying rates.

Figure 4–5

Under normal resting conditions, blood moves through the alveolar-capillary membrane in about 0.75 second. The oxygen pressure (P_{O_2}) and carbon dioxide pressure (P_{CO_2}) reach equilibrium in about 0.25 second—one-third of the time available. $P\bar{v}_{O_2}$ = partial pressure of oxygen in mixed venous blood; $P\bar{v}_{CO_2}$ = partial pressure of carbon dioxide in mixed venous blood; PA_{O_2} = partial pressure of oxygen in alveolar gas; PA_{CO_2} = partial pressure of carbon dioxide in alveolar gas; Pa_{O_2} = partial pressure of oxygen in arterial blood; Pa_{CO_2} = partial pressure of carbon dioxide in arterial blood.

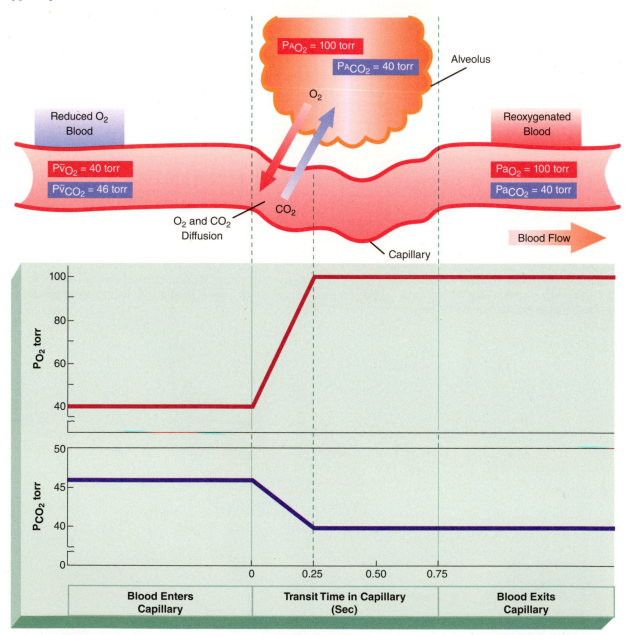

In exercise, however, blood passes through the alveolar-capillary system at a much faster rate and, therefore, the time for gas diffusion decreases (i.e., the time available for gas diffusion is <0.75 second). In the healthy lung, oxygen equilibrium usually occurs in the alveolar-capillary system during exercise—in spite of the shortened transit time (Figure 4–6). In the presence of certain pulmonary diseases, however, the time available to achieve oxygen equilibrium in the alveolar-capillary system may not be adequate. Such diseases include pulmonary edema, pneumonia (alveolar consolidation), and interstitial lung diseases (Figure 4–7 on page 192).

Figure 4–6

During exercise or stress, the total transit time for blood through the alveolar-capillary membrane is less than normal (normal = 0.75 second). In the healthy individual, however, oxygen equilibrium usually occurs. $P\overline{v}_{O_2}$ = partial pressure of oxygen in mixed venous blood; PA_{O_2} = partial pressure of oxygen in alveolar gas; Pa_{O_2} = partial pressure of oxygen in arterial blood.

© Cengage Learning 2013

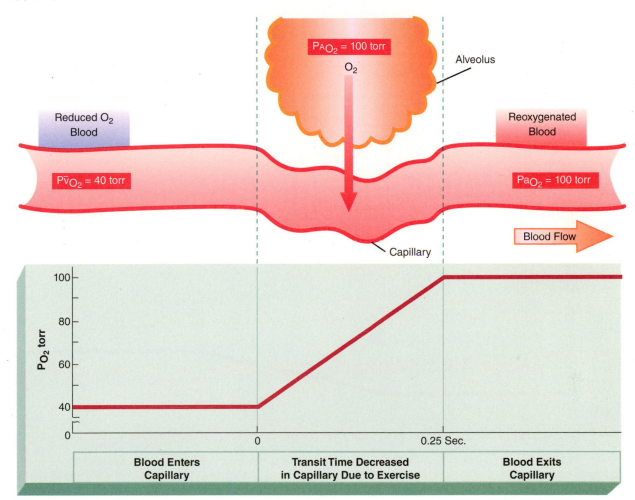

Clinical Connection—4-3

Oxygen Toxicity

Although breathing high concentrations of oxygen is safe for short periods of time, what is called **oxygen toxicity** can develop within 24 hours in response to high partial pressures of inspired oxygen (P_{O_2}), and with longer exposure times to inspired oxygen concentrations (FI_{O_2}) above 0.50. In other words, the higher the inspired P_{O_2} and the longer the exposure, the more likely oxygen toxicity will develop. Oxygen toxicity affects the lungs and the central nervous system. Pulmonary effects include tracheobronchitis, substernal chest pain, atelectasis, decreased vital capacity, decreased lung compliance, and decreased diffusing capacity. Central nervous system effects include tremors, twitching, convulsions, coma, and death. Central nervous system effects tend to occur only when a patient is breathing oxygen at pressures greater than 1 atm (hyperbaric medicine).

When the rate of diffusion is decreased because of alveolar thickening, oxygen equilibrium will likely not occur when the total transit time is decreased as a result of exercise or stress. $P\bar{v}_{O_2}$ = partial pressure of oxygen in mixed venous blood; PA_{O_2} = partial pressure of oxygen in alveolar gas; Pa_{O_2} = partial pressure of oxygen in arterial blood.

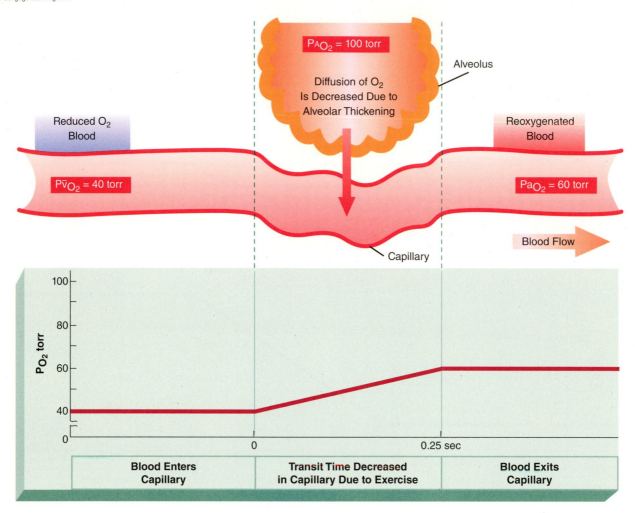

Gas Diffusion

Fick's Law

The diffusion of gas takes place according to Fick's law, which is written as follows:

$$\dot{V}gas \approx \frac{A \cdot D \cdot (P_1 - P_2)}{T}$$

where $\dot{V}gas$ is the amount of gas that diffuses from one point to another, A is surface area, D is diffusion constant, $P_1 - P_2$ is the difference in partial pressure between two points, and T is thickness.

The law states that the rate of gas transfer across a sheet of tissue is directly proportional to the surface area of the tissue, to the diffusion constants,

© Cengage Learning 2013

Figure 4–8

Fick's law.

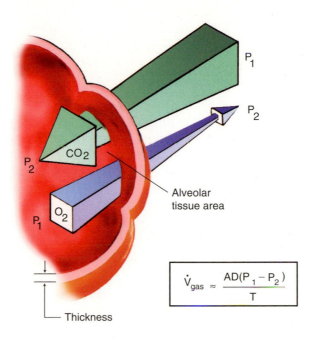

$$\dot{V}_{gas} \approx \frac{AD(P_1 - P_2)}{T}$$

and to the difference in partial pressure of the gas between the two sides of the tissue, and it is inversely proportional to the thickness of the tissue (Figure 4–8).

The diffusion constant (D), noted in Fick's, law is determined by Henry's law and Graham's law.

Henry's Law

Henry's law states that the amount of a gas that dissolves in a liquid at a given temperature is proportional to the partial pressure of the gas. The amount of gas that can be dissolved by 1 mL of a given liquid at standard pressure (760 mm Hg) and specified temperature is known as the *solubility coefficient* of the liquid. At 37°C and 760 mm Hg pressure, the solubility coefficient of oxygen is 0.0244 mL/mm Hg/mL H_2O. The solubility coefficient of carbon dioxide is 0.592 mL/mm Hg/mL H_2O. The solubility coefficient varies inversely with temperature (i.e., if the temperature rises, the solubility coefficient decreases in value).

On the basis of the solubility coefficients of oxygen and carbon dioxide, it can be seen that in a liquid medium (e.g., alveolar-capillary membrane) carbon dioxide is more soluble than oxygen:

$$\frac{\text{Solubility } CO_2}{\text{Solubility } O_2} = \frac{0.592}{0.0244} = \frac{24}{1}$$

Graham's Law

Graham's law states that the rate of diffusion of a gas through a liquid is (1) directly proportional to the solubility coefficient of the gas and (2) indirectly proportional to the square root of the gram-molecular weight (GMW) of the gas. In comparing the relative rates of diffusion to oxygen (GMW = 32) and carbon dioxide (GMW = 44), it can be seen that, because oxygen is the lighter gas, it moves faster than carbon dioxide:

$$\frac{\text{Diffusion rate for } CO_2}{\text{Diffusion rate for } O_2} = \frac{\sqrt{GMW\ O_2}}{\sqrt{GMW\ CO_2}} = \frac{\sqrt{32}}{\sqrt{44}}$$

$$= \frac{5.6}{6.6}$$

By combining Graham's and Henry's laws, it can be said that the rates of diffusion of two gases are directly proportional to the ratio of their solubility coefficients, and inversely proportional to the ratio of their gram-molecular weights. For example, when the two laws are used to determine the relative rates of diffusion of carbon dioxide and oxygen, it can be seen that carbon dioxide diffuses about 20 times faster than oxygen.

$$\frac{\text{Diffusion rate for } CO_2}{\text{Diffusion rate for } O_2} = \frac{5.6 \times 0.592}{6.6 \times 0.0244} = \frac{20}{1}$$

To summarize, the diffusion constant (D) for a particular gas is directly proportional to the solubility coefficients (S) of the gas, and inversely proportional to the square root of the GMW of the gas:

$$D = \frac{S}{\sqrt{GMW}}$$

Mathematically, by substituting the diffusion constant,

$$D = \frac{S}{\sqrt{GMW}}$$

into Fick's law

$$\dot{V} \text{ gas} \approx \frac{A \cdot D \cdot (P_1 - P_2)}{T}$$

then Fick's law can be rewritten as:

$$\dot{V} \text{ gas} \approx \frac{A \cdot S \cdot (P_1 - P_2)}{\sqrt{GMW} \times T}$$

Clinical Application of Fick's Law

Clinically, Fick's law applies to the following general statements:

- The area (A) component of the law is verified in that a decreased alveolar surface area (e.g., caused by alveolar collapse or alveolar fluid) decreases the ability of oxygen to enter the pulmonary capillary blood.
- The $P_1 - P_2$ portion of the law is confirmed in that a decreased alveolar oxygen pressure ($P_{A_{O_2}}$ or P_1) (e.g., caused by high altitudes or alveolar hypoventilation) reduces the diffusion of oxygen into the pulmonary capillary blood.

- The thickness (T) factor is confirmed in that an increased alveolar tissue thickness (e.g., caused by alveolar fibrosis or alveolar edema) reduces the movement of oxygen across the alveolar-capillary membrane.

Fick's law also suggests how certain adverse pulmonary conditions may be improved. For example, when a patient's oxygen diffusion rate is decreased because of alveolar thickening, the administration of oxygen therapy will be beneficial. As the patient's fractional concentration of inspired oxygen ($F_{I_{O_2}}$) increases, the patient's alveolar oxygen pressure (i.e., $P_{A_{O_2}}$ or the P_1) also increases, causing the movement of oxygen across the alveolar-capillary membrane to increase.

Clinical Connection—4-4

The Clinical Case Applications of Fick's Law

In the Clinical Application Section—Case 1 (page 202), the respiratory therapist is called to care for a 68-year-old man in severe left ventricular heart failure and pulmonary edema (see Figure 4–13). This case illustrates both the undesirable effects, and the therapeutic effects, associated with Fick's law. This clinical event describes how the pathologic changes associated with pulmonary edema increase the thickness of the alveolar-capillary (AC) membrane. Because gas diffusion ($\dot{V}$) is indirectly related to thickness (T), the diffusion of oxygen across the AC membrane decreases. Case 1 further describes how the respiratory therapist treats the patient's low oxygenation status

by increasing the patient's alveolar oxygen pressure ($P_{A_{O_2}}$) or P_1 of Fick's law. Because gas diffusion is directly related to $P_1 - P_2$, the diffusion of gas across the patient's AC membrane is enhanced.

In the Clinical Application Section—Case 2 (page 204), the respiratory therapist is called to treat a 78-year-old woman with a long history of chronic interstitial lung disease (alveolar thickening and fibrosis) who is in respiratory distress. This case illustrates both the acute and chronic harmful effects of an increased AC-membrane thickness (T), and the therapeutic benefits of increasing the patient's $P_{A_{O_2}}$ (P_1).

Clinical Connection—4-5

Respiratory Disorders That Decrease the Alveolar Surface Area

A number of respiratory disorders can drastically reduce the alveolar surface area (the "A" component in Fick's law). For example, because emphysema breaks down the walls of adjacent alveoli and pulmonary capillaries, the alveoli merge together into large air sacs (called *bullae*). Because emphysema destroys both the alveoli and pulmonary capillaries, the alveolar surface

area decreases. Increasing the patient's $P_{A_{O_2}}$ (P_1) can be helpful with these patients. The alveolar surface area is also reduced in pulmonary disorders associated with excessive tracheobronchial tree secretions or tumors, which block air flow to the alveoli, and alveolar collapse (e.g., pleural effusion, pneumothorax, or excessive airway secretions).

Perfusion-Limited Gas Flow

Perfusion limited means that the transfer of gas across the alveolar wall is a function of the amount of blood that flows past the alveoli. Nitrous oxide (N_2O) is an excellent gas to illustrate this concept. When N_2O moves across the alveolar wall and into the blood, it does not chemically combine with hemoglobin. Because of this, the partial pressure of N_2O in the blood plasma rises very quickly. It is estimated that the partial pressure of N_2O will equal that of the alveolar gas when the blood is only about one-tenth of the way through the alveolar-capillary system (Figure 4–9). Once the partial pressures of the N_2O in the blood and in the alveolar gas are equal, the diffusion of N_2O stops. In order for the diffusion of N_2O to resume, additional blood must enter the alveolar-capillary system. The rate of perfusion, therefore, determines the amount of diffusion of N_2O.

Figure 4–9

Nitrous oxide (N_2O) quickly equilibrates with pulmonary blood. When equilibrium occurs, the diffusion of N_2O stops. In order for the diffusion of N_2O to resume, fresh blood (pulmonary artery blood) must enter the alveolar-capillary system. This phenomenon is called *perfusion limited*. P_{N_2O} = partial pressure of N_2O in the blood.

© Cengage Learning 2013

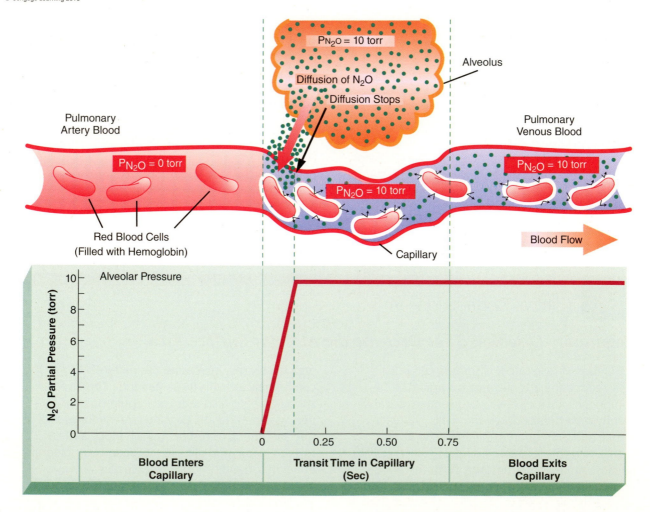

Clinical Connection—4-6

Decreased $D_{L_{CO}}$—The Classic Pulmonary Function Diagnostic Sign of Emphysema

Clinically, the signs and symptoms associated with emphysema appear very similar to other chronic obstructive pulmonary disorders. For example, at the bedside, patients with emphysema, chronic bronchitis, or cystic fibrosis may all demonstrate a barrel chest, digital clubbing, or diminished breath sounds. Their arterial blood gas values generally reveal low oxygenation levels and high carbon dioxide levels. All patients with significant COPD demonstrate elevated RVs and FRC (caused by air trapping) and decreased FVC and FEV_1 values (caused by increased airway resistance). However, the classic pulmonary function diagnostic test that verifies that a patient has emphysema is a decreased $D_{L_{CO}}$. This is because of the alveolar-capillary destruction (decreased alveolar surface area) associated with emphysema. Alveolar-capillary destruction is not associated with the other chronic obstructive pulmonary disorders.

In addition to emphysema, there other lung disorders associated with a decreased $D_{L_{CO}}$ value. The following table provides three useful ways to correlate a patient's $D_{L_{CO}}$ value, lung volumes (usually the FRC), and specific lung abnormalities:

Lung Abnormality	$D_{L_{CO}}$ and FRC	Pulmonary Disorder
Hyperinflation and decreased $D_{L_{CO}}$	Decreased $D_{L_{CO}}$ Increased FRC	Emphysema, etc. (COPD)
Hypoinflation and decreased $D_{L_{CO}}$	Decreased $D_{L_{CO}}$ Decreased FRC	Restrictive lung disease (e.g., pulmonary edema, chronic interstitial lung disease)
Normal lung volume and decreased $D_{L_{CO}}$	Decreased $D_{L_{CO}}$ Normal FRC	Pulmonary embolism

Diffusion-Limited Gas Flow

Diffusion limited means that the movement of gas across the alveolar wall is a function of the integrity of the alveolar-capillary membrane itself. Carbon monoxide (CO) is an excellent gas to illustrate this concept. When CO moves across the alveolar wall and into the blood, it rapidly enters the red blood cells (RBCs) and tightly bonds to hemoglobin (CO has an affinity for hemoglobin that is about 210 times greater than that of oxygen).

Note that when gases are in chemical combination with hemoglobin, they no longer exert a partial pressure. Thus, because CO has a strong chemical attraction to hemoglobin, most of the CO enters the RBCs, combines with hemoglobin, and no longer exerts a partial pressure in the blood plasma. Because there is no appreciable partial pressure of CO in the blood plasma at any time (i.e., $P_1 - P_2$ stays constant), only the diffusion characteristics of the alveolar-capillary membrane, not the amount of blood flowing through the capillary, limit the diffusion of CO (Figure 4–10 on page 198).

Figure 4–10

Carbon monoxide (CO) rapidly bonds to hemoglobin and, thus, does not generate an appreciable partial pressure (P_{CO}) in the plasma. As a result of this chemical relationship, blood flow (perfusion) does not limit the rate of CO diffusion. When the alveolar-capillary membrane is abnormal (e.g., in alveolar fibrosis), however, the rate of CO diffusion decreases. This phenomenon is called *diffusion limited*. In essence, diffusion limited means that the structure of the alveolar-capillary membrane alone limits the rate of gas diffusion.

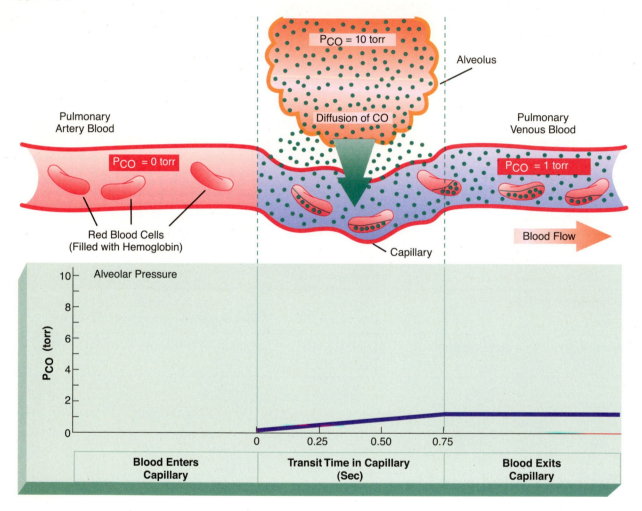

This property makes CO an excellent gas for evaluating the lung's ability to diffuse gases and is used in what is called the *diffusion capacity of carbon monoxide* (DL_{CO}) test. The DL_{CO} test measures the amount of CO that moves across the alveolar-capillary membrane into the blood in a given time. In essence, this test measures the physiologic effectiveness of the alveolar-capillary membrane. The normal diffusion capacity of CO is 25 mL/min/mm Hg. Figure 4–11 shows clinical conditions that may cause problems in diffusion. See Figure 4–7 for an illustration of the diffusion of oxygen during a diffusion-limited state. Table 4–3 on page 200 presents factors that affect measured DL_{CO}.

Clinical conditions that decrease the rate of gas diffusion. These conditions are known as *diffusion-limited problems.*

© Cengage Learning 2013

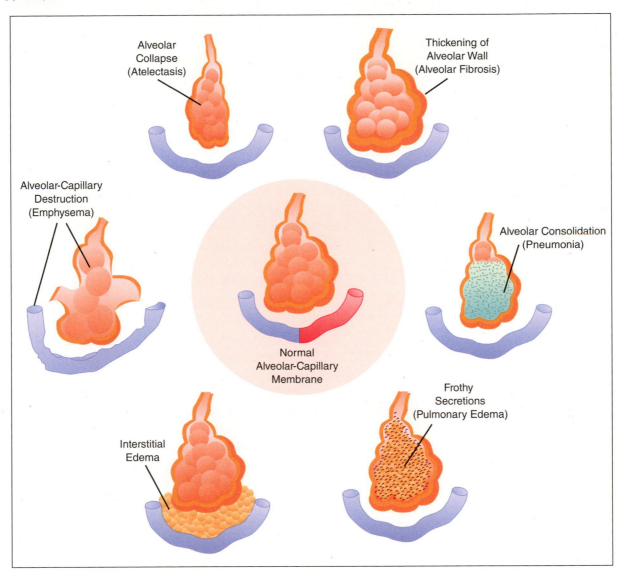

How Oxygen Can Be Either Perfusion or Diffusion Limited

When oxygen diffuses across the alveolar wall and into the blood, it enters the RBCs and combines with hemoglobin—but not with the same avidity as does carbon monoxide. Hemoglobin quickly becomes saturated with oxygen and, once this occurs, oxygen molecules in the plasma can no longer enter the RBCs. This, in turn, causes the partial pressure of oxygen in the plasma to increase.

Table 4–3	
Factors That Affect Measured $D_{L_{CO}}$	
Age	The $D_{L_{CO}}$ progressively increases between birth and 20 years of age. After age 20, the $D_{L_{CO}}$ decreases as a result of the normal anatomic alterations of the lungs that reduce the overall alveolar-capillary surface area.
Lung volume	The $D_{L_{CO}}$ is directly related to an individual's lung size. Thus, the greater the subject's lung volume, the greater the $D_{L_{CO}}$.
Body size	As a general rule, the $D_{L_{CO}}$ increases with body size. The size of the lungs is directly related to the subject's ideal body size. Thus, the larger the subject, the greater the lung size and the higher the $D_{L_{CO}}$.
Body position	The $D_{L_{CO}}$ is about 15% to 20% greater when the individual is in the supine position, compared with the upright position.
Exercise	The $D_{L_{CO}}$ increases with exercise. This is most likely because of the increased cardiac output, and capillary recruitment and distention, associated with exercise.*
Alveolar P_{O_2} ($P_{A_{O_2}}$)	The $D_{L_{CO}}$ decreases in response to a high $P_{A_{O_2}}$. This is because O_2 and CO both compete for the same hemoglobin sites.[†]
Hemoglobin concentration	*Anemia:* Patients with low hemoglobin content have a low CO-carrying capacity and, therefore, a low $D_{L_{CO}}$ value. *Polycythemia:* Patients with high hemoglobin content have a high CO-carrying capacity and, therefore, a high $D_{L_{CO}}$ value.
Carboxyhemoglobin	Individuals who already have CO bound to their hemoglobin (e.g., smokers or fire fighters overcome by smoke inhalation) generate a "back pressure" to alveolar P_{CO}. This condition decreases the pressure gradient between the alveolar CO and the blood CO, which in turn reduces the $D_{L_{CO}}$ (see discussion of Fick's law).

© Cengage Learning 2013

* Refer to Chapter 5.
† Refer to Chapter 6.

Under normal resting conditions, the partial pressure of oxygen in the capillary blood equals the partial pressure of oxygen in the alveolar gas when the blood is about one-third of the way through the capillary. Beyond this point, the transfer of oxygen is perfusion limited (Figure 4–12). When the patient has either a decreased cardiac output or a decreased hemoglobin level (anemia), the effects of perfusion limitation may become significant.

When the diffusion properties of the lungs are impaired (see Figure 4–11), however, the partial pressure of oxygen in the capillary blood may never equal the partial pressure of the oxygen in the alveolar gas during the normal alveolar-capillary transit time. Thus, under normal circumstances the diffusion of oxygen is perfusion limited, but under certain abnormal pulmonary conditions the transfer of oxygen may become diffusion limited.

Under normal resting conditions, the diffusion of oxygen across the alveolar-capillary membrane stops when blood is about one-third of the way through the capillary. This occurs because the partial pressure of oxygen in the capillary blood (P_{O_2}) equals the partial pressure of oxygen in the alveolus ($P_{A_{O_2}}$). Once oxygen equilibrium occurs between the alveolus and capillary blood, the diffusion of oxygen is *perfusion limited.*

© Cengage Learning 2013

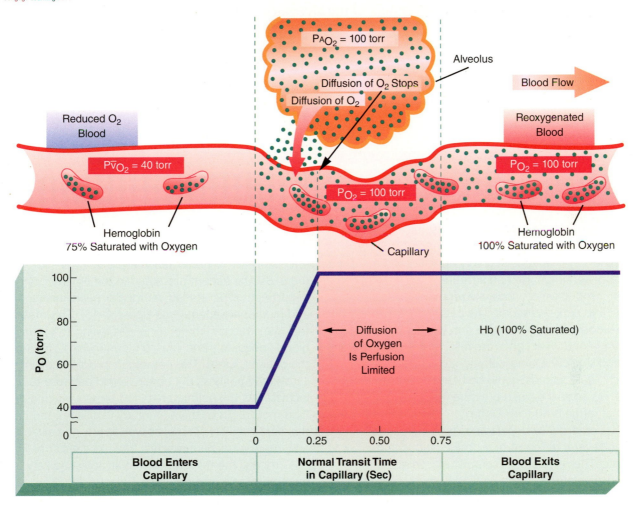

Chapter Summary

Diffusion is the movement of gas molecules from an area of relatively high concentration of gas (high-pressure) to one of low concentration (low-pressure). When several different gases are mixed together, each gas in the mixture diffuses according to its own individual pressure gradient. Diffusion continues until all gases in the two areas are in equilibrium. Fundamental to the understanding of the diffusion of gases is Dalton's law. Dalton's law provides the basic foundation to understand (1) the gases that compose the barometric pressure, (2) the partial pressure of these gases in the air, alveoli, and blood, and (3) the ideal alveolar gas equation.

Essential to the knowledge base of gas diffusion is the understanding of (1) the diffusion of oxygen and carbon dioxide across the alveolar-capillary membrane; (2) Fick's law, including how Henry's law and Graham's law are used in Fick's law; (3) perfusion-limited gas flow; (4) diffusion-limited gas flow; and (5) how oxygen can be either perfusion or diffusion limited. Clinical connections associated with these topics include (1) pulmonary disorders that increase the thickness of the alveolar-capillary thickness, (2) hyperbaric oxygen therapy, (3) oxygen toxicity, (4) Fick's law applied to patients suffering from increased alveolar-capillary membranes, (5) respiratory disorders that reduce alveolar surface area, and (6) why a decreased $D_{L_{CO}}$ is a classic diagnostic sign of emphysema.

1 Clinical Application Case

This 68-year-old man entered the hospital in severe left ventricular heart failure and pulmonary edema (Figure 4–13).[5] He appeared very anxious, and his lips and skin were blue. He had a frequent and strong cough, productive of moderate amounts of frothy, white, and pink secretions. The patient's vital signs were blood pressure—140/88 mm Hg, heart rate—93 beats/min and weak, and respiratory rate—28 breaths/min and shallow. On auscultation, crackles and rhonchi (fluid sounds) could be heard over both lung fields. His arterial oxygen pressure (Pa_{O_2}) was 53 torr (normal range is 80 to 100 torr).

The emergency department physician administered several different heart medications and a diuretic. The respiratory therapist placed a continuous positive airway pressure (CPAP) mask over the patient's nose and mouth and set the pressure at +10 cm H_2O and the fractional concentration of inspired oxygen (FI_{O_2}) at 0.4. One hour later, the patient was breathing comfortably. His lips and skin no longer appeared blue, and his cough was less frequent. No frothy or pink sputum was noted at this time. His vital signs were blood pressure—126/78 mm Hg, heart rate—77 beats/min, and respiratory rate—16 breaths/min. On auscultation, his breath sounds were improved. His arterial oxygen pressure (Pa_{O_2}) was 86 torr.

Discussion

This case illustrates both the adverse and therapeutic effects of factors presented in Fick's law (see Figure 4–8). The patient presented in the emergency department in severe left ventricular heart failure and pulmonary edema (see Figure 4–13). This means that the patient's left ventricle was failing to pump blood adequately and caused blood to back up into the patient's lungs. This pathologic process, in turn, caused the patient's pulmonary blood pressure to increase. As the pulmonary blood pressure increased, fluid moved out of the pulmonary capillaries and into the extra-capillary spaces, as well as into the alveoli and into the tracheobronchial tree. As a result of this process, the thickness of the alveolar-capillary membrane also increased (see Figure 4–3).

Because gas diffusion ($\dot{V}$) is *indirectly* related to thickness (T), the diffusion of oxygen across the alveolar-capillary membrane decreased (Fick's law). This fact was illustrated by the low Pa_{O_2} of 53 torr when the patient first entered the hospital. The physician treated the original cause of this condition—the failing heart and fluid overload—with medications. As the cardiac function and fluid overload improved, the thickness of the alveolar-capillary membrane returned to normal. As the thickness of the alveolar-capillary membrane decreased, the diffusion of oxygen increased.

While the physician was treating the patient's failing heart, the respiratory therapist worked to offset the patient's poor oxygenation by increasing the patient's PA_{O_2} (P_1 of Fick's law). As Fick's law shows, the diffusion of gas is *directly* related to $P_1 - P_2$. The therapist increased the patient's PA_{O_2} by (1) increasing

---

[5] Pulmonary edema refers to fluid accumulation in the alveoli and airways. Pulmonary edema is commonly associated with congestive heart failure (CHF).

Clinical Application Case 1 (continued)

Figure 4–13

Cross-sectional view of alveoli with pulmonary edema. Pathology includes (1) interstitial edema, (2) fluid engorgement throughout the alveolar wall interstitium, and (3) frothy white secretions in the alveoli.

© Cengage Learning 2013

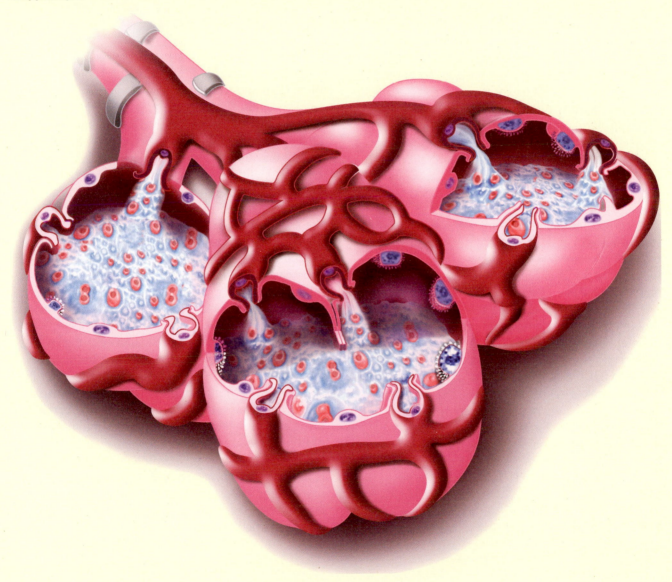

the pressure at the level of the patient's alveoli with the CPAP mask and (2) increasing the inspired F_{IO_2} to 0.4.

Thus, the reduction in alveolar-capillary membrane thickness (decreased via medications), the increased pressure at the level of the alveoli (produced via CPAP), and the increased F_{IO_2} (increased P_1) all worked to enhance the diffusion of oxygen, as shown by the Pa_{O_2} of 86 torr achieved 1 hour later. The patient's cardiac condition progressively improved and he was discharged from the hospital 2 days later.

A 78-year-old woman with a long history of chronic interstitial lung disease (alveolar thickening and fibrosis) was admitted to the hospital because of respiratory distress. She was well known to the hospital staff. She had been admitted to the hospital on several occasions, and for the 2 years prior to this admission, she had been on continuous oxygen at home (2 L/min by nasal cannula). The home care respiratory therapist made regular visits to the patient's home to check on her equipment and to assess her respiratory status. In fact, it was the respiratory therapist who alerted the physician about the patient's poor respiratory status that prompted this hospitalization.

On admission, the patient appeared anxious and agitated. Her skin was pale and blue and felt cool and clammy. Her vital signs were blood pressure—166/91 mm Hg, heart rate—105 beats/min, and respiratory rate—24 breaths/min. Her breath sounds were clear and loud. Although chest X-ray regularly showed signs of increased alveolar density (white appearance) because of her lung fibrosis, this day's chest X-ray was markedly worse.

The physician on duty felt that the chest X-ray showed an acute inflammatory condition from an undetermined cause. The physician started the patient on corticosteroids. The respiratory therapist noted that even though the patient's alveolar oxygen pressure ($P_{A_{O_2}}$) was calculated to be 165 torr, the patient's arterial oxygen pressure (Pa_{O_2}) was only 57 torr (normal, 80 to 100 torr). In response to the low Pa_{O_2}, the therapist increased the patient's inspired oxygen concentration ($F_{I_{O_2}}$) from 2 L/min via nasal cannula (an $F_{I_{O_2}}$ of about 0.28) to 0.5 via an oxygen Venturi mask.

Over the next 24 hours, the patient's condition progressively improved. She stated that she was breathing much better. Her skin color returned to normal and no longer felt cold or wet. Her vital signs were blood pressure—128/86 mm Hg, heart rate—76 beats/min, and respiratory rate—14 breaths/min. A second chest X-ray showed improvement, compared with the previous day's chest X-ray, and her Pa_{O_2} was 89 torr, within normal limits.

Discussion

This case illustrates both the acute and chronic effects of an increased alveolar-capillary membrane. As Fick's law states, the diffusion of gas is *indirectly* related to the thickness of the alveolar-capillary membrane, and *directly* related to $P_1 - P_2$ (see Figure 4–8). Because the patient had chronic alveolar fibrosis and thickening, her oxygen diffusion was low. This is why continuous oxygen (2 L/min) administered via nasal cannula at home was needed to offset this condition. Increasing the alveolar oxygen level (i.e., increasing the $P_{A_{O_2}}$ or P_1) enhanced oxygen diffusion. When the patient's usual chronic status was stable, the 2 L/min oxygen via cannula at home was usually adequate to oxygenate her alveolar-capillary blood.

Because the patient had an acute alveolar inflammatory condition overlying her chronic problem, her alveolar-capillary membrane became even thicker. As a result, her usual home oxygen administration was not enough to meet the new challenge. Over the course of her hospitalization, however, the steroid therapy reduced her alveolar inflammation. As the acute alveolar inflammation improved, the thickness of her alveolar-capillary membrane decreased. While this process was taking place, the increased oxygen concentration (P_1) worked to offset the patient's poor oxygenation status and thus worked to make her comfortable. The patient continued to improve and was discharged on day 5 of her hospital stay. She continued to use oxygen via nasal cannula at home.

Review Questions

1. Assuming a normal barometric pressure of 760 mm Hg, if the percentage of oxygen is 0.4, the partial pressure of oxygen would be:
   A. 159 mm Hg
   B. 215 mm Hg
   C. 304 mm Hg
   D. 560 mm Hg

2. How many feet below sea level must an individual descend to exert a total pressure on the body of 3 atmospheres (2280 mm Hg)?
  A. 13 feet
  B. 33 feet
  C. 66 feet
  D. 99 feet

3. Which of the following gas laws states that in a mixture of gases the total pressure is equal to the sum of the partial pressure of each gas?
  A. Dalton's law
  B. Gay-Lussac's law
  C. Charles' law
  D. Boyle's law

4. At sea level, the normal percentage of carbon dioxide (CO_2) in the atmosphere is
  A. 5%
  B. 40%
  C. 78%
  D. 0.03%

5. At sea level, the alveolar water vapor pressure is normally about
  A. 0.2 torr
  B. 47 torr
  C. 0.0 torr
  D. 40 torr

6. If a patient is receiving an $F_{I_{O_2}}$ of 0.60 on a day when the barometric pressure is 725 mm Hg, and if the Pa_{CO_2} is 50 torr, what is the patient's alveolar oxygen tension (PA_{O_2})?
  A. 177 torr
  B. 233 torr
  C. 344 torr
  D. 415 torr

7. The normal transit time for blood through the alveolar-capillary system is about
  A. 0.25 second
  B. 0.50 second
  C. 0.75 second
  D. 1.0 second

8. Under normal resting conditions, the diffusion of oxygen and carbon dioxide is usually completed in about
  1. 0.25 second
  2. 0.50 second
  3. 0.75 second
  4. 1.0 second
  5. one-third of the time available
    A. 2 only
    B. 3 only
    C. 4 and 5 only
    D. 1 and 5 only

9. Which of the following states that the rate of gas diffusion is inversely proportional to the weight of the gas?
   A. Graham's law
   B. Charles' law
   C. Henry's law
   D. Gay-Lussac's law

10. According to Fick's law, gas diffusion is
    1. directly proportional to the thickness of the tissue
    2. indirectly proportional to the diffusion constants
    3. directly proportional to the difference in partial pressure of the gas between the two sides
    4. indirectly proportional to the tissue area
       A. 1 only   C. 4 only
       B. 3 only   D. 2 and 3 only

Clinical Application Questions

Case 1

1. As a result of the severe left heart failure and increased pulmonary blood pressure in the case, fluid moved out of the pulmonary capillaries and into the extracapillary spaces. The pathologic process caused the thickness of the alveolar-capillary membrane to _____ _____.

2. Because gas diffusion is indirectly related to the thickness, the diffusion of oxygen across the alveolar-capillary membrane in this case _____.

3. While the physician was treating the patient's failing heart, the respiratory therapist worked to offset the patient's poor oxygenation by increasing the patient's _____, which is _____ of Fick's law.

4. The therapist achieved the goal in question 3 by increasing the patient's overall _____, and increasing the inspired _____.

Case 2

1. Which factor in Fick's law confirmed why the patient's oxygenation status was chronically low in this case?

   _____

2. Which factor in Fick's law was used therapeutically to improve the patient's oxygenation status?

   _____

3. Which factor in Fick's law caused the patient's oxygenation status to acutely worsen in this case?

   _____

4. In addition to the corticosteroid therapy, what factor in Fick's law was used therapeutically to improve the patient's oxygenation status?

   _____

Chapter 5

The Anatomy and Physiology of the Circulatory System

Objectives

By the end of this chapter, the student should be able to:

1. Describe the function of the following specialized cells (formed elements) in the plasma:
   —Red blood cells (Erythrocytes)
   —White blood cells (Leukocytes)
   —Platelets (Thrombocytes)
2. Describe the clinical connection associated with anemia.
3. Explain the clinical connection associated with complete blood cell count.
4. List the chemical components of plasma.
5. Describe the structure and function of the following components of the heart:
   —Inferior vena cava and superior vena cava
   —Right and left atria
   —Right and left ventricles
   —Pulmonary trunk
   —Pulmonary arteries
   —Pulmonary semilunar valve
   —Pulmonary veins
   —Tricuspid valve
   —Bicuspid valve (or mitral valve)
   —Aortic valve
   —Chordae tendineae
   —Papillary muscles
6. Describe the function of the major components of the pericardium.
7. Describe the clinical connection associated with pericarditis.
8. Describe the clinical connection associated with cardiac tamponade.
9. Describe the major components of the heart wall, including:
   —Epicardium
   —Myocardium
   —Endocardium

10. Describe the blood supply of the heart, including:
    —Left coronary artery
    • Circumflex branch
    • Anterior interventricular branch
    —Right coronary artery
    • Marginal branch
    • Posterior interventricular branch
    —Venous drainage
    • Great cardiac veins
    • Middle cardiac vein
    • Coronary sinus
    • Thebesian vein
11. Describe the clinical connection associated with myocardial infarction and treatment interventions of blocked arteries.
12. Describe how blood flows through the heart.
13. Describe the following components of the pulmonary and systemic vascular systems:
    —Arteries
    —Arterioles
    —Capillaries
    —Venules
    —Veins
14. Explain the neural control of the vascular system.
15. Describe the clinical connection associated with carotid sinus massage.
16. Describe the function of the baroreceptors.
17. Describe the clinical connection associated with the automobile accident victim with massive blood loss.
18. Define the following types of *pressures:*
    —Intravascular pressure
    —Transmural pressure
    —Driving pressure

(continues)

207

19. Describe how the following relate to the *cardiac cycle* and *blood pressure:*
    —Ventricular systole
    —Ventricular diastole
20. List the *intraluminal blood pressures* throughout the pulmonary and systemic vascular systems.
21. Describe how blood volume affects blood pressure, and include the following:
    —Stroke volume
    —Heart rate
    —Cardiac output
22. Identify the percentage of blood found throughout the various parts of the pulmonary and systemic systems.
23. Describe the influence of *gravity* on blood flow, and include how it relates to
    —Zone 1
    —Zone 2
    —Zone 3
24. Define the following *determinants of cardiac output:*
    —Ventricular preload
    —Ventricular afterload
    —Myocardial contractility
25. Describe the clinical connection associated with congestive heart failure.

26. Describe the clinical connection associated with left ventricular heart failure and pulmonary edema.
27. Define *vascular resistance*.
28. Describe how the following affect the pulmonary vascular resistance:
    —Active mechanisms
      • Abnormal blood gas values
      • Pharmacologic stimulation
      • Pathologic conditions
    —Passive mechanisms
      • Increased pulmonary arterial pressure
      • Increased left atrial pressure
      • Lung volume and transpulmonary pressure changes
      • Blood volume changes
      • Blood viscosity changes
29. Describe the clinical connection associated with cor pulmonale.
30. Describe the clinical connection associated with the cardiopulmonary hazards of positive pressure ventilation.
31. Complete the review questions at the end of this chapter.

The transport of oxygen from the lungs to the cells of the body and the transport of carbon dioxide from the tissue cells to the lungs is a function of blood flow. Thus, when the flow of blood is inadequate, good alveolar ventilation is of little value. The circulatory system consists of the **blood**, the **heart** (pump), and the **vascular system**.

The Blood

As shown in Figure 5–1, whole **blood** consists of a variety of specialized cells, called **formed elements**, which are suspended in a liquid matrix called **plasma**. Blood makes up about 8 percent of the total body weight. The average total blood volume in the adult male is about 5 to 6 liters and about 4 to 5 liters in the adult female. The *formed elements* make up about 45 percent, and the plasma makes up about 55 percent of the total blood volume. The formed elements are composed of the **red blood cells**, the **white blood cells** (neutrophils, lymphocytes, monocytes, eosinophils, and basophils), and **platelets**. The *plasma* is composed of about 91 percent water, 7 percent proteins (albumins, globulins, and fibrinogen), and 2 percent other substances (electrolytes, nutrients, respiratory, gases, waste products, and regulatory substances).

The functions of blood are to (1) transport oxygen to the tissue cells and carbon dioxide to the lungs; (2) transport nutrients and waste products;

Figure 5–1

Composition of whole blood.

© Cengage Learning 2013

Composition of whole blood

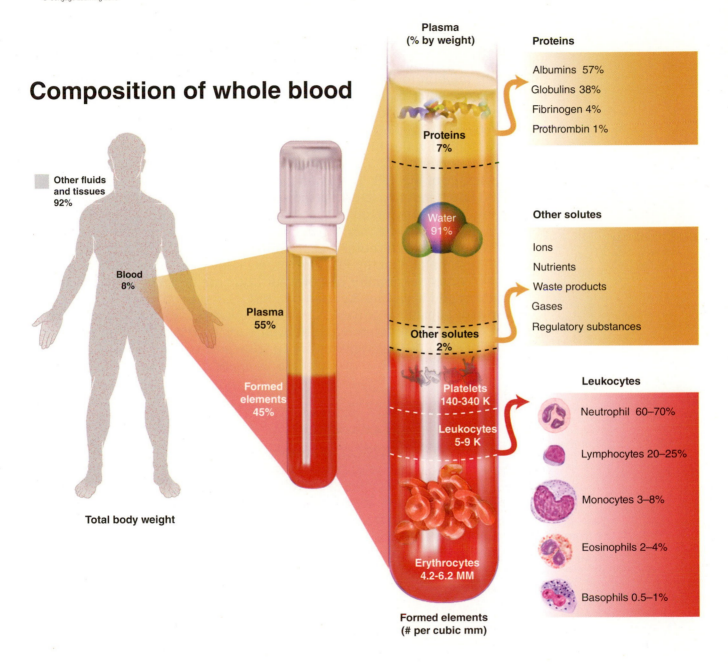

Plasma (% by weight)

Proteins
Albumins 57%
Globulins 38%
Fibrinogen 4%
Prothrombin 1%

Proteins 7%

Water 91%

Other solutes
Ions
Nutrients
Waste products
Gases
Regulatory substances

Other solutes 2%

Leukocytes
Neutrophil 60–70%
Lymphocytes 20–25%
Monocytes 3–8%
Eosinophils 2–4%
Basophils 0.5–1%

Platelets 140–340 K
Leukocytes 5-9 K
Erythrocytes 4.2-6.2 MM

Formed elements (# per cubic mm)

Other fluids and tissues 92%

Blood 8%

Plasma 55%

Formed elements 45%

Total body weight

(3) transport processed molecules from one part of the body to another—for example, lactic acid is carried by the blood to the liver, where it is converted into glucose; (4) transport regulatory hormones and enzymes; (5) regulate the pH and osmosis; (6) maintain body temperature; (7) protect against foreign substance; and (8) form clots.

Red Blood Cells (Erythrocytes)

The primary function of red blood cells (RBCs), or erythrocytes, is to transport oxygen from the lungs to the tissues and to transport carbon dioxide from the tissue cells to the lungs. In the normal adult, the number of RBCs ranges between 4.2 and 6.2 million per each millimeter of blood (mm^3). The average RBC count for the adult male is about 5.8 million per mm^3, and the average adult female is about 4.8 million per mm^3. The percentage of RBCs in relation to the total blood volume is known as the hematocrit. In the normal adult male, the hematocrit is about 45 percent, and about 42 percent in the normal adult female. In the healthy newborn, the hematocrit ranges between 45 and 60 percent.

Microscopically, the RBCs appear as biconcave discs, averaging about 7.5 μm in diameter and 2.5 μm in thickness, with the edges that are thicker than the center of the cell. The biconcave shape increases the surface area of the RBC compared to a flat shaped disc the same size. The greater surface area enhances the movement of gases into and out of the RBC. The RBCs are produced in the red bone marrow in the spongy bone of the cranium, bodies of vertebrae, ribs, sternum, and proximal epiphyses of the humerus and femur. It is estimated that the RBCs are produced at the rate of 2 million cells per second. An equal number of worn-out RBCs are destroyed each second by the spleen and liver. The life span of a RBC is about 120 days.

The major substance of the RBCs is hemoglobin, which occupies about one-third of the cells' volume and accounts for its red color. The primary functions of the RBC hemoglobin are to transport oxygen from the lungs to the tissue cells, and to transport carbon dioxide from the tissue cells to the lung.[1]

White Blood Cells (Leukocytes)

The white blood cells (WBCs), or leukocytes, protect the body against invading microorganism—for example, bacteria, viruses, parasites, toxins, and tumors—and work to remove dead cells and debris from the body. There are five different types of WBCs, which are classified as either *granulocytes* or *agranulocytes*, according to (1) the presence or absence of granules and (2) the staining characteristics of their cytoplasm:

Granulocytes include the following three WBCs—named according to their cytoplasmic staining properties—that have large granules embedded in their cytoplasm:

- Neutropils
- Eosinophils
- Basophils

Agranulocytes include the following two WBCs—leukocytes without cytoplasmic granules:

- Lymphocytes
- Monocytes

---

[1] The role of hemoglobin in the transport of oxygen and carbon dioxide is discussed in detail in Chapter 6.

Clinical Connection—5-1

Anemia

Anemia is defined as a deficiency of hemoglobin in the blood. It can be caused by a reduced number of red blood cells, a decrease in the amount of hemoglobin in each red blood cell, or both. A decreased hemoglobin level decreases the ability of blood to transport oxygen. Common causes of anemia include:

- **Nutritional deficiency (iron deficiency anemia)** is caused by a reduced intake or absorption of iron. This form of anemia results in a reduced hemoglobin production and smaller red blood cells (microcytic).

- **Hemorrhagic anemia** is caused by a blood loss, such as can result from trauma, ulcers, or excessive menstrual bleeding. Chronic blood loss, in which small amounts of blood are lost over a period of time, can also cause iron-deficiency anemia.

- **Folate deficiency**—an inadequate intake of folate in the diet—can cause anemia. Common sources of folate include brewer's yeast, lentils, romaine lettuce, pinto beans, okra, black beans, black-eye peas, spinach, and kidney beans. Folate deficiency is commonly seen in pregnant women, the poor, and chronic alcoholics.

- **Pernicious anemia** is caused by an inadequate dietary intake of vitamin B_{12}. Vitamin B_{12} is important for folate synthesis. A vitamin B_{12} deficiency causes a secondary folate deficiency. Thus, a vitamin B_{12} deficiency also causes a decreased production of red blood cells that are larger than normal.

- **Hemolytic anemia** can develop when the red blood cells rupture or are destroyed at an excessive rate. Causes of hemolytic anemia include inherited defects within the red blood cells, drugs, snake venom, artificial heart valves, autoimmune disease, or hemolytic disease of the newborn.

- **Aplastic anemia** is caused by the inability of the bone marrow to produce red blood cells. Causes of aplastic anemia include chemicals (e.g., benzene), drugs (e.g., certain antibiotics and sedatives), or radiation.

- **Sickle-cell anemia** is an autosomal recessive hereditary disorder found mostly in people of African ancestry, and occasionally among people of Mediterranean heritage. The hemoglobin in a person with sickle-cell anemia causes the red blood cells to become sickle-shaped and rigid—resulting in plugging of small blood vessels. They are also more fragile than normal red blood cells. In severe cases, sickle-cell anemia is usually fatal before the person is 30 years of age.

Unlike the red blood cells, which are confined to the blood vessels, the WBCs are able to leave the blood vessels—a process called **diapedesis**—when needed for inflammatory or immune responses. Diapedesis is activated by chemical signals released by the damaged cells (**positive chemotaxis**). Once the WBCs are out of the blood stream, they form cytoplasmic extensions that are used to migrate through the tissue spaces toward the damaged cells. This unique WBC motility is called **ameboid movement**.

The normal average number of WBCs ranges between 5000 and 9000 cells/mm³. An overall increase in the number of WBCs is called **leukocytosis**. An overall decrease in the number of WBCs is called **leukopenia.** A patient's WBC count is obtained from the **differential WBC count**, which is a component of one of the most useful and frequently performed diagnostic blood test called the **complete blood cell count**, or simple the **CBC** (see Clinical Connection 5–2: Complete Blood Cell Count, page 212). In a differential

Table 5–1		
Differential Count of White Blood Cells*		
Class	**Normal Range (%)**	**Typical Value (%)****
Neutrophils	65–75	65
Lymphocytes	20–25	25
Monocytes	3–8	6
Eosinophils	2–5	3
Basophils	0.5–1	1
Total	100	100

© Cengage Learning 2013

* The sum of the percentage of any differential count must, of course, always be 100%.

** A good mnemonic phrase to help remember percent values in decreasing order is the following: "**N**ever **L**et **M**onkeys **E**at **B**ananas."

WBC count, the proportions of each type of white blood cell are reported as percentages of the total WBC count. Because these numbers change certain abnormal conditions, they have clinical significance. For example, during an asthmatic episode, the percentage of eosinophils is elevated. Table 5–1 provides the WBC percentages.

Granulocytes

Neutrophils. The neutrophils cytoplasmic granules are numerous and stain light purple. Because the nuclei of the neutrophils have two, three, or more lobes, they are also called polymorphoneuclear leukocytes. Under normal conditions, the neutrophil numbers average about 65 percent of the total WBC count. The neutrophils are very mobile, active phagocytic cells. The cytoplasmic granules in the neutrophils contain powerful lysosomes, which are digestivelike enzymes that phagocytize invading bacteria.

Eosinophils. The eosinophils contain cytoplasmic granules that are large, numerous, and coarse in appearance. The cytoplasmic granules stain orangered. Their nuclei usually have two lobes. Normally, the esosinophils make up about 2 to 5 percent of the circulating WBCs. The eosinophils are numerous in the tissue lining the respiratory and digestive tracts. Eosinophils destroy protozoa and parasitic worms, and release antinflammatory substances in

Clinical Connection—5-2

Complete Blood Cell Count

The **complete blood cell count (CBC)** is one of the most useful and frequently ordered blood tests. The CBC consists of a battery of tests that measures the patient's standard red blood cell, white blood cell, and thrombocyte counts; the differential white blood cell count; hematocrit; hemoglobin content; and other characteristics of the formed blood elements. The respiratory therapist often reviews the patient's CBC when assessing the patient's red blood cell count, differential white blood cell count, hematocrit, and hemoglobin level.

antigen–antibody reactions. An elevated eosinophil count is commonly seen in asthmatic patients.

Basophils. The basophils are the least numerous of the WBCs, accounting for 0.5 to 1 percent of the total WBC count. The cytoplasmic granules are sparse, relatively large, and stain blue to dark purple. The nuclei of the basophils appear S-shaped and the cytoplasmic granules contain histamine and heparin. *Histamine* is an inflammatory substance that causes vasodilation and attracts other WBCs to the inflamed site. The *heparin* inhibits blood clotting (an anticoagulant). The basophils increase in number in both allergic and inflammatory reactions.

Agranulocytes

Lymphocytes. Lymphocytes are the second most numerous leukocytes in the blood, accounting for 25 percent of the total WBC count. The lymphocytes stain darkpurple and their nuclei are usually spherical in shape and surrounded by a thin rim of paleblue cytoplasm. Although large numbers of lymphocytes exist in the body, only a small amount is found in the bloodstream. Most of the lymphocytes are found in the lymphoid tissues (lymph nodes), where they play a number of important roles in immunity. For example, the T lymphocytes (T cells) function in the immune response by acting directly against virus-infected cells and tumors. The B lymphocytes (B cells) give rise to *plasma cells*, which produce antibodies (immunoglobulins) that work to inactivate invading antigens.

Monocytes. Monocytes are the largest of the WBCs and account for 4 to 8 percent of the WBCs. They have paleblue cytoplasm and a darkly stained U-shaped or kidney-shaped nucleus. In the tissue, monocytes differentiate into highly mobile macrophages with large appetites. They phagocytize bacteria, dead cells, cell fragments, and viral-infected cells. An increase in the number of monocytes is associated with chronic infections, such as tuberculosis.

Platelets

Platelets, or thrombocytes, are the smallest of the formed elements in the plasma. Platelets are roughly disk-shaped and average about 3 μm in diameter. The normal platelet count ranges from 250,000 to 500,000/mm³ of blood. The platelets play an important role in preventing blood loss from a traumatized area by (1) forming platelet plugs that seal holes in small blood vessels and (2) forming blood clots, which work to seal off larger tears in the blood vessels. The platelets also contain *serotonin*, which, when released, causes smooth-muscle constriction and reduced blood flow.

Table 5–2 on page 214 summarizes the formed elements of the blood.

Plasma

Plasma is the liquid part of the blood—whole blood without the formed elements. Plasma constitutes about 55 percent of the total blood volume (see Figure 5–1). Plasma is a pale yellow fluid that consists of about 91 percent water and 7 percent proteins (albumins, globulins, fibrinogen, and prothrombin) with other solutes (electrolytes, nutrients, respiratory, gases, waste products, and regulatory substances). Table 5–3 on page 215 outlines the chemical composition of plasma.

Table 5–2

Formed Elements of the Blood

Cell Type	Illustration	Description	Number of Cells/mm³ of Blood	Duration of Development (D) and Life Span (LS)	Function
Erythrocytes (red blood cells, RBCs)		Biconcave, anucleate disc; salmon-colored; diameter 7–8 μm	4–6 million	D: 5–7 days LS: 100–120 days	Transport oxygen and carbon dioxide
Leukocytes (white blood cells, WBCs)		Spherical, nucleated cells	4,000–11,000		
Neutrophils		Nucleus multilobed; inconspicuous cytoplasmic granules; diameter 10–14 μm	3000–7000	D: 6–9 days LS: 6 hours to a few days	Phagocytize bacteria
Eosinophils		Nucleus bilobed; red cytoplasmic granules; diameter 10–14 μm	100–400	D: 6–9 days LS: 8–12 days	Kill parasitic worms; destroy antigen-antibody complexes; inactivate some inflammatory chemicals of allergy
Basophils		Nucleus lobed; large blue-purple cytoplasmic granules; diameter 10–12 μm	20–50	D: 3–7 days LS: a few hours to a few days	Release histamine and other mediators of inflammation; contain heparin, an anticoagulant
Agranulocytes Lymphocytes		Nucleus spherical or indented; pale blue cytoplasm; diameter 5–17 μm	1500–3000	D: days to weeks LS: hours to years	Mount immune response by direct cell attack or via antibodies
Monocytes		Nucleus, U or kidney-shaped; gray-blue cytoplasm; diameter 14–24 μm	100–700	D: 2–3 days LS: months	Phagocytosis; develop into macrophages in tissues
Platelets		Discoid cytoplasmic fragments containing granules; stain deep purple; diameter 2–4 μm	250,000–500,000	D: 4–5 days LS: 5–10 days	Seal small tears in blood vessels; instrumental in blood clotting

Table 5–3

Chemical Composition of Plasma

Water		Food Subtances	
	93% of plasma weight	Amino acids	40 mg/100 mL
		Glucose/carbohydrates	100 mg/100 mL
Proteins		Lipids	500 mg/100 mL
Albumins	4.5 g/100 mL	Individual vitamins	0.0001–2.5 mg/100 mL
Globulins	2.5 g/100 mL		
Fibrinogen	0.3 g/100 mL	**Respiratory Gases**	
Prothrombin	< 0.1 g/100 mL	O_2	0.3 mL/100 mL
		CO_2	2 mL/100 mL
Electrolytes		N_2	0.9 mL/100 mL
Cations			
Na$^+$	143 mEq/L		
K$^+$	4 mEq/L	**Individual Hormones**	
Ca^{2+}	2.5 mEq/L		0.000001–0.05 mg/100 mL
Mg^{2+}	1.5 mEq/L		
Anions		**Waste Products**	
Cl$^-$	103 mEq/L	Urea	34 mg/100 mL
PO$_4$$^{3-}$	1 mEq/L	Creatinine	1 mg/100 mL
SO$_4$$^{2-}$	0.5 mEq/L	Uric acid	5 mg/100 mL
HCO$_3$$^-$	27 mEq/L	Bilirubin	0.2–1.2 mg/100 mL

The Heart

The **heart** is a hollow, four-chambered, muscular organ that consists of the upper right and left **atria** and the lower right and left **ventricles** (Figure 5–2 on page 216). The atria are separated by a thin muscular wall called the **interatrial septum**; the ventricles are separated by a thick muscular wall called the **interventricular septum**. The heart actually functions as two separate pumps. The right atrium and ventricle act as one pump to propel unoxygenated blood to the lungs. At the same time, the left atrium and ventricle act as another pump to propel oxygenated blood throughout the systemic circulation. Compared with the ventricles, the atria are small, thin-walled chambers. As a rule, they contribute little to the propulsive pumping activity of the heart.

Externally, the heart appears as a cone-shaped structure, weighing between 250 and 350 grams. It is enclosed in the **mediastinum** and extends obliquely between the second rib and the fifth intercostal space (Figure 5–3A on page 217). The heart rests on the superior surface of the diaphragm, anterior to the vertebral column and posterior to the sternum (Figure 5–3B). Both the left and right lateral portions of the heart are flanked by the lungs, which partially obscure it (Figure 5–3C). Approximately two-thirds of the heart lies to the left of the midsternal line; the balance extends to the right.

The **base** of the heart is broad and flat, about 9 cm, and points toward the right shoulder. The **apex** points inferiorly toward the left hip. When fingers are pressed between the fifth and sixth ribs just below the left nipple, the heart beat can be felt where the apex is in contact with the internal chest wall. This site is called the **point of maximal intensity (PMI)**.

Figure 5–2

A. Anterior view of the heart; **B.** posterior view of the heart.

© Cengage Learning 2013

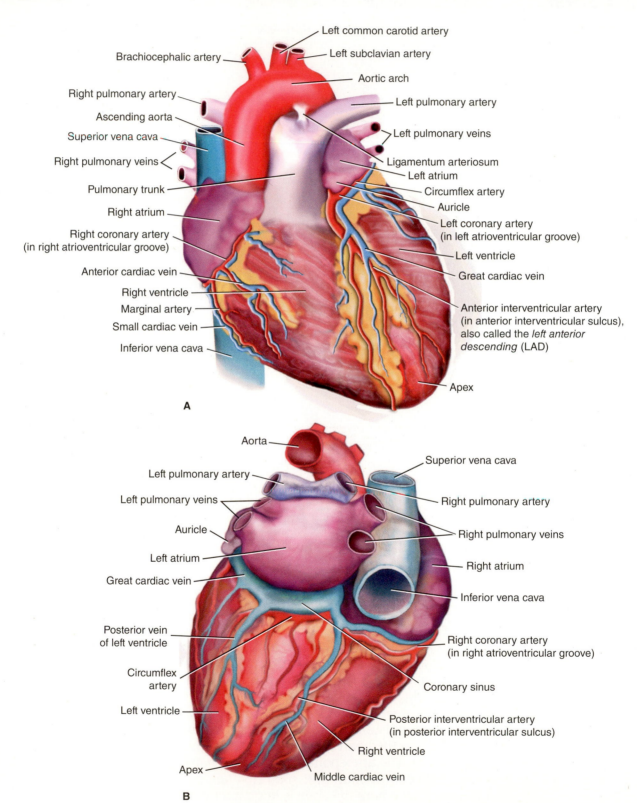

Figure 5–3

The relationship of the heart to the thorax: **A.** the relationship of the heart to the sternum, ribs, and diaphragm; **B.** across-sectional view showing the relationship of the heart to the thorax; and **C.** the relationship of the heart to the lungs and great vessels.

© Cengage Learning 2013

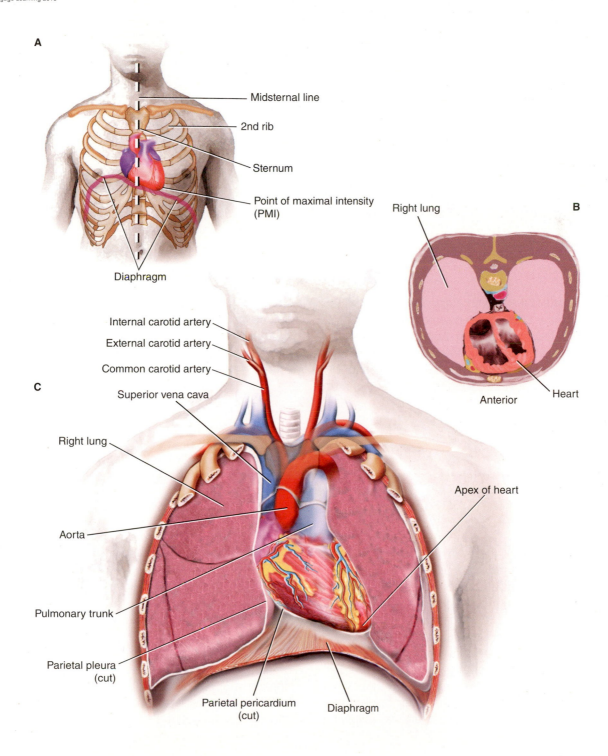

The Pericardium

The heart is enclosed in a double-walled sac called the pericardium (Figure 5–5). The outer wall, the fibrous pericardium, is a tough, dense, connective tissue layer. Its primary function is to (1) protect the heart; (2) anchor the heart to surrounding structures, such as the diaphragm and the great vessels; and (3) prevent the heart from overfilling. The inner wall, the serous pericardium, is a thin, slippery, serous membrane. The serous pericardium is composed of two layers: the parietal layer, which lines the internal surface of the fibrous pericardium, and the visceral layer (also called the epicardium). The epicardium is an integral part of the heart often described as the outermost layer of the heart. Between the two layers of the serous pericardium there is a film of serous fluid, which allows the parietal and visceral membranes to glide smoothly against one another, which in turn permits the heart to work in a relatively friction-free environment.

Clinical Connection—5-3

Pericarditis

Pericarditis is an inflammation of the pericardium. Although the cause is often unknown, it is associated with trauma, infection, myocardial infarction, and malignant neoplastic disease. Pericarditis can be extremely painful, with sensations radiating between the patient's back and chest—sometimes being confused with the pain of myocardial infarction (heart attack). Pericarditis can result in excessive fluid accumulation within the pericardial sac—a **cardiac tamponade** (see Clinical Connection 5–4: Cardiac Tamponade).

Clinical Connection—5-4

Cardiac Tamponade

A **cardiac tamponade** (also called cardiac compression or pericardial tamponade) is a potential medical emergency in which a large volume of fluid or blood collects in the pericardial sac. Because the fluid compresses the heart from the outside, the heart cannot adequately fill with blood during relaxation (diastole). Consequently, the patient's cardiac output and blood pressure rapidly decrease, causing the patient to die. Causes of a cardiac tamponade include trauma, rupture of the heart wall following a myocardial infarction, rupture of blood vessels caused by a malignant tumor, and radiation therapy. Treatment includes the insertion of a needle into the pericardial cavity and a syringe to drain the fluid.

Figure 5–4 shows the chest X-ray and CT scan of a 2-year-old boy who developed a cardiac tamponade after being accidently shot in right ventricle by his 4-year-old sister with their father's nail gun—and lived to tell about it!

Clinical Connection—5-4, continued

Figure 5–4

The chest X-ray and CT scan of a 2-year-old boy who developed a cardiac tamponade. **A.** Nail in a lateral chest X-ray. **B.** CT scan shows the nail lodged in the right ventricle.

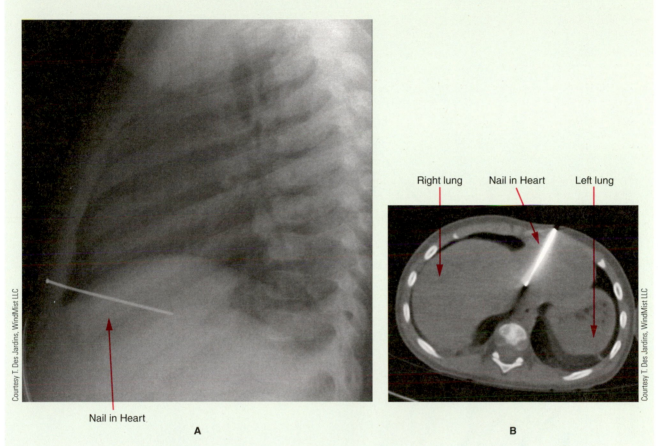

Right lung   Nail in Heart   Left lung

Nail in Heart

Courtesy T. Des Jardins, WindMist LLC

Courtesy T. Des Jardins, WindMist LLC

A

B

The Wall of the Heart

The heart wall is composed of the following three layers: epicardium (visceral pericardium), myocardium, and endocardium (see Figure 5–5 on page 220).

The **epicardium**, or visceral layer of the pericardium, is composed of a single sheet of squamous epithelial cells overlying delicate connective tissue. In older patients, the epicardium layer is often infiltrated with fat.

The **myocardium** is a thick contractile middle layer of uniquely constructed and arranged muscle cells. The myocardium forms the bulk of the heart. It is the layer that actually contracts. The contractile tissue of the myocardium is composed of fibers with the characteristic cross-striations of muscular tissue. The cardiac muscle cells are interconnected to form a network spiral or circular bundles (Figure 5–6 on page 221). These interlacing circular bundles effectively connect all the parts of the heart together. Collectively, the spiral bundles form a dense network called the **fibrous skeleton of the heart**, which reinforces the internal portion of the myocardium. Specifically modified tissue fibers of the myocardium constitute the conduction system of the heart (i.e., the sinoatrial [SA] node, the atrioventricular [AV] node, the AV bundle of His, and the Purkinje fibers) (discussed in more detail in Chapter 12).

Figure 5–5

The layers of the pericardium and the heart wall.

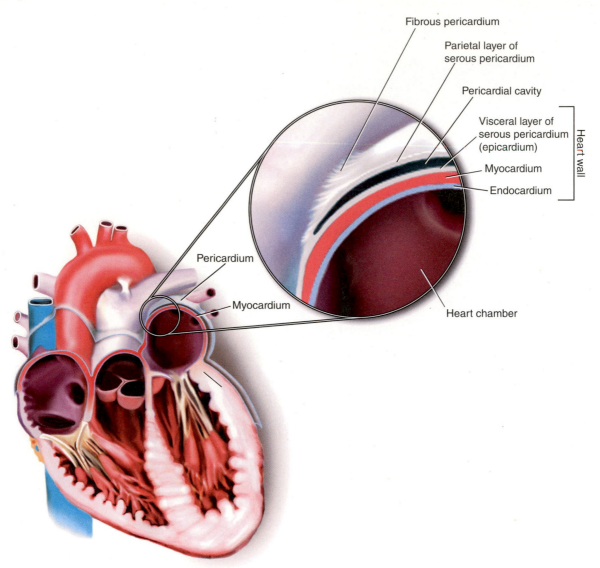

The **endocardium** is a glistening white sheet of squamous epithelium that rests on a thin connective tissue layer. Located in the inner myocardial surface, it lines the heart's chambers. It contains small blood vessels and a few bundles of smooth muscles. It is continuous with the endothelium of the great blood vessels—the superior and inferior vena cava.

Blood Supply of the Heart

Arterial Supply

The blood supply of the heart originates directly from the aorta by means of two arteries: the **left coronary artery** and the **right coronary artery**.

The left coronary artery divides into the **circumflex branch** and the **anterior interventricular branch** (Figure 5–7A). The circumflex branch runs posteriorly and supplies the left atrium and the posterior wall of the left

Figure 5–6

View of the spiral and circular arrangement of the cardiac muscle bundles.

© Cengage Learning 2013

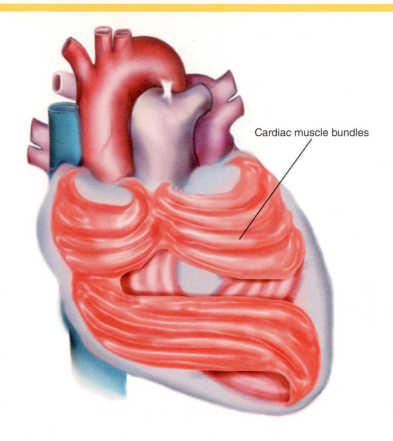

Cardiac muscle bundles

Figure 5–7

Coronary circulation: **A.** arterial vessels; **B.** venous vessels.

© Cengage Learning 2013

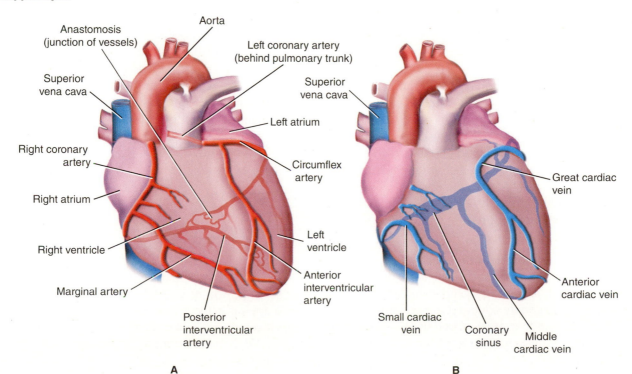

Anastomosis (junction of vessels)

Aorta

Left coronary artery (behind pulmonary trunk)

Superior vena cava

Superior vena cava

Right coronary artery

Left atrium

Circumflex artery

Right atrium

Left ventricle

Right ventricle

Anterior interventricular artery

Marginal artery

Great cardiac vein

Anterior cardiac vein

Posterior interventricular artery

Small cardiac vein

Coronary sinus

Middle cardiac vein

A

B

ventricle. The anterior interventricular branch travels toward the apex of the heart and supplies the anterior walls of both ventricles and the interventricular septum. The right coronary artery supplies the right atrium and then divides into the **marginal branch** and the **posterior interventricular branch**. The marginal branch supplies the lateral walls of the right atrium and right ventricle. The posterior interventricular branch supplies the posterior wall of both ventricles.

Venous Drainage

The venous system of the heart parallels the coronary arteries. Venous blood from the anterior side of the heart empties into the **great cardiac veins**; venous blood from the posterior portion of the heart is collected by the **middle cardiac vein** (see Figure 5–7B). The great and middle cardiac veins merge and empty into a large venous cavity within the posterior wall of the right atrium called the **coronary sinus**. A small amount of venous blood is collected by the **thebesian veins**, which empties directly into both the right and left atrium. The venous drainage that flows into the left atrium contributes to the normal anatomic shunt, the phenomenon whereby oxygenated blood mixes with deoxygenated blood (this concept is discussed in more detail in Chapter 6).

Clinical Connection—5-5

Myocardial Infarction—Common Diagnostic and Treatments Interventions for Blocked Coronary Arteries

Myocardial infarction (heart attack) is caused by a prolonged lack of blood flow—and oxygen delivery—to a part of the cardiac muscle. The most common cause of a myocardial infarction is a thrombus formation (blood clot) that blocks the coronary artery. Coronary arteries narrowed by atheroscleratic lesions increase the chances of myocardial infarction. If the blood supply to the heart is reestablished in about 20 minutes, no permanent tissue cell damage occurs. When the lack of oxygen is longer, cell death results. Common diagnostic and treatment interventions for a blocked coronary artery include the following:

1. **Cardiac catheterization** entails the insertion of a small plastic tube into an artery or vein and advancing it into the chambers of the heart or into the coronary arteries. Cardiac catheterization is used to examine blood flow to the heart, measure the oxygen concentration in the blood,

and determine how well the heart is pumping blood. The catheter is also used to inject a radiopaque dye into the coronary arteries—a procedure called **coronary angiography** (also called **coronary ateriography**). As the dye circulates throughout the arteries, a radiograph called an **angiogram** (also called an **arteriogram**) reveals the outline of the arteries as if they were made of bone.

2. **Angioplasty** entails inserting a long, small-diameter catheter with a small balloon tip into an artery (usually the femoral artery). It is threaded through the aorta and into each of the coronary arteries. During this procedure, the catheter movement is viewed on an X-ray screen. Once the catheter is in a coronary artery, a dye is injected into it. The dye, which can be viewed on the X-ray machine, reveals any blockages that may be present. At this point, there

Clinical Connection—5-5, continued

are several types of interventional procedures the doctor may perform, including the following:

- **Balloon angioplasty**—once the balloon tip has entered the partially occluded coronary artery, it is inflated to compress and flatten the fatty deposits against the vessel walls—resulting is a wider coronary artery and an increased blood flow to the heart.

- **Stent**—a small metal mesh tube, called a stent, can be inserted into the artery to help prevent future blockage. The stent acts as a scaffold to provide support inside the coronary artery. Over a several-week period, the artery heals around the stent. Some stents contain medicine to reduce the risk of reblockage. See Figure 5–8, which illustrates pre- and post-stent.

3. A **coronary bypass** is a surgical procedure that entails harvesting healthy blood vessels from other parts of the patient's body (usually leg veins) and using them to bypass obstructions in the coronary arteries. The respiratory therapist routinely manages the mechanical ventilator for coronary bypass patients after surgery.

Figure 5–8

Angiogram showing **A.** pre-stent and **B.** post-stent. Note the wires used to close the chest after a past open heart surgery.

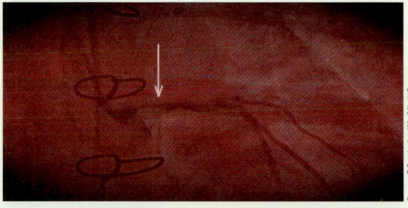

A

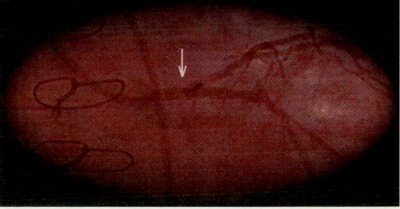

B

Courtesy T. Des Jardins, WindMist LLC

Blood Flow through the Heart

As shown in Figure 5–9, the right atrium receives venous blood from the inferior vena cava and superior vena cava. A small amount of cardiac venous blood enters the right atrium by means of the thebesian veins. This blood is low in oxygen and high in carbon dioxide. A one-way valve, the tricuspid valve, lies between the right atrium and the right ventricle. The tricuspid valve gets it name from its three valve leaflets, or cusps. The tricuspid leaflets are held in place by tendinous cords called chordae tendinae, which are secured to the ventricular wall by the papillary muscles. When the ventricles contract, the tricuspid valve closes and blood leaves the right ventricle through the pulmonary trunk and enters the lungs by way of the right and left pulmonary arteries. The pulmonary semilunar valve separates the right ventricle from the pulmonary trunk.

After blood passes through the lungs, it returns to the left atrium by way of the pulmonary veins. These vessels are best seen in a posterior view of the heart (see Figure 5–2B). The returning blood is high in oxygen and low in carbon dioxide. The bicuspid valve (also called the mitral valve) lies between the left atrium and the left ventricle. This valve, which consists of two cusps, prevents blood from returning to the left atrium during ventricular contraction. Similar to the tricuspid valve, the bicuspid valve is also held in position by chordae tendinae and papillary muscles. The left ventricle pumps blood through the ascending aorta. The aortic valve, which lies at the base of the ascending aorta, has semilunar cusps (valves) that close when the ventricles relax. The closure of the semilunar valves prevent the backflow of blood into the left ventricle (see Figure 5–9).

Figure 5–9

Internal chambers and valves of the heart.

© Cengage Learning 2013

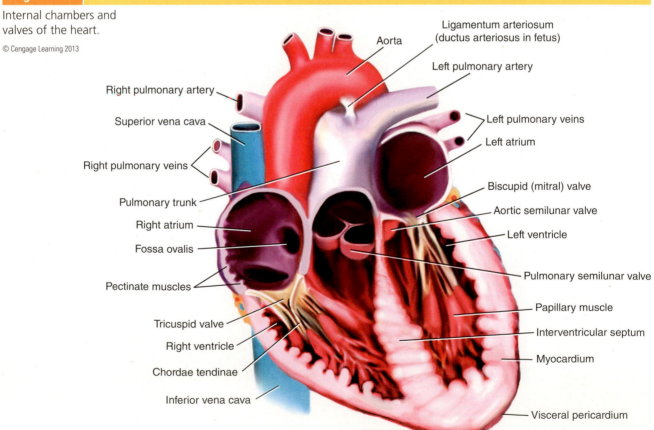

The Pulmonary and Systemic Vascular Systems

The vascular network of the circulatory system is composed of two major subdivisions: the systemic system and the pulmonary system (Figure 5–10). The pulmonary system begins with the pulmonary trunk and ends in the left atrium. The systemic system begins with the aorta and ends in the right atrium. Both systems are composed of arteries, arterioles, capillaries, venules, and veins (refer to Figure 1–33).

Figure 5–10

Pulmonary and systemic circulation. Pulmonary circulation is indicated by pink arrows; systemic circulation is indicated by blue arrows.

© Cengage Learning 2013

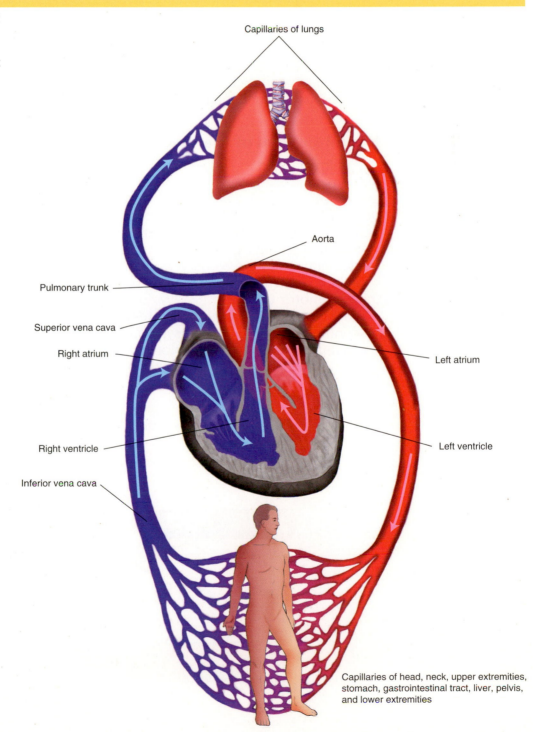

Capillaries of lungs

Aorta

Pulmonary trunk

Superior vena cava

Right atrium

Left atrium

Right ventricle

Left ventricle

Inferior vena cava

Capillaries of head, neck, upper extremities, stomach, gastrointestinal tract, liver, pelvis, and lower extremities

Arteries are vessels that carry blood away from the heart. The arteries are strong, elastic vessels that are well suited for carrying blood under high pressure in the systemic system. The arteries subdivide as they move away from the heart into smaller vessels and, eventually, into vessels called arterioles. Arterioles play a major role in the distribution and regulation of blood pressure and are referred to as the resistance vessels.

Gas exchange occurs in the capillaries. In the capillaries of the pulmonary system, gas exchange is called external respiration (gas exchange between blood and air). In the capillaries of the systemic system, gas exchange is called internal respiration (gas exchange between blood and tissues).

The venules are tiny veins continuous with the capillaries. The venules empty into the veins, which carry blood back to the heart. The veins differ from the arteries in that they are capable of holding a large amount of blood with very little pressure change. Because of this unique feature, the veins are called capacitance vessels. Approximately 60 percent of the body's total blood volume is contained within the venous system.

Neural Control of the Vascular System

The pulmonary arterioles and most of the arterioles in the systemic circulation are controlled by sympathetic impulses. Sympathetic fibers are found in the arteries, arterioles and, to a lesser degree, in the veins (Figure 5–11). The vasomotor center, which is located in the medulla oblongata, governs the number of sympathetic impulses sent to the vascular systems. Under normal circumstances, the vasomotor center transmits a continual stream of sympathetic impulses to the blood vessels, maintaining the vessels in a moderate state of constriction all the time. This state of vascular contraction is called the vasomotor tone.

The vasomotor center coordinates both vasoconstriction and vasodilation by controlling the number of sympathetic impulses that leave the medulla. For example, when the vasomotor center is activated to constrict a particular

Figure 5–11

Neural control of the vascular system. Sympathetic neural fibers to the arterioles are especially abundant.

© Cengage Learning 2013

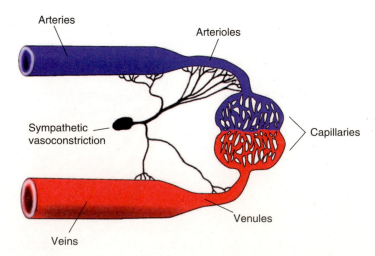

vascular region (i.e., more than the normal state of constriction), it does so by increasing the number of sympathetic impulses to that vascular area. In contrast, the vasomotor center initiates vasodilation by reducing the number of sympathetic impulses sent to a certain vascular region. (The major vascular beds in the systemic system that are *not* controlled by this mechanism are the arterioles of the heart, brain, and skeletal muscles. Sympathetic impulses to these vessels cause vasodilation.) In addition to the sympathetic control, blood flow through the large veins can be affected by abdominal and intrathoracic pressure changes.

Working together, the vasomotor center and the cardiac centers in the medulla oblongata regulate the arterial blood pressure in response to signals received from special pressure receptors located throughout the body. These pressure receptors are called **arterial baroreceptors**.

The Baroreceptor Reflex

Specialized stretch receptors called **baroreceptors** (also called *pressoreceptors*) are located in the walls of the carotid arteries and the aorta. In the **carotid arteries**, the baroreceptors are found in the carotid sinuses located high in the neck where the common carotid arteries divide into the external and internal carotid arteries (Figure 5–12 on page 228). The walls of the carotid sinuses are thin and contain a large number of branching, vinelike nerve endings that are sensitive to stretch or distortion. The afferent fibers from the carotid sinuses travel with the **glossopharyngeal nerve** (ninth cranial) to the medulla. In the aorta, the baroreceptors are located in the **aortic arch** (see Figure 5–12). The afferent fibers from the aortic arch baroreceptors travel with the **vagus nerve** (tenth cranial).

The baroreceptors regulate the arterial blood pressure by initiating reflex adjustments to changes in blood pressure. For example, when the arterial pressure decreases, the neural impulses transmitted from the baroreceptors to the vasomotor and cardiac centers in the medulla also decrease. This causes the medulla to increase its sympathetic activity, which in turn causes an increase in the following:

- Heart rate.
- Myocardial force of contraction.
- Arterial constriction.
- Venous constriction.

The net result is (1) an increased cardiac output (because of an increased heart rate and stroke volume), (2) an increase in the total peripheral resistance (primarily induced by arterial constriction), and (3) the return of blood pressure toward normal. The vascular constriction occurs primarily in the abdominal region (including the liver, spleen, pancreas, stomach, intestine, kidneys, skin, and skeletal muscles).

In contrast, when the blood pressure increases, the neural impulses from the arterial baroreceptors increase. This causes the medulla to decrease its sympathetic activity, which in turn reduces both the cardiac output and the total peripheral resistance.

Finally, the baroreceptors function as short-term regulators of arterial blood pressure. That is, they respond instantly to any blood pressure change to restore the blood pressure toward normal (to the degree possible in the situation). If, however, the factors responsible for moving the arterial pressure

Location of the arterial baroreceptors.

away from normal persist for more than a few days, the arterial barorecep-tors will eventually come to "accept" the new pressure as normal. For exam-ple, in individuals who have chronically high blood pressure (*hypertension*), the baroreceptors still operate, but at a higher level—in short, their operating point is reset at a higher level.

Other Baroreceptors

Baroreceptors are also found in the large arteries, large veins, and pulmonary vessels and in the cardiac walls themselves. Functionally, most of these receptors are similar to the baroreceptors in the carotid sinuses and aortic arch in that they send an increased rate of neural transmissions to the medulla in response to increased pressure. By means of these additional receptors, the medulla gains a further degree of sensitivity to venous, atrial, and ventricular pressures. For example, a slight decrease in atrial pressure initiates sympathetic activity even before there is a decrease in cardiac output and, therefore, a decrease in the arterial blood pressure great enough to be detected by the aortic and carotid baroreceptors.

Clinical Connection—5-6

Carotid Sinus Massage

In the emergency department and critcal care areas, the respiratory therapist will commonly work alongside the attending physician who is performing carotid sinus massage on a patient experiencing cardiac arrhymthmias. **Carotid sinus massage** involves the firm rubbing of the patient's neck over the bifurcation of the carotid artery at the angle of the jaw (see Figure 5–13). The carotid sinus contains numerous baroeceptors that monitor and maintain normal blood pressure. Massaging the carotid sinus stimulates the nerve endings located in the carotid artery walls that are capable of slowing the heart rate. Carotid sinus massage is used to slow a patient's heart rate during episodes of atrial flutter, fibrillation, and some tachycardias. It may stop the arrthymia completely. Carotid sinus message may also make the discomfort of angina pertoris disappear. Do not attempt to do this on yourself or others.

Figure 5–13

Carotid sinus massage.

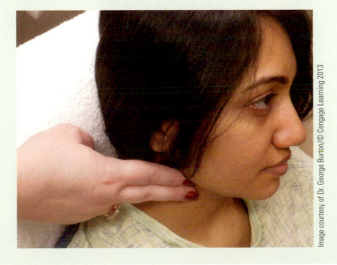

Image courtesy of Dr. George Burton/© Cengage Learning 2013

Schematic of a blood vessel and an alveolus, showing the types of blood pressures used to study blood flow. Within the blood vessel, the intravascular pressure at point A is 15 mm Hg, and the intravascular pressure at point B is 5 mm Hg. The pressure within the alveolus (which represents the pressure surrounding the blood vessel) is zero. In view of these numbers, the following can be stated: (1) The transmural pressure at point A is +15 mm Hg, (2) the transmural pressure at point B is +5 mm Hg, and (3) the driving pressure between point A and point B is 10 mm Hg.

© Cengage Learning 2013

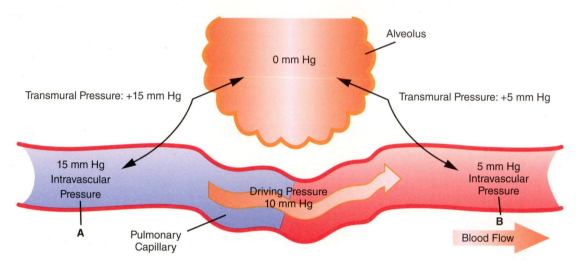

Pressures in the Pulmonary and Systemic Vascular Systems

Three different types of pressures are used to study the blood flow: intravascular, transmural, and driving.

Intravascular pressure is the actual blood pressure in the lumen of any vessel at any point, relative to the barometric pressure. This pressure is also known as the intraluminal pressure.

Transmural pressure is the difference between the intravascular pressure of a vessel and the pressure surrounding the vessel. The transmural pressure is *positive* when the pressure inside the vessel exceeds the pressure outside the vessel and *negative* when the pressure inside the vessel is less than the pressure surrounding the vessel.

Driving pressure is the difference between the pressure at one point in a vessel and the pressure at any other point downstream in the vessel.

Figure 5–14 illustrates the different types of pressures used to study the flow of blood.

Clinical Connection—5-7

Case Study—Automobile Accident Victim with Massive Blood Loss

In the **Clinical Application Section—Case 1** (Page 248), the respiratory therapists is called to help care for a 16-year-old girl involved in an automobile accident. In the emergency room, the patient is unconscious and hypotensive from massive blood loss. The case illustrates (1) the activation of the barorreceptor reflex, (2) hypovolemia and how it relates to preload, (3) negative transmural pressure, and (4) the effects of gravity blood flow. This case further illustrates how these mechanisms can be offset by lowering the patient's head and elevating the legs and replacing the volume of blood loss with Ringer's solution.

The Cardiac Cycle and Its Effect on Blood Pressure

The arterial blood pressure rises and falls in a pattern that corresponds to the phases of the cardiac cycle. When the ventricles contract (ventricular systole), blood is forced into the pulmonary artery and the aorta, and the pressure in these arteries rises sharply. The maximum pressure generated during ventricular contraction is the **systolic pressure**. When the ventricles relax (ventricular diastole), the arterial pressure drops. The lowest pressure that remains in the arteries prior to the next ventricular contraction is the **diastolic pressure** (Figure 5–15). In the systemic system, normal systolic pressure is about 120 mm Hg and normal diastolic pressure is about 80 mm Hg. In the pulmonary system, the normal systolic pressure is about 25 mm Hg and the normal diastolic pressure is about 8 mm Hg (Figure 5–16 on page 232).

The mean arterial blood pressure (MAP) can be estimated by measuring the systolic blood pressure (SBP) and the diastolic blood pressure (DBP) and using the following formula:

$$MAP = \frac{SBP + (2 \times DBP)}{3}$$

For example, the mean arterial blood pressure of the systemic system, which has a systolic pressure of 120 mm Hg and a diastolic pressure of 80 mm Hg, would be calculated as follows:

$$MAP = \frac{SBP + (2 \times DBP)}{3}$$
$$= \frac{120 + (2 \times 80)}{3}$$
$$= \frac{280}{3}$$
$$= 93 \text{ mm Hg}$$

In the normal adult, the MAP ranges between 80 to 100 mm Hg. When the MAP falls below 60 mm Hg, the blood flow through the brain and kidneys is significantly reduced. Organ deterioration and failure may occur in minutes.

The pulmonary circulation is a low-pressure system. The mean pressure in the pulmonary artery is about 15 mm Hg and the mean pressure in the left atrium is about 5 mm Hg. Thus, the driving pressure needed to move blood through

Figure 5–15

Sequence of cardiac contraction: **A.** ventricular diastole and atrial systole; **B.** ventricular systole and atrial diastole.

© Cengage Learning 2013

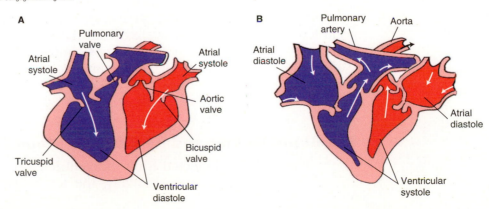

Figure 5–16

Summary of diastolic and systolic pressures in various segments of the circulatory system. Red vessels: oxygenated blood. Blue vessels: Deoxygenated blood.

© Cengage Learning 2013

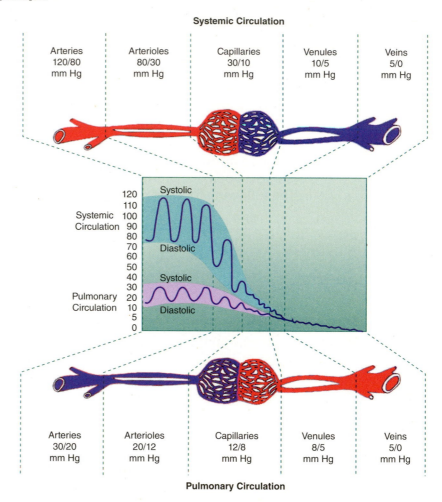

the lungs is 10 mm Hg. In contrast, the mean intraluminal pressure in the aorta is about 100 mm Hg and the mean right atrial pressure is about 2 mm Hg, making the driving pressure through the systemic system about 98 mm Hg. Compared with the pulmonary circulation, the pressure in the systemic system is about 10 times greater. Figure 5–17 shows the mean intraluminal blood pressures throughout both the pulmonary and systemic vascular systems.

The surge of blood rushing into the arterial system during each ventricular contraction causes the elastic walls of the arteries to expand. When the ventricular contraction stops, the pressure drops almost immediately and the arterial walls recoil. This alternating expansion and recoil of the arterial wall can be felt as a pulse in systemic arteries that run close to the skin's surface. Figure 5–18 on page 234 shows the major sites where a pulse can be detected by palpation.

The Blood Volume and Its Effect on Blood Pressure

The volume of blood ejected from the ventricle during each contraction is called the **stroke volume**. Normally, the stroke volume ranges between

Figure 5–17

Mean intraluminal blood pressure (in mm Hg) at various points in the pulmonary and systemic vascular systems.

© Cengage Learning 2013

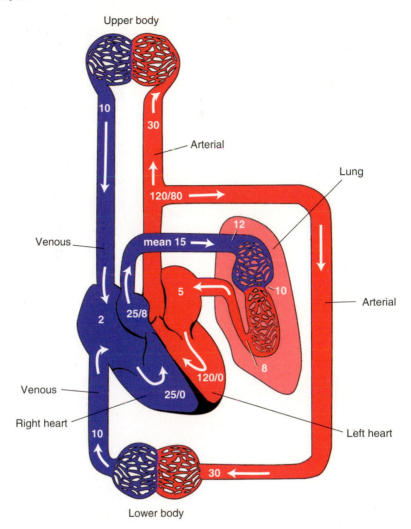

Upper body

10

30

Arterial

Lung

120/80

12

Venous

mean 15

10

5

Arterial

2

25/8

8

120/0

Venous

25/0

Right heart

Left heart

10

30

Lower body

40 and 80 mL. The total volume of blood discharged from the ventricles per minute is called **cardiac output**. The cardiac output (CO) is calculated by multiplying the stroke volume (SV) by the heart rate (HR) per minute (CO = SV × HR). Thus, if the stroke volume is 70 mL, and the heart rate is 72 beats per minute (bpm), the cardiac output is 5040 mL/min.

Under normal circumstances, the cardiac output directly influences blood pressure. In other words, *when either the stroke volume or heart rate increases, the blood pressure increases.* Conversely, when the stroke volume or heart rate decreases, the blood pressure decreases.

Although the total blood volume varies with age, body size, and sex, the normal adult volume is about 5 L. Of this volume, about 75 percent is in the systemic circulation, 15 percent in the heart, and 10 percent in the pulmonary circulation. Overall, about 60 percent of the total blood volume is in the veins, and about 10 percent is in the arteries. Normally, the pulmonary capillary bed contains about 75 mL of blood, although it has the capacity of about 200 mL.

Figure 5–18

Major sites where an arterial pulse can be detected.

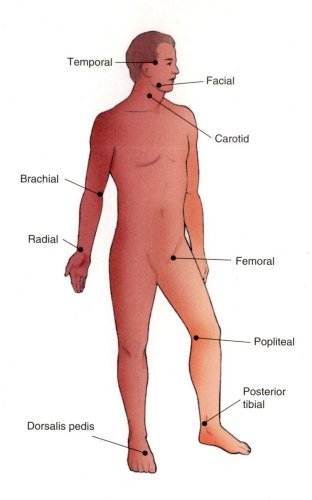

Temporal

Facial

Carotid

Brachial

Radial

Femoral

Popliteal

Posterior tibial

Dorsalis pedis

The Distribution of Pulmonary Blood Flow

In the upright lung, blood flow progressively decreases from the base to the apex (Figure 5–19). This linear distribution of blood is a function of (1) **gravity**, (2) **cardiac output**, and (3) **pulmonary vascular resistance**.

Gravity

Because blood is a relatively heavy substance, it is **gravity dependent**; that is, it naturally moves to the portion of the body, or portion of the organ, that is closest to the ground. In the average lung, there is a distance of about 30 cm between the base and the apex. The blood that fills the lung from the bottom to the top is analogous to a column of water 30 cm long and, therefore, exerts a pressure of about 30 cm H_2O (22 mm Hg) between the base and apex. Because the pulmonary artery enters each lung about midway between the top and bottom of the lung, the pulmonary artery pressure must be greater than 15 cm H_2O (11 mm Hg) to overcome the gravitational force and, thereby, supply blood to the lung apex. For this reason, most of the blood flows through (or falls into) the lower half of the lung—the gravity-dependent portion of the lung.

Figure 5–19

Distribution of pulmonary blood flow. In the upright lung, blood flow steadily increases from the apex to the base.

© Cengage Learning 2013

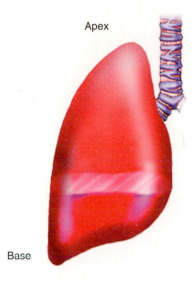

Apex

Base

As a result of the gravitational effect on blood flow, the intraluminal pressures of the vessels in the gravity-dependent area (lower lung region) are greater than the intraluminal pressures in the least gravity-dependent area (upper lung region). The high intraluminal pressure of the vessels in the gravity-dependent area causes the vessels to distend. As the vessels widen, the vascular resistance decreases and, thus, permits blood flow to increase. The fact that blood flow is enhanced as the vascular system widens is according to Poiseuille's law for flow ($\dot{V} = Pr^4$)

The position of the body can significantly change the gravity-dependent portion of the lungs. For example, when an individual is in the supine position (lying on the back), the gravity-dependent area is the posterior portion of the lungs; when an individual is in the prone position (lying on the stomach), the gravity-dependent region is the anterior portion of the lungs; when the person is lying on the side, the lower, lateral half of the lung nearest the ground is gravity dependent; when an individual is suspended upside down, the apices of the lungs become gravity dependent (Figure 5–20 on page 236).

Figure 5–21 on page 237 uses a three-zone model to illustrate the effects of gravity and alveolar pressure on the distribution of pulmonary blood flow.

In **Zone 1** (the least gravity-dependent area), the alveolar pressure is sometimes greater than both the arterial and the venous intraluminal pressures. As a result, the pulmonary capillaries can be compressed and blood is prevented from flowing through this region. Under normal circumstances, this situation does not occur, because the pulmonary arterial pressure (generated by the cardiac output) is usually sufficient to raise the blood to the top of the lungs and to overcome the alveolar pressure. There are, however, a variety of conditions—such as severe hemorrhage, dehydration, and positive pressure ventilation—that can result in the alveolar pressure being higher than the arterial and venous pressures. When the alveoli are ventilated but not perfused, no gas exchange can occur and **alveolar dead space** is said to exist (refer to Figure 2–40).

Figure 5–20

Blood flow normally moves into the gravity-dependent areas of the lungs. Thus, body position affects the distribution of the pulmonary blood flow as illustrated in the **A.** erect, **B.** supine, **C.** lateral, and **D.** upside-down positions.

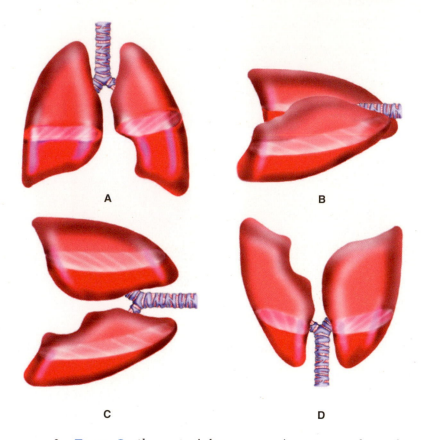

In **Zone 2**, the arterial pressure is greater than the alveolar pressure and, therefore, the pulmonary capillaries are perfused. Because the alveolar pressure is greater than the venous pressure, the effective driving pressure for blood flow is determined by the pulmonary arterial pressure minus the alveolar pressure—not the normal arterial-venous pressure difference. Thus, because the alveolar pressure is essentially the same throughout all the lung regions, and because the arterial pressure progressively increases toward the gravity-dependent areas of the lung, the effective driving pressure (arterial pressure minus alveolar pressure) steadily increases down the vertical axis of Zone 2. As a result, from the beginning of the upper portion of Zone 2 (the point at which the arterial pressure equals the alveolar pressure) to the lower portion of Zone 2 (the point at which the venous pressure equals the alveolar pressure) the flow of blood progressively increases.

In **Zone 3** (gravity-dependent area), both the arterial and the venous pressures are greater than the alveolar pressure and, therefore, blood flow through this region is constant. Because the arterial pressure and venous pressure both increase equally downward in Zone 3, the arterial-venous pressure difference and, therefore, blood flow is essentially the same throughout all of Zone 3.

Determinants of Cardiac Output

As described earlier, the cardiac output is equal to the stroke volume times the heart rate (CO = SV × HR). The stroke volume is determined by (1) ventricular preload, (2) ventricular afterload, and (3) myocardial contractility.

Figure 5–21

Relationship among gravity, alveolar pressure (P_A), pulmonary arterial pressure (P_a), and pulmonary venous pressure (P_v) in different lung zones. Note: The +2 cm H_2O pressure in the alveoli (e.g., during expiration) was arbitrarily selected for this illustration.

© Cengage Learning 2013

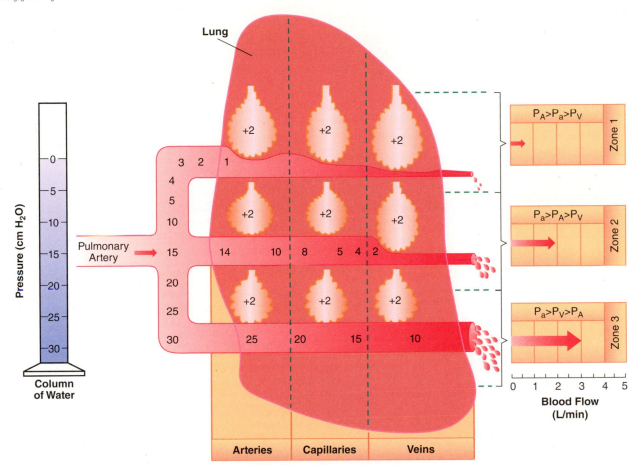

Ventricular Preload

Ventricular preload refers to the degree that the myocardial fiber is stretched prior to contraction (*end-diastole*). Within limits, the more the myocardial fiber is stretched during diastole (*preload*), the more strongly it will contract during systole and, therefore, the greater the myocardial contractility will be. This mechanism enables the heart to convert an increased venous return into an increased stroke volume. Beyond a certain point, however, the cardiac output does not increase as the preload increases.

Because the degree of myocardial fiber stretch (preload) is a function of the pressure generated by the volume of blood returning to the ventricle during diastole, ventricular preload is reflected in the **ventricular end-diastolic pressure (VEDP)**—which, in essence, reflects the **ventricular end-diastolic volume (VEDV)**. In other words, as the VEDV increases or decreases, the VEDP (and, therefore, the cardiac output) increases or decreases, respectively. It should be noted, however, that similar to lung compliance (C_L), VEDP and VEDV are also influenced by ventricular compliance. For example, when the ventricular compliance is decreased as a result of disease, the VEDP increases significantly more than the VEDV.

The relationship between the VEDP (degree of myocardial stretch) and cardiac output (stroke volume) is known as the **Frank-Starling curve** (Figure 5–22).

Ventricular Afterload

Ventricular afterload is defined as the force against which the ventricles must work to pump blood. It is determined by several factors, including (1) the volume and viscosity of the blood ejected, (2) the peripheral vascular resistance, and (3) the total cross-sectional area of the vascular space into which blood is ejected. The arterial systolic blood pressure best reflects the ventricular afterload. For example, as the arterial systolic pressure increases, the resistance (against which the heart must work to eject blood) also increases. Clinically, this condition is particularly serious in the patient with congestive heart failure and low stroke volume. By reducing the peripheral resistance (*afterload reduction*) in such patients, the stroke volume increases with little or no change in the blood pressure. This is because blood pressure (BP) is a function of the cardiac output (CO) times the systemic vascular resistance (SVR): BP = CO × SVR.

Figure 5–22

Frank-Starling curve. The Frank-Starling curve shows that the more the myocardial fiber is stretched as a result of the blood pressure that develops as blood returns to the chambers of the heart during diastole, the more the heart muscle will contract during systole. In addition, the heart muscle will contract with greater force. The stretch produced within the myocardium at end-diastole is called preload. Clinically, it would be best to determine the preload of the left ventricle by measuring the end-diastolic pressure of the left ventricle or left atrium. However, because this practice would be impractical at the patient's bedside, the best preload approximation of the left heart is the pulmonary capillary wedge pressure (PCWP). As shown here, the relationship of the PCWP (preload) to the left ventricular stroke work index (LVSWI) (force of contraction) may appear in four quadrants: (1) hypovolemia, (2) optimal function, (3) hypervolemia, and (4) cardiac failure.

© Cengage Learning 2013

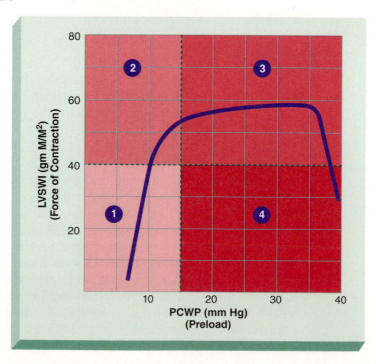

Clinical Connection—5-8

Congestive Heart Failure

Congestive heart failure (CHF) (also called left-heart failure) is the inability of the *left* ventricle to pump blood effectively. When a patient has CHF, the right ventricle continues to pump blood to the lungs, but the left ventricle does not adequately pump the returning blood from the lungs into the systemic circulation. As a result, the vascular system in the lungs become engorged with blood, the pulmonary capillary blood pressure increases, and fluid leaks out of the capillaries into the alveoli—causing the condition known as **pulmonary edema**. The respiratory therapist will frequently treat patients suffering from pulmonary edema. These patients are difficult to oxygenate—even on 100 percent oxygen. Additional therapy includes diuretics to reduce excess fluids, and **bi-level positive airway pressure (BiPAP)** ventilation until sufficient fluid has been eliminated by the kidneys.

Myocardial Contractility

Myocardial contractility may be regarded as the force generated by the myocardium when the ventricular muscle fibers shorten. In general, when the contractility of the heart increases or decreases, the cardiac output increases or decreases, respectively.

There is no single measurement that defines contractility in the clinical setting. Changes in contractility, however, can be inferred through clinical assessment (e.g., pulse, blood pressure, skin temperature) and serial hemodynamic measurements (discussed in Chapter 15). An increase in myocardial contractility is referred to as positive inotropism. A decrease in myocardial contractility is referred to as negative inotropism.

Vascular Resistance

Circulatory resistance is approximated by dividing the mean arterial pressure (MAP) by the cardiac output (CO):

$$\text{Resistance} = \frac{\text{MAP}}{\text{CO}}$$

In general, when the vascular resistance increases, the blood pressure increases (which in turn increases the ventricular afterload). Because of this relationship, blood pressure monitoring can be used to reflect pulmonary

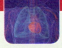

Clinical Connection—5-9

Case Study—Left Ventricular Heart Failure and Pulmonary Edema

In the **Clinical Application Section—Case 2** (page 249), the respiratory therapist is called to help care for a 72-year-old woman with left ventricular heart failure and pulmonary edema (congestive heart failure). The case illustrates the effects of high blood pressure on (1) ventricular afterload, (2) ventricular contractility, (3) ventricular preload, and (4) transmural pressure. This case further illustrates how positive inotropic vasodilators and diuretic agents work to offset the adverse affects of left ventricular heart failure.

or systemic resistance. That is, when resistance increases or decreases, the blood pressure will increase or decrease.

In the pulmonary system, there are several known mechanisms that change the vascular resistance. Such mechanisms are classified as either *active* or *passive mechanisms.*

Active Mechanisms Affecting Vascular Resistance

Active mechanisms that affect vascular resistance include abnormal blood gases, pharmacologic stimulation, and pathologic conditions that have a direct effect on the vascular system.

Abnormal Blood Gases.

- Decreased P_{O_2} (hypoxia).
- Increased P_{CO_2} (hypercapnia).
- Decreased pH (acidemia).

The pulmonary vascular system constricts in response to a decreased alveolar oxygen pressure (**hypoxia**). The exact mechanism of this phenomenon is unknown. Some investigators suggest that alveolar hypoxia causes the lung parenchyma to release a substance that produces vasoconstriction. It is known, however, that the partial pressure of oxygen in the *alveoli* (PA_{O_2})—not the partial pressure of oxygen of the *capillary blood* P_{CO_2}—controls this response. The effect of hypoxic vasoconstriction is to direct blood away from the hypoxic lung regions to lung areas that have a higher partial pressure of oxygen.

Clinically, when the number of hypoxic regions becomes significant (e.g., in the advanced stages of emphysema or chronic bronchitis), generalized pulmonary vasoconstriction can develop. This can cause a substantial increase in the pulmonary vascular resistance and in the work of the right heart. This in turn leads to right ventricular hypertrophy, or *cor pulmonale.*

Pulmonary vascular resistance increases in response to an acute increase in the P_{CO_2} level (**hypercapnia**). It is believed, however, that the vasoconstriction that occurs is most likely due to the increased hydrogen ion (H^+) concentration (*respiratory acidosis*) that develops from a sudden increase in the P_{CO_2} level, rather than to the P_{CO_2} itself. This is supported by the fact that pulmonary vasoconstriction does not occur when hypercapnia is accompanied by a normal pH (*compensated respiratory acidosis*).

 Clinical Connection—5-10

Cor Pulmonale

Cor pulmonale is the enlargement of the *right* ventricle caused by primary lung disease. Cor pulmonale eventually results in the inability of the right ventricle to pump blood effectively to the lungs (also called right-heart failure). When the right ventricle starts to fail, blood returning to the heart backs up and pools throughout the peripheral vascular system—for example, in the liver, legs, neck veins, ankles, feet, and hands. Pulmonary emboli (clots in the pulmonary artery) and end-stage COPD are a common causes of cor pulmonale. Treatment includes oxygen therapy for hypoxemia and blood thinners to prevent blood clots.

Pulmonary vasoconstriction develops in response to decreased pH (increased H$^+$ concentration), or **acidemia**, of either metabolic or respiratory origin.

Pharmacologic Stimulation. The pulmonary vessels constrict in response to various pharmacologic agents, including:

- Epinephrine.
- Norepinephrine.
- Dobutamine.
- Dopamine.
- Phenylephrine.

Constricted pulmonary vessels relax in response to the following agents:

- Oxygen.
- Isoproterenol.
- Aminophylline.
- Calcium-channel blocking agents.

Pathologic Conditions. Pulmonary vascular resistance increases in response to a number of pathologic conditions. Some of the more common ones are:

- Vessel blockage or obstruction (e.g., caused by a thrombus or an embolus, such as a blood clot, fat cell, air bubble, or tumor mass).
- Vessel wall diseases (e.g., sclerosis, polyarteritis, or scleroderma).
- Vessel destruction or obliteration (e.g., emphysema or pulmonary interstitial fibrosis).
- Vessel compression (e.g., pneumothorax, hemothorax, or tumor mass).

Pathologic disturbances in the pulmonary vasculary system can develop in the arteries, arterioles, capillaries, venules, or veins. When increased vascular resistance originates in the venules or veins, the transmural pressure increases and, in severe cases, causes the capillary fluid to spill into the alveoli. This is called **pulmonary edema**. Left ventricular failure will cause the same pathologic disturbances. When the resistance originates in the arteries or arterioles, the pulmonary artery pressure will increase but the pulmonary capillary pressure will be normal or low. Regardless of the origin of the pathologic disturbance, a severe and persistent pulmonary vascular resistance is ultimately followed by an elevated right ventricular pressure, right ventricular strain, right ventricular hypertrophy, and right heart failure.

Passive Mechanisms Affecting Vascular Resistance

The term *passive mechanism* refers to a secondary change in pulmonary vascular resistance that occurs in response to another mechanical change. In other words, when a mechanical factor in the respiratory system changes, a passive increase or decrease in the caliber of the pulmonary blood vessels also occurs. Some of the more common passive mechanisms are discussed next.

Pulmonary Arterial Pressure Changes. As pulmonary arterial pressure increases, the pulmonary vascular resistance decreases (Figure 5–23 on page 242). This is assuming that lung volume and left atrial pressure remain constant. The pulmonary vascular resistance decreases because of the increase in intraluminal distending pressure, which increases the total cross-sectional areas of the pulmonary vascular system through the mechanisms of **recruitment** and **distention**.

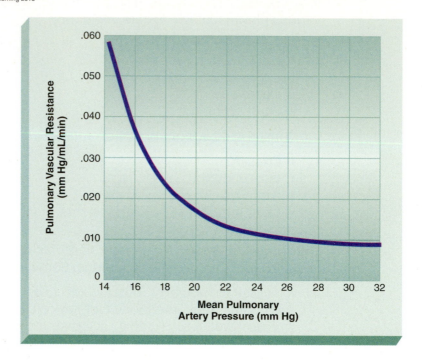

Figure 5–23

Increased mean pulmonary arterial pressure decreases pulmonary vascular resistance.

© Cengage Learning 2013

As shown in Figure 5–24, *recruitment* means the opening of vessels that were closed or not being utilized for blood flow before the vascular pressure increased. *Distention,* on the other hand, means the stretching or widening of vessels that were open, but not to their full capacity. Both of these mechanisms increase the total cross-sectional area of the vascular system, which in turn reduces the vascular resistance. These mechanisms, however, have their limits.

Left Atrial Pressure Changes. As the left atrial pressure increases, while the lung volume and pulmonary arterial pressure are held constant, pulmonary vascular resistance decreases.

Lung Volume Changes. The effect of changes in lung volume on pulmonary vascular resistance varies according to the location of the vessel. Two major groups of vessels must be considered: (1) **alveolar vessels**—those vessels that surround the alveoli (*pulmonary capillaries*)—and (2) **extra-alveolar vessels**—the larger arteries and veins.

Alveolar Vessels. Because the pulmonary capillary vessels are so thin, intrapleural pressure changes directly affect the anatomy of the capillaries. During normal inspiration, the alveolar vessels progressively stretch and flatten. During expiration, the alveolar vessels shorten and widen. Thus, as the lungs are inflated, the resistance offered by the alveolar vessels progressively increases (Figure 5–25). During the inspiratory phase of mechanical ventilation (*positive pressure phase*), moreover, the resistance generated by the alveolar vessels may become excessively high and, as a result, restrict the flow of pulmonary blood. The pressure difference between the alveoli and the lumen of the pulmonary capillaries is called the *transmural pressure* (see Figure 5–14).

Figure 5–24

Schematic of the mechanisms that may be activated to decrease pulmonary vascular resistance when the mean pulmonary artery pressure increases. **A.** A group of pulmonary capillaries, one-half of which are not perfused; **B.** the previously unperfused capillaries shown in A are recruited (i.e., opened) in response to the increased pulmonary artery pressure; **C.** the increased blood pressure has distended the capillaries that are already open.

© Cengage Learning 2013

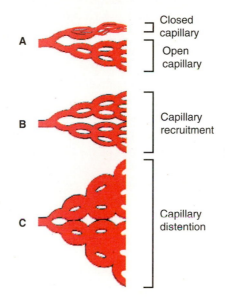

Figure 5–25

Schematic of pulmonary vessels during inspiration. The alveolar vessels (pulmonary capillaries) are exposed to the intrapleural pressure change and are stretched and flattened. The extra-alveolar vessels expand as the intrapleural pressure becomes increasingly negative during inspiration.

© Cengage Learning 2013

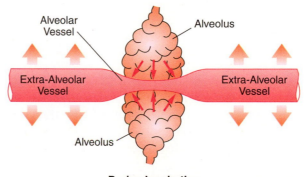

During Inspiration

Extra-Alveolar Vessels. The extra-alveolar vessels (the large arterioles and veins) are also exposed to the intrapleural pressure. They behave differently, however, from the pulmonary capillaries (alveolar vessels) when subjected to volume and pressure changes. That is, as the lung volume increases in response to a more negative intrapleural pressure during inspiration, the transmural pressure increases (i.e., the pressure within the vessels becomes more positive) and the extra-alveolar vessels distend (see Figure 5–25). A second factor that dilates the extra-alveolar vessels at higher lung volumes is the radial traction generated by the connective tissue and by the alveolar septa that hold the larger vessels in place throughout the lung.

Clinical Connection—5-11

The Cardiopulmonary Hazards of Positive-Pressure Ventilation

A hazard of positive-pressure ventilation (PPV) is a decreased cardiac output and arterial blood pressure. This can occur because of the increased alveolar pressures that are transmitted to the intrapleural space and to the great vessels (the inferior and superior vena cava) of the thorax. The increased intrathoracic pressure compresses the great vessels and reduces the venous return to the right atrium and right ventricle. The reduced right ventriclar stroke volume leads to a decreased left ventriclar stroke volume—which, in turn, decreases cardiac output and arterial blood pressure.

In addition, PPV causes the mean airway pressure (P_{aw}), alveolar pressure, and intrapleural pressure to increase. The increased alveolar pressure stretches and narrows the pulmonary capillaries that surround the alveoli. This action increases the pulmonary vascular resistance. This increases the right ventricular afterload. In normal individuals, the right ventricular stroke volume is usually maintained by the heart's ability to overcome reasonable increases in pulmonary vascular resistance. However, in the patient with a preexisting cardiovascular disease, the right ventricle may not be able to overcome these increases in pulmonary resistance. Furthermore, an increased pulmonary vascular resistance can cause overdistention of the right ventricle (cor pulmonale)—which further reduces the right ventricle's output. This action

further decreases the left ventricular output and arterial blood pressure.

Finally, if **positive end-expiratory pressure (PEEP)** is added to the PPV, the patient's P_{aw} is increased even more. It is reasonable to assume that the adverse effects of positive pressure on the patient's venous return and cardiac output will be greater with PPV with PEEP than with PPV alone. Oftentimes, the respiratory therapist will perform what is called **optimal** or **best PEEP** studies to determine the point of maximum oxygenation with minimal reduction in blood pressures. Optimal PEEP can be defined as the PEEP that maximizes oxygen delivery ($D_{O_2} = Q_T \times [Ca_{O_2} \times 10]$—refer to Chapter 6). In general, the PEEP level is progressively increased in increments of 2 cm H_2O until there is a decline in the oxygen delivery. The PEEP is then turned down to the previous level—or the "best" PEEP in terms of oxygen delivery. Although the optimal PEEP level must be specifically determined for each patient, the level of PEEP typically falls in the 8 to 15 cm H_2O range.

In view of the possible hazards of PPV, the respiratory therapist must monitor all patients for signs of cardiovascular instability and closely monitor patients with preexisting cardiovascular disease for signs of decreased cardiac output and blood pressure.

Another type of extra-alveolar vessel is the so-called corner vessel, located at the junction of the alveolar septa. As the lung volume increases, the corner vessels are also pulled open (dilated) by the radial traction force created by the expansion of the alveoli (Figure 5–26).

To summarize, at low lung volumes (low distending pressures), the extra-alveolar vessels narrow and cause the vascular resistance to increase. The alveolar vessels, however, widen and cause the vascular resistance to decrease. In contrast, at high lung volumes (high distending pressures), the extra-alveolar vessels dilate and cause the vascular resistance to decrease. The alveolar vessels, however, flatten and cause the vascular resistance to increase.

Finally, because the alveolar and extra-alveolar vessels are all part of the same vascular system, the resistance generated by the two groups of vessels is additive at any lung volume. The effect of changes in lung volume on the total pulmonary vascular resistance is a U-shaped curve (Figure 5–27). Thus, the pulmonary vascular resistance (PVR) is lowest near the functional residual capacity (FRC) and increases in response to both high and low lung volumes.

Figure 5–26

Schematic of the extra-alveolar "corner vessels" found at the junction of the alveolar septa. Expansion of the alveoli generates radial traction on the corner vessels, causing them to dilate. The alveolar vessels are compressed and flattened at high lung volumes.

© Cengage Learning 2013

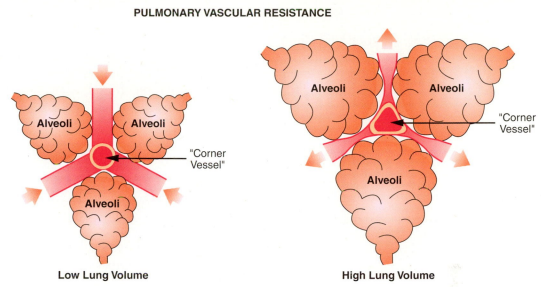

PULMONARY VASCULAR RESISTANCE

Low Lung Volume

High Lung Volume

Figure 5–27

At low lung volumes, the extra-alveolar vessels generate a greater resistance to pulmonary blood flow; at high lung volumes, the alveolar vessels generate a greater resistance to pulmonary blood flow. When added together, the resistances of the extra-alveolar and alveolar vessels demonstrate a U-shaped curve. Pulmonary vascular resistance (PVR) is lowest near the functional residual capacity (FRC) and increases at both high and low lung volumes. RV = residual volume; TLC = total lung capacity.

© Cengage Learning 2013

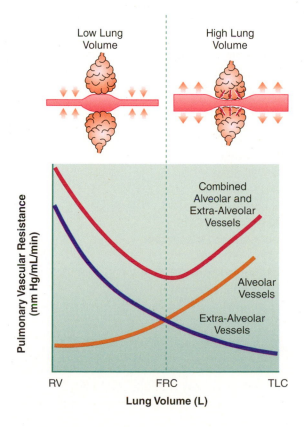

Blood Volume Changes. As blood volume increases, the recruitment and distention of pulmonary vessels will ensue, and pulmonary vascular resistance will tend to decrease (see Figure 5–24).

Blood Viscosity Changes. The viscosity of blood is derived from the hematocrit, the integrity of red blood cells, and the composition of plasma. As blood viscosity increases, the pulmonary vascular resistance increases. Table 5–4 summarizes the active and passive mechanisms of vascular resistance.

Table 5–4		
Summary of the Effects of Active and Passive Mechanisms on Vascular Resistance		
	↑ **Resistance (vascular constriction)**	↓ **Resistance (vascular dilation)**
ACTIVE MECHANISMS		
Abnormal Blood Gases		
$\downarrow P_{O_2}$	X	
$\uparrow P_{CO_2}$	X	
$\downarrow$pH	X	
Pharmacologic Stimulation		
Epinephrine	X	
Norepinephrine	X	
Dobutamine	X	
Dopamine	X	
Phenylephrine	X	
Oxygen		X
Isoproterenol		X
Aminophylline		X
Calcium-channel blocking agents		X
Pathologic Conditions		
Vessel blockage/obstruction	X	
Vessel wall disease	X	
Vessel destruction	X	
Vessel compression	X	
PASSIVE MECHANISMS		
↑Pulmonary arterial pressure		X
↑Left atrial pressure		X
↑Lung volume (extreme)	X	
↓Lung volume (extreme)	X	
↑Blood volume		X
↑Blood viscosity	X	

↑ = increased; ↓ = decreased.

Chapter Summary

The transport of oxygen from the lungs to the cells of the body and to transport carbon dioxide from the tissue cells to the lungs is a function of the circulatory system. The essential components of the circulatory system consist of the blood, the heart, and the pulmonary and systemic vascular systems. *Blood* consists of a variety of specialized cells called formed elements that are suspended in a fluid called *plasma*. The formed elements in the plasma are the red blood cells, white cells, and platelets. The white cells include the neutrophils, eosinphils, basophils, lymphocytes, and monocytes.

Essential components of the *heart* include the right and left atria, right and left ventricles, the interventricular septum, the pericardium, the walls of the heart (i.e., epicardium, myocardium, endocardium), the arterial supply of the heart (the left and right coronary artery), the venous drainage (i.e., the great cardiac veins, middle cardiac vein, coronary sinus, and thebesian veins), and the blood flow through the heart.

The *pulmonary* and *systemic vascular systems* are composed of the arteries, arterioles, capillaries, venules, and veins. The pulmonary arterioles and most of the arterioles in the systemic circulation are controlled by sympathetic impulses. Specialized stretch receptors called *baroreceptors* regulate the arterial blood pressure by initiating reflex adjustments to deviations in blood pressure.

The following three types of pressures are used to study the blood flow in the pulmonary and systemic vascular systems: intravascular, transmural, and driving. During each cardiac cycle, the ventricular systole and diastole have a direct relationship to the blood pressure. During ventricular systole, the arterial blood pressure sharply increases; during ventricular diastole, the arterial blood pressure decreases. The high and low blood pressures generated by ventricular systole and diastole result in mean intraluminal blood pressures throughout the pulmonary and systemic circulation. The mean systemic vascular pressure is about 10 times that of the pulmonary vascular system.

The distribution of pulmonary blood flow is a function of (1) gravity, (2) cardiac output, and (3) pulmonary vascular resistance. The influence of gravity in the upper right lung is described in terms of zones 1, 2, and 3; zone 3 is the most gravity-dependent area. Determinants of cardiac output are a function of ventricular preload, ventricular afterload, and myocardial contractility.

Finally, the pulmonary vascular resistance may increase or decrease as a result of active and passive mechanisms. Active mechanisms include abnormal blood gases, pharmacologic stimulation, and pathologic conditions. Passive mechanisms include increased pulmonary arterial pressure, increased left atrial pressure, lung volume changes, and blood volume and blood viscosity changes

Clinical connections associated with the topics discussed in this chapter include (1) anemia, (2) complete blood cell count, (3) pericarditis, (4) cardiac tamponade, (5) myocardial infarction—common diagnostic and treatment interventions of blocked coronary arteries, (6) carotid sinus massage, (7) a case study illustrating an automobile accident victim with massive blood loss, (8) congestive heart failure, (9) a case study illustrating left ventricular heart failure and pulmonary edema, (10) cor pulmonale, and (11) the cardiopulmonary hazards of positivepressure ventilation.

A 16-year-old girl was involved in an automobile accident on the way home from school during a freezing rain. As she drove over a bridge, her car hit a patch of ice, spun out of control, and hit a cement embankment. It took the emergency rescue team almost an hour to cut her out of her car with the "Jaws of Life." She was stabilized at the accident scene and then transported to the trauma center.

In the emergency department, the patient was unconscious and hypotensive. It was obvious that she had lost a lot of blood; her shirt and pants were soaked with blood. She had several large lacerations on her forehead, face, neck, left arm, and left leg. The patient's head was lowered and her legs were elevated. The emergency department nurse started an intravenous infusion of Ringer's lactated solution. The respiratory therapist placed a nonrebreathing oxygen mask on the patient's face and drew an arterial blood sample. The radiologic technician took several portable X-rays.

The patient had several large bruises and abrasions over her left anterior chest that were most likely caused by the steering wheel when her car hit the cement embankment. Her four upper front teeth were broken off at the gum line. Her skin was pale and blue. Her vital signs were blood pressure—78/42 mm Hg, heart rate—145 beats/min and weak, and respirations—22 breaths/min and shallow. Her breath sounds were diminished bilaterally. Her arterial oxygen pressure (Pa_{O_2}) was 72 torr.

Although chest X-ray showed no broken ribs, patches of pulmonary infiltrates (increased alveolar density) could be seen over the left anterior lung. Additional X-rays showed that she had a broken left humerus and left tibia. She was taken to surgery to repair her lacerations and broken bones. Five hours later, she was transferred to the surgical intensive care unit with her left arm and left leg in a cast.

To offset the increased alveolar density noted on the chest X-ray, the respiratory therapist administered continuous positive airway pressure (CPAP) via a face mask for 20 minutes every hour. Between the CPAP treatments, the patient continued to receive oxygen via a non-rebreathing mask. Two hours later, the patient was conscious and talking to her parents. Her skin appeared normal and her vital signs were blood pressure—115/82 mm Hg, heart rate—75 beats/min

and strong, and respirations—14 breaths/min. Normal vesicular breath sounds were heard throughout both lungs. Her fractional concentration of inspired oxygen FI_{O_2} was decreased to 0.4, and her Pa_{O_2} on this setting was 94 torr.

The patient's cardiopulmonary status progressively improved and she was discharged on the sixth day of hospitalization. Although her broken bones healed adequately, she had trouble walking normally for some time after the accident. Because of this problem, she continued to receive physical therapy twice a week for 6 months on an outpatient basis. At the time of her high school graduation, she had completely recovered.

Discussion

This case study illustrates (1) the activation of the baroreceptor reflex, (2) hypovolemia and how it relates to preload, (3) negative transmural pressure, and (4) the effects of gravity on blood flow.

As shown in this chapter, the specialized stretch receptors called *baroreceptors* (see Figure 5–12) regulate the arterial blood pressure by initiating reflex adjustments to changes in blood pressure. In this case, as the patient's blood pressure decreased from the loss of blood, neural impulses transmitted from the baroreceptors to the vasomotor and cardiac centers in the medulla decreased. This action, in turn, likely caused the patient's medulla to increase its sympathetic activity, which increased the heart rate (her pulse was 145 beats/min in the emergency department).

Because *ventricular preload* is a function of the blood pressure generated by the volume of blood returning to the left or right ventricle during diastole, it can easily be seen why the patient's ventricular preload decreased as she became hypovolemic from the loss of blood. In the emergency department, the fact that the patient's ventricular preload was low was reflected by her low blood pressure (78/42 mm Hg). It should be noted that as preload decreases, cardiac output decreases.

Finally, as the patient's preload decreased (from blood loss), the *transmural pressure* in her least gravity-dependent lung areas became increasingly negative. *Transmural pressure* is the difference between the intraluminal pressure of a vessel and the pressure surrounding the vessel (see Figure 5–14). The transmural pressure is negative when the pressure surrounding the vessel is greater than the pressure inside the vessel. In this case, this pathophysiologic process was offset by (1) lowering the patient's head and elevating her legs, which used the effects of gravity to move blood to the patient's lungs, and (2)

replacing the volume of blood lost by administering Ringer's lactated solution. These two procedures worked to change the negative transmural pressures to positive transmural pressures in the lung regions.

2   Clinical Application Case

A 72-year-old woman presented in the intensive care unit with left ventricular heart failure and pulmonary edema (also called congestive heart failure). She had no history of respiratory disease. The patient's husband stated that she had gone to bed with no remarkable problems but awoke with severe dyspnea after several hours of sleep. Concerned, her husband called 911.

On observation, the patient's skin was cyanotic and she was in obvious respiratory distress. Her neck veins were distended and her ankles were swollen. Her vital signs were blood pressure—214/106 mm Hg, heart rate—90 beats/min, and respirations—28 breaths/min. On auscultation, rales and rhonchi were heard over both lung fields. She had a frequent, productive cough with frothy white secretions. Her arterial oxygen pressure (Pa_{O_2}) on 3 L/min oxygen via nasal cannula was 48 torr. A portable chest X-ray showed dense, fluffy opacities (white areas) that spread outward from the hilar areas to the peripheral borders of the lungs. The chest X-ray also showed that the left ventricle was enlarged (ventricular hypertrophy).

The physician prescribed *positive inotropic agents* (refer to Table 15–3) to improve the strength of the left ventricular contraction and cardiac output and a systemic *vasodilator* (refer to Table 15–6) to decrease the patient's elevated blood pressure. Diuretic agents were also administered to promote fluid excretion. The respiratory therapist increased the patient's oxygen levels using a partial rebreathing mask.

Two hours later, the patient's cardiopulmonary status had significantly improved. Her skin appeared normal and her neck veins were no longer distended. Her peripheral edema was no longer present. Her vital signs were blood pressure—130/87 mm Hg, heart rate—81 beats/min, and respirations—14 breaths/min. Her Pa_{O_2}, on 2 L/min oxygen via nasal cannula, was

103 torr. A second chest X-ray showed that her lungs were clear and the left ventricle had returned to normal size.

Discussion

This case illustrates the effects of high blood pressure on (1) ventricular afterload, (2) ventricular contractility, (3) ventricular preload, and (4) transmural pressure.

Ventricular afterload is defined as the force against which the ventricles must work to pump blood. In this case, the patient's left ventricular afterload was very high because of increased peripheral vascular resistance. Clinically, this was reflected by the patient's high blood pressure of 214/106 mm Hg. Because of the high blood pressure and high left ventricular afterload, the patient's left ventricle eventually weakened and began to fail. As the ability of the left ventricle to pump blood decreased, the blood volume (and pressure) in the left ventricle increased. Even though the preload was increased, the left ventricle was unable to meet the increased demands created by the increased blood volume.

As this condition worsened, blood backed up into the patient's lungs, causing the *transmural pressure* in the pulmonary capillary to increase significantly. As a result of the excessively high transmural pressure, fluid leaked out of the pulmonary capillaries and into the alveoli and airways. Clinically, this was verified by the rales and rhonchi heard during auscultation, and by the white, frothy secretions produced when the patient coughed. As fluid accumulated in the patient's alveoli, the diffusion of oxygen into the pulmonary capillaries decreased. This was verified by the decreased Pa_{O_2} of 48 torr.

Finally, as the blood volume and the transmural pressure in the pulmonary capillaries increased, the

(continues)

right ventricular afterload increased, which in turn decreased the ability of the right ventricle to pump blood despite the fact that the preload increased. This condition was reflected by the patient's distended neck veins and peripheral edema.

Fortunately, in this case the patient responded well to the positive inotropic vasodilator and diuretic agents. The vasodilator and diuretics worked to reduce the right and left ventricular afterloads, and the inotropic agents increased the ability of the ventricles to pump blood. The patient rapidly improved and was discharged on the fourth day of her hospital stay. Presently, she is seen by her family physician every 2 months.

Review Questions

1. Which of the following are granulocytes?
1. Neutrophils
2. Monocytes
3. Eosinophils
4. Lymphocytes
5. Basophils
   a. 2 only
   b. 5 only
   c. 2 and 4 only
   d. 1, 3, and 5 only

2. In healthy men, the hematocrit is about
   a. 25 percent
   b. 35 percent
   c. 45 percent
   d. 65 percent

3. Which of the following agents cause pulmonary vascular constriction?
1. Isoproterenol
2. Epinephrine
3. Oxygen
4. Dopamine
   a. 3 only
   b. 2 and 4 only
   c. 1, 2, and 4 only
   d. 1, 2, 3, and 4

4. If the pressure in the pulmonary artery is 34 mm Hg and the pressure in the left atrium is 9 mm Hg, what is the driving pressure?
   a. 9 mm Hg
   b. 17 mm Hg
   c. 25 mm Hg
   d. 34 mm Hg

5. The tricuspid valve lies between the
   a. right atrium and the right ventricle
   b. left ventricle and the aorta
   c. right ventricle and the pulmonary artery
   d. left atrium and the left ventricle

6. Which of the following is usually elevated in patients with asthma?
- a. Lymphocytes
- b. Neutrophils
- c. Basophils
- d. Eosinophils

7. The mean intraluminal pressure in the pulmonary capillaries is
- a. 5 mm Hg
- b. 10 mm Hg
- c. 15 mm Hg
- d. 20 mm Hg

8. An increase in the number of which of the following suggests a bacterial infection?
- a. Lymphocytes
- b. Neutrophils
- c. Monocytes
- d. Eosinophils

9. The force the ventricles must work against to pump blood is called
- a. myocardial contractility
- b. ventricular afterload
- c. negative inotropism
- d. ventricular preload

10. Compared with the systemic circulation, the pressure in the pulmonary circulation is about
- a. $\frac{1}{10}$ the pressure
- b. $\frac{1}{4}$ the pressure
- c. $\frac{1}{3}$ the pressure
- d. $\frac{1}{2}$ the pressure

11. The difference between the pressure in the lumen of a vessel and that of the pressure surrounding the vessel is called the
- a. driving pressure
- b. transmural pressure
- c. diastolic pressure
- d. intravascular pressure

12. Which of the following cause(s) pulmonary vasoconstriction?
1. Hypercapnia
2. Hypoxia
3. Acidemia
4. Increased H^+ concentration
- a. 3 only
- b. 2 and 4 only
- c. 2, 3, and 4 only
- d. 1, 2, 3, and 4

13. The cardioinhibitor center of the medulla slows the heart by sending neural impulses by way of the
   1. tenth cranial nerve
   2. parasympathetic nervous system
   3. sympathetic nervous system
   4. vagus nerve
      a. 4 only
      b. 3 only
      c. 1 and 4 only
      d. 1, 2, and 4 only

14. Which of the following cause(s) passive changes in the pulmonary vascular resistance?
   1. pH changes
   2. Transpulmonary pressure changes
   3. P_{CO_2} changes
   4. Blood viscosity changes
      a. 2 only
      b. 3 only
      c. 1 and 3 only
      d. 2 and 4 only

15. Which of the following cause blood clotting at a traumatized site?
      a. Thrombocytes
      b. Basophils
      c. Monocytes
      d. Eosinophils

Clinical Application Questions

Case 1

1. As the patient's blood pressure decreased from the loss of blood, neural impulses transmitted from _____ to the vasomotor and cardiac centers in the medulla (decreased ___; increased ___).

2. In the emergency department, the patient's low preload was reflected by her low _____.

3. As the preload decreases, the cardiac output _____.

4. The negative transmural pressure in this case was offset by (1) _____ _____ and (2) _____ _____ _____.

Case 2

1. In this case, the patient's left ventricular afterload was very high. This condition was reflected by the patient's _____.

2. As a result of the excessively high transmural pressure, fluid leaked out of the pulmonary capillaries and into the alveoli and airways. Clinically, this was verified by the _____ and _____ heard on auscultation.

3. As fluid accumulated in the patient's alveoli, the diffusion of oxygen into the pulmonary capillaries decreased. This was verified by the

   _____.

4. The increased right ventricular afterload was reflected by the patient's

   _____.

5. The vasodilator and diuretic agents worked to reduce the right and left ventricular _____.

Chapter 6

Oxygen and Carbon Dioxide Transport

Objectives

By the end of this chapter, the student should be able to:

1. Calculate the quantity of oxygen that *dissolves in the plasma* of the blood.
2. Describe the major features of *hemoglobin,* including:
   —Heme portion
   • Iron
   —Globin portion
   • Four amino acid chains
      ○ Two alpha chains
      ○ Two beta chains
   —Ferrous state versus ferric state
   —Normal hemoglobin concentrations in the adult male and female and in the infant
3. Calculate the quantity of oxygen that *combines with hemoglobin.*
4. Calculate the *total amount* of oxygen in the blood.
5. Identify the abbreviations for the following:
   —Oxygen content of arterial blood
   —Oxygen content of mixed venous blood
   —Oxygen content of pulmonary capillary blood
6. Describe how the following relate to the *oxyhemoglobin dissociation curve:*
   —Percentage of hemoglobin bound to oxygen
   —Oxygen pressure
   —Oxygen content
7. Describe the clinical connection associated with the importance of hemoglobin in oxygen transport.
8. Describe the clinical connection associated with polycythemia.
9. Describe the clinical significance of the
   —Flat portion of the oxyhemoglobin dissociation curve
   —Steep portion of the oxyhemoglobin dissociation curve
   —P_{50}

10. Describe the clinical connection associated with the pulse oximeter and the Pa_{O_2} and Sa_{O_2} relationship.
11. Identify the factors that shift the oxyhemoglobin dissociation curve to the right.
12. Identify the factors that shift the oxyhemoglobin dissociation curve to the left.
13. Explain the clinical significance of a right or left shift of the oxyhemoglobin dissociation curve with regard to the
    —Loading of oxygen in the lungs
    —Unloading of oxygen at the tissues
14. Describe the clinical connection associated with the clinical significance of a right shift in the oxyhemoglobin dissociation curve.
15. Perform the following oxygen transport calculations:
    —Total oxygen delivery
    —Arterial-venous oxygen content difference
    —Oxygen consumption
    —Oxygen extraction ratio
    —Mixed venous oxygen saturation
16. Describe the clinical connection associated with the importance of starting cardiopulmonary resuscitation (CPR) as soon as possible.
17. Identify the factors that increase and decrease the *oxygen transport* calculations.
18. Differentiate between the following forms of *pulmonary shunting:*
    —Absolute shunts
    • Anatomic shunt
    • Capillary shunt
    —Relative shunt (shunt-like effect)
19. Explain the meaning of *venous admixture.*
20. Calculate the *shunt equation.*
21. Describe the clinical significance of pulmonary shunting.

(continues)

22. Describe the differences between *hypoxemia* and *hypoxia*.
23. Define the four main types of tissue hypoxia:
    —Hypoxic hypoxia
    —Anemic hypoxia
    —Circulatory hypoxia
    —Histotoxic hypoxia
24. Describe the clinical connection associated with hemoglobin and carbon monoxide poisoning.
25. Explain the meaning of cyanosis.
26. Describe the clinical connection associated with blood doping.
27. List the three ways in which carbon dioxide is transported in the *plasma*.
28. List the three ways in which carbon dioxide is transported in the *red blood cells*.
29. Describe how carbon dioxide is converted to HCO_3^- at the tissue sites and then transported in the plasma to the lungs.
30. Explain how carbon dioxide is eliminated in the lungs.
31. Describe how the *carbon dioxide dissociation curve* differs from the *oxyhemoglobin dissociation curve*.
32. Explain how the *Haldane effect* relates to the carbon dioxide dissociation curve.
33. Complete the review questions at the end of this chapter.

An understanding of oxygen and carbon dioxide transport is essential to the study of pulmonary physiology and to the clinical interpretation of arterial and venous blood gases (see Figure 6–1). Table 6–1 lists the normal blood gas values.[1,2] To fully understand this subject, the student must understand (1) how oxygen is transported from the lungs to the tissues, (2) the oxyhemoglobin dissociation curve and its clinical significance, (3) how various oxygen transport calculations are used to identify the patient's cardiac and ventilatory status, (4) the major forms of tissue hypoxia, and (5) how carbon dioxide is transported from the tissues to the lungs.

Oxygen Transport

The transport of oxygen between the lungs and the cells of the body is a function of the blood and the heart. Oxygen is carried in the blood in two forms: (1) as dissolved oxygen in the blood plasma and (2) chemically bound to the hemoglobin (Hb) that is encased in the erythrocytes or red blood cells (RBCs).

Oxygen Dissolved in the Blood Plasma

As oxygen diffuses from the alveoli into the pulmonary capillary blood, it dissolves in the plasma of the blood. The term **dissolve** means that when a

---

[1] See Appendix V for a representative example of a cardiopulmonary profile sheet used to monitor the blood gas values of the critically ill patient.

[2] It should be noted that it is common to use either **mm Hg** or **torr** gas pressure values (e.g, P_{O_2}, P_{CO_2}, N_2). The *torr* was named after Evangelista Torricelli, an Italian physicist and mathematician, who discovered the principle of the mercury barometer in 1644. In honor of Torricelli, the torr was defined as a unit of pressure equal to 1 mm Hg—i.e., 1 torr = 1 mm Hg.

The **National Board for Respiratory Care (NBRC)** uses the following on national board exams:

- **torr** is used for blood gases values (e.g., Pa_{O_2} or Pa_{CO_2}).

- **mm Hg** is used for blood pressure and barometric values.

© sfam_photo/www.Shutterstock.com

Figure 6–1

Radial-arterial blood gas stick. An arterial blood gas sample being obtained from a three-way stopcock, which is connected to an indwelling arterial catheter line. Common sites for indwelling arterial lines are the radial and brachial arteries.

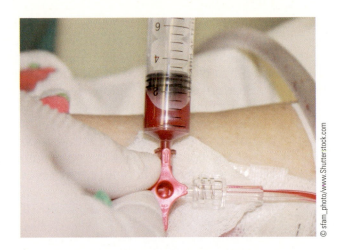

Table 6–1

Normal Blood Gas Value Ranges

Blood Gas Value*	Arterial	Venous
pH	7.35–7.45	7.30–7.40
P_{CO_2}	35–45 torr (Pa_{CO_2})	42–48 torr $(P\overline{v}_{CO_2})$
HCO_3^-	22–28 mEq/L	24–30 mEq/L
P_{O_2}	80–100 torr (Pa_{O_2})	35–45 torr $(P\overline{v}_{O_2})$

* Technically, only the oxygen (P_{O_2}) and carbon dioxide (P_{CO_2}) pressure readings are "true" blood gas values. The pH indicates the balance between the bases and acids in the blood. The bicarbonate (HCO_3^-) reading is an indirect measurement that is calculated from the pH and P_{CO_2} levels.

© Cengage Learning 2013

gas like oxygen enters the plasma, it maintains its precise molecular structure (in this case, O_2) and moves freely throughout the plasma in its normal gaseous state. Clinically, it is this portion of the oxygen that is measured to assess the patient's partial pressure of oxygen (P_{O_2}) (see Table 6–1).

The quantity of oxygen that dissolves in the plasma is a function of Henry's law, which states that the amount of gas that dissolves in a liquid (in this case, plasma) at a given temperature is proportional to the partial pressure of the gas. At normal body temperature, about 0.003 mL of oxygen will dissolve in 100 mL of blood for every 1 torr of P_{O_2}. Thus, in the healthy individual with an arterial oxygen partial pressure (Pa_{O_2}) of 100 torr, approximately 0.3 mL of oxygen is dissolved in every 100 mL of plasma (0.003 × 100 torr = 0.3 mL). This is written as 0.3 volume percent (vol%). Volume percent represents the amount of O_2 in milliliters that is in 100 mL of blood (vol% = mL O_2/100 mL blood). For example, 10 vol% of O_2 means that there are 10 mL of O_2 in 100 mL of blood. In terms of total oxygen transport, a relatively small percentage of oxygen is transported in the form of dissolved oxygen.

Oxygen Bound to Hemoglobin

Hemoglobin

Most of the oxygen that diffuses into the pulmonary capillary blood rapidly moves into the RBCs and chemically attaches to the hemoglobin. Each RBC contains approximately 280 million hemoglobin molecules, which are highly specialized to transport oxygen and carbon dioxide.

Normal adult hemoglobin, which is designated Hb A, consists of (1) four heme groups, which are the pigmented, iron-containing nonprotein portions of the hemoglobin molecule, and (2) four amino acid chains (polypeptide chains) that collectively constitute globin (a protein) (Figure 6–2).

At the center of each heme group, the iron molecule can combine with one oxygen molecule in an easily reversible reaction to form oxyhemoglobin:

$$Hb + O_2 \rightleftharpoons Hb_{O_2}$$

| Reduced hemoglobin (uncombined or deoxygenated hemoglobin) | Oxygen | Oxyhemoglobin (combined or oxygenated hemoglobin) |

Because there are four heme/iron groups in each Hb molecule, a total of four oxygen molecules can combine with each Hb molecule. When four oxygen molecules are bound to one Hb molecule, the Hb is said to be 100 percent saturated with oxygen; an Hb molecule with three oxygen molecules is 75 percent saturated; and so forth. Hemoglobin bound with oxygen (Hb_{O_2}) is called **oxyhemoglobin**. Hemoglobin not bound with oxygen (Hb) is called **reduced hemoglobin** or **deoxyhemoglobin**. The amount of oxygen bound to Hb is directly related to the partial pressure of oxygen.

The globin portion of each Hb molecule consists of two identical alpha (α) chains, each with 141 amino acids, and two identical beta (β) chains,

---

| **Figure 6–2** |

Schematic of a hemoglobin molecule. The globin (protein) portion consists of two identical alpha (α) chains and two beta (β) chains. The four heme (iron-containing) portions are in the center of each globin molecule.

© Cengage Learning 2013

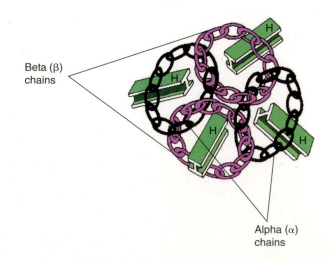

Beta (β) chains

Alpha (α) chains

each with 146 amino acids ($\alpha_2\beta_2$). Normal fetal hemoglobin (Hb F) has two alpha (α) chains and two gamma (γ) chains ($\alpha_2\gamma_2$). This increases hemoglobin's attraction to oxygen and facilitates transfer of maternal oxygen across the placenta. Fetal hemoglobin is gradually replaced with Hb A over the first year of postnatal life.

When the precise number, sequence, or spatial arrangement of the globin amino acid chains is altered, the hemoglobin will be abnormal. For example, sickle cell hemoglobin (Hb S) has a different amino acid substituted into the β chain. This causes the deoxygenated hemoglobin molecule (hemoglobin not bound to oxygen) to change the RBC shape from biconcave to a crescent or sickle form that has a tendency to form thrombi (clots). Various drugs and chemicals, such as nitrites, can change the iron molecule in the heme from the *ferrous state* to the *ferric state*, eliminating the ability of hemoglobin to transport oxygen. This type of hemoglobin is known as *methemoglobin*.

The normal hemoglobin value for the adult male is 14 to 16 g/100 mL of blood. In other words, if all the hemoglobin were to be extracted from all the RBCs in 100 mL of blood, the hemoglobin would actually weigh between 14 and 16 g. Clinically, the weight measurement of hemoglobin, in reference to 100 mL of blood, is referred to as either the *gram percent of hemoglobin* (g% Hb) or *grams per deciliter* (g/dL). The average adult female hemoglobin value is 12 to 15 g%. The average infant hemoglobin value is 14 to 20 g%. Hemoglobin constitutes about 33 percent of the RBC weight.

Quantity of Oxygen Bound to Hemoglobin

Each g% of Hb is capable of carrying approximately 1.34 mL[3] of oxygen. Thus, if the hemoglobin level is 15 g%, and if the hemoglobin is fully saturated, about 20.1 vol% of oxygen will be bound to the hemoglobin. The 20.1 value is calculated using the following formula:

$$O_2 \text{ bound to Hb} = 1.34 \text{ mL } O_2 \times 15 \text{ g\% Hb}$$
$$= 20.1 \text{ vol\% } O_2$$

At a normal arterial oxygen pressure (Pa$_{O_2}$) of 100 torr, however, the hemoglobin saturation (Sa$_{O_2}$) is only about 97 percent because of these normal physiologic shunts:

- Thebesian venous drainage into the left atrium
- Bronchial venous drainage into the pulmonary veins
- Alveoli that are underventilated relative to pulmonary blood flow

Thus, the amount of arterial oxygen in the preceding equation must be adjusted to 97 percent. The equation is written as follows:

$$\begin{array}{r} 20.1 \text{ vol\% } O_2 \\ \times\ 0.97 \\ \hline 19.5 \text{ vol\% } O_2 \end{array}$$

---

[3] The literature also reports values of 1.36, 1.38, and 1.39. The figure 1.34 is the most commonly used factor and is used in this textbook.

Clinical Connection—6-1

Case Study—The Importance of Hemoglobin in Oxygen Transport

In the **Clinical Application Section—Case 1** (page 298), the respiratory therapist is called to assist in the care of a 12-year-old female victim of a drive-by shooting. This case demonstrates the importance of hemoglobin in the transport of oxygen. As a result of the gunshot wound to the chest, the patient has a significant amount of blood loss—causing the patient to lose consciousness, become cyanotic, and be damp to the touch. Even though the patient's Pa_{O_2} is very high in the emergency department (>500 torr), her tissue oxygenation is seriously impaired because of a very low Hb concentration (4 g%). This case nicely illustrates how the Pa_{O_2} and Sa_{O_2} can be very misleading—and dangerous—when the hemoglobin level is not entered into the patient's oxygen transport calculations. Note that a unit of "life-saving" blood was started immediately on the patient's arrival in the emergency department.

Total Oxygen Content

To determine the total amount of oxygen in 100 mL of blood, the dissolved oxygen and the oxygen bound to hemoglobin must be added together. The following case study summarizes the calculations required to compute an individual's total oxygen content.

Case Study: Anemic Patient

A 27-year-old woman with a long history of anemia (decreased hemoglobin concentration) is showing signs of respiratory distress. Her respiratory rate is 36 breaths/min, heart rate 130 beats/minute, and blood pressure 155/90 mm Hg. Her hemoglobin concentration is 6 g%, and her Pa_{O_2} is 80 torr (Sa_{O_2} 90%).

Based on this information, the patient's total oxygen content is computed as follows:

1. Dissolved O_2:

$$\begin{array}{r} 80 \ Pa_{O_2} \\ \times \ 0.003 \ \text{(dissolved } O_2 \text{ factor)} \\ \hline 0.24 \ \text{vol\% } O_2 \end{array}$$

2. Oxygen bound to hemoglobin:

$$\begin{array}{r} 6 \ \text{g\% Hb} \\ \times \ 1.34 \ \text{(}O_2 \text{ bound to Hb factor)} \\ \hline 8.04 \ \text{vol\% } O_2 \ \text{(at } Sa_{O_2} \text{ of 100\%)} \end{array}$$

$$\begin{array}{r} 8.04 \ \text{vol\% } O_2 \\ \times \ 0.90 \ Sa_{O_2} \\ \hline 7.236 \ \text{vol\% } O_2 \end{array}$$

3. Total oxygen content:

$$\begin{array}{r} 7.236 \ \text{vol\% } O_2 \ \text{(bound to hemoglobin)} \\ + \ 0.24 \ \text{vol\% } O_2 \ \text{(dissolved } O_2) \\ \hline 7.476 \ \text{vol\% } O_2 \ \text{(total amount of } O_2/100 \ \text{mL of blood)} \end{array}$$

Note that the patient's total arterial oxygen content is less than 50 percent of normal. Her hemoglobin concentration, which is the primary mechanism for transporting oxygen, is very low. Once this problem is corrected, the clinical manifestations of respiratory distress should no longer be present.

The total oxygen content of the arterial blood (Ca_{O_2}), mixed venous blood ($C\bar{v}_{O_2}$), and pulmonary capillary blood (Cc_{O_2}) is calculated as follows:

- Ca_{O_2}: Oxygen content of arterial blood
  $$(Hb \times 1.34 + Sa_{O_2}) + (Pa_{O_2} \times 0.003)$$

- $C\bar{v}_{O_2}$: Oxygen content of mixed venous blood
  $$(Hb \times 1.34 \times S\bar{v}_{O_2}) + (P\bar{v}_{O_2} \times 0.003)$$

- Cc_{O_2}: Oxygen content of pulmonary capillary blood
  $$(Hb \times 1.34)* + (P_{A_{O_2}}** \times 0.003)$$

It will be shown later in this chapter how various mathematical manipulations of the Ca_{O_2}, $C\bar{v}_{O_2}$, and Cc_{O_2} values are used in different oxygen transport calculations to reflect important factors concerning the patient's cardiac and ventilatory status.

Clinical Connection—6-2

Polycythemia

An abnormally high red blood cell (RBC) count is known as **polycythemia**. It commonly occurs when the bone marrow is stimulated to make more RBCs in response to chronically low arterial blood oxygen levels—which is referred to as **secondary polycythemia**. Polycythemia helps to offset the adverse affects of a chronically low oxygen level in the blood by increasing the oxygen-carrying capacity of the blood.

The hallmark of polycythemia is an elevated hematocrit or hemoglobin. Polycythemia is identified when the hematocrit is greather than 52 percent in men (normal: 45 percent) and 48 percent in women (normal: 42 percent). When using the hemoglobin level, polycythemia is present when the hemoglobin level is greater than 18.5 g% in men (normal: 14 to 16 g%), and 16.5 g% in women (normal 12 to 15 g%).

The respiratory therapist will frequently treat patients with polycythemia who are suffering from chronically low P_{O_2} levels caused by chronic pulmonary disorders—such as emphysema, bronchitis, and cystic fibrosis. For example, consider

the following representative case study of a typical patient with polycythemia:

Case Study: COPD Patient with Polycythemia

A 71-year-old male with a long history of emphysema and chronic bronchitis (COPD) enters the hospital for a routine evaluation. The patient is well known to the respiratory care team. He has a 45-year history of smoking two packs of cigarettes a day. He has a history of high blood pressure and a number of episodes of congestive heart failure. Inspection reveals a barrel chest, clubbing of the fingers and toes, cyanotic skin, and pitting edema around the ankles. He is experiencing pursed-lip breathing, and he is using his accessory muscles of respiration. Vital signs are: blood pressure 135/90, heart rate 85 bpm, respiratory rate 10/min, and oral temperature 37°C (98.6°F).

On room air, the patient's Pa_{O_2} is 45 torr and the Sa_{O_2} is 75 percent. The patient's CBCs reveal an Hb level of 19 g%. When evaluating the patient's Pa_{O_2} and Sa_{O_2} values, the oxygenation status

(continues)

---

* It is assumed that the hemoglobin saturation with oxygen in the pulmonary capillary blood (Sc_{O_2}) is 100 percent or 1.0.

** Refer to "Ideal Alveolar Gas Equation" in Chapter 4.

Clinical Connection—6-2, continued

appears severely low. However, when the patient's total oxygen content is computed—with an Hb level of 19 g%—the patient's total oxygen delivery status is actually quite good—see the following calculation:

1. **Dissolved O_2**

$$\frac{\begin{array}{r}45\ Pa_{O_2}\\ \times\ 0.003\ (\text{dissolved }O_2\text{ factor})\end{array}}{0.135}$$

2. **Oxygen bound to hemoglobin**

$$\frac{\begin{array}{r}19\ g\%\ Hg\\ \times\ 1.34\ (O_2\text{ bound to Hb factor})\end{array}}{25.46\ \text{vol}\%\ O_2\ (\text{at }Sa_{O_2}\text{ of }100\%)}$$

$$\frac{\begin{array}{r}25.46\ \text{vol}\%\ O_2\\ \times\ 0.75\ Sa_{O_2}\end{array}}{19.095\ \text{vol}\%\ O_2}$$

3. **Total oxygen content**

$$\frac{\begin{array}{r}19.095\ \text{vol}\%\ O_2\ (\text{bound to hemoglobin})\\ +\ 0.135\end{array}}{\begin{array}{l}19.23\ \text{vol}\%\ O_2\ (\text{total amount of }O_2/100\ mL\\ \text{of blood})\end{array}}$$

Note that the patient's "total arterial oxygen content" is normal (19.23 vol% O_2)—in spite of the fact the the Pa_{O_2} is only 45 torr. This is because the patient's hemoglobin concentration, which is one of the major mechanisms for transporting oxygen, is very high: the patient has polycythemia.

Unfortunately, the advantage of the increased oxygen-carrying capacity in polycythemia is often offset by the increased viscosity of the blood when the hematocrit reaches about 55 to 60 percent. Because of the increased viscosity of the blood, a greater driving pressure is needed to maintain a given flow. The work on the right and left ventricle must increase in order to generate the pressure needed to overcome the increased viscosity. This can ultimately lead to left ventricular hypertrophy and failure and to right ventricular hypertrophy and cor pulmonale. The general clinical manifestations of polycythemia include weakness and fatigue, headaches, lightheadedness, and dizziness, digital clubbing, and low Pa_{O_2} levels.

Oxyhemoglobin Dissociation Curve

As shown in Figure 6–3, the **oxyhemoglobin dissociation curve** (Hb_{O_2} curve), also known as the **oxyhemoglobin equilibrium curve**, is part of a nomogram that graphically illustrates the *percentage of hemoglobin* (left-hand side of the graph) that is chemically bound to oxygen at each *oxygen pressure* (bottom portion of the graph). On the right-hand side of the graph, a second scale is included that gives the precise *oxygen content* that is carried by the hemoglobin at each oxygen pressure.

The curve is S-shaped with a steep slope between 10 and 60 torr and a flat portion between 70 and 100 torr. The steep portion of the curve shows that oxygen rapidly combines with hemoglobin as the P_{O_2} increases. Beyond this point (60 torr), a further increase in the P_{O_2} produces only a slight increase in oxygen-hemoglobin bonding. In fact, because the hemoglobin is already 90 percent saturated at a P_{O_2} of 60 torr, an increase in the P_{O_2} from 60 to 100 torr elevates the total saturation of the hemoglobin by only 7 percent (see Figure 6–3).

Clinical Significance of the Flat Portion of the Curve

The P_{O_2} can fall from 100 to 60 torr and the hemoglobin will still be 90 percent saturated with oxygen. Thus, the upper curve plateau illustrates that hemoglobin has an excellent safety zone for the loading of oxygen in the lungs.

Figure 6–3

Oxyhemoglobin dissociation curve.

© Cengage Learning 2013

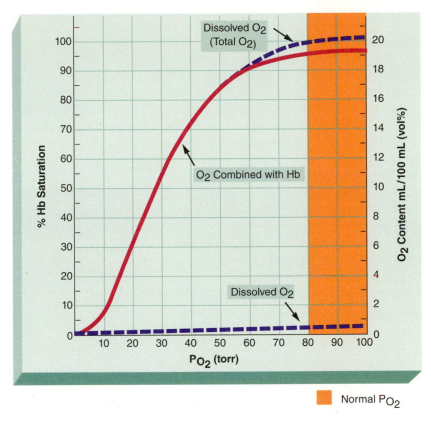

Normal P_{O_2}

As the hemoglobin moves through the alveolar-capillary system to pick up oxygen, a significant partial pressure difference continues to exist between the alveolar gas and the blood, even after most of the oxygen is transferred. This mechanism enhances the diffusion of oxygen during the transit time of the hemoglobin in the alveolar-capillary system.

The flat portion also means that increasing the P_{O_2} beyond 100 torr adds very little additional oxygen to the blood. In fact, once the P_{O_2} increases enough to saturate 100 percent of the hemoglobin with oxygen, the hemoglobin will no longer accept any additional oxygen molecules. However, a small additional amount of oxygen continues to dissolve in the plasma as the P_{O_2} rises $\left(P_{O_2} \times 0.003 = \text{dissolved } P_{O_2}\right)$

Clinical Significance of the Steep Portion of the Curve

A reduction of P_{O_2} to below 60 torr produces a rapid decrease in the amount of oxygen bound to hemoglobin. Clinically, therefore, when the P_{O_2} continues to fall below 60 torr, the quantity of oxygen delivered to the tissue cells may be significantly reduced.

The steep portion of the curve also shows that as the hemoglobin moves through the capillaries of the tissue cells, a large amount of oxygen is released from the hemoglobin for only a small decrease in P_{O_2}. Thus, the diffusion of oxygen from the hemoglobin to the tissue cells is enhanced.

Clinical Connection—6-3

The Pulse Oximeter—The Pa_{O_2} and Sa_{O_2} Relationship

The **pulse oximeter** is a clip-like medical device that indirectly monitors the patient's arterial oxyhemoglobin saturation (see Figure 6–4). When a pulse oximeter is used, the oxygen saturation value is reported as Sp_{O_2} (the "p" represents pulse)—as opposed to measuring the oxygen saturation directly by means of an arterial blood gas sample, which is reported as Sa_{O_2} (the "a" represents direct arterial blood).

The pulse oximeter measures oxygen saturation by reflecting light off the hemoglobin. The color change in hemoglobin is directly related to its oxygen saturation. To prevent measuring capillary or venous blood, the oximeter assesses only the pulsing waveforms. The pulse oximeter is easily connected to the patient's fingertip, toe, or earlobe. Most monitors also display the pulse rate. The pulse oximeter is routinely used to follow a patient's

oxygen saturation tends—and, importantly, to identify potentially dangerous drops in the patient's partial pressure of arterial oxygenation (Pa_{O_2}) status.

For example, by using the general rule of thumb called the **40-50-60/70-80-90 Pa_{O_2}/Sa_{O_2} rule** in the following box, the patient's Sa_{O_2} value can readily provide a good estimate of the patient's Pa_{O_2} value.

The 40-50-60/70-80-90 Rule (General Pa_{O_2}/Sa_{O_2} Relationship)	
Approximate Pa_{O_2} (torr)	**Approximate Sa_{O_2} (%)**
40	70
50	80
60	90

Thus, if a patient's pulse oximeter reading is 90 percent or greater, the patient should have a Pa_{O_2} of 60 torr or greater. It should be stressed, however, that this rule is only a general guideline. The 40-50-60/70-80-90 rule works best when (1) the pH, Pa_{CO_2}, and Hb values are within the normal range, and (2) the patient's Pa_{O_2} value is on the steep portion of the oxyhemoglobin dissociation curve (see Figure 6–3). Whenever the respiratory therapist suspects the patient's oxygenation status is moving in a harmful direction, an arterial blood gas should be performed to fully evaluate the patient's pH, Pa_{CO_2}, HCO_3^-, Pa_{O_2}, and Sa_{O_2} values. Most pulse oximeter measurements below 70 percent are considered inaccurate and unreliable.

Figure 6–4

A pulse oximeter.

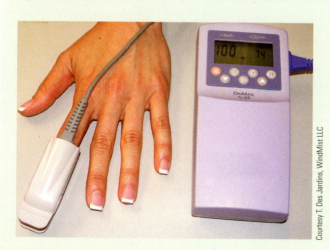

Courtesy T. Des Jardins, WindMist LLC

The P_{50}

A point of reference on the oxyhemoglobin dissociation curve is the P_{50} (Figure 6–5). The P_{50} represents the partial pressure at which the hemoglobin is 50 percent saturated with oxygen—that is, when there are two oxygen molecules on each hemoglobin molecule. Normally, the P_{50} is about 27 torr. Clinically, however, there are a variety of abnormal conditions that can shift the oxyhemoglobin dissociation curve to either the right or left.

When this happens, the P_{50} changes. For example, when the curve shifts to the right, the affinity of hemoglobin for oxygen decreases, causing the hemoglobin to be less saturated at a given P_{O_2}. Thus, *when the curve shifts to the right, the P_{50} increases.* On the other hand, when the curve moves to the left, the affinity of hemoglobin for oxygen increases, causing the hemoglobin to be more saturated at a given P_{O_2}. Thus, *when the curve shifts to the left, the P_{50} decreases* (see Figure 6–5).

Factors That Shift the Oxyhemoglobin Dissociation Curve

pH

As the blood hydrogen ion concentration increases (decreased pH), the oxyhemoglobin dissociation curve shifts to the right. This mechanism enhances the unloading of oxygen at the cellular level, because the pH decreases in this area as carbon dioxide (the acidic end-product of cellular metabolism) moves into the blood. In contrast, as the blood hydrogen ion (H^+) concentration decreases, the curve shifts to the left. This mechanism facilitates the loading of oxygen onto hemoglobin as blood passes through the lungs, because the pH increases as carbon dioxide moves out of the blood and into the alveoli.

Figure 6–5

The P_{50} represents the partial pressure at which hemoglobin is 50 percent saturated with oxygen. When the oxyhemoglobin dissociation curve shifts to the right, the P_{50} increases. When the oxyhemoglobin dissociation curve shifts to the left, the P_{50} decreases.

© Cengage Learning 2013

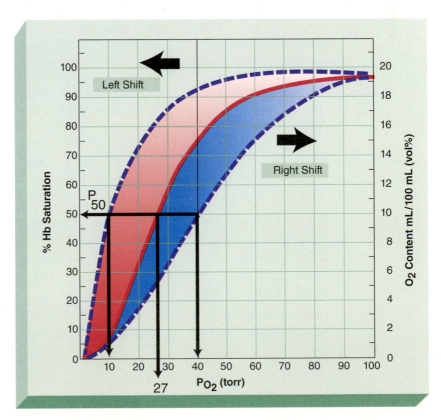

Temperature

As the body temperature increases, the curve moves to the right. Thus, exercise, which produces an elevated temperature, enhances the release of oxygen as blood flows through the muscle capillaries. Conversely, as the body temperature decreases, the curve shifts to the left. This mechanism partly explains why an individual's lips, ears, and fingers appear blue while swimming in very cold water. That is, their Pa_{O_2} is normal, but oxygen is not readily released from the hemoglobin at the cold tissue sites.

Carbon Dioxide

As the P_{CO_2} level increases (increased H^+ concentration), the oxyhemoglobin saturation decreases, shifting the oxyhemoglobin dissociation curve to the right, whereas decreasing Pa_{O_2} levels (decreased H^+ concentrations) shift the curve to the left. The effect of Pa_{O_2} and pH on the oxyhemoglobin curve is known as the **Bohr effect**. The Bohr effect is most active in the capillaries of working muscles, particularly the myocardium.

2,3-Biphosphoglycerate (formally called 2,3-Diphosphoglycerate)

The RBCs contain a large quantity (about 15 mol/g Hb) of the substance 2,3-biphosphoglycerate (2,3-BPG). 2,3-BPG is a metabolic intermediary that is formed by the RBCs during anaerobic glycolysis. Hemoglobin's affinity for oxygen decreases as the 2,3-BPG level increases. Thus, the effect of an elevated concentration of 2,3-BPG is to shift the oxyhemoglobin dissociation curve to the right. Clinically, a variety of conditions affect the level of 2,3-BPG.

Hypoxia. Regardless of the cause, hypoxia increases the 2,3-BPG level.

Anemia. The 2,3-BPG level increases as the hemoglobin concentration decreases. This mechanism may explain why individuals with anemia frequently do not manifest the signs or symptoms associated with hypoxia.

pH Changes. As the pH increases, the 2,3-BPG concentration increases. Thus, the shift of the oxyhemoglobin dissociation curve to the left by the increased pH is offset somewhat by the increased 2,3-BPG level, which shifts the curve to the right. Conversely, as the pH decreases, the 2,3-BPG concentration decreases. Thus, while the decreased pH shifts the curve to the right, the decreased 2,3-BPG level works to shift the curve to the left.

Stored Blood. Blood stored for as little as 1 week has been shown to have very low concentrations of 2,3-BPG. Thus, when patients receive stored blood, the oxygen unloading in their tissues may be reduced because of the decreased 2,3-BPG level.

Fetal Hemoglobin

Fetal hemoglobin (Hb F) is chemically different from adult hemoglobin. Hb F has a greater affinity for oxygen and, therefore, shifts the oxyhemoglobin dissociation curve to the left (reducing the P_{50}). During fetal development, the higher affinity of Hb F enhances the transfer of oxygen from maternal blood to fetal blood. After birth, Hb F progressively disappears and is completely absent after about 1 year.

© Cengage Learning 2013

Figure 6–6

Factors that shift the oxyhemoglobin dissociation curve to the right and left. (BPG = 2,3-biphosphoglycerate; for other abbreviations, see text)

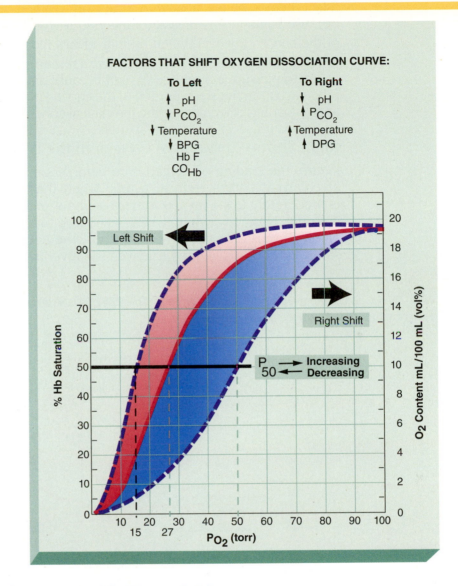

Carbon Monoxide Hemoglobin

Carbon monoxide (CO) has about 210 times the affinity of oxygen for hemoglobin. Because of this, a small amount of CO can tie up a large amount of hemoglobin and, as a result, prevent oxygen molecules from bonding to hemoglobin. When CO bonds with hemoglobin it is called **carboxyhemoglobin (CO_{Hb})**.

CO_{Hb} can seriously reduce the amount of oxygen transferred to the tissue cells. In addition, when CO_{Hb} is present, the affinity of hemoglobin for oxygen increases and shifts the oxyhemoglobin dissociation curve to the left. Thus, the oxygen molecules that do manage to combine with hemoglobin are unable to unload easily in the tissues.

Figure 6–6 summarizes factors that shift the oxyhemoglobin dissociation curve to the right and left and how the P_{50} is affected by these shifts.

Clinical Significance of Shifts in the Oxyhemoglobin Dissociation Curve

When an individual's blood Pa_{O_2} is within normal limits (80 to 100 torr), a shift of the oxyhemoglobin dissociation curve to the right or left does not significantly affect hemoglobin's ability to transport oxygen to the peripheral tissues, because shifts in this pressure range (80 to 100 torr) occur on the flat portion of the curve. However, when an individual's blood Pa_{O_2} falls below the normal range, a shift to the right or left can have a remarkable effect on the hemoglobin's ability to pick up and release oxygen because shifts below the normal pressure range occur on the steep portion of the curve. For example, consider the loading and unloading of oxygen during the clinical conditions discussed next.

Right Shifts—Loading of Oxygen in the Lungs

Picture the loading of oxygen onto hemoglobin as blood passes through the alveolar-capillary system at a time when the alveolar oxygen tension Pa_{O_2} is moderately low—say, 60 torr (caused, for example, by an acute asthmatic episode). Normally, when the Pa_{O_2} is 60 torr, the P_{O_2} of the pulmonary capillary blood (P_{CO_2}) is also about 60 torr. Thus, the hemoglobin is about 90 percent saturated with oxygen as it leaves the alveoli (Figure 6–7). If, however, the

Figure 6–7

Normally, when the Pa_{O_2} is 60 torr, the plasma P_{O_2} of the alveolar-capillary blood is also about 60 torr and the hemoglobin is about 90 percent saturated with oxygen as it leaves the alveoli.

© Cengage Learning 2013

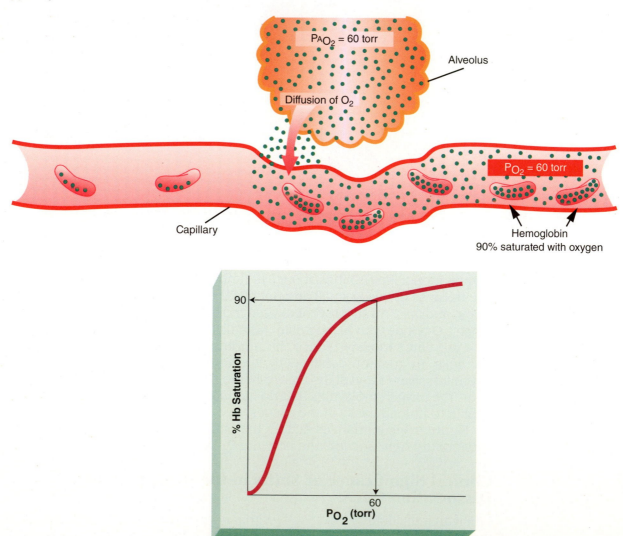

oxyhemoglobin dissociation curve shifts to the right, as indicated in Figure 6–8 (caused by a pH of about 7.1), the hemoglobin will be only about 75 percent saturated with oxygen as it leaves the alveoli—despite the fact that the patient's plasma P_{O_2} is still 60 torr.

In view of this gas transport phenomenon, therefore, it should be stressed that *the total oxygen delivery may be much lower than indicated by a particular Pa_{O_2} value when a disease process is present that causes the oxyhemoglobin dissociation curve to shift to the right* (see Figure 6–6). However, as discussed later, the unloading of oxygen at the tissue sites is actually enhanced when the oxyhemoglobin dissociation curse is shifted to the right. This action helps to offset the decreased loading of oxygen between the alveoli and pulmonary capillaries when the curve is shifted to the right. Note also that when a right shift is accompanied by either a decreased cardiac output or a reduced level of hemoglobin, the patient's ability to transport oxygen will be jeopardized even more.

Figure 6–8

When the Pa_{O_2} is 60 torr at a time when the oxyhemoglobin dissociation curve has shifted to the right because of a pH of 7.1, the hemoglobin will be only about 75 percent saturated with oxygen as it leaves the alveoli.

© Cengage Learning 2013

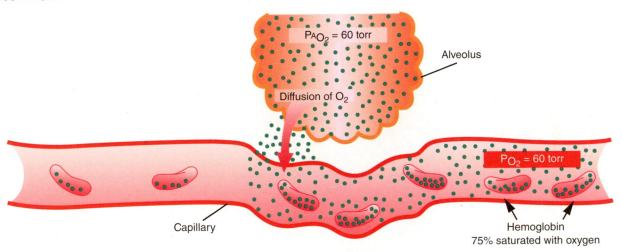

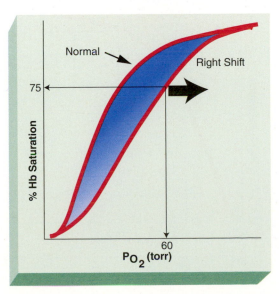

Right Shifts—Unloading of Oxygen at the Tissues

Although the total oxygen delivery may decrease in the above situation, the plasma P_{O_2} at the tissue sites does not have to fall as much to unload oxygen from the hemoglobin. For example, if the tissue cells metabolize 5 vol% oxygen at a time when the oxyhemoglobin dissociation curve is in its normal position, the plasma P_{O_2} must fall from 60 torr to about 35 torr to free 5 vol% oxygen from the hemoglobin (Figure 6–9). If, however, the curve shifts to the right in response to a pH of 7.1, the plasma P_{O_2} at the tissue sites would only have to fall from 60 torr to about 40 torr to unload 5 vol% oxygen from the hemoglobin (Figure 6–10).

Figure 6–9

Normally, when the plasma P_{O_2} is 60 torr, the P_{O_2} must fall from 60 torr to about 35 torr to free 5 vol% oxygen from the hemoglobin for tissue metabolism.

© Cengage Learning 2013

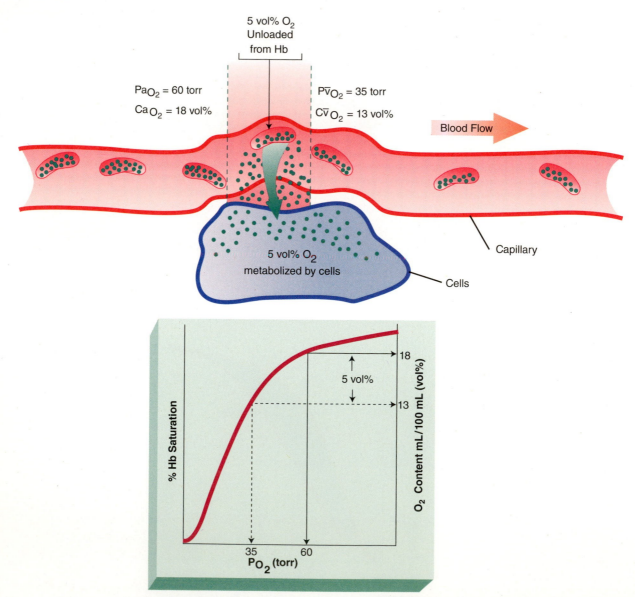

Figure 6–10

When the Pa_{O_2} is 60 torr at a time when the oxyhemoglobin dissociation curve has shifted to the right because of a pH of 7.1, the plasma P_{O_2} at the tissue site would have to fall from 60 torr to about 40 torr to unload 5 vol% oxygen from the hemoglobin.

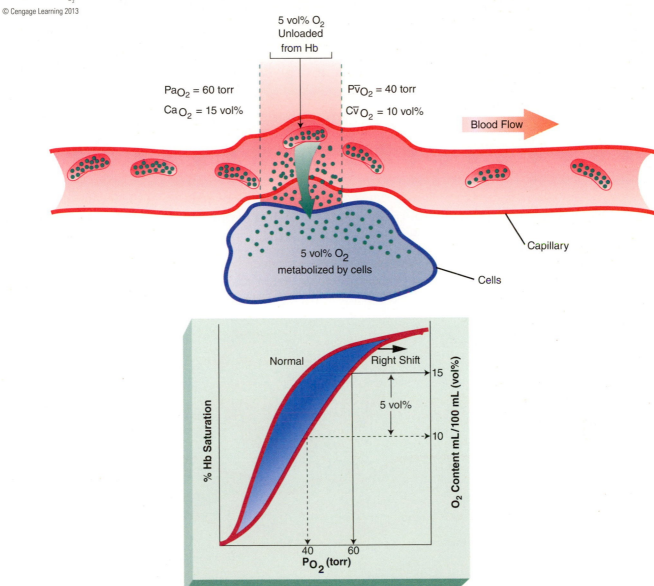

Clinical Connection—6-4

Case Study—The Significance of a Right Shift in the Oxyhemoglobin Dissociation Curve

In the **Clinical Application Section—Case 2** (page 299), the respiratory therapist is called to assist in the care of an 18-year-old woman who presents in the emergency department in severe respiratory distress during an asthmatic episode. This case illustrates how a right shift in the oxygen dissociation—produced by a decreased pH and an increased Pa_{CO_2} level—causes (1) a decrease in the loading of oxygen as hemoglobin passes through the lungs and (2) a decrease in the patient's total oxygen delivery. This case effectively highlights that when additional clinical factors are present—that shift the oxygen dissociation curve to the right, or left—the respiratory therapist must take into account these factors in the final analysis of the patient's overall oxygenation status.

Left Shifts—Loading of Oxygen in the Lungs

If the oxyhemoglobin dissociation curve shifts to the left, as indicated in Figure 6–11 (caused by a pH of about 7.6), at a time when the $P_{A_{O_2}}$ is 60 torr, the hemoglobin will be about 95 percent saturated with oxygen as it leaves the alveoli, even though the patient's plasma P_{O_2} is only 60 torr.

Left Shifts—Unloading of Oxygen at the Tissues

Although the total oxygen delivery increases in the previously mentioned situation, the plasma P_{O_2} at the tissue sites must decrease more than normal in order for oxygen to dissociate from the hemoglobin. For example, if the tissue cells require 5 vol% oxygen at a time when the oxyhemoglobin dissociation curve is normal, the plasma P_{O_2} will fall from 60 torr to about 35 torr to free 5 vol% of oxygen from the hemoglobin (see Figure 6–9). If, however, the curve shifts to the left because of a pH of 7.6, the plasma P_{O_2} at the tissue sites would have to fall from 60 torr to about 30 torr in order to unload 5 vol% oxygen from the hemoglobin (Figure 6–12).

Figure 6–11

When the $P_{A_{O_2}}$ is 60 torr at a time when the oxyhemoglobin dissociation curve has shifted to the left because of a pH of 7.6, the hemoglobin will be about 95 percent saturated with oxygen as it leaves the alveoli.

© Cengage Learning 2013

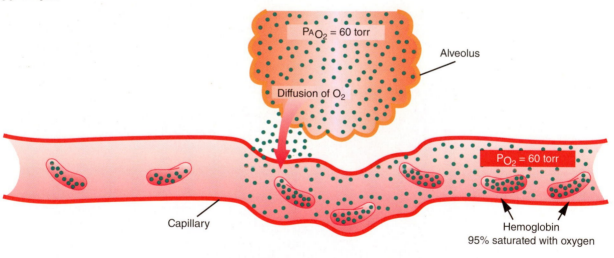

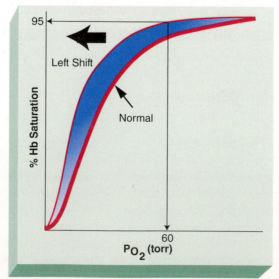

Figure 6–12

When the Pa_{O_2} is 60 torr at a time when the oxyhemoglobin dissociation curve has shifted to the left because of a pH of 7.6, the plasma P_{O_2} at the tissue sites would have to fall from 60 torr to about 30 torr to unload 5 vol% oxygen from the hemoglobin.

© Cengage Learning 2013

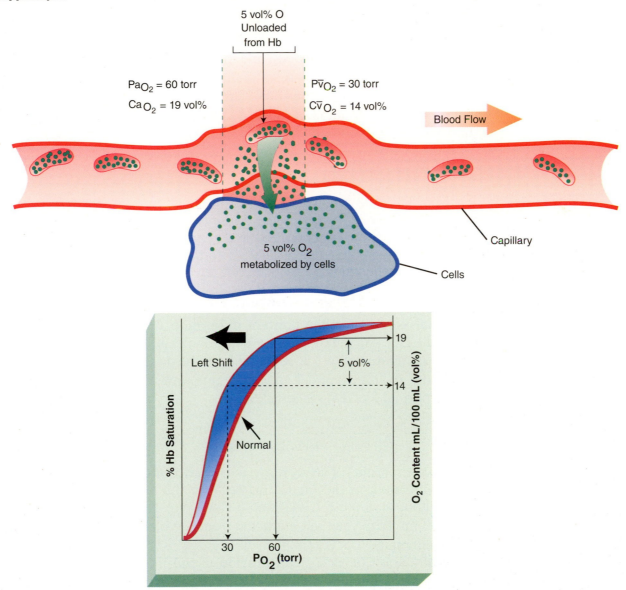

Oxygen Transport Calculations

Various mathematical manipulations of the Ca_{O_2}, $C\bar{v}_{O_2}$ and Cc_{O_2} values can serve as excellent indicators of an individual's cardiac and ventilatory status. Clinically, the most common oxygen transport studies performed are (1) total oxygen delivery, (2) arterial-venous oxygen content difference, (3) oxygen consumption, (4) oxygen extraction ratio, (5) mixed venous oxygen saturation, and (6) pulmonary shunting.[4]

---

[4] See Appendix V for a representative example of a cardiopulmonary profile sheet used to monitor the oxygen transport status of the critically ill patient.

Total Oxygen Delivery

The total amount of oxygen delivered or transported to the peripheral tissues is dependent on (1) the body's ability to oxygenate blood, (2) the hemoglobin concentration, and (3) the cardiac output ($\dot{Q}$). **Total oxygen delivery** (D_{O_2}) is calculated as follows:

$$D_{O_2} = \dot{Q}_T \times \left(Ca_{O_2} \times 10\right)$$

where $\dot{Q}_T$ is total cardiac output (L/min); Ca_{O_2} is the oxygen content of arterial blood (mL oxygen/100 mL blood); and the factor 10 is needed to convert the Ca_{O_2} to mL O_2/L blood.

For example, if an individual has a cardiac output of 5 L/min and a Ca_{O_2} of 20 vol%, the total amount of oxygen delivered to the peripheral tissues will be about 1000 mL of oxygen per minute:

$$\begin{aligned} D_{O_2} &= \dot{Q}_T \times \left(Ca_{O_2} \times 10\right) \\ &= 5\,L \times (20\text{ vol\%} \times 10) \\ &= 1000\text{ mL } O_2/\text{min} \end{aligned}$$

Oxygen delivery decreases when there is a decline in (1) blood oxygenation, (2) hemoglobin concentration, or (3) cardiac output. When possible, an individual's hemoglobin concentration or cardiac output will often increase in an effort to compensate for a reduced oxygen delivery.

Arterial-Venous Oxygen Content Difference

The **arterial-venous oxygen content difference**, $C(a - \bar{v})_{O_2}$ is the difference between the Ca_{O_2} and the $C\bar{v}_{O_2}$ $\left(Ca_{O_2} - C\bar{v}_{O_2}\right)$. Clinically, the mixed venous blood needed to compute the $C\bar{v}_{O_2}$ is obtained from the patient's pulmonary artery.

Normally, the Ca_{O_2} is about 20 vol% and the $C\bar{v}_{O_2}$ is 15 vol% (Figure 6–13). Thus, the normal $C(a - \bar{v})_{O_2}$ is about 5 vol%:

$$\begin{aligned} C(a - \bar{v})_{O_2} &= Ca_{O_2} - C\bar{v}_{O_2} \\ &= 20\text{ vol\%} - 15\text{ vol\%} = 5\text{ vol\%} \end{aligned}$$

In other words, 5 mL of oxygen are extracted from each 100 mL of blood for tissue metabolism (50 mL O_2/L). Because the average individual has a cardiac output of about 5 L/min and a $C(a - \bar{v})_{O_2}$ of about 5 vol%, approximately 250 mL of oxygen are extracted from the blood during the course of 1 minute (50 mL O_2/L $\times$ 5 L/min).

Clinically, the $C(a - \bar{v})_{O_2}$ can provide useful information regarding the patient's cardiopulmonary status, because oxygen changes in mixed venous blood can occur earlier than oxygen changes in an arterial blood gas. Table 6–2 lists factors that can cause the $C(a - \bar{v})_{O_2}$ to increase. Factors that can cause the $C(a - \bar{v})_{O_2}$ to decrease are listed in Table 6–3.

Oxygen Consumption

The amount of oxygen extracted by the peripheral tissues during the period of 1 minute is called **oxygen consumption**, or *oxygen uptake* $\left(\dot{V}_{O_2}\right)$. An individual's oxygen consumption is calculated by using this formula:

$$\dot{V}_{O_2} = \dot{Q}_T \left[C(a - \bar{v})_{O_2} \times 10\right]$$

where $\dot{Q}_T$ is the total cardiac output (L/min); $C(a - \bar{v})_{O_2}$ is the arterial-venous oxygen content difference $\left(Ca_{O_2} - C\bar{v}_{O_2}\right)$ and the factor 10 is needed to convert the $C(a - \bar{v})_{O_2}$ to mL O_2/L.

Figure 6–13

Oxyhemoglobin dissociation curve. The normal oxygen content difference between arterial and venous blood is about 5 vol%. Note that both the right side and the left side of the graph illustrate that approximately 25 percent of the available oxygen is used for tissue metabolism and, therefore, the hemoglobin returning to the lungs is normally about 75 percent saturated with oxygen.

© Cengage Learning 2013

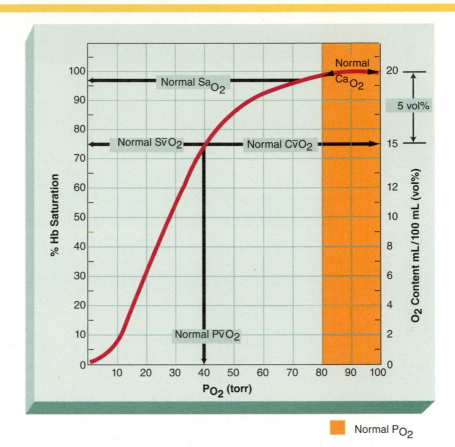

Normal P_{O_2}

Table 6–2

Factors That Increase the $C(a - \bar{v})_{O_2}$

Decreased cardiac output
Periods of increased oxygen consumption
    Exercise
    Seizures
    Shivering
    Hyperthermia

© Cengage Learning 2013

Table 6–3

Factors That Decrease the $C(a - \bar{v})_{O_2}$

Increased cardiac output
Skeletal muscle relaxation (e.g., induced by drugs)
Peripheral shunting (e.g., sepsis, trauma)
Certain poisons (e.g., cyanide prevents cellular metabolism)
Hypothermia

© Cengage Learning 2013

Table 6–4	
Factors That Increase $\dot{V}_{O_2}$	
Exercise	
Seizures	
Shivering	
Hyperthermia	

© Cengage Learning 2013

Table 6–5	
Factors That Decrease $\dot{V}_{O_2}$	
Skeletal muscle relaxation (e.g., induced by drugs)	
Peripheral shunting (e.g., sepsis, trauma)	
Certain poisons (e.g., cyanide prevents cellular metabolism)	
Hypothermia	

© Cengage Learning 2013

For example, if an individual has a cardiac output of 5 L/min and a $C(a - \bar{v})_{O_2}$ of 5 vol%, the total amount of oxygen metabolized by the tissues in 1 minute will be 250 mL:

$$\dot{V}_{O_2} = \dot{Q}_T \, [C(a - \bar{v})_{O_2} \times 10]$$
$$= 5 \text{ L/min} \times 5 \text{ vol\%} \times 10$$
$$= 250 \text{ mL } O_2/\text{min}$$

Clinically, the oxygen consumption is usually related to the patient's body surface area (BSA) (see Appendix IV), because the amount of oxygen extracted by the peripheral cells varies with an individual's height and weight. The patient's oxygen consumption index is derived by dividing the $\dot{V}_{O_2}$ by the BSA. The average oxygen consumption index ranges between 125 to 165 mL O_2/m^2.

Factors that cause an increase in oxygen consumption are listed in Table 6–4. Table 6–5 lists factors that cause a decrease in oxygen consumption.

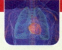 Clinical Connection—6-5

Cardiopulmonary Resuscitation (CPR)—Start as Early as Possible!

In sudden cardiac arrest, permanent brain damage can begin in as little as 4 minutes—and death can follow minutes later. When reflecting on the oxygen tranport calculations—especially the **total oxygen delivery (D_{O_2})** and the **oxygen consumption ($\dot{V}_{O_2}$)** equations—the respiratory therapist can quickly develop a whole new appreciation for the basic cardiopulmonary physiology that supports the importance of starting CPR as early as possible— *ideally, within the first 4 minutes!*

For example, let's first consider the relationship between the D_{O_2} equation and the $\dot{V}_{O_2}$ equation under normal, healthy conditions: The D_{O_2} calculation—the O_2 supply system equation— illustrates that about 1000 mL of oxygen are transported to the tissue cells each minute. On the other hand, the $\dot{V}_{O_2}$ calculation—the O_2 demand system equation—illustrates that of this 1000 mL, about 250 mL of oxygen are consumed by the tissue cells in the course of the metabolic process. Using the normal D_{O_2} and $\dot{V}_{O_2}$ relationship, let's consider the following basic math, time sequence, and oxygen consumption that typically occurs during a 4-minute period:

Clinical Connection—6-5, continued

Normal Oxygen Consumption over a 4-Minute Period

Time	Oxygen Metabolism by Tissue Cells
Minute 1	As the $\dot{V}_{O_2}$ calculation illustrates, the body normally consumes about **250 mL of O_2** each minute.
Minute 2	During the 2nd minute, the body continues to consume another 250 mL of O_2—for a **total 500 mL O_2**.
Minute 3	During the 3rd minute, the body continues to consume another 250 mL O_2—for a **total of 750 mL O_2**.
Minute 4	During the 4th minute, the body continues to consume another 250 mL of O_2—for a **total of 1000 mL O_2**.

Thus, in just 4 minutes—under normal healthy conditions—the body consumes about 1000 mL O_2—a liter of oxygen.

Now let's consider what happens to the oxygen transport system during a sudden cardiac arrest: immediately, the patient's entire blood flow throughout the body stops—and, the blood pressure rapidly falls. In other words, the patient's entire blood volume—an average of about 5 L—becomes motionless when the heart stops beating. It is estimated that *only* about 5 percent of an individual's total blood volume is contained in the systemic capillary system at any given moment—that is, in the tissue oxygen utilization area. (Approximately 65 percent of the total blood volume is contained in the systemic veins and venules, about 15 percent is contained in the systemic arteries and arterioles, and about 15 percent is contained in the heart and pulmonary vessels.)

The bottom line is this: when the heart stops beating, only a small amount of the total blood volume—about 5 percent—is in the systemic capillary system. Only the oxygen contained in the systemic capillary blood is available for tissue metabolism. Once this oxygen is consumed, anerobic metabolism, tissue cell damage, and death will quickly ensue.

Although it is impossible to determine the precise amount of oxygen in the sytemic capillary system at any given moment and the rate at which the oxygen is being metabolized immediately after a cardiac arrest, it is known that a number of unfavorable mechanisms rapidly develop that adversely affect the patient's oxygenation status—including the following:

- The immediate stoppage of the oxygen delivery system—which, in turn, leads to anaerobic metabolism and lactic acidosis.

- The sudden stoppage of transporting the tissue CO_2 to the lungs for elimination—which, in turn, lead to a rapid accumulation of CO_2 throughout the body.

- The abrupt drop in pH—which is caused by the CO_2 accumulation and lactic acid accumulation.

Additional confounding factors may include (1) the patient's initial baseline oxygenation level, which may be low; (2) the patient's general health, which may be poor; and (3) the patient's age.

Thus, as one can easily see, the initiation of CPR as soon as possible in the cardiac arrest patient is absolutely critical! The tissue cells will continue to consume any available oxygen in the stagnated blood as long as possible. When it comes to CPR—and the administration of 100 percent oxygen—the earlier the better! The following box provides an overview of the generally accepted likelihood of brain damage or death after a cardiac arrest.

Brain Damage after Cardiac Arrest

Time after Cardiac Arrest	Chances of Brain Damage
0–4 minutes	Minimal
4–6 minutes	Possible
6–10 minutes	Likely
>10 minutes	Brain death likely

Oxygen Extraction Ratio

The oxygen extraction ratio (O_2ER) is the amount of oxygen extracted by the peripheral tissues divided by the amount of oxygen delivered to the peripheral cells. The O_2ER is also known as the *oxygen coefficient ratio* or the *oxygen utilization ratio.*

The O_2ER is easily calculated by dividing the $C(a - \bar{v})_{O_2}$ by the Ca_{O_2}. In considering the normal Ca_{O_2} of 20 vol%, and the normal $C\bar{v}_{O_2}$ of 15 vol% (see Figure 6–11), the O_2ER ratio of the healthy individual is about 25 percent:

$$O_2ER = \frac{Ca_{O_2} - C\bar{v}_{O_2}}{Ca_{O_2}}$$

$$= \frac{20 \text{ vol\%} - 15 \text{ vol\%}}{20 \text{ vol\%}}$$

$$= \frac{5 \text{ vol\%}}{20 \text{ vol\%}}$$

$$= 0.25$$

Under normal circumstances, therefore, an individual's hemoglobin returns to the alveoli approximately 75 percent saturated with oxygen (see Figure 6–13). In an individual with a total oxygen delivery of 1000 mL/min, an extraction ratio of 25 percent would mean that during the course of 1 minute, 250 mL of oxygen are metabolized by the tissues and 750 mL of oxygen are returned to the lungs.

Factors that cause the O_2ER to increase are listed in Table 6–6. Table 6–7 lists factors that cause the O_2ER to decrease.

Table 6–6
Factors That Increase the O_2ER
Decreased cardiac output
Periods of increased oxygen consumption
Exercise
Seizures
Shivering
Hyperthermia
Anemia
Decreased arterial oxygenation

© Cengage Learning 2013

Table 6–7
Factors That Decrease the O_2ER
Increased cardiac output
Skeletal muscle relaxation (e.g., induced by drugs)
Peripheral shunting (e.g., sepsis, trauma)
Certain poisons (e.g., cyanide prevents cellular metabolism)
Hypothermia (slows cellular metabolism)
Increased hemoglobin concentration
Increased arterial oxygenation

© Cengage Learning 2013

The O_2ER provides an important view of an individual's oxygen transport status that is not readily available from other oxygen transport measurements. For example, in an individual with normal Ca_{O_2} and normal $C\bar{v}_{O_2}$:

$$
\begin{array}{ll}
Ca_{O_2}: & 20\ vol\% \\
-\ C\bar{v}_{O_2}: & 15\ vol\% \\
\hline
C(a - \bar{v})_{O_2} & =\ 5\ vol\%
\end{array}
$$

the $C(a - \bar{v}_{O_2})$ is 5 vol% and the O_2ER is 25 percent (normal). However, in an individual with reduced Ca_{O_2} and reduced $C\bar{v}_{O_2}$:

$$
\begin{array}{ll}
Ca_{O_2}: & 10\ vol\% \\
-\ C\bar{v}_{O_2}: & 5\ vol\% \\
\hline
C(a - \bar{v})_{O_2} & =\ 5\ vol\%
\end{array}
$$

the $C(a - \bar{v}_{O_2})$ is still 5 vol% (assuming O_2 consumption remains constant), but the extraction ratio (O_2ER) is now 50 percent—clinically, a potentially dangerous situation.

Mixed Venous Oxygen Saturation

In the presence of a normal arterial oxygen saturation level Sa_{O_2} and hemoglobin concentration, the continuous monitoring of mixed venous oxygen saturation $(S\bar{v}_{O_2})$ is often used in the clinical setting to detect changes in the patient's $C(a - \bar{v})_{O_2}$, $\dot{V}_{O_2}$, and O_2ER. Normally, the $(S\bar{v}_{O_2})$ is about 75 percent (see Figure 6–13). Clinically, an $(S\bar{v}_{O_2})$ of about 65 percent is acceptable.

Factors that can cause the $(S\bar{v}_{O_2})$ to decrease are listed in Table 6–8. Table 6–9 lists factors that can cause the $(S\bar{v}_{O_2})$ to increase.

Table 6–8

Factors That Decrease the $S\bar{v}_{O_2}$*

Decreased cardiac output
Periods of increased oxygen consumption
    Exercise
    Seizures
    Shivering
    Hyperthermia

* A decreased $S\bar{v}_{O_2}$ indicates that the $C(a - \bar{v})_{O_2}$, $\dot{V}_{O_2}$, and O_2ER are increasing.
© Cengage Learning 2013

Table 6–9

Factors That Increase the $S\bar{v}_{O_2}$*

Increased cardiac output
Skeletal muscle relaxation (e.g., induced by drugs)
Peripheral shunting (e.g., sepsis, trauma)
Certain poisons (e.g., cyanide prevents cellular metabolism)
Hypothermia

* An increased $S\bar{v}_{O_2}$ indicates that the $C(a - \bar{v})_{O_2}$, $\dot{V}_{O_2}$, and O_2ER are decreasing.
© Cengage Learning 2013

Table 6–10

Clinical Factors Affecting Various Oxygen Transport Calculation Values

Clinical Factors	Oxygen Transport Calculations				
	D_{O_2} (1000 mL O_2/min)	$\dot{V}_{O_2}$ (250 mL O_2/min)	$C(a-\bar{v})_{O_2}$ (5 vol%)	O_2ER (25%)	$S\bar{v}_{O_2}$ (75%)
↑ **O_2 Loading in the lungs** ↑ Hb ↑ Pa_{O_2} ↓ Pa_{CO_2} ↑ pH ↓ Temperature	↑	Same	Same	↓	↑
↓ **O_2 Loading in the lungs** ↓ Hb ↑ Pa_{CO_2} ↓ pH ↓ Pa_{O_2} Anemia ↑ Temperature	↓	Same	Same	↑	↓
↑ **Metabolism** Exercise Seizures Hyperthermia Shivering	Same	↑	↑	↑	↓
↓ **Metabolism** Hypothermia Skeletal muscle relaxation (e.g., drug induced)	Same	↓	↓	↓	↑
↓ **Cardiac output**	↓	Same	↑	↑	↓
↑ **Cardiac output**	↑	Same	↓	↓	↑
Peripheral shunting (e.g., sepsis, trauma)	Same	↓	↓	↓	↑
Certain poisons (e.g., cyanide)	Same	↓	↓	↓	↑

↑ = increased; ↓ = decreased.

Continuous $S\bar{v}_{O_2}$ monitoring can signal changes in the patient's $C(a-\bar{v})_{O_2}$, $\dot{V}_{O_2}$, and O_2ER earlier than routine arterial blood gas monitoring, because the Pa_{O_2} and Sa_{O_2} levels are often normal during early $C(a-\bar{v})_{O_2}$, $\dot{V}_{O_2}$, and O_2ER changes. Table 6–10 summarizes how various clinical factors may alter an individual's D_{O_2}, $\dot{V}_{O_2}$, $C(a-\bar{v})_{O_2}$, O_2ER, and $S\bar{v}_{O_2}$.

Pulmonary Shunting

Pulmonary shunting is defined as that portion of the cardiac output that moves from the right side to the left side of the heart without being exposed to alveolar oxygen ($P_{A_{O_2}}$) Clinically, pulmonary shunting can be subdivided into (1) *absolute shunts* (also called *true shunt*) and (2) *relative shunts* (also called *shunt-like effects*).

Absolute Shunt

Absolute shunts (also called *true shunts*) can be grouped under two major categories: *anatomic shunts* and *capillary shunts.*

Anatomic Shunts. An **anatomic shunt** exists when blood flows from the right side of the heart to the left side without coming in contact with an alveolus for gas exchange (see Figures 6–14A and B on page 282). In the healthy lung, there is a normal anatomic shunt of about 3 percent of the cardiac output. This normal shunting is caused by nonoxygenated blood completely bypassing the alveoli and entering (1) the pulmonary vascular system by means of the bronchial venous drainage and (2) the left atrium by way of the thebesian veins. The following are common abnormalities that cause anatomic shunting:

- Congenital heart disease.
- Intrapulmonary fistula.
- Vacular lung tumors.

Congenital Heart Disease. Certain congenital defects permit blood to flow directly from the right side of the heart to the left side without going through the alveolar capillary system for gas exchange. Congenital heart defects include ventricular septum defect or newborns with persistent fetal circulation.

Intrapulmonary Fistula. In this type of anatomic shunting, a right-to-left flow of pulmonary blood does not pass through the alveolar-capillary system. It may be caused by chest trauma or disease. For example, a penetrating chest wound that damages both the arteries and veins of the lung can leave an arterial-venous shunt as a result of the healing process.

Vascular Lung Tumors. Some lung tumors can become very vascular. Some permit pulmonary arterial blood to move through the tumor mass and into the pulmonary veins without passing through the alveolar-capillary system.

Capillary Shunts. A **capillary shunt** is commonly caused by (1) alveolar collapse or atelectasis, (2) alveolar fluid accumulation, or (3) alveolar consolidation (Figure 6–14C).

The sum of the anatomic shunt and capillary shunt is referred to as the *absolute*, or *true, shunt*. Clinically, patients with absolute shunting respond poorly to oxygen therapy, because alveolar oxygen does not come in contact with the shunted blood. Absolute shunting is *refractory* to oxygen therapy; that is, the reduced arterial oxygen level produced by this form of pulmonary shunting cannot be treated simply by increasing the concentration of inspired oxygen, because (1) the alveoli are unable to accommodate any form of ventilation and (2) the blood that bypasses functional alveoli cannot carry more oxygen once it has become fully saturated—except for a very small amount that dissolves in the plasma ($P_{O_2} \times 0.003 =$ dissolved O_2).

Relative Shunt

When pulmonary capillary perfusion is in excess of alveolar ventilation, a **relative shunt**, or **shunt-like effect**, is said to exist (Figure 6–14D). Common causes of this form of shunting include (1) hypoventilation,

Figure 6–14

Pulmonary shunting: **A.** normal alveolar-capillary unit; **B.** anatomic shunt; **C.** types of capillary shunts; and **D.** types of shunt-like effects.

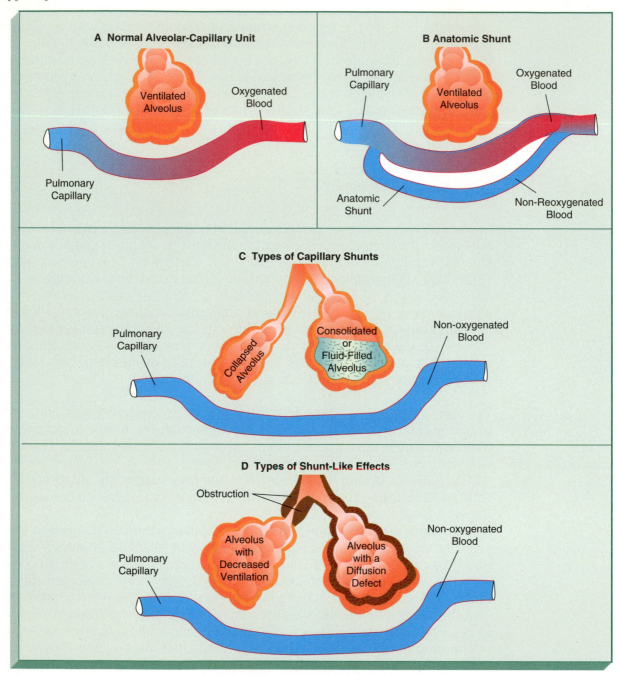

(2) ventilation/perfusion mismatches (e.g., chronic emphysema, bronchitis, asthma, and excessive airway secretions), and (3) alveolar-capillary diffusion defects (e.g., alveolar fibrosis or alveolar edema).

Even though the alveolus may be ventilated in the presence of an alveolar-capillary defect, the blood passing by the alveolus does not have enough time to equilibrate with the alveolar oxygen tension. If the diffusion defect is severe enough to completely block gas exchange across the alveolar-capillary membrane, the shunt is referred to as an *absolute* or *true shunt* (see preceding section). Relative shunting may also occur following the administration of drugs that cause an increase in cardiac output or dilation of the pulmonary vessels. Conditions that cause a shunt-like effect are readily corrected by oxygen therapy. In other words, they are not refractory to oxygen therapy.

Venous Admixture

The end result of pulmonary shunting is **venous admixture**. Venous admixture is the mixing of shunted, *non-reoxygenated blood* with *reoxygenated blood* distal to the alveoli (i.e., downstream in the pulmonary venous system) (Figure 6–15). When venous admixture occurs, the shunted, non-reoxygenated blood gains oxygen molecules while, at the same time, the reoxygenated blood loses oxygen molecules.

This process continues until (1) the P_{O_2} throughout all of the plasma of the newly mixed blood is in equilibrium, and (2) all of the hemoglobin molecules carry the same number of oxygen molecules. The end result is a blood mixture that has a higher P_{O_2} and oxygen content than the original shunted, non-reoxygenated blood, but a lower P_{O_2} and oxygen content than the original reoxygenated blood. The final outcome of venous admixture is a reduced Pa_{O_2} and Ca_{O_2} returning to the left side of the heart. Clinically, it is this oxygen mixture that is evaluated downstream (e.g., from the radial artery) to determine an individual's arterial blood gases (see Table 6–1).

Figure 6–15

Venous admixture occurs when reoxygenated blood mixes with non-reoxygenated blood distal to the alveoli.

© Cengage Learning 2013

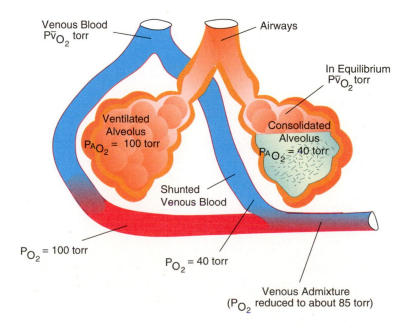

Shunt Equation

Because pulmonary shunting and venous admixture are common complications in respiratory disorders, knowledge of the degree of shunting is often desirable when developing patient care plans. The amount of intrapulmonary shunting can be calculated by using the **classic shunt equation**, which is written as follows:

$$\frac{\dot{Q}s}{\dot{Q}_T} = \frac{Cc_{O_2} - Ca_{O_2}}{Cc_{O_2} - C\bar{v}_{O_2}}$$

where $\dot{Q}s$ is cardiac output that is shunted, $\dot{Q}_T$ is total cardiac output, Cc_{O_2} is oxygen content of capillary blood, Ca_{O_2} is oxygen content of arterial blood, and $C\bar{v}_{O_2}$ is oxygen content of mixed venous blood.

To obtain the data necessary to calculate the degree of pulmonary shunting, the following clinical information must be gathered:

- P_B (barometric pressure).
- Pa_{O_2} (partial pressure of arterial oxygen).
- Pa_{CO_2} (partial pressure of arterial carbon dioxide).
- $P\bar{v}_{O_2}$ (partial pressure of mixed venous oxygen).
- Hb (hemoglobin concentration).
- PA_{O_2} (partial pressure of alveolar oxygen).
- FI_{O_2} (fractional concentration of inspired oxygen).

Case Study: Motorcycle Crash Victim

A 38-year-old man is on a volume-cycled mechanical ventilator on a day when the barometric pressure is 750 mm Hg. The patient is receiving an FI_{O_2} of 0.70. The following clinical data are obtained:

Hb:	13 g%
Pa_{O_2}:	50 torr (Sa_{O_2} = 85%)
Pa_{CO_2}:	43 torr
$P\bar{v}_{O_2}$:	37 torr ($S\bar{v}_{O_2}$ = 65%)

With this information, the patient's PA_{O_2}, Cc_{O_2}, Ca_{O_2}, and $C\bar{v}_{O_2}$ can now be calculated. (Remember: P_{H_2O} represents alveolar water vapor pressure and is always considered to be 47 torr.)

1. $PA_{O_2} = \left(P_B - P_{H_2O}\right) FI_{O_2} - Pa_{CO_2}(1.25)$
   $= (750 - 47)0.70 - 43(1.25)$
   $= (703)0.70 - 53.75$
   $= 492.1 - 53.75$
   $= 438.35$ torr

2. $Cc_{O_2} = (Hb \times 1.34)^* + (PA_{O_2}^{**} \times 0.003)$
   $= (13 \times 1.34) + (438.35 \times 0.003)$
   $= 17.42 + 1.315$
   $= 18.735$ (vol% O_2)

---

* It is assumed that the hemoglobin saturation with oxygen in the pulmonary capillary blood is 100 percent or 1.0.

**Refer to "Ideal Alveolar Gas Equation" section in Chapter 4.

3. $Ca_{O_2} = (Hb \times 1.34 \times Sa_{O_2}) + (Pa_{O_2} \times 0.003)$
   $\quad = (13 \times 1.34 \times 0.85) + (50 \times 0.003)$
   $\quad = 14.807 + 0.15$
   $\quad = 14.957 \text{ (vol\% } O_2)$

4. $C\bar{v}_{O_2} = (Hb \times 1.34 \times S\bar{v}_{O_2}) + (P\bar{v}_{O_2} \times 0.003)$
   $\quad = (13 \times 1.34 \times 0.65) + (37 \times 0.003)$
   $\quad = 11.323 + 0.111$
   $\quad = 11.434 \text{ (vol\% } O_2)$

Based on these calculations, the patient's degree of pulmonary shunting can now be calculated:

$$\frac{\dot{Q}s}{\dot{Q}_T} = \frac{Cc_{O_2} - Ca_{O_2}}{Cc_{O_2} - C\bar{v}_{O_2}}$$

$$= \frac{18.735 - 14.957}{18.735 - 11.434}$$

$$= \frac{3.778}{7.301}$$

$$= 0.517$$

Thus, in this case, 51.7 percent of the patient's pulmonary blood flow is perfusing lung tissue that is not being ventilated.

Today, most critical care units have programmed the oxygen transport calculations into inexpensive personal computers. What was once a time-consuming, error-prone task is now quickly and accurately performed.

The Clinical Significance of Pulmonary Shunting

Pulmonary shunting below 10 percent reflects normal lung status. A shunt between 10 and 20 percent is indicative of an intrapulmonary abnormality but is seldom of clinical significance. Pulmonary shunting between 20 and 30 percent denotes significant intrapulmonary disease and may be life threatening in patients with limited cardiovascular function.

When the pulmonary shunting is greater than 30 percent, a potentially life-threatening situation exists and aggressive cardiopulmonary supportive measures are almost always necessary.

Calculating the degree of pulmonary shunting is not reliable in patients who demonstrate (1) a questionable perfusion status, (2) a decreased myocardial output, or (3) an unstable oxygen consumption demand. This is because these conditions directly affect a patient's Ca_{O_2} and $C\bar{v}_{O_2}$ values—two major components of the shunt equation.

Hypoxia

Hypoxemia versus Hypoxia

Hypoxemia refers to an abnormally low arterial oxygen tension (Pa_{O_2}) and is frequently associated with *hypoxia,* which is an inadequate level of tissue oxygenation (see following discussion). Although the presence of hypoxemia strongly suggests tissue hypoxia, it does not necessarily mean the absolute

Table 6–11	
Hypoxemia Classification*	
Classification	**Pa$_{O_2}$ (torr) (Rule of Thumb)**
Normal	80–100
Mild hypoxemia	60–80
Moderate hypoxemia	40–60
Severe hypoxemia	<40

*The hypoxemia classifications presented in this table are generally accepted classifications. Minor variations on these values are found in the literature. In addition, a number of clinical factors often require some changes in these values (e.g., a Pa$_{O_2}$ less than 60 torr may be called severe in the patient with a very low blood volume or anemia). Nevertheless, the hypoxemia classifications and Pa$_{O_2}$ range(s) provided in this table are useful guidelines.

© Cengage Learning 2013

existence of tissue hypoxia. For example, the reduced level of oxygen in the arterial blood may be offset by an increased cardiac output. Hypoxemia is commonly classified as mild, moderate, or severe hypoxemia (Table 6–11). As will be discussed in Chapter 9, the presence of mild hypoxemia generally stimulates the oxygen peripheral chemoreceptors to increase the patient's breathing rate and heart rate.

Hypoxia refers to low or inadequate oxygen for aerobic cellular metabolism. Hypoxia is characterized by tachycardia, hypertension, peripheral vasoconstriction, dizziness, and mental confusion. There are four main types of hypoxia: (1) hypoxic hypoxia, (2) anemic hypoxia, (3) circulatory hypoxia, and (4) histotoxic hypoxia (Table 6–12).

When hypoxia exists, alternate anaerobic mechanisms are activated in the tissues that produce dangerous metabolites—such as lactic acid—as a waste product. Lactic acid is a nonvolatile acid and causes the pH to decrease.

Hypoxic Hypoxia

Clinically, hypoxic hypoxia (also called hypoxemic hypoxia) refers to the condition in which there is inadequate oxygen at the tissue cells caused by low arterial oxygen tension (Pa$_{O_2}$). Common causes of a decreased Pa$_{O_2}$ are (1) a low alveolar oxygen tension (PA$_{O_2}$), (2) diffusion defects, (3) ventilation-perfusion mismatches, and (4) pulmonary shunting. The following sections describe the common causes of hypoxic hypoxia in more detail.

Low Alveolar Oxygen Tension (Decreased PA$_{O_2}$)

Because the arterial oxygen pressure (Pa$_{O_2}$) is determined by the alveolar oxygen pressure (PA$_{O_2}$), any condition that leads to a decreased PA$_{O_2}$ will result in a reduction of the patient's Pa$_{O_2}$—and, subsequently, to an inadequate Ca$_{O_2}$. A low PA$_{O_2}$ can develop from a variety of conditions, including (1) hypoventilation, (2) high altitudes, (3) diffusion defects, and (4) pulmonary shunting—either absolute or relative shunts.

Table 6–12
Types of Hypoxia

Hypoxia	Descriptions	Common Causes
Hypoxic hypoxia (also called hypoxemic hypoxia)	Inadequate oxygen at the tissue cells caused by low arterial oxygen tension (Pa_{O_2})	Low PA_{O_2} caused by: • Hypoventilation • High altitude Diffusion impairment • Interstitial fibrosis • Interstitial lung disease • Pulmonary edema • Pneumoconiosis Ventilation-perfusion mismatch Pulmonary shunting
Anemic hypoxia	Pa_{O_2} is normal, but the oxygen-carrying capacity of the hemoglobin is inadequate	Decreased hemoglobin concentration • Anemia • Hemorrhage Abnormal hemoglobin • Carboxyhemoglobin • Methemoglobin
Circulatory hypoxia (also called stagnant or hypoperfusion hypoxia)	Blood flow to the tissue cells is inadequate; thus, oxygen is not adequate to meet tissue needs	Slow or stagnant (pooling) peripheral blood flow Arterial-venous shunts
Histotoxic hypoxia	Impaired ability of the tissue cells to metabolize oxygen	Cyanide poisoning

© Cengage Learning 2013

Hypoventilation is caused by numerous conditions, such as chronic obstructive pulmonary disease, central nervous system depressants, head trauma, and neuromuscular disorders (e.g., myasthenia gravis or Guillain-Barré syndrome).

High altitude can cause hypoxic hypoxia to develop. This is because the barometric pressure progressively decreases as altitude increases. As the barometric pressure decreases, the atmospheric oxygen tension (P_{O_2}) also decreases. In other words, the higher the altitude, the lower the oxygen pressure. Thus, the higher an individual hikes up a mountain, the lower the oxygen pressure (P_{O_2}) the person is inhaling—which, in turn, leads to a decreased PA_{O_2} and Pa_{O_2}.

Diffusion Defects

Diffusion defects are abnormal anatomic alterations of the lungs that result in an impedance of oxygen transfer across the alveolar-capillary membrane. When a diffusion defect is present, the time available for oxygen equilibrium between the alveolus and pulmonary capillary is not adequate. Common causes of diffusion defects are chronic interstitial lung diseases, pulmonary edema, and pneumoconiosis.

Ventilation-Perfusion ($\dot{V}/\dot{Q}$ Ratio) Mismatch

When the pulmonary capillary blood is in excess of the alveolar ventilation, a decreased $\dot{V}/\dot{Q}$ ratio is said to exist. This condition causes pulmonary shunting, which in turn causes the Pa_{O_2} and Ca_{O_2} to decrease. Common causes of a decreased $\dot{V}/\dot{Q}$ ratio include chronic obstructive pulmonary disease, pneumonia, and pulmonary edema. The effects of different $\dot{V}/\dot{Q}$ relationships are discussed in greater detail in Chapter 8.

Pulmonary Shunting

The end result of pulmonary shunting and venous admixture is a decreased Pa_{O_2} and Ca_{O_2} (see earlier "Pulmonary Shunting" and "Venous Admixture" sections).

Anemic Hypoxia

In this type of hypoxia, the oxygen tension in the arterial blood is normal but the oxygen-carrying capacity of the blood is inadequate. This form of hypoxia can develop from (1) a low amount of hemoglobin in the blood or (2) a deficiency in the ability of hemoglobin to carry oxygen, as occurs in carbon monoxide poisoning or methemoglobinemia.

Anemic hypoxia develops in carbon monoxide poisoning because the affinity of carbon monoxide for hemoglobin is about 210 times greater than that of oxygen. As carbon monoxide combines with hemoglobin, the ability of hemoglobin to carry oxygen diminishes and tissue hypoxia may ensue. In methemoglobinemia, iron atoms in the hemoglobin are oxidized to the ferric state, which in turn eliminates the hemoglobin's ability to carry oxygen. Increased cardiac output is the main compensatory mechanism for anemic hypoxia.

Clinical Connection—6-6

Hemoglobin and Carbon Monoxide Poisoning

Carbon monoxide (CO) is a colorless, odorless gas produced by all internal combustion engines—including gasoline, diesel, and propane-powered engines. CO is also produced by furnaces; by burning wood, paper, or plastic products; and by welding when carbon dioxide shielding gas is used. CO is also is also found in cigarette smoke and is produced by kerosene space heaters. CO has an attraction for hemoglobin that is more than 200 times greater than that of oxygen—forming a relatively stable compound called **carboxyhemoblobin (CO_{Hb})**. In essence, CO_{Hb} "blocks" oxygen from binding with hemoglobin.

The more an individual is exposed to CO, the more CO_{Hb} that is formed—which, in turn, means less oxygen that is being carried by the blood to the tissue cells—a life-threatening situation! At lower exposure levels, individuals sometimes mistake the symptoms of CO exposure (e.g., headache, dizziness, nausea) as the flu. In addition, the fetus of the smoking pregnant woman can be adversely affected by the CO she inhales.

It should be noted that when a patient is known or suspected to have CO poisoning, a standard pulse oximeter does not correct for the presence of carboxyhemoblobin—it overestimates the true oxygen saturation level. In addition, a standard blood gas analyzer should not be used, because it will give a falsely high Pa_{O_2} and Sa_{O_2} reading. The only way to acurratly meaure the Pa_{O_2} and Sa_{O_2} in the patient with CO poisoning is by running the patient's blood through a special laboratory machine called a **CO-oximter/hemoximeter**.

Treatment for CO poisoning is 100 percent oxygen, usually by a nonrebreather oxygen mask. (Oftentimes, the respiratory therapist working in the emergency department appropriately "overoxygenates" the patient who is suspected of CO poisoning—e.g., the fireman or victim overcome by smoke.) One therapeutic strategy used to remove the CO is to place the patient in a hyperbaric oxygen chamber—high P_{O_2} pressures can "knock off" the CO from the Hb, allowing the oxygen to form oxyhemoglobin (Hb_{O_2}).

Circulatory Hypoxia

In *circulatory hypoxia,* also called *stagnant* or *hypoperfusion hypoxia,* the arterial blood that reaches the tissue cells may have a normal oxygen tension and content, but the amount of blood—and, therefore, the amount of oxygen—is not adequate to meet tissue needs. The two main causes of circulating hypoxia are (1) slow or stagnant peripheral blood flow and (2) arterial-venous shunting.

Stagnant (hypoperfusion) hypoxia can occur when the peripheral capillary blood flow is slow or stagnant (*pooling*). This condition can be caused by (1) a decreased cardiac output, (2) vascular insufficiency, or (3) neurochemical abnormalities. When blood flow through the tissue capillaries is sluggish, the time needed for oxygen exchange increases while, at the same time, the oxygen supply decreases. Because tissue metabolism continues at a steady rate, the oxygen pressure gradient between the blood and the tissue cells can become insufficient, causing tissue hypoxia. Stagnant hypoxia is primarily associated with cardiovascular disorders and often occurs in the absence of arterial hypoxemia. It is commonly associated with a decreased $S\overline{v}_{O_2}$.

When arterial blood completely bypasses the tissue cells and moves into the venous system, an *arterial-venous shunt* is said to exist. This condition can also cause tissue hypoxia, because arterial blood is prevented from delivering oxygen to the tissue cells. Localized arterial or venous obstruction can cause a similar form of tissue hypoxia because the flow of blood into or out of the tissue capillaries is impeded. Circulatory hypoxia can also develop when the tissues' need for oxygen exceeds the available oxygen supply.

Histotoxic Hypoxia

Histotoxic hypoxia develops in any condition that impairs the ability of tissue cells to utilize oxygen. Cyanide poisoning produces this form of hypoxia. Clinically, the Pa_{O_2} and Ca_{O_2} in the blood are normal, but the tissue cells are extremely hypoxic. The $P\overline{v}_{O_2}$, $C\overline{v}_{O_2}$, and $S\overline{v}_{O_2}$ are elevated because oxygen is not utilized.

Figure 6–16

Cyanosis may appear whenever the blood contains at least 5 g% (g/dL) of reduced hemoglobin. In the normal individual with 15 g% hemoglobin, a Pa_{O_2} of about 30 torr will produce 5 g% of reduced hemoglobin. Overall, however, the hemoglobin is still about 60 percent saturated with oxygen.

© Cengage Learning 2013

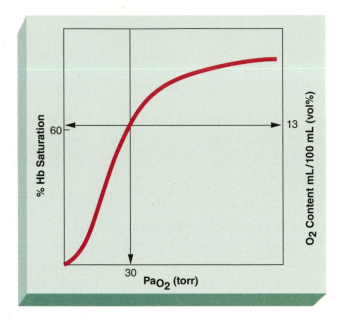

Cyanosis

When hypoxemia is severe, signs of cyanosis may develop. *Cyanosis* is the term used to describe the blue-gray or purplish discoloration seen on the mucous membranes, fingertips, and toes whenever the blood in these areas contains at least 5 g% of reduced hemoglobin per dL (100 mL). When the normal 14 to 15 g% of hemoglobin is fully saturated, the Pa_{O_2} will be about 97 to 100 torr, and there will be about 20 vol% of oxygen in the blood. In the patient with cyanosis with one-third (5 g%) of the hemoglobin reduced, the Pa_{O_2} will be about 30 torr, and there will be about 13 vol% of oxygen in the blood (Figure 6–16). In the patient with polycythemia, however, cyanosis may be present at a Pa_{O_2} well above 30 torr, because the amount of reduced hemoglobin is often greater than 5 g% in these patients—even when their total oxygen transport is within normal limits (about 20 vol% of O_2).

The detection and interpretation of cyanosis is difficult, and there is wide individual variation among observers. The recognition of cyanosis depends on the acuity of the observer, the lighting conditions in the examining room, and the pigmentation of the patient. Cyanosis of the nail beds is also influenced by the temperature, because vasoconstriction induced by cold may slow circulation to the point where the blood becomes bluish in the surface capillaries, even though the arterial blood in the major vessels is not oxygen poor.

Clinical Connection—6-7

Blood Doping

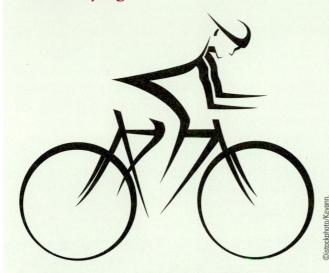

©istockphoto/Kayann.

Blood doping (also called **blood packing** or **blood boosting**) is the illegal practice of increasing the number of red blood cells (RBCs) in the bloodstream in order to enhance athletic performance. In theory, more RBCs—thus, more hemoglobin—will carry more oxygen to the muscles—thus, giving the athlete an unfair edge during competition. Since the 1970s, blood doping has been commonly associated with Olympic athletes who compete in high-endurance races—such as cycling, long-distance running, or cross-country skiing. In 1985, the U.S. Olympic Committee banned the practice of blood doping.

In general, blood doping involves the havesting of the athlete's own blood a few weeks before competition. The blood is usually processed down to a high concentration of RBCs and then stored. A day or two before the sports event, the stored RBCs are then re-injected into the athlete's bloodsteam—thus, increasing the overall number of RBCs (and hemoglobin).

More recently, the advances in medicine have led to an entirely new form of blood doping—the use of the **hormone erythropoietin (EPO)**. EPO is a naturally occuring hormone that stimulates the formation of RBCs. As the science of sports medicine continues to advance, the issues associated with blood doping (e.g., ethics, health, and competitive fairness) will likely be debated for many years to come.

Finally, in addition to being illegal for Olympic competition, there are many negative consequences associated with the practice of blood doping—including possible transfusion problems (e.g., infections, receiving tainted blood, hepatitis, or AIDS), increased blood viscosity, increased blood pressure, heart attack, blood clots, stroke, and pulmonary embolism. On the other hand, it is legal for athletes to train in areas of high altitude—such as Denver, Colorado. Such training may stimulate a natural increase of RBCs because the atmospheric pressure of oxygen is less at high altitudes. In other words, the body generates more RBCs to compensate for the decreased arterial oxygen content. Likewise, athletes who compete in Denver will be at a disadvantage if their training occurred at sea level.

Carbon Dioxide Transport

An understanding of carbon dioxide (CO_2) transport is also essential to the study of pulmonary physiology and to the clinical interpretation of arterial blood gases (see Table 6–1). To fully comprehend this subject, a basic understanding of (1) the six ways carbon dioxide is transported from the tissues to the lungs, (2) how carbon dioxide is eliminated at the lungs, and (3) carbon dioxide dissociation curve is necessary.

The Six Ways Carbon Dioxide is Transported to the Lungs

At rest, the metabolizing tissue cells consume about 250 mL of oxygen and produce about 200 mL of carbon dioxide each minute. The newly formed carbon dioxide is transported from the tissue cells to the lungs by six different mechanisms—three are in the plasma and three in the red blood cells (RBCs) (Figure 6–17).

In Plasma

- Carbamino compound (bound to protein).
- Bicarbonate.
- Dissolved CO_2.

Although relatively insignificant, about 1 percent of the CO_2 that dissolves in the plasma chemically combines with free amino groups of protein molecules and forms a **carbamino compound** (see Figure 6–17).

Approximately 5 percent of the CO_2 that dissolves in the plasma ionizes as **bicarbonate** (HCO_3^-). Initially, CO_2 combines with water in a process called *hydrolysis*. The hydrolysis of CO_2 and water forms carbonic acid (H_2CO_3), which in turn rapidly ionizes into HCO_3^- and H^+ ions.

$$CO_2 + H_2O \leftrightarrows H_2CO_3 \leftrightarrows HCO_3^- + H^+$$

The resulting H^+ ions are buffered by the plasma proteins. The rate of this hydrolysis reaction in the plasma is very slow and, therefore, the amount of HCO_3^- and H^+ ions that form by this mechanism is small.

Dissolved carbon dioxide (CO_2) in the plasma accounts for about 5 percent of the total CO_2 released at the lungs. It is this portion of the CO_2 transport system in the venous blood that is measured to assess the patient's partial pressure of CO_2 (P_{CO_2}) (see Table 6–13).

Note also that the concentration of H_2CO_3 that forms in the plasma is about 1/1000 that of the physically dissolved CO_2 (P_{CO_2}) and, therefore, is proportional to the partial pressure of the CO_2. The H_2CO_3 concentration can be determined by multiplying the partial pressure of CO_2 by the factor 0.03.

Table 6–13		
Carbon Dioxide (CO_2) Transport Mechanisms		
CO_2 Transport Mechanisms	**Approx. % of Total CO_2 Transported to the Lungs**	**Approx. Quantity of Total CO_2 Transported to the Lungs (mL/min)**
In Plasma		
Carbamino compound	1	2
Bicarbonate	5	10
Dissolved CO_2	5	10
In Red Blood Cells		
Dissolved CO_2	5	10
Carbamino-Hb	21	42
Bicarbonate	63	126
Total	**100**	**200**

Figure 6–17

How CO_2 is converted to HCO_3^- at the tissue sites. Most of the CO_2 that is produced at the tissue cells is carried to the lungs in the form of HCO_3^-.

© Cengage Learning 2013

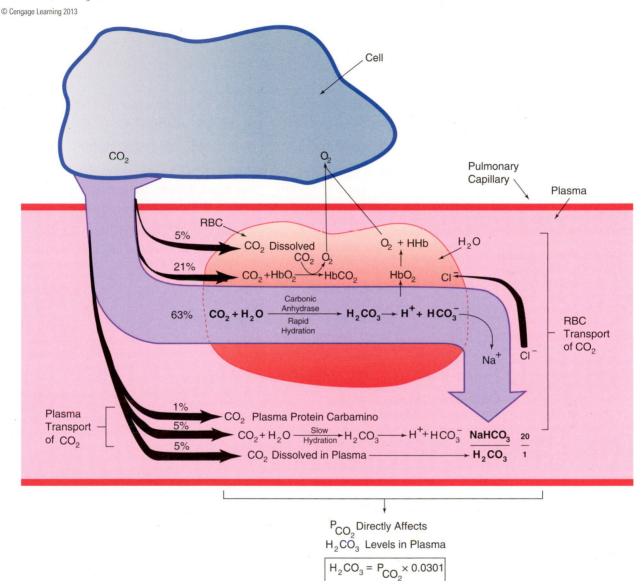

For example, a P_{CO_2} of 40 torr generates an H_2CO_3 concentration of 1.2 mEq/L ($0.03 \times 40 = 1.2$) (see Figure 6–17).

In Red Blood Cells

- Dissolved CO_2.
- Carbamino-Hb.
- Bicarbonate.

Dissolved carbon dioxide (CO_2) in the intracellular fluid of the red blood cells accounts for about 5 percent of the total CO_2 released at the lungs (see Figure 6–17).

About 21 percent of the CO_2 combines with hemoglobin to form a compound called **carbamino-Hb**. The O_2 that is released by this reaction is available for tissue metabolism (see Figure 6–17).

Most of the CO_2 (about 63 percent) is transported from the tissue cells to the lungs in the form of HCO_3^-. The major portion of the dissolved CO_2 that enters the RBCs is converted to HCO_3^- by the following reactions (see Figure 6–17):

1. The bulk of dissolved CO_2 that enters the RBC undergoes hydrolysis according to the following reaction (CA = carbonic anhydrase):

$$CO_2 + H_2O \overset{\text{CA}}{\leftrightarrows} H_2CO_3 \leftrightarrows H^+ + HCO_3^-$$

This reaction, which is normally a very slow process in the plasma, is greatly enhanced in the RBC by the enzyme carbonic anhydrase.

2. The resulting H^+ ions are buffered by the reduced hemoglobin.

3. The rapid hydrolysis of CO_2 causes the RBC to become saturated with HCO_3^-. To maintain a concentration equilibrium between the RBC and plasma, the excess HCO_3^- diffuses out of the RBC.

4. Once in the plasma, the HCO_3^- combines with sodium (Na^+), which is normally in the plasma in the form of sodium chloride (NaCl). The HCO_3^- is then transported to the lungs as $NaHCO_3$ in the plasma of the venous blood.

5. As HCO_3^- moves out of the RBC, the Cl^- (which has been liberated from NaCl) moves into the RBC to maintain electric neutrality. This movement is known as the **chloride shift**, or the **Hamburger phenomenon**, or as an **anionic shift to equilibrium**. During the chloride shift, some water moves into the RBC to preserve the osmotic equilibrium. This action causes the RBC to slightly swell in the venous blood.

6. In the plasma, the ratio of HCO_3^- and H_2CO_3 is normally maintained at 20:1. This ratio keeps the blood pH level within the normal range of 7.35 to 7.45. The pH of the blood becomes more alkaline as the ratio increases and less alkaline as the ratio decreases.

Carbon Dioxide Elimination at the Lungs

As shown in Figure 6–18, as the venous blood enters the alveolar capillaries, the chemical reactions occurring at the tissue level are reversed. These chemical processes continue until the CO_2 pressure is equal throughout the entire system. Table 6–13 summarizes the percentage and quantity of the total CO_2 that is transported from the tissue cells to the lungs by the six CO_2 mechanisms each minute.

Carbon Dioxide Dissociation Curve

Similar to the oxyhemoglobin dissociation curve, the loading and unloading of CO_2 in the blood can be illustrated in graphic form (Figure 6–19 on page 296). Unlike the S-shaped oxygen dissociation curve, however, the carbon dioxide curve is almost linear. This means that compared with the oxyhemoglobin dissociation curve, there is a more direct relationship between the partial pressure of CO_2 (P_{CO_2}) and the amount of CO_2 (CO_2 content) in the blood. For example, when the P_{CO_2} increases from 40 to 46 torr between the arterial and venous blood,

Figure 6–18

How HCO_3^- is transformed back into CO_2 and eliminated in the alveoli.

© Cengage Learning 2013

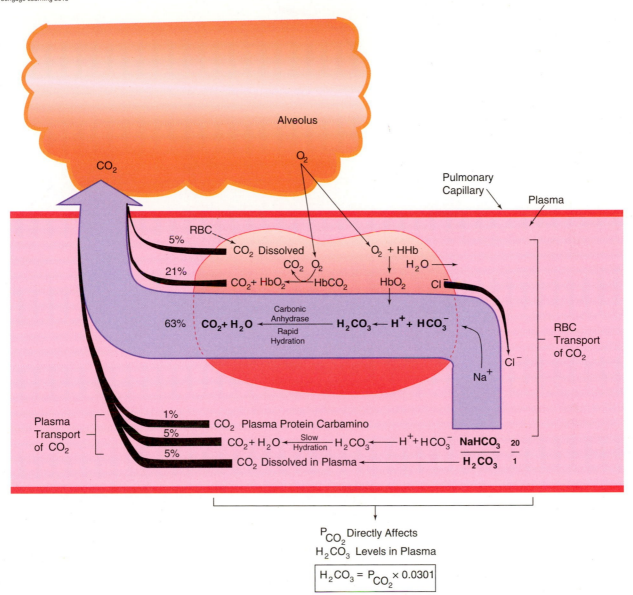

$$H_2CO_3 = P_{CO_2} \times 0.0301$$

the CO_2 content increases by about 5 vol% (Figure 6–20 on page 296). The same partial pressure change of oxygen would increase the oxygen content only by about 2 vol% (see Figure 6–3).

The level of saturation of hemoglobin with oxygen (e.g., Sa_{O_2} or $S\bar{v}_{O_2}$) also affects the carbon dioxide dissociation curve. When the hemoglobin is 97 percent saturated with oxygen, for example, there is less CO_2 content for any given P_{CO_2} than if the hemoglobin is, say, 75 percent saturated with oxygen (Figure 6–21 on page 297). The fact that deoxygenated blood enhances the loading of CO_2 is called the **Haldane effect**. Note also that the Haldane effect works the other way—that is, the oxygenation of blood enhances the unloading of CO_2.

Carbon dioxide
dissociation curve.

© Cengage Learning 2013

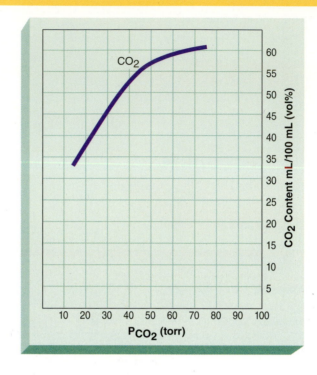

Carbon dioxide dissociation curve. An increase in the P_{CO_2} from 40 to 46 torr raises the CO_2 content by about 5 vol%.
P_{CO_2} changes have a greater effect on CO_2 content levels than P_{O_2} changes have on O_2 levels.

© Cengage Learning 2013

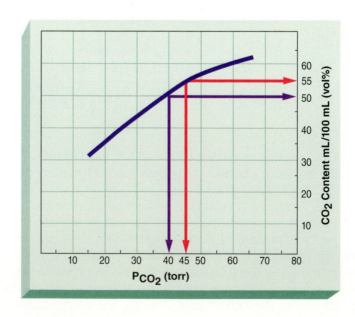

Figure 6–22 compares both the oxygen and the carbon dioxide dissociation curves in terms of partial pressure, content, and shape.

Figure 6–21

Carbon dioxide dissociation curve at two different oxygen/hemoglobin saturation levels (Sa_{O_2} of 97 and 75 percent). When the saturation of O_2 increases in the blood, the CO_2 content decreases at any given P_{CO_2}. This is known as the Haldane effect.

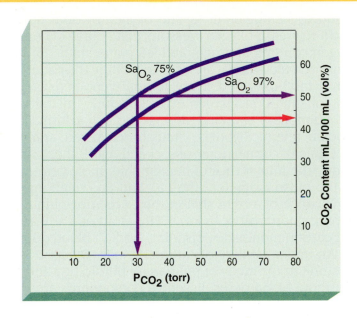

Figure 6–22

Comparison of the oxygen and carbon dioxide dissociation curves in terms of partial pressure, content, and shape.

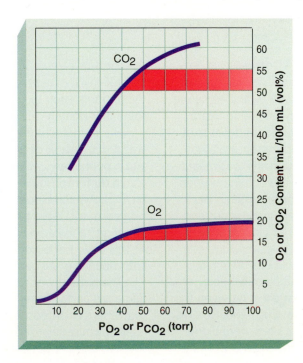

Chapter Summary

The understanding of oxygen transport is a fundamental cornerstone to the clinical interpretation of arterial and venous blood gases. Essential components are (1) how oxygen is transported from the lungs to the tissue, including the calculation of the quantity of oxygen that is dissolved in the plasma and bound to hemoglobin; (2) the oxyhemoglobin dissociation nomogram and how it relates to oxygen pressure, percentage of hemoglobin bound to oxygen, oxygen content, and right and left curve shifts; (3) how the following oxygen transport calculations are used to identify the patient's cardiac and ventilatory status: total oxygen delivery, arterial-venous oxygen content difference, oxygen consumption, oxygen extraction ratio, mixed venous oxygen saturation, and pulmonary shunting; and (4) the major forms of tissue hypoxia: hypoxic hypoxia, anemic hypoxia, circulatory hypoxia, and histotoxic hypoxia.

Clinical connections associated with these topics include (1) a case study—the importance of hemoglobin in oxygen transport, (2) polycythemia, (3) the pulse oximeter—the Pa_{O_2} and Sa_{O_2} relationship, (4) a case study—the significance of a right shift of the oxyhemoglobin dissociation curve, (5) cardiopulmonary resuscitation (CPR)—start as early as possible, (6) hemoglobin and carbon monoxide poisoning, and (7) blood doping.

An understanding of carbon dioxide transport is also a fundamental cornerstone to the study of pulmonary physiology and the clinical interpretation of arterial blood gases. Essential components are the transport of carbon dioxide from the tissues to the lungs, including the three ways in which carbon dioxide is transported in the plasma and three ways in the red blood cells, the elimination of carbon dioxide at the lung, and how the carbon dioxide dissociation curves differ from the oxyhemoglobin dissociation curves.

1 Clinical Application Case

A 12-year-old girl was a victim of a "drive-by" shooting. She was standing in line outside a movie theater with some friends when a car passed by and someone inside began shooting at three boys standing nearby. Two of the boys died immediately, the third was shot in the shoulder and lower jaw, and the girl was shot in the upper anterior chest. Although she was breathing spontaneously through a non-rebreathing oxygen mask when she was brought to the emergency department 25 minutes later, she was unconscious and had obviously lost a lot of blood. Her clothes were completely soaked with blood.

The patient's skin, lips, and nail beds were blue. Her skin felt cool and clammy. A small bullet hole could be seen over the left anterior chest between the second and third rib at the mid-clavicular line. No exit bullet hole could be seen. Her vital signs were blood pressure—55/35 mm Hg, heart rate—120 beats/min, and respiratory rate—22 breaths/min. Auscultation of

the chest revealed normal breath sounds. A portable chest X-ray showed that the bullet had passed through the upper portion of the aorta and lodged near the spine. Fortunately, the bullet did not damage her lung.

Her hematocrit was 15 percent and hemoglobin was 4 g%. A unit of blood was started immediately, and a pulmonary catheter and arterial line were inserted (Refer to Figure 15–1). Cardiac output was 6 L/min. Arterial blood gas values (on a nonrebreathing oxygen mask) were pH—7.47, Pa_{CO_2}—31 torr, HCO_3—23 mEq/L, and Pa_{O_2}—503 torr. Her Sa_{O_2} was 98 percent. At this time, her oxygen indices were assessed (see accompanying Oxygen Transport Study 1).

The patient was rushed to surgery to repair her damaged aorta. Three hours later, she was transferred to the surgical intensive care unit and placed on a mechanical ventilator. The surgery was considered a success, and the patient's parents were relieved to learn that a full recovery was expected. The patient was conscious and appeared comfortable and her skin felt warm and dry. Her vital signs were blood pressure—125/83 mm Hg, heart rate—76 beats/min, respiratory rate—12 breaths/min (i.e., the ventilator rate was set at 12), and temperature 37°C. Auscultation revealed normal bronchovesicular breath sounds.

Oxygen Transport Study 1					
D_{O_2}	$\dot{V}_{O_2}$	$C(a-\bar{v})_{O_2}$	O_2ER	$S\bar{v}_{O_2}$	$\dot{Q}s/\dot{Q}_T$
316 mL	214 mL	3.58 vol%	68%	32%	3%

Oxygen Transport Study 2					
D_{O_2}	$\dot{V}_{O_2}$	$C(a-\bar{v})_{O_2}$	O_2ER	$S\bar{v}_{O_2}$	$\dot{Q}s/\dot{Q}_T$
935 mL	245 mL	5 vol%	25%	75%	3%

D_{O_2} = total oxygen delivery; $\dot{V}_{O_2}$ = oxygen consumption; $C(a-\bar{v})_{O_2}$ = arterial-venous oxygen content difference; O_2ER = oxygen extraction ratio; $S\bar{v}_{O_2}$ = mixed venous oxygen saturation; $\dot{Q}s/\dot{Q}_T$ = the amount of intrapulmonary shunting.

A portable chest X-ray showed no cardiopulmonary problems. Laboratory blood work showed a hematocrit of 41 percent and hemoglobin was 12 g%. Arterial blood gas values (while on the mechanical ventilation and on an inspired oxygen concentration [$F_{I_{O_2}}$] of 0.4) were pH—7.43, Pa_{CO_2}—38 torr, HCO_3—24 mEq/L, and Pa_{O_2}—109 torr. Sa_{O_2} was 97 percent. A second oxygen transport study showed significant improvement (see accompanying Oxygen Transport Study 2). Over the

next 4 days, the patient was weaned from the ventilator and transferred from the surgical intensive care unit to the medical ward. A week later the patient was discharged from the hospital.

Discussion

This case illustrates the importance of *hemoglobin* in the oxygen transport system. As a result of the gunshot wound to the chest, the patient lost a great deal of blood—her hemoglobin was only 4 g%. Because of the excessive blood loss, the patient was unconscious, cyanotic, and hypotensive, and her skin was cool and damp to the touch. Despite the fact that the patient had an elevated Pa_{O_2} of 503 torr (normal, 80–100 torr) and an Sa_{O_2} of 98 percent in the emergency department, her tissue oxygenation was seriously impaired. In fact, the patient's Pa_{O_2} and Sa_{O_2} in this case were very misleading. Clinically, this was verified by the oxygen transport studies. For example, her D_{O_2} was only 316 mL (normal, about 1000 mL).

Furthermore, note that the patient's $\dot{V}_{O_2}$ was 214 mL/min and O_2ER was 68 percent (the normal extraction ratio is 25 percent). In other words, the patient was consuming 68 percent of the D_{O_2} (214 mL of oxygen out of a possible 316 mL of oxygen per minute). Her oxygen reserve was only about 30 percent. If this condition had not been treated immediately, she would not have survived much longer. It should be stressed that the patient's Pa_{O_2} of 503 torr and Sa_{O_2} of 98 percent were very misleading—and dangerous.

2 Clinical Application Case

An 18-year-old woman presented in the emergency department in severe respiratory distress. She was well known to the respiratory care team. She had suffered from asthma all of her life (Figure 6–23). Over the years, she had been admitted to the hospital on numerous occasions, averaging about three admissions per year. Five separate asthmatic episodes had required mechanical ventilation. Although she was usually weaned from the ventilator within 48 hours, on one occasion she was on the ventilator for 7 days. At the time of this admission, it had been more than 4 years since she was last placed on mechanical ventilation.

Upon observation, the patient appeared fatigued and cyanotic, and she was using her accessory muscles of inspiration. She was in obvious respiratory distress. Her vital signs were blood pressure—177/110 mm Hg, heart rate—160 beats/min, and respiratory rate—32 breaths/min and shallow. Her breath sounds were diminished and wheezing could be heard bilaterally. A portable chest X-ray showed that her lungs were hyperinflated and her diaphragm was depressed. Arterial blood gas values on 4 L/min oxygen via cannula were pH—7.25, Pa_{CO_2}—71, HCO_3^-—27, Pa_{O_2}—27, and Sa_{O_2}—42 percent.

(continues)

Figure 6–23

Asthma. Pathology includes (1) bronchial smooth muscle constriction, (2) inflammation and excessive production of thick, whitish bronchial secretions, and (3) alveolar hyperinflation.

© Cengage Learning 2013

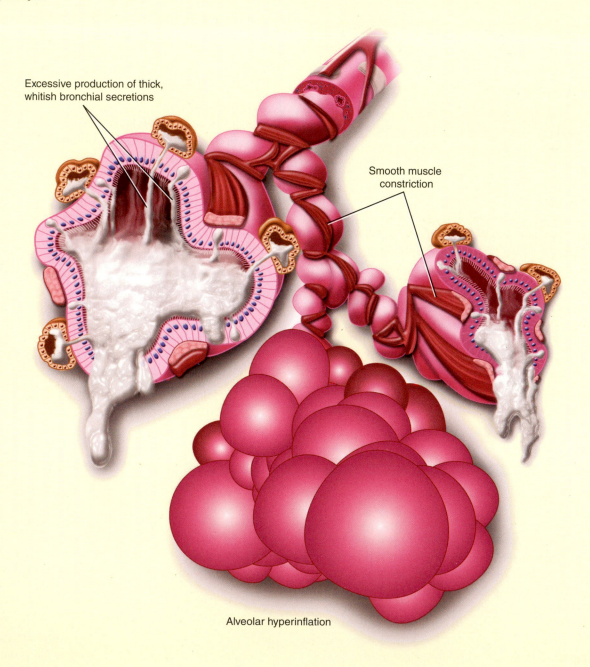

Excessive production of thick, whitish bronchial secretions

Smooth muscle constriction

Alveolar hyperinflation

Because she was in acute ventilatory failure with severe hypoxemia and was clearly fatigued, the patient was immediately transferred to the intensive care unit, intubated, and placed on mechanical ventilation at a rate of 3 breaths/min. A pulmonary catheter and arterial line were inserted. An intravenous infusion was started and medications to treat her bronchoconstriction were administered. A hemodynamic study showed that her cardiac output ($\dot{Q}_T$) was 6.5 L/min. Her hemoglobin was 13 g%. An oxygen transport study was performed at this time (see accompany Oxygen Transport Studies, Study 1).

Oxygen Transport Study 1					
D_{O_2}	$\dot{V}_{O_2}$	$C(a-\bar{v})_{O_2}$	O_2ER	$S\bar{v}_{O_2}$	$\dot{Q}s/\dot{Q}_T$
523 mL	314 mL	4.83 vol%	58%	24%	47%

Oxygen Transport Study 2					
D_{O_2}	$\dot{V}_{O_2}$	$C(a-\bar{v})_{O_2}$	O_2ER	$S\bar{v}_{O_2}$	$\dot{Q}s/\dot{Q}_T$
990 mL	255 mL	5 vol%	24%	75%	3%

D_{O_2} = total oxygen delivery; $\dot{V}_{O_2}$ = oxygen consumption; $C(a-\bar{v})_{O_2}$ = arterial-venous oxygen content difference; O_2ER = oxygen extraction ratio; $S\bar{v}_{O_2}$ = mixed venous oxygen saturation; $\dot{Q}s/\dot{Q}_T$ = the amount of intrapulmonary shunting.

Although the patient's first day in the intensive care unit was a stormy one, her asthma progressively improved over the second day. On the morning of the third day, her skin was pink and dry and she was resting comfortably on the mechanical ventilator. Although she was receiving 3 mechanical breaths/min, the patient was breathing primarily on her own. Her vital signs were blood pressure—125/76 mm Hg, heart rate—70 beats/min, and respiratory rate—10 breaths/min (10 spontaneous breaths between the 3 mechanical ventilations per minute). Auscultation revealed normal bronchovesicular breath sounds, and portable chest X-ray no longer showed hyperinflated lungs or a flattened diaphragm. Arterial blood gas values on an inspired oxygen concentration ($F_{I_{O_2}}$) of 0.25 were pH—7.42, Pa_{CO_2}—37, HCO_3^-—24, Pa_{O_2}—115, and Sa_{O_2}—97 percent. An oxygen transport study was performed at this time (see accompanying Oxygen Transport Study 2). The patient was weaned from the ventilator and was discharged from the hospital the next day.

Discussion

This case illustrates the clinical significance of a *right shift* in the *oxyhemoglobin dissociation curve* on (1) the loading of oxygen on hemoglobin in the lungs, and (2) the patient's total oxygen delivery (D_{O_2}). As a result of the asthmatic episode (i.e., bronchial smooth muscle constriction, inflammation, and excessive secretions, the patient's alveolar ventilation was very poor in the emergency department. Clinically, this was verified on chest X-ray showing alveolar hyperinflation and a flattened diaphragm and by arterial blood gas analysis and the oxygen indices.

Note that alveolar "hyperinflation" does not mean the lungs are being excessively ventilated. In fact, they are being underventilated. The lungs become hyperinflated during a severe asthmatic episode because gas is unable to leave the lungs during exhalation. As a result, "fresh" ventilation is impeded on subsequent inspirations. This condition causes the alveolar oxygen (PA_{O_2}) to decrease and the alveolar carbon dioxide (PA_{CO_2}) to increase. As the PA_{O_2} declined, the patient's intrapulmonary shunting ($\dot{Q}s \div \dot{Q}_T$) and oxygen extraction ratio (O_2ER) increased and total oxygen delivery (D_{O_2}) decreased (see Oxygen Transport Study 1).

In addition, as shown by the first arterial blood gas analysis, her condition was further compromised by the presence of a decreased pH (7.25) and an increased Pa_{CO_2} (72 torr), which caused the oxyhemoglobin dissociation curve to shift to the right. A right shift of the oxyhemoglobin dissociation curve reduces the ability of oxygen to move across the alveolar-capillary membrane and bond to hemoglobin (see Figure 6–8). Because of this, the patient's hemoglobin saturation was lower than expected for a particular Pa_{O_2} level. In this case, the patient's Sa_{O_2} was only 42 percent at a time when the Pa_{O_2} was 27 torr. Normally, when the Pa_{O_2} is 27 torr, the hemoglobin saturation is 50 percent (see Figure 6–6). Thus, it should be emphasized that when additional factors are present that shift the oxyhemoglobin dissociation curve to the right or left, the respiratory practitioner should consider these factors in the final analysis of the patient's total oxygenation status.

Review Questions

1. If a patient has a Hb level of 14 g% and a Pa_{O_2} of 55 torr (85 percent saturated with oxygen), approximately how much oxygen is transported to the peripheral tissues in each 100 mL of blood?
   A. 16 vol%
   B. 17 vol%
   C. 18 vol%
   D. 19 vol%

2. When the blood pH decreases, the oxyhemoglobin dissociation curve shifts to the
   A. right and the P_{50} decreases
   B. left and the P_{50} increases
   C. right and the P_{50} increases
   D. left and the P_{50} decreases

3. When shunted, non-reoxygenated blood mixes with reoxygenated blood distal to the alveoli (*venous admixture*), the
   1. P_{O_2} of the non-reoxygenated blood increases
   2. Ca_{O_2} of the reoxygenated blood decreases
   3. P_{O_2} of the reoxygenated blood increases
   4. Ca_{O_2} of the non-reoxygenated blood decreases
      A. 1 only
      B. 4 only
      C. 1 and 2 only
      D. 3 and 4 only

4. The normal arterial HCO_3^- range is
   A. 18–22 mEq/L
   B. 22–28 mEq/L
   C. 28–35 mEq/L
   D. 35–45 mEq/L

5. The normal calculated anatomic shunt is about
   A. 0.5–1 percent
   B. 2–5 percent
   C. 6–9 percent
   D. 10–12 percent

6. In which of the following types of hypoxia is the oxygen pressure of the arterial blood $\left(Pa_{O_2}\right)$ usually normal?
   1. Hypoxic hypoxia
   2. Anemic hypoxia
   3. Circulatory hypoxia
   4. Histotoxic hypoxia
      A. 1 only
      B. 2 only
      C. 3 and 4 only
      D. 2, 3, and 4 only

7. If a patient normally has a 12 g% Hb, cyanosis will likely appear when
   A. 10 g% Hb is saturated with oxygen
   B. 9 g% Hb is saturated with oxygen
   C. 8 g% Hb is saturated with oxygen
   D. 7 g% Hb is saturated with oxygen

8. The advantages of polycythemia begin to be offset by the increased blood viscosity when the hematocrit reaches about
    A. 30–40 percent
    B. 40–50 percent
    C. 55–60 percent
    D. 60–70 percent

9. Assuming everything else remains the same, when an individual's cardiac output decreases, the
    1. $C(a - \bar{v})_{O_2}$ increases
    2. O_2ER decreases
    3. $\dot{V}_{O_2}$ increases
    4. $S\bar{v}_{O_2}$ decreases
        A. 1 only
        B. 4 only
        C. 2 and 3 only
        D. 1 and 4 only

10. Under normal conditions, the O_2ER is about
    A. 10 percent
    B. 15 percent
    C. 20 percent
    D. 25 percent

11. Case Study: Automobile Collision Victim
    A 37-year-old woman is on a volume-cycled mechanical ventilator on a day when the barometric pressure is 745 mm Hg. The patient is receiving an $F_{I_{O_2}}$ of 0.50. The following clinical data are obtained:

    Hb: 11 g%
    Pa_{O_2} 60 torr $\left(Sa_{O_2} = 90\%\right)$
    $P\bar{v}_{O_2}$ 35 torr $\left(S\bar{v}_{O_2} = 65\%\right)$
    Pa_{CO_2} 38 torr

    Cardiac output: 6 L/min

    Based on this information, calculate the patient's
    A. Total oxygen delivery

    _____

    B. Arterial-venous oxygen content difference

    _____

    C. Intrapulmonary shunting

    _____

    D. Oxygen consumption

    _____

    E. Oxygen extraction ratio

    _____

Clinical Application Questions

Case 1

1. As a result of the gunshot wound to the chest, the patient lost a large amount of blood. Because of the excessive blood loss, the patient was

_____

_____

2. As a result of the excessive blood loss, the patient's Pa_{O_2} of 503 torr and Sa_{O_2} of 98 percent were very misleading. Which oxygen transport studies verified this fact?

_____

_____

3. In the first oxygen transport study, the patient's $\dot{D}_{O_2}$ was only 316 mL. Her $\dot{V}_{O_2}$ was 214 mL. What was her O_2ER?

_____

_____

Case 2

1. As a result of the asthmatic episode, the patient's $P_{A_{O_2}}$ (decreased _____, increased _____), and the alveolar carbon dioxide $(P_{A_{CO_2}})$ (decreased _____, increased _____).

2. As the preceding condition worsened, the patient's intrapulmonary shunting $(\dot{Q}s/\dot{Q}_T)$ (decreased _____, increased _____), the oxygen extraction ratio (O_2ER) (decreased _____, increased _____), and the total oxygen delivery (D_{O_2}) (decreased _____, increased_____).

3. The patient's condition was compromised by the presence of a decreased pH (7.25) and an increased Pa_{CO_2} (72 torr), which caused the oxyhemoglobin dissociation curve to shift to the _____ _____.

4. Because of the condition described in question 3, the patient's hemoglobin saturation was (higher _____, lower _____) than expected for a particular Pa_{O_2} level.

Chapter 7

Acid–Base Balance and Regulation

Objectives

By the end of this chapter, the student should be able to:

1. Describe how the following relate to the acid–base balance and regulation of the body:
   —Acids
   - Hydrogen ions
   - Proton donors
   - Strong and weak acids
   —Bases
   - Proton acceptors
   - Bicarbonate ions
   - Strong and weak bases
   —pH: acid–base concentration
   —The chemical buffer system's role in acid–base balance
   - Carbonic acid–bicarbonate buffer system
     - Henderson-Hasselbalch equation
     - Clinical application of the H-H equation
   - Phosphate buffer system
   - Protein buffer system
   —The respiratory system's role in acid–base balance
   —The renal system's role in acid–base balance

2. Identify the following acid–base disturbances on the P_{CO_2}/HCO_3^-/pH nomogram:
   —Acute ventilatory failure (respiratory acidosis)
   —Acute ventilatory failure (with partial renal compensation)
   —Chronic ventilatory failure (with complete renal compensation)

3. Identify common causes of acute ventilatory failure.

4. Describe the clinical connection associated with the P_{CO_2}/HCO_3^-/pH relationship—the general rule of thumb.

5. Describe the clinical connection associated with the case study example for acute ventilatory failure (acute respiratory acidosis).

6. Describe the clinical connection associated with the case study example for chronic ventilatory failure (compensated respiratory acidosis).

7. Identify the following acid–base disturbances on the P_{CO_2}/HCO_3^-/pH nomogram:
   —Acute alveolar hyperventilation (respiratory alkalosis)
   —Acute alveolar hyperventilation (with partial renal compensation)
   —Chronic alveolar hyperventilation (with complete renal compensation)

8. Identify common causes of acute alveolar hyperventilation.

9. Describe the clinical connection associated with the case study example for acute alveolar hyperventilation (acute respiratory alkalosis).

10. Describe the clinical connection associated with the case study example for chronic alveolar hyperventilation (compensated respiratory alkalosis).

11. Describe the clinical connection associated with the case study that illustrates the application of the P_{CO_2}/HCO_3^-/pH nomogram to a victim of carbon monoxide poisoning.

12. Identify the following acid–base disturbances on the P_{CO_2}/HCO_3^-/pH nomogram:
    —Metabolic acidosis, and include the anion gap
    —Metabolic acidosis (with partial respiratory compensation)
    —Metabolic acidosis (with complete respiratory compensation)
    —Combined metabolic and respiratory acidosis

13. Identify common causes of metabolic acidosis.

14. Describe the clinical connection associated with the case study example for metabolic acidosis.

(continues)

15. Describe the clinical connection associated with the case study example for combined metabolic and respiratory acidosis.
16. Describe the clinical connection associated with the case study that illustrates the application of the P_{CO_2}/HCO_3^-/pH nomogram to a patient with both respiratory and metabolic acidosis.
17. Identify the following acid–base disturbances on the P_{CO_2}/HCO_3^-/pH nomogram:
   —Metabolic alkalosis
   —Metabolic alkalosis (with partial respiratory compensation)
   —Metabolic alkalosis (with complete respiratory compensation)
   —Combined metabolic and respiratory alkalosis
18. Identify common causes of metabolic alkalosis.
19. Describe the clinical connection associated with the case study example for metabolic alkalosis.
20. Describe the clinical connection associated with the case study example for combined metabolic and respiratory alkalosis.
21. Describe base excess/deficit.
22. Complete the review questions at the end of this chapter.

Introduction

Nearly all biochemical reactions in the body are influenced by the acid–base balance of their fluid environment. When the pH is either too high or too low, essentially nothing in the body functions properly. Under normal conditions, the blood pH remains within a very narrow range. The normal arterial pH range is 7.35 to 7.45. The normal venous pH range is 7.30 to 7.40. When the pH of the arterial blood is greater than 7.45, **alkalosis** or **alkalemia** is said to exist; the blood has an excess amount of bicarbonate ions (HCO_3^-). When the pH falls below 7.35, **acidosis** or **acidemia** is said to be present; the blood has an excess amount of hydrogen ions (H^+).

Most H^+ ions in the body originate from (1) the breakdown of phosphorous-containing proteins (phosphoric acid), (2) the anaerobic metabolism of glucose (lactic acid), (3) the metabolism of body fats (fatty and ketone acids), and (4) the transport of CO_2 in the blood as HCO_3^- liberates H^+ ions. Under normal conditions, both the H^+ and HCO_3^- ion concentrations in the blood are regulated by the following three major systems: the *chemical buffer system*, the *respiratory system*, and the *renal system*.

The **chemical buffer system** responds within a fraction of a second to resist pH changes, and is called the *first line of defense*. This system is composed of (1) the *carbonic acid-bicarbonate buffer system*, (2) the *phosphate buffer system*, and (3) the *protein buffer system*. The chemical buffer system inactivates H^+ ions and liberates HCO_3^- ions in response to acidosis, or generates more H^+ ions and decreases the concentration of HCO_3^- ions in response to alkalosis.

The **respiratory system** acts within 1 to 3 minutes by increasing or decreasing the breathing depth and rate to offset acidosis or alkalosis, respectively. For example, in response to metabolic acidosis, the respiratory system causes the depth and rate of breathing to increase, causing the body's CO_2 to decrease and the pH to increase. In response to metabolic alkalosis, the respiratory system causes the depth and rate of breathing to decrease, causing the body's CO_2 to increase and the pH to decrease.

The renal system is the body's most effective acid–base balance monitor and regulator. The renal system requires a day or more to correct abnormal pH concentrations. When the extracellular fluids become acidic, the renal system retains HCO_3^- and excretes H^+ ions into the urine, causing the blood pH to increase. On the other hand, when the extracellular fluids become alkaline, the renal system retains H^+ and excretes basic substances (primarily HCO_3^-) into the urine, causing the blood pH to decrease.

To fully appreciate acid–base balance, and how it is normally regulated, a fundamental understanding of acids and bases, and their influences on pH, is essential.

The Basic Principles of Acid–Base Reactions and pH

Acids and Bases

Similar to salts, acids and bases are electrolytes. Thus, both acids and bases can ionize and dissociate in water and conduct an electrical current.

Acids

Acids are sour tasting, can react with many metals, and can "burn" a hole through clothing. With regard to acid–base physiology, however, an acid is a substance that releases hydrogen ions [H^+] in measurable amounts. Because a hydrogen ion is only a hydrogen nucleus proton, acids are defined as proton donors. Thus, when acids dissolve in a water solution, they release hydrogen ions (protons) and anions.

The acidity of a solution is directly related to the concentration of protons. In other words, the acidity of a solution reflects only the free hydrogen ions, not those bound to anions. For example, *hydrochloric acid* (HCl), the acid found in the stomach that works to aid digestion, dissociates into a proton and a chloride ion:

$$HCl \rightarrow \underset{\text{proton}}{H^+} \underset{\text{anion}}{Cl^-}$$

Other acids in the body include acetic acid ($HC_2H_3O_2$), often abbreviated as [HAc], and carbonic acid (H_2CO_3). The molecular formula for common acids is easy to identify because it begins with the hydrogen ion.

Strong and Weak Acids. First, it is important to remember that the acidity of a solution reflects only the free hydrogen ions—not the hydrogen ions still combined with anions. Thus, strong acids, which dissociate completely (i.e., they liberate all the H^+) and irreversibly in water, dramatically change the pH of the solution. For example, if 100 hydrochloric (HCl) acid molecules were placed in 1 mL of water, the hydrochloric acid would dissociate into 100 H^+ and 100 Cl^- ions. There would be no undissociated hydrochloric acid molecules in the solution.

Weak acids, on the other hand, do not dissociate completely in a solution and, therefore, have a much smaller effect on pH. However, even though weak acids have a relatively small effect on changing pH levels, they have a very important role in resisting sudden pH changes. Examples of weak acids are carbonic acid (H_2CO_3) and acetic acid ($HC_2H_3O_2$). If 100 acetic acid molecules were placed in 1 mL of water, only one acidic acid molecule would likely be ionized at any given moment as shown in the following reaction:

$$100\ HC_2H_3O_2 \rightarrow 99\ HC_2H_3O_2 + \underset{\text{(hydrogen ions)}}{1H^+} + \underset{\text{(acetate ions)}}{1\ C_2H_3O_2}$$

Because undissociated acids do not alter the pH, the acidic solution will not be as acidic as the HCl solution discussed earlier. Because the dissociation of weak acids is predictable, and because the molecules of intact acids are in constant dynamic equilibrium with the dissociated ions, the dissociation of acetic acid can be written as follows:

$$HC_2H_3O_2 \leftrightharpoons H^+ + C_2H_3O_2^-$$

Using this equation, it can be seen that when H^+ (released by a strong acid) is added to the acetic acid solution, the equilibrium moves to the left as some of the additional H^+ bonds with $C_2H_3O_2^-$ to form $HC_2H_3O_2$. On the other hand, when a strong base is added to the solution (adding additional OH^- and causing the pH to increase), the equilibrium shifts to the right. This occurs because the additional OH^- consumes the H^+. This causes more $HC_2H_3O_2$ molecules to dissociate and replenish the H^+. Weak acids play a very important role in the chemical buffer systems of the human body.

Bases

Bases are **proton acceptors**. Bases taste bitter and feel slippery. With regard to acid–base physiology, a base is a substance that takes up hydrogen ions [H^+] in measurable amounts. Common inorganic bases include the hydroxides, for example, magnesium hydroxide (milk of magnesia) and sodium hydroxide (lye). Similar to acids, when dissolved in water, hydroxides dissociate into **hydroxide ions** (OH^-) and cations. For example, ionization of sodium hydroxide (NaOH) results in a hydroxide ion and a sodium ion. The liberated hydroxide ion then bonds, or accepts, a proton present in the solution. This reaction produces water and, at the same time, decreases the acidity [H^+ concentration] of the solution:

$$NaOH \rightarrow \underset{\text{cation}}{Na^+} + \underset{\text{hydroxide ion}}{OH^-}$$

and then

$$OH^- + H^+ \rightarrow \underset{\text{water}}{H_2O}$$

The **bicarbonate ion (HCO_3^-)** is an important base in the body and is especially abundant in the blood. **Ammonia** (NH_3), a natural waste product of protein breakdown, is also a base. Ammonia has a pair of unshared electrons that strongly attract protons. When accepting a proton, ammonia becomes an ammonium ion:

$$NH_3 + H^+ \rightarrow \underset{\text{ammonium ion}}{NH_4^+}$$

Strong and Weak Bases. With regard to strong and weak bases, it is important to remember that bases are proton acceptors. Strong bases (e.g., hydroxides) dissociate easily in water and quickly tie up H^+. In contrast, weak bases (e.g., sodium bicarbonate or baking soda) dissociate incompletely and reversibly and are slower to accept protons. Because sodium bicarbonate accepts a relatively small amount of protons, its released bicarbonate ion is described as a weak base.

pH: Acid–Base Concentration

As the concentration of hydrogen ions in a solution increases, the solution becomes more acidic. On the other hand, as the level of hydroxide ions increases, the solution becomes more basic, or alkaline. Clinically, the concentration of hydrogen ions in the body is measured in units called *pH units*. The pH scale runs from 0 to 14 and is logarithmic, which means each successive unit change in pH represents a tenfold change in hydrogen ion concentration. The pH of a solution, therefore, *is defined as the negative logarithm, to the base 10, of the hydrogen ion concentration [H^+] in moles per liter, or −log H^+:*

$$pH = -\log_{10} [H^+]$$

When the pH is 7 ($H^+ = 10^{-7}$ mol/L), the number of hydrogen ions precisely equals the number of hydroxide ions (OH^-), and the solution is neutral—that is, neither acidic nor basic. Pure water has a neutral pH of 7, or 10^{-7} mol/L (0.0000001 mol/L) of hydrogen ions. A solution with a pH below 7, is acidic—that is, there are more hydrogen ions than hydroxide ions. For example, a solution with a pH of 6 has 10 times more hydrogen ions than a solution with a pH of 7.

A solution with a pH greater than 7 is alkaline—that is, the hydroxide ions outnumber the hydrogen ions. For example, a solution with a pH of 8 has 10 times more hydroxyl ions than a solution with a pH of 7. Thus, as the hydrogen ion concentration increases, the hydroxide ion concentration falls, and vice versa. Figure 7–1 on page 310 provides the approximate pH values of several human fluids and common household substances.

The Chemical Buffer Systems and Acid–Base Balance

Chemical buffers resist pH changes and are the body's first line of defense. The ability of an acid–base mixture to resist sudden changes in pH is called its buffer action. The tissue cells and vital organs of the body are extremely sensitive to even the slightest change in the pH environment. In high concentrations, both acids and bases can be extremely damaging to living cells—essentially every biological process within the body is disrupted.

Buffers work against sudden and large changes in the pH of body fluids by releasing hydrogen ions (acting as acids) when the pH increases and binding hydrogen ions (acting as bases) when the pH decreases. The three major chemical buffer systems in the body are the *carbonic acid-bicarbonate buffer system, phosphate buffer system*, and the *protein buffer system*.

Figure 7–1

The pH values of representative substances. The pH scale represents the number of hydrogen ions in a substance. The concentration of hydrogen ions (H^+) and the corresponding hydroxyl concentration (OH^-) for each representative substance is also provided. Note that when the pH is 7.0, the amounts of H^+ and OH^- are equal and the solution is neutral.

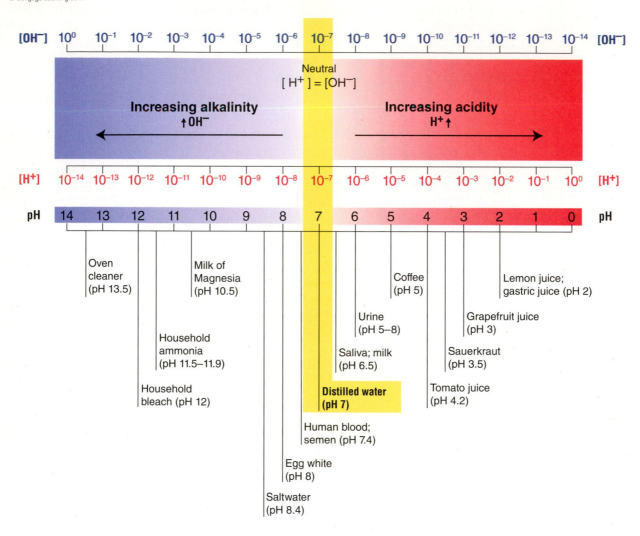

Carbonic Acid–Bicarbonate Buffer System and Acid–Base Balance

The carbonic acid–bicarbonate buffer system plays an extremely important role in maintaining pH homeostasis of the blood. Carbonic acid (H_2CO_3) dissociates reversibly and releases bicarbonate ions (HCO_3^-) and protons (H^+) as follows:

$$
\underset{\substack{H^+\ \text{donor}\\(\text{weak acid})}}{H_2CO_3}
\quad
\underset{\text{Response to a decrease in pH}}{\overset{\text{Response to an increase in pH}}{\rightleftharpoons}}
\quad
\underset{\substack{H^+\ \text{acceptor}\\(\text{weak proton})}}{HCO_3^-}
\ +\
\underset{\text{proton}}{H^+}
$$

Under normal conditions, the ratio between HCO_3^- and H_2CO_3 in the blood is 20:1 (refer to Figure 6–17). The chemical equilibrium between carbonic acid (weak acid) and bicarbonate ion (weak base) works to resist sudden changes in blood pH. For example, when the blood pH increases (i.e., becomes more alkaline from the addition of a strong base), the equilibrium shifts to the right. A right shift forces more carbonic acid to dissociate, which in turn causes the pH to decrease.

In contrast, when the blood pH decreases (i.e., becomes more acidic from the addition of a strong acid), the equilibrium moves to the left. A left shift forces more bicarbonate to bind with protons. In short, the carbonic acid–bicarbonate buffer system converts strong bases to a weak base (bicarbonate ion) and strong acids to a weak acid (carbonic acid). As a result, blood pH changes are much less than they would be if this buffering system did not exist.

The Henderson-Hasselbalch Equation

The **Henderson-Hasselbalch (H-H) equation** mathematically illustrates how the pH of a solution is influenced by the HCO_3^- to H_2CO_3 ratio (base to acid ratio). The H-H equation is written as follows:

$$pH = pK + \log \frac{[HCO_3^-] \text{ (base)}}{[H_2CO_3] \text{ (acid)}}$$

The pK is derived from the dissociation constant of the acid portion of the buffer combination. The pK is 6:1 and, under normal conditions, the HCO_3^- to H_2CO_3 ratio is 20:1.

Clinically, the dissolved CO_2 ($P_{CO_2} \times 0.03$) can be used for the denominator of the H-H equation, instead of the H_2CO_3. This is possible because the dissolved carbon dioxide is in equilibrium with, and directly proportional to, the blood $[H_2CO_3]$. This is handy, because the patient's value can easily be obtained from an arterial blood gas. Thus, the H-H equation can be written as follows:

$$pH = pK + \log \frac{[HCO_3^-]}{[P_{CO_2} \times 0.03]}$$

H-H Equation Applied during Normal Conditions. When the HCO_3^- is 24 mEq/L, and the Pa_{CO_2} is 40 torr, the base to acid ratio is 20:1 and the pH is 7.4 (normal). The H-H equation confirms the 20:1 ratio and pH of 7.4 as follows:

$$pH = pK + \log \frac{[HCO_3^-]}{[P_{CO_2} \times 0.03]}$$

$$= 6.1 + \log \frac{24 \text{ mEq/L}}{(40 \times 0.03)}$$

$$= 6.1 + \log \frac{24 \text{ mEq/L}}{(1.2 \text{ mEq/L})}$$

$$= 6.1 + \log \frac{20}{1} \quad \text{(20:1 ratio)}$$

$$= 6.1 + 1.3$$

$$= 7.4$$

H-H Equation Applied during Abnormal Conditions. When the HCO_3^- is 29 mEq/L, and the Pa_{CO_2} is 80 torr, the base to acid ratio decreases to 12:1 and the pH is 7.18 (acidic). The H-H equation confirms the 12:1 ratio and the pH of 7.18 as follows:

$$pH = pK + \log\frac{[HCO_3^-]}{[P_{CO_2} \times 0.03]}$$

$$= 6.1 + \log\frac{29 \text{ mEq/L}}{(80 \times 0.03)}$$

$$= 6.1 + \log\frac{29 \text{ mEq/L}}{(2.4 \text{ mEq/L})}$$

$$= 6.1 + \log\frac{12}{1} \qquad (12:1 \text{ ratio})$$

$$= 6.1 + 1.08$$

$$= 7.18$$

In contrast, when the HCO_3^- is 20 mEq/L, and the Pa_{CO_2} is 20 torr, the base to acid ratio increases to 33:1 and the pH is 7.62 (alkalotic). The H-H equation confirms the 33:1 ratio and the pH of 7.62 as follows:

$$pH = pK + \log\frac{[HCO_3^-]}{[P_{CO_2} \times 0.03]}$$

$$= 6.1 + \log\frac{20 \text{ mEq/L}}{(20 \times 0.03)}$$

$$= 6.1 + \log\frac{20 \text{ mEq/L}}{(0.6 \text{ mEq/L})}$$

$$= 6.1 + \log\frac{33}{1} \qquad (33:1 \text{ ratio})$$

$$= 6.1 + 1.52$$

$$= 7.62$$

Clinical Application of the H-H Equation

Clinically, the Henderson-Hasselbalch equation can be used to calculate the pH, $[HCO_3^-]$, or Pa_{CO_2} when any two of these three variables are known. $[HCO_3^-]$ is solved as follows:

$$[HCO_3^-] = \text{antilog}(7.40 - 6.1) \times (P_{CO_2} \times 0.03)$$

P_{CO_2} is determined as follows:

$$P_{CO_2} = \frac{[HCO_3^-]}{(\text{antilog } [pH - 6.1] \times 0.03)}$$

The H-H equation may be helpful in cross-checking the validity of the blood gas reports when the pH, P_{CO_2}, and $[HCO_3^-]$ values appear out of line. It may also be useful in estimating what changes to expect when any one of the H-H equation components is altered. For example, consider the case example that follows.

Case. A mechanically ventilated patient has a pH of 7.54, a Pa_{CO_2} of 26 torr, and a HCO_3^- of 22 mEq/L. The physician asks the respiratory practitioner to adjust the patient's Pa_{CO_2} to a level that will decrease the pH to 7.45. Using the H-H equation, the Pa_{CO_2} change needed to decrease the pH to 7.45 can be estimated as follows:

$$P_{CO_2} = \frac{[HCO_3^-]}{(antilog\ [pH - 6.1] \times 0.03)}$$

$$= \frac{22}{antilog\ (7.45 - 6.1) \times 0.03}$$

$$= \frac{22}{antilog\ (1.35) \times 0.03}$$

$$= \frac{22}{22.38 \times 0.03}$$

$$= \frac{22}{0.67}$$

$$= 32.8\ or\ 33\ torr$$

Thus, increasing the to about 33 torr should move the patient's pH level close to 7.45. In this case, the respiratory practitioner would begin by either decreasing the tidal volume, or the respiratory rate, on the mechanical ventilator. After the ventilator changes are made, another arterial blood gas should be obtained in about 20 minutes. The pH and should be reevaluated, and followed by appropriate ventilator adjustments if necessary.

Phosphate Buffer System and Acid–Base Balance

The function of the phosphate buffer system is almost identical to that of the carbonic acid–bicarbonate buffer system. The primary components of the phosphate buffer system are the sodium salts of dihydrogen phosphate ($H_2PO_4^-$) and monohydrogen phosphate (HPO_4^-). NaH_2PO_4 is a weak acid. Na_2HPO_4, which has one less hydrogen atom, is a weak base. When H^+ ions are released by a strong acid, the phosphate buffer system works to inactivate the acidic effects of the H^+ as follows:

HCl	+ Na_2HPO_4	→	NaH_2PO_4	+	NaCl
strong acid	weak base		weak acid		Salt

On the other hand, strong bases are converted to weak bases as follows:

NaOH	+ NaH_2PO_4	→	Na_2HPO_4	+	H_2O
strong base	weak acid		weak base		water

Because the phosphate buffer system is only about one-sixth as effective as that of the carbonic acid-bicarbonate buffer system in the extracellular fluid, it is not an effective buffer for blood plasma. However, it is an effective buffer system in urine and in intracellular fluid where the phosphate levels are typically greater.

Protein Buffer System and Acid–Base Balance

The body's most abundant and influential supply of buffers is the protein buffer system. Its buffers are found in the proteins in the plasma and cells. In fact, about 75 percent of the buffering power of body fluids is found in the intracellular proteins. Proteins are polymers of amino acids. Some of the amino acids have exposed groups of atoms known as organic acid (carboxyl) groups (—COOH), which dissociate and liberate H^+ in response to a rising pH:

$$R^1—COOH \rightarrow —COO^- + H^+$$

In contrast, other amino acids consist of exposed groups that can function as bases and accept H^+. For example, an exposed—NH_2 group can bond with hydrogen ions to form—NH_3^+:

$$R—NH_2 + H^+ \rightarrow R—NH_3^+$$

Because this reaction ties up free hydrogen ions, it prevents the solution from becoming too acidic. In addition, a single protein molecule can function as either an acid or a base relative to its pH environment. Protein molecules that have a reversible ability are called amphoteric molecules.

The hemoglobin in red blood cells is a good example of a protein that works as an intracellular buffer. As discussed earlier, CO_2 released at the tissue cells quickly forms H_2CO_3, and then dissociates into H^+ and HCO_3^- ions (refer to Figure 6-17). At the same time, the hemoglobin is unloading oxygen at the tissue sites and becoming *reduced hemoglobin*. Because reduced hemoglobin carries a negative charge, the free H^+ ions quickly bond to the hemoglobin anions. This action reduces the acidic effects of the H^+ on the pH. In essence, the H_2CO_3, which is a weak acid, is buffered by an even weaker acid—the hemoglobin protein.

The Respiratory System and Acid–Base Balance

Although the respiratory system does not respond as fast as the chemical buffer systems, it has up to two times the buffering power of all of the chemical buffer systems combined. As discussed earlier, the respiratory system eliminates CO_2 from the body while at the same time replenishing it with O_2. The CO_2 produced at the tissue cells enters the red blood cells and is converted to HCO_3^- ions as follows:

$$CO_2 + H_2O \leftrightarrows H_2CO_3 \leftrightarrows H^+ + HCO_3^-$$

The first set of double arrows illustrates a reversible equilibrium between the dissolved carbon dioxide and the water on the left and carbonic acid on the right. The second set of arrows shows a reversible equilibrium between carbonic acid on the left and hydrogen and bicarbonate ions on the right. Because of this relationship, an increase in any of these chemicals causes a shift in the opposite direction. Note also that the right side of this equation is the same as that for the carbonic acid-bicarbonate buffer system.

Under normal conditions, the volume of CO_2 eliminated at the lung is equal to the amount of CO_2 produced at the tissues. When the CO_2 is unloaded at the lungs, the preceding equation flows to the left, and causes the H^+ generated from the carbonic acid to transform back to water (refer to Figure 6–18). Because of the protein buffer system (discussed earlier), the H^+ generated by the CO_2 transport system is not permitted to increase and, therefore, has little or no effect on blood pH.

However, under abnormal conditions, the respiratory system quickly responds by either increasing or decreasing the rate and depth of breathing

---

[1] R represents the entire organic molecule, which is composed of many atoms.

to compensate for acidosis or alkalosis, respectively. For example, when the pH declines (e.g., metabolic acidosis caused by lactic acids), the respiratory system responds by increasing the breathing depth and rate. This action causes more CO_2 to be eliminated from the lungs and, therefore, pushes the preceding reaction to the left and reduces the H^+ concentration. This process works to return the acidic pH back to normal. On the other hand, when the pH rises (e.g., metabolic alkalosis caused by hypokalemia), the respiratory system responds by decreasing the breathing depth and rate. This action causes less CO_2 to be eliminated from the lungs and, thus, moves the preceding reaction to the right and increases the H^+ concentration. This works to pull the alkalotic pH back to normal.

Finally, note that when the respiratory system is impaired for any reason, a serious acid–base imbalance can develop. For example, severe head trauma can cause a dramatic increase in the depth and rate of breathing that is completely unrelated to the CO_2 concentration. When this happens, the volume of CO_2 expelled from the lungs will be greater than the amount of CO_2 produced at the tissue cells. In other words, hyperventilation is present. This condition causes the pH to increase and respiratory alkalosis is said to exist. In contrast, the ingestion of barbiturates can cause a dramatic decrease in the depth and rate of breathing. When this occurs, the volume of CO_2 eliminated from the lungs is less than the amount of CO_2 produced at the tissue cells. In this case, hypoventilation is present. This condition causes the pH to fall and respiratory acidosis is said to exist. The control of ventilation is presented in Chapter 9.

The Renal System and Acid–Base Balance

Even though the chemical buffer systems can inactivate excess acids and bases momentarily, they are unable to eliminate them from the body. Similarly, although the respiratory system can expel the volatile carbonic acid by eliminating CO_2, it cannot expel other acids generated by cellular metabolism. Only the *renal system* can rid the body of acids such as phosphoric acids, uric acids, lactic acids, and ketone acids (also called fixed acids).

In addition, only the renal system can regulate alkaline substances in the blood and restore chemical buffers that are used up in managing the H^+ levels in the extracellular fluids. (For example, some HCO_3^-, which helps to adjust H^+ concentrations, is lost from the body when CO_2 is expelled from the lungs.) Basically, when the extracellular fluids become acidic, the renal system retains HCO_3^- and excretes H^+ ions into the urine, causing the blood pH to increase. On the other hand, when the extracellular fluids become alkaline, the renal system retains H^+ and excretes basic substances (primarily HCO_3^-) into the urine, causing the blood pH to decrease.

The Role of the P_{CO_2}/HCO_3^-/pH Relationship in Acid–Base Balance

Acid–Base Balance Disturbances

As shown earlier in this chapter, the normal bicarbonate (HCO_3^-) to carbonic acid (H_2CO_3) ratio in the blood plasma is 20:1. In other words, for every H_2CO_3 ion produced in blood plasma, 20 HCO_3^- ions must be formed to maintain a 20:1 ratio (normal pH). Or, for every H_2CO_3 ion loss in the blood plasma, 20 HCO_3^- ions must be eliminated to maintain a normal pH. In other words, the H_2CO_3 ion is 20 times more powerful than the HCO_3^- ion in changing the blood pH.

Figure 7–2

Alveolar hypoventilation causes the $P_{A_{CO_2}}$ and the plasma P_{CO_2}, H_2CO_3, and HCO_3^- to increase. This action decreases the HCO_3^-/H_2CO_3 ratio, which in turn decreases the blood pH.

© Cengage Learning 2013

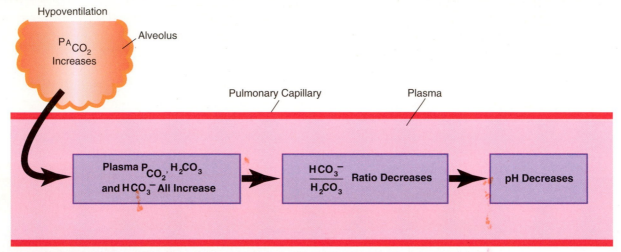

Figure 7–3

Alveolar hyperventilation causes the $P_{A_{CO_2}}$ and the plasma P_{CO_2}, H_2CO_3, and HCO_3^- to decrease. This action increases the HCO_3^-/H_2CO_3 ratio, which in turn increases the blood pH.

© Cengage Learning 2013

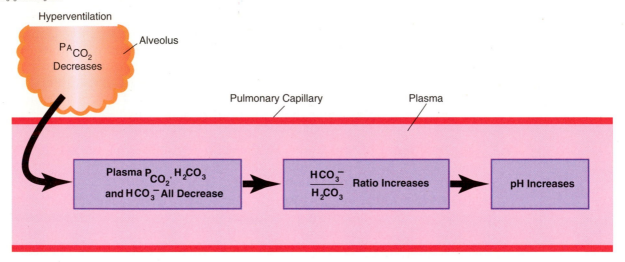

Under normal conditions, the 20:1 acid–base balance in the body is automatically regulated by the chemical buffer systems, the respiratory system, and the renal system. However, these normal acid–base regulating systems have their limits. The bottom line is this: The body's normal acid–base watchdog systems cannot adequately respond to sudden, large changes in H^+ and HCO_3^- concentrations—regardless of the cause.

For example, hypoventilation causes the partial pressure of the alveolar carbon dioxide ($P_{A_{CO_2}}$) to increase, which in turn causes the plasma P_{CO_2}, HCO_3^-, and H_2CO_3 to all increase. This chemical chain of events causes the HCO_3^- to H_2CO_3 ratio to decrease, and the pH to fall (Figure 7–2). Or, when the $P_{A_{CO_2}}$ decreases, as a result of alveolar hyperventilation, the plasma P_{CO_2}, HCO_3^-, and H_2CO_3 all decrease—which, in turn, causes the HCO_3^- to H_2CO_3 ratio to increase, and the pH to rise (Figure 7–3).

The relationship between acute P_{CO_2} changes, and the resultant pH and HCO_3^- changes that occur, is graphically illustrated in the $P_{CO_2}/HCO_3^-/pH$ nomogram (Figure 7–4). The $P_{CO_2}/HCO_3^-/pH$ nomogram is an excellent clinical tool that can be used to identify a specific acid–base disturbance[2].Table 7–1 on page 318 provides an overview of the common acid–base balance disturbances that can be identified on the $P_{CO_2}/HCO_3^-/pH$ nomogram. The following sections describe the common acid–base disturbances and how to identify them on the $P_{CO_2}/HCO_3^-/pH$ nomogram.

Figure 7–4

Nomogram of $P_{CO_2}/HCO_3^-/pH$ relationship.

© Cengage Learning 2013

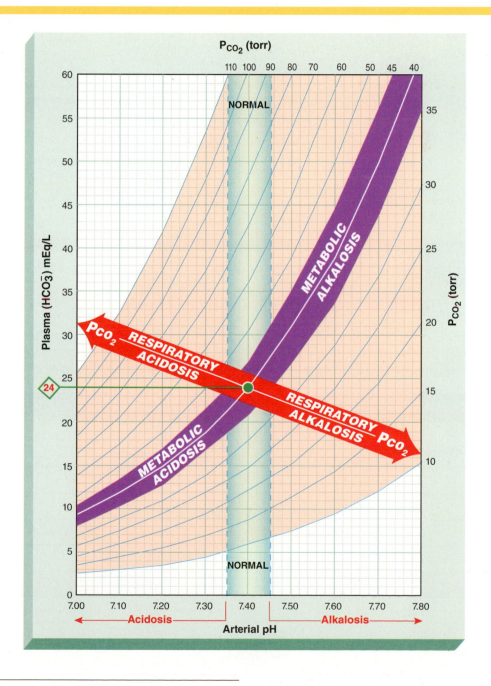

---

[2] See Appendix VI for a pocket-size $P_{CO_2}/HCO_3^-/pH$ nomogram card that can be cut out, laminated, and used as a handy arterial blood gas reference tool in the clinical setting.

Table 7-1
Common Acid–Base Disturbance Classifications

- Respiratory Acid–Base Disturbances
  - Acute ventilatory failure (respiratory acidosis)
  - Acute ventilatory failure with partial renal compensation
  - Chronic ventilatory failure with complete renal compensation

  - Acute alveolar hyperventilation (respiratory alkalosis)
  - Acute alveolar hyperventilation with partial renal compensation
  - Chronic alveolar hyperventilation with complete renal compensation

- Metabolic Acid–Base Disturbances
  - Metabolic acidosis
  - Metabolic acidosis with partial respiratory compensation
  - Metabolic acidosis with complete respiratory compensation
  - Combined metabolic and respiratory acidosis

  - Metabolic alkalosis
  - Metabolic alkalosis with partial respiratory compensation
  - Metabolic alkalosis with complete respiratory compensation
  - Combined metabolic and respiratory alkalosis

© Cengage Learning 2013

Clinical Connection—7-1

$P_{CO_2}/HCO_3^-/pH$ Relationship—Rule of Thumb

Clinically, the respiratory therapist will find the following general rules—based on the $P_{CO_2}/HCO_3^-/pH$ nomogram presented in Figure 7–4—helpful when working to confirm the expected pH and HCO_3^- changes that occur in response to an "acute" increase or decrease in the P_{CO_2} level.

General Rules for the $P_{CO_2}/HCO_3^-/pH$ Relationship		
pH (Approximate)	**P_{CO_2}** (Approximate)	**HCO_3^-** (Approximate)
7.60	20	20
7.55	25	21
7.50	30	22
7.45	35	23
7.40	40	24
7.35	50	25
7.30	60	26
7.25	70	27
7.20	80	28

Respiratory Acid–Base Disturbances
Acute Ventilatory Failure (Respiratory Acidosis)

During **acute ventilatory failure** (e.g., acute hypoventilation caused by an overdose of narcotics or barbiturates), the $P_{A_{CO_2}}$ progressively increases. This action simultaneously causes an increase in the blood P_{CO_2}, H_2CO_3, and HCO_3^- levels. Because acute changes in H_2CO_3 levels are more significant than acute changes in HCO_3^- levels, a decreased HCO_3^- to H_2CO_3 ratio develops (a ratio less than 20:1), which in turn causes the blood pH to decrease, or become acidic (see Figure 7–2). The resultant pH and HCO_3^- changes, caused by a sudden increase in the P_{CO_2} level, can be easily identified by using the left side of the red-colored normal P_{CO_2} blood buffer bar located on the $P_{CO_2}/HCO_3^-/pH$ nomogram—titled "Respiratory Acidosis" in Figure 7–5 on page 320.

Acute ventilatory failure is confirmed when the reported P_{CO_2}, pH, and HCO_3^- values all intersect within the red-colored "Respiratory Acidosis" bar. For example, when the reported P_{CO_2} is 80 torr, at a time when the pH is 7.18 and the HCO_3^- is 28 mEq/L, acute ventilatory failure is confirmed (see Figure 7–5). This is because all reported values (i.e., P_{CO_2}, HCO_3^-, and pH) intersect within the red-colored normal P_{CO_2} blood buffer bar, and the pH and HCO_3^- readings are precisely what is expected for an acute increase in the P_{CO_2} to 80 torr (see Figure 7–5). Table 7–2 lists common causes of acute ventilatory failure.

Table 7–2	
Common Causes of Acute Ventilatory Failure	
Chronic obstructive pulmonary disorders	Pulmonary disorders such as chronic emphysema and chronic bronchitis can lead to acute ventilatory failure
Drug overdose	Drugs such as narcotics or barbiturates can depress ventilation.
General anesthesia	General anesthetics can cause ventilatory failure.
Head trauma	Severe trauma to the brain can cause acute ventilatory failure.
Neurologic disorders	Neurologic disorders such as Guillain-Barré syndrome and myasthenia gravis can lead to acute ventilatory failure.

© Cengage Learning 2013

Figure 7–5

Acute ventilatory failure is confirmed when the reported P_{CO_2}, pH, and HCO_3^- values all intersect within the red-colored "Respiratory Acidosis" bar. For example, when the reported P_{CO_2} is 80 torr, at a time when the pH is 7.18 and the HCO_3^- is 28 mEq/L, acute ventilatory failure is confirmed.

© Cengage Learning 2013

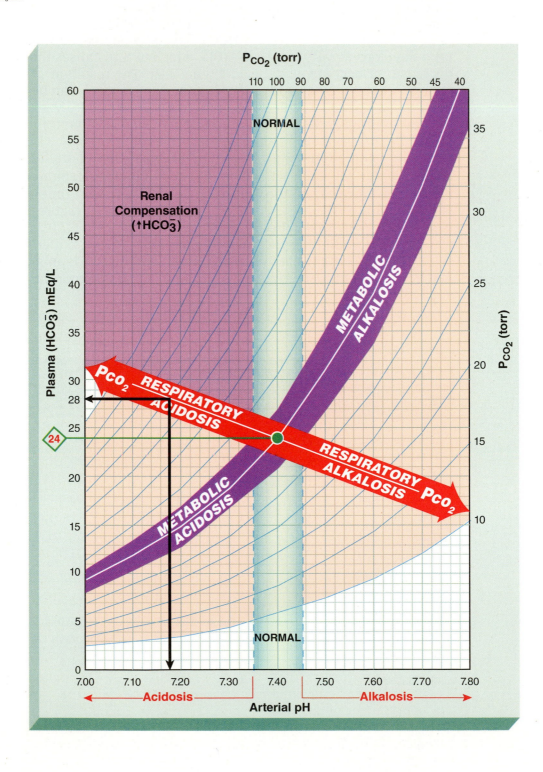

Clinical Connection—7-2

Case Study—Acute Ventilatory Failure (Acute Respiratory Acidosis)

Acute ventilatory failure—also called *acute respiratory acidosis* is a medical emergency! The patient requires immediate ventilatory assistance—for example, mouth-to-mouth ventilation, manual bag-and-mask ventilation, or mechanical ventilation. For example, consider the following case scenario.

CASE: A 20-year-old-female presents in the emergency room as a result of a drug overdose from snorting heroin. She is unconscious, unresponsive, and appears cyanotic. Her pupils are dilated and fixed, and her breath sounds are diminished. Room air arterial blood gases (ABGs) and vital signs are as follows:

ABGs		Vital Signs	
pH:	7.22	Blood pressure:	145/95
Pa_{CO_2}:	78	Heart rate:	115
HCO_3^-:	28	Respiratory rate:	7 and shallow
Pa_{O_2}:	38	Temperature:	98.6°F

The clinical interpretation of the preceding ABG is **acute ventilatory failure**—with **severe hypoxemia** (see Figure 7–5). Clinically, this ABG confirms the immediate need to provide this patient with

mechanical ventilation. In fact, while the ventilator is being set up, the respiratory therapist should manually ventilate this patient with 100 percent oxygen. Once the patient is appropriately secured to a mechanical ventilator, a repeat ABG should be performed to make the appropriate ventilator adjustments to maintain the patient's ABG values in the normal range (i.e., pH—7.35–7.45, Pa_{CO_2}—35–45, HCO_3^-—24, Pa_{O_2}—80–100).

Acute ventilatory failure can be seen in any patient—young or old. It is not associated with a particular ventilatory pattern—for example, apnea, hyperpnea, or tachypnea. The bottom line is that acute ventilatory failure can develop in any condition that does not provide adequate alveolar ventilation—when an increased Pa_{CO_2} level is accompanied with a decreased pH (acidemia), acute ventilatory failure is said to be present. In this case, the patient's ability to adequately ventilate her lungs was seriously compromised by an overdose of heroin. The respiratory therapist commonly provides care for patients who are in acute ventilatory failure. Other causes of acute ventilatory failure include COPD, general anesthesia, head trauma, and neurologic disorders (e.g., Guillain-Barré syndrome and myasthenia gravis).

Renal Compensation

In the patient who hypoventilates for a long period of time (e.g., because of chronic obstructive pulmonary disease), the kidneys will work to correct the decreased pH by retaining HCO_3^- in the blood. The presence of renal compensation is verified when the reported P_{CO_2}, HCO_3^-, and pH values all intersect in the purple-colored area shown in the upper left-hand corner of the P_{CO_2}/HCO_3^-/pH nomogram of Figure 7–6 on page 322.

Acute ventilatory failure with partial renal compensation (also called partially compensated respiratory acidosis) is present when the reported pH and HCO_3^- are both above the normal red-colored P_{CO_2} blood buffer bar (in the purple-colored area), but the pH is still less than normal. For example, when the P_{CO_2} is 80 torr, at a time when the pH is 7.30 and the HCO_3^- is 37 mEq/L, ventilatory failure with partial renal compensation is confirmed (see Figure 7–6).

Chronic ventilatory failure with complete renal compensation (also called compensated respiratory acidosis) is present when the HCO_3^- increases enough to cause the acidic pH to move back into the normal range (7.35 or higher), which, in this case, would be above 42 mEq/L (see Figure 7–6).

Figure 7–6

Acute ventilatory failure with partial renal compensation (also called partially compensated respiratory acidosis) is present when the reported pH and HCO_3^- are both above the normal red-colored P_{CO_2} blood buffer bar (in the purple-colored area), but the pH is still less than normal. For example, when the P_{CO_2} is 80 torr, at a time when the pH is 7.30 and the HCO_3^- is 37 mEq/L, ventilatory failure with partial renal compensation is confirmed.

© Cengage Learning 2013

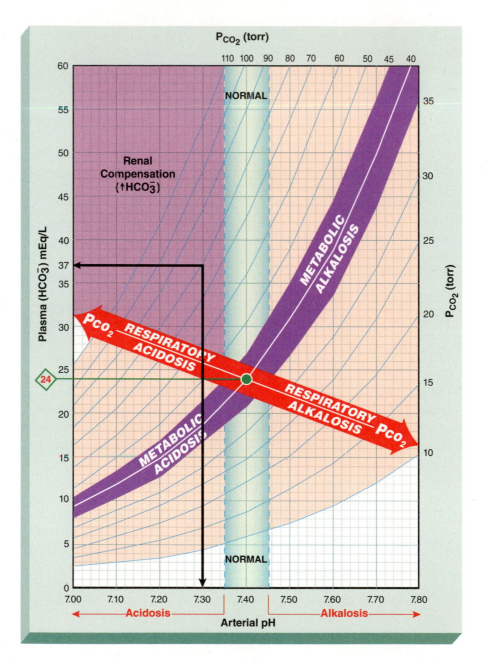

Acute Alveolar Hyperventilation (Respiratory Alkalosis)

During **acute alveolar hyperventilation** (e.g., hyperventilation due to pain and/ or anxiety), the $P_{A_{CO_2}}$ will decrease and allow more CO_2 molecules to leave the pulmonary blood. This action simultaneously causes a decrease in the blood P_{CO_2}, H_2CO_3, and HCO_3^- levels. Because acute changes in H_2CO_3 levels are more significant than acute changes in HCO_3^- levels, an increased HCO_3^- to H_2CO_3 ratio develops (a ratio greater than 20:1), which, in turn, causes the blood pH to increase, or become more alkaline (see Figure 7–3). The resultant pH and

Clinical Connection—7-3

Case Study—Chronic Ventilatory Failure (Compensated Respiratory Acidosis)

Chronic ventilatory failure—also called *compensated respiratory acidosis* is defined as a higher than normal Pa_{CO_2}, an elevated HCO_3^- level (which compensates for the high Pa_{CO_2} level), a normal pH, and a lower than normal Pa_{O_2} level. For example, consider the following case scenario.

CASE: A 76-year-old-female with a long history of chronic obstructive pulmonary disorder (COPD) enters the hospital for a routine stress test. Upon general inspection, she has a barrel chest, digital clubbing, and appears cyanotic. She is using her accessory muscles of inspiration and is pursed-lip breathing. She has a frequent cough and produces a small amount of yellow and green sputum with each coughing episode. On auscultation, she has diminished breath and heart sounds. Her past pulmonary function study records reveal severe obstructive lung function. Room air arterial blood gases (ABGs) and vital signs are as follows:

ABGs		Vital Signs	
pH:	7.37	Blood pressure:	130/85
Pa_{CO_2}:	76	Heart rate:	72
HCO_3^-:	44	Respiratory rate:	10
Pa_{O_2}:	56	Temperature:	98.6°F

The clinical interpretation of the preceding ABG is **chronic ventilatory failure**—with **moderate hypoxemia** (see discussion for Figure 7–6). Although chronic ventilator failure is most commonly associated with chronic obstructive pulmonary disorders (e.g., emphysema, chronic bronchitis, bronchiectasis, and cystic fibrosis), it may also be seen in severe restrictive lung disorders. For example, chronic ventilatory failure is commonly associated with chronic tuberculosis, fungal disorders (e.g., histoplasmosis or coccidioidomycosis), kyphoscoliosis, and bronchopulmonary dysplasia.

Note the patient's low Pa_{O_2} (in this case, 56). Patients suffering from chronic ventilator failure commonly learn to live with low oxygen levels— as do normal individuals living at extremely high altitudes (e.g., in the Andes mountains that peak at 22,841 feet, or the Himalayas mountains that exceed 23,622 feet). In fact, it is common for these patients to function just fine with their day-to-day activities with this low oxygen level. For short physical excursions, however—such as going to the grocery store—they may require some low-flow oxygen via a nasal cannula and portable oxygen tank. COPD is the fourth leading cause of death, claiming more than 100,000 Americans each year. It is estimated that COPD will become the third leading cause of death by 2030.

Finally, as will be discussed in further detail in Chapter 9, chronically high Pa_{CO_2} levels can disrupt the ability of the CO_2 receptors, located in the medulla, to stimulate breathing. Patients with chronically high CO_2 levels often rely on their special oxygen-sensitive receptors—the peripheral chemoreceptors—to trigger respirations. Caution must be taken to not over oxygenate these patients. Oxygen therapy that raises the Pa_{O_2} level above 50 to 60 torr can result in apnea. Clinically, these patients are commonly referred to as CO_2 retainers and are identified by a Pa_{CO_2} above 50 torr and a HCO_3^- above normal— which corrects the pH to within the normal range.

HCO_3^- changes caused by an acute decrease in the P_{CO_2} level can be easily identified by using the right side of the red-colored normal blood buffer bar located on the P_{CO_2}/HCO_3^-/pH nomogram titled "Respiratory Alkalosis" (Figure 7–7 on page 324). Acute alveolar hyperventilation is confirmed when the reported P_{CO_2}, pH, and HCO_3^- values all intersect within the red-colored "Respiratory Alkalosis" bar. For example, when the reported P_{CO_2} is 25 torr, at a time when the pH is 7.55 and the HCO_3^- is 21 mEq/L, acute alveolar hyperventilation is confirmed (see Figure 7–7). This is because all the reported values (i.e., P_{CO_2}, HCO_3^-, and pH) intersect within the red-colored normal P_{CO_2} blood buffer bar, and the pH and HCO_3^- readings are precisely what is expected for an acute decrease in the P_{CO_2} to 25 torr (see Figure 7–7). Table 7–3 lists common causes of acute alveolar hyperventilation.

Renal Compensation

In the patient who hyperventilates for a long period of time (e.g., a patient who has been overly mechanically hyperventilated for more than 24 to 48 hours),

---

Figure 7–7

Acute alveolar hyperventilation is confirmed when the reported P_{CO_2}, pH, and HCO_3^- values all intersect within the red-colored "Respiratory Alkalosis" bar. For example, when the reported P_{CO_2} is 25 torr, at a time when the pH is 7.55 and the HCO_3 is 21 mEq/L, acute alveolar hyperventilation is confirmed.

© Cengage Learning 2013

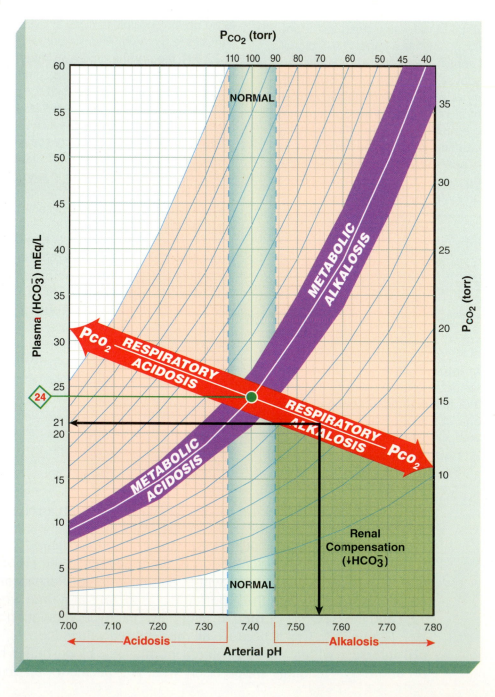

Table 7–3

Common Causes of Acute Alveolar Hyperventilation

Hypoxia	Any cause of hypoxia (e.g., lung disorders, high altitudes, and heart disease) can cause acute alveolar hyperventilation.
Pain, anxiety, and fever	Relative to the degree of pain, anxiety, and fever, hyperventilation may be seen.
Brain inflammation	Relative to the degree of cerebral inflammation, hyperventilation may be seen.
Stimulant drugs	Agents such as amphetamines can cause alveolar hyperventilation.

© Cengage Learning 2013

Clinical Connection—7-4

Case Study—Acute Alveolar Hyperventilation (Acute Respiratory Alkalosis)

Acute alveolar hyperventilation—also called *acute respiratory alkalosis* is most commonly caused by **hypoxemia**. For example, consider the following case scenario.

CASE: A 16-year-old female enters the emergency room in severe respiratory distress caused by an asthmatic episode. Room air arterial blood gases (ABGs) and vital signs are as follows:

ABGs		Vital Signs	
pH:	7.54	Blood pressure:	145/95
Pa_{CO_2}:	27	Heart rate:	115
HCO_3^-:	22	Respiratory rate:	28
Pa_{O_2}:	58	Temperature:	98.6°F

The clinical interpretation of the above ABG is **acute alveolar hyperventilation**—with **moderate hypoxemia** (see Figure 7–7). In this case, the patient's hypoxemia—produced by the acute asthmatic episode—caused the patient's respiratory rate to increase.

The increased respiratory rate, in turn, caused a secondary decrease in the patient's Pa_{CO_2} (in this case, 27)—which caused an acute increase in the patient's pH (in this case, 7.54). The HCO_3^- normally decreases about 2 mEq/L for every acute 10 torr decrease in the P_{CO_2} level—in this case 22 (see Clinical

Connection 7-1: P_{CO_2}/HCO_3^-/pH Relationship—Rule of Thumb, page 318).

When the cause of acute alveolar ventilation is hypoxemia, the patient's ABGs usually return to normal once the Pa_{O_2} is therapeutically adjusted back to the patient's normal oxygen range (80 to 100 torr). Also note that the patient's blood pressure, heart rate, and respiratory rate are increased. These are common vital sign findings when there is an acute decrease in the Pa_{O_2} level. The patient's vital signs should also return back to normal once the Pa_{O_2} is corrected.

In addition to asthma, other common respiratory disorders that cause acute alveolar hyperventilation *with* hypoxemia include pneumonia, postoperative atelectasis, pulmonary edema, pneumothorax, pleural effusion, and acute respiratory distress syndrome.[3] Common causes of acute alveolar hyperventilation *without* hypoxemia include pain, anxiety, fear, brain inflammation, stimulant drugs, and metabolic acidosis. When acute alveolar hyperventilation is caused by one of these conditions, the ABG will show a normal Pa_{O_2}.

---

[3] When the patient becomes overly fatigued, he or she may not be able to maintain the acute alveolar hyperventilation—and, therefore, may begin to hypoventilate! In these cases, the patient's ABGs will reveal the following trends: increasing Pa_{CO_2}, decreasing pH, and decreasing Pa_{O_2}—that is, acute ventilatory failure with hypoxemia (acute respiratory acidosis with hypoxemia).

the kidneys will work to correct the increased pH by excreting excess HCO_3^- in the urine. The presence of renal compensation is verified when the reported P_{CO_2}, HCO_3^-, and pH values all intersect in the green-colored area shown in the lower right-hand corner of the $P_{CO_2}/HCO_3^-/pH$ nomogram of Figure 7–8.

Alveolar hyperventilation with partial renal compensation (also called partially compensated respiratory alkalosis) is present when the reported pH and HCO_3^- are both below the normal red-colored P_{CO_2} blood buffer bar (in the green-colored area), but the pH is still greater than normal. For example, when the P_{CO_2} is 20 torr, at a time when the pH is 7.50 and the HCO_3^- is 15 mEq/L, alveolar hyperventilation with partial renal compensation is confirmed (see Figure 7–8).

Chronic alveolar hyperventilation with complete renal compensation (also called compensated respiratory alkalosis) is present when the HCO_3^- level decreases enough to return the alkalotic pH to normal (7.45 or lower), which, in this case, would be below 14 mEq/L (see Figure 7–8).

General Comments

As a general rule, the kidneys do not overcompensate for an abnormal pH. That is, if the patient's blood pH becomes acidic for a long period of time due

---

Clinical Connection—7-5

Case Study—Chronic Alveolar Hyperventilation (Compensated Respiratory Alkalosis)

Chronic alveolar hyperventilation—also called *compensated respiratory alkalosis*—is a common baseline arterial blood gas (ABG) in the normal female during the third trimester of pregnancy. For example, consider the following case scenario.

CASE: A 27-year-old female in her third trimester of pregnancy enters the emergency room in with a fractured left tibia caused by a fall on the ice. She appears short of breath, is agitated, and is complaining of severe pain. Room air ABGs and vital signs are as follows:

ABGs		Vital Signs	
pH:	7.43	Blood pressure:	130/85
Pa_{CO_2}:	31	Heart rate:	75
HCO_3^-:	22	Respiratory rate:	18
Pa_{O_2}:	74	Temperature:	98.6°F

The clinical interpretation of the above ABG is **chronic alveolar hyperventilation**—with **mild**

hypoxemia (see discussion for Figure 7–8). During the first and second trimesters of pregnancy, it is not unusual for the Pa_{CO_2} to fall to the low 30s—e.g., while exercising, walking briskly or climbing a flight of stairs. During the third trimester of pregnancy, the Pa_{CO_2} is often consistently in the low 30s.

The chronic alveolar hyperventilation seen during the third trimester of pregnancy is most likely explained by the baby's size limiting the mother's lung expansion (which can cause a reduced Pa_{O_2} level) and the normal hormonally induced increases in ventilatory drive associated with pregnancy. Even though this patient appears short of breath, oxygen therapy is not really indicated (although is would not hurt the patient). Her agitation and appearance of respiratory distress is most likely caused by pain.

Chronic alveolar hyperventilation is also seen in patients during the early stages of chronic pulmonary disease, chronic heart failure, and in people who reside in areas of high altitudes.

Figure 7–8

Alveolar hyperventilation with partial renal compensation (also called partially compensated respiratory alkalosis) is present when the reported pH and HCO_3^- are both below the normal red-colored P_{CO_2} blood buffer bar (in the green-colored area), but the pH is still greater than normal. For example, when the P_{CO_2} is 20 torr, at a time when the pH is 7.50 and the HCO_3^- is 15 mEq/L, alveolar hyperventilation with partial renal compensation is confirmed.

© Cengage Learning 2013

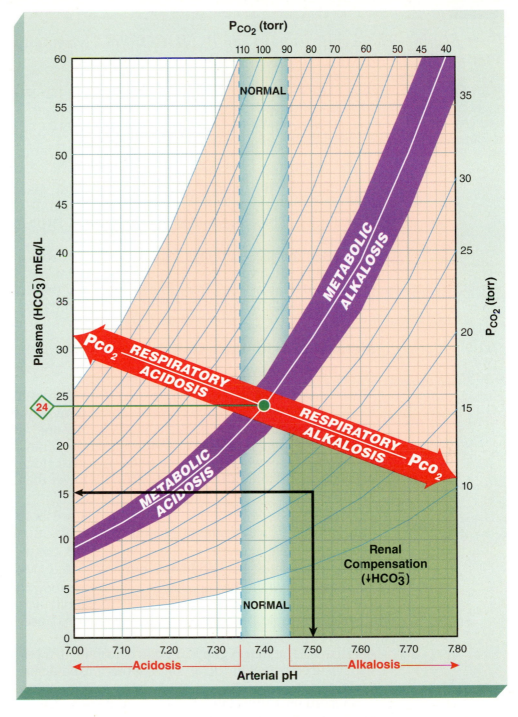

to hypoventilation, the kidneys will not retain enough HCO_3^- for the pH to climb higher than 7.40. The opposite is also true: Should the blood pH become alkalotic for a long period of time due to hyperventilation, the kidneys will not excrete enough HCO_3^- for the pH to fall below 7.40.

However, there is one important exception to this rule. In persons who chronically hypoventilate for a long period of time (e.g., patients with chronic emphysema or chronic bronchitis), it is not uncommon to find a pH greater than 7.40 (e.g., 7.43 or 7.44). This is due to water and chloride ion shifts that

Clinical Connection—7-6

Case Study—The Application of the $P_{CO_2}/HCO_3^-/pH$ Nomogram to a Victim of Carbon Monoxide Poisoning

In the **Clinical Application Section—Case 1** (page 343), the respiratory therapist is called to help care for a 36-year-old man who is overcome by carbon monoxide poisoning. The case illustrates how clinical signs and symptoms can be very misleading and how the $P_{CO_2}/HCO_3^-/pH$ nomogram can be used to help verify the cause of certain arterial blood gas findings.

occur between the intercellular and extracellular spaces when the renal system works to compensate for a decreased blood pH. This action causes an overall loss of blood chloride (hypochloremia). Hypochloremia increases the blood pH.

To summarize, the lungs play an important role in maintaining the P_{CO_2}, HCO_3^-, and pH levels on a moment-to-moment basis. The kidneys, on the other hand, play an important role in balancing the HCO_3^- and pH levels during long periods of hyperventilation or hypoventilation.

Metabolic Acid–Base Imbalances

Metabolic Acidosis

The presence of other acids, not related to an increased P_{CO_2} level, can also be identified on the $P_{CO_2}/HCO_3^-/pH$ nomogram. Clinically, this condition is called **metabolic acidosis**. Metabolic acidosis is present when the P_{CO_2} reading is within the normal range (35 to 45 torr), but not within the red-colored normal blood buffer line when compared to the reported HCO_3^- and pH levels. This is because the pH and HCO_3^- readings are both lower than expected for a normal P_{CO_2} level.

When the reported pH and HCO_3^- levels are both lower than expected for a normal P_{CO_2} level, the P_{CO_2} reading will drop into the purple-colored bar titled "Metabolic Acidosis" (Figure 7–9). In short, the pH, HCO_3^-, and P_{CO_2} readings will all intersect within the purple-colored "Metabolic Acidosis" bar. For example, when the reported P_{CO_2} is 40 torr (normal), at a time when the pH is 7.25 and the HCO_3^- is 17 mEq/L, metabolic acidosis is confirmed (see Figure 7–9). Table 7–4 on page 330 lists common causes of metabolic acidosis.

Anion Gap. The **anion gap** is used to determine if a patient's metabolic acidosis is caused by either the accumulation of fixed acids (e.g., lactic acids, keto acids, or salicylate intoxication) or by an excessive loss of HCO_3^-.

According to the **law of electroneutrality**, the total number of plasma positively charged ions (cations) must equal the total number of plasma negatively charged ions (anions) in the body fluids. To determine the anion gap, the most commonly measured cations are sodium (Na^+) ions. The most commonly measured anions are the chloride (Cl^-) ions and bicarbonate (HCO_3^-) ions. The normal plasma concentrations of these cations and anions are as follows:

Na^+ :   140 mEq/L
Cl^- :   105 mEq/L
HCO_3^- : 24 mEq/L

Figure 7–9

When the reported pH and HCO$_3^-$ levels are both lower than expected for a normal P$_{CO_2}$ level, the P$_{CO_2}$ reading will drop into the purple-colored bar titled "Metabolic Acidosis." For example, when the reported P$_{CO_2}$ is 40 torr (normal), at a time when the pH is 7.25 and the HCO$_3^-$ is 17 mEq/L, metabolic acidosis is confirmed.

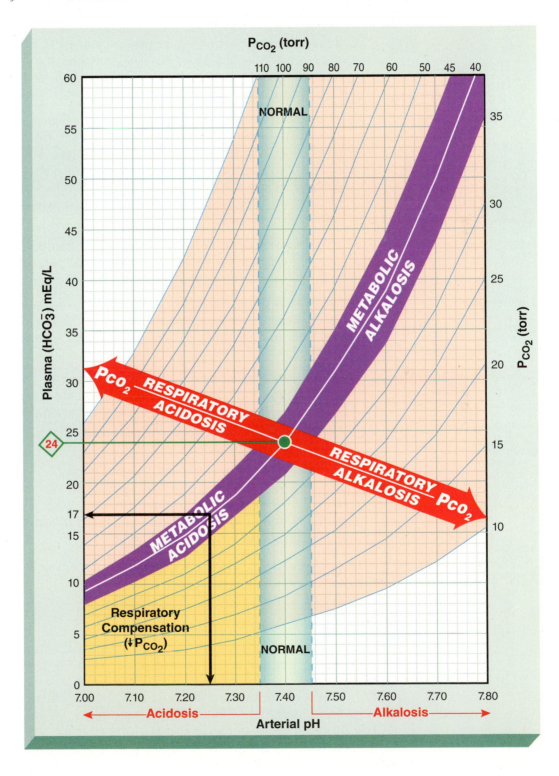

Table 7–4	
Common Causes of Metabolic Acidosis	
Lactic acidosis (fixed acids)	When the oxygen level is inadequate to meet tissue needs, alternate biochemical reactions are activated that do not utilize oxygen. This is known as **anaerobic metabolism** (non–oxygen-utilizing). Lactic acid is the end-product of this process. When these ions move into the blood, the pH decreases. Whenever an acute hypoxemia is present, the presence of lactic acids should be suspected. Lactic acids cause the anion gap to increase.
Ketoacidosis (fixed acids)	When blood insulin is low in the patient with diabetes, serum glucose cannot easily enter the tissue cells for metabolism. This condition activates alternate metabolic processes that produce **ketones** as metabolites. Ketone accumulation in the blood causes ketoacidosis. The absence of glucose because of starvation can also cause ketoacidosis. Ketoacidosis may also be seen in patients with excessive alcohol intake. The presence of ketone acids causes the anion gap to increase.
Salicylate intoxication (aspirin overdose) (fixed acids)	The excessive ingestion of aspirin leads to an increased level of salicylic acids in the blood and metabolic acidosis. Metabolic acidosis caused by salicylate intoxication causes the anion gap to increase.
Renal failure	Renal failure causes the HCO_3^- concentration to decrease and the H^+ concentration to increase. This action leads to metabolic acidosis. Metabolic acidosis caused by renal failure is associated with a normal anion gap.
Uncontrolled diarrhea	Uncontrolled diarrhea causes a loss of HCO_3^- and an increased concentration of H^+. This action leads to metabolic acidosis. Metabolic acidosis caused by severe diarrhea is associated with a normal anion gap.

© Cengage Learning 2013

Mathematically, the anion gap is the calculated difference between the Na^+ ions and the sum of the HCO_3^- and Cl^- ions:

$$\text{Anion gap} = [Na^+] - ([Cl^-] + [HCO_3^-])$$
$$= 140 - (105 + 24)$$
$$= 140 - 129$$
$$= 11 \text{ mEq/L}$$

The normal anion gap range (or the range of the unmeasured ions) is 9 to 14 mEq/L. An anion gap greater than 14 mEq/L represents metabolic acidosis.

An elevated anion gap is most commonly caused by the accumulation of fixed acids (e.g., lactic acids, ketoacids, or salicylate intoxication) in the blood. This is because the H^+ ions that are generated by the fixed acids chemically react with—and are buffered by—the plasma HCO_3^-. This action causes the HCO_3^- concentration to decrease and the anion gap to increase.

Clinical Connection—7-7

Case Study—Metabolic Acidosis

Metabolic acidosis is caused by either the loss of HCO_3^- or the accumulation of **nonvolatile acids**. *Nonvolatile acids* (also called **fixed acids** or **metabolic acids**) are produced from sources other than carbon dioxide—for example, ketone acids, which are commonly associated with diabetes or starvation. The lungs do not excrete nonvolatile acids; only the renal system can excrete fixed acids. Metabolic acidosis usually stimulates a compensatory alveolar hyperventilation to lower the patient's Pa_{CO_2}—which, in turn, decreases the H^+ concentration. For example, consider the following case scenario.

CASE: A 31-year-old female with known insulin-dependent diabetes mellitus presented in the emergency department. She is semi-conscious and is Kussmaul breathing. Her skin is dry and her breath has a sweet, fruity smell. Room air arterial blood gases (ABGs) and vital signs were as follows:

ABGs		Vital Signs	
pH:	7.26	Blood pressure:	115/70
Pa_{CO_2}:	28	Heart rate:	90
HCO_3^-:	13	Respiratory rate:	16
Pa_{O_2}:	105	Temperature:	98.6°F

The clinical interpretation of the preceding ABG is **metabolic acidosis** (see Figure 7–9). Clinically, it is not always immediately apparent what may be causing a patient's metabolic acidosis. In this case, however, based on the patient's history, the preceding ABGs, the Kussmaul breathing, and the sweet smelling breath, it can be readily assured that the patient is suffering from **ketoacidosis**—because of her diabetic crisis. The lack of insulin or a low glucose level usually causes a diabetic crisis. When the body must use stored fats for energy—as opposed to sugars—ketones (acids) are a by-product. Ketoacidosis is commonly seen in the diabetic patient who is not eating properly or not taking his or her insulin at regular intervals.

A classic symptom of ketoacidosis is a sweet, fruity smelling breath. Another classic symptom of ketoacidosis is Kussmaul's breathing (the typical "hyperventilation" of diabetic acidosis). As discussed in Chapter 2, Kussmaul's breathing is both an increased breathing depth (hyperpnea) and an increased rate of breathing (tachypnea). This breathing pattern causes the patient's PA_{CO_2} and Pa_{CO_2} to decrease—decreasing the patient's overall concentration of H^+ caused by the ketone acids.

In this case, it is also interesting to note that the patient is *not* hyperventilating because of a low arterial oxygenation level. In fact, the patient's Pa_{O_2} is 105. A greater than normal Pa_{O_2}—even as high as 115 to 120 torr—is not unusual in the patient with ketoacidosis—even on room air! This is because the decreased Pa_{CO_2}—caused by the Kussmaul' breathing—allow more oxygen to enter the alveoli (refer to Chapter 4, "The Partial Pressures of Gases in the Air, Alveoli, and Blood," page 186).

Other causes of metabolic acidosis include lactic acidosis (caused by inadequate oxygen for tissue metabolism), renal failure, salicylate intoxication (aspirin overdose), and uncontrolled diarrhea.

Finally, it should be mentioned that when the metabolic acidosis is caused by lactic acids, the patient's ABG would reveal a low Pa_{O_2}. The basic cause of lactic acidosis is this: When the patient's arterial oxygen level is inadequate to meet the needs of tissue metabolism, an alternative biochemical reaction occurs that does not use oxygen. This process is called **anaerobic metabolism** (non-oxygen-using). Lactic acid is the by-product of this process. Once the patient is adequately oxygenated, the metabolic acidosis (caused by lactic acids) usually dissipates rapidly. The respiratory therapist commonly cares for patients who have lactic acidosis.

Clinically, when the patient presents with both metabolic acidosis and an increased anion gap, the respiratory care practitioner must investigate further to determine the source of the fixed acids. This needs to be done in order to appropriately treat the patient. For example, a metabolic acidosis caused by lactic acids justifies the need for oxygen therapy (to reverse the accumulation of the lactic acids) or one caused by ketone acids justifies the need for insulin (to reverse the accumulation of the ketone acids).

Interestingly, metabolic acidosis caused by an excessive loss of HCO_3^- (e.g., renal disease or severe diarrhea) does not cause the anion gap to increase. This is because, as the HCO_3^- concentration decreases, the Cl^- concentration routinely increases to maintain electroneutrality. In other words, for each HCO_3^- that is lost, a Cl^- anion takes its place (i.e., law of electroneutrality). This action maintains a normal anion gap. Metabolic acidosis caused by a decreased HCO_3^- is often called **hyperchloremic metabolic acidosis**.

To summarize, when metabolic acidosis is accompanied by an increased anion gap, the most likely cause of the acidosis is fixed acids (e.g., lactic acids, ketoacids, or salicylate intoxication). Or, when a metabolic acidosis is seen with a normal anion gap, the most likely cause of the acidosis is an excessive lose of HCO_3^- (e.g., caused by renal disease or severe diarrhea).

Metabolic Acidosis with Respiratory Compensation

Under normal conditions, the immediate compensatory response to metabolic acidosis is an increased ventilatory rate (respiratory compensation). This action causes the Pa_{CO_2} to decline. As the P_{CO_2} decreases, the H^+ concentration decreases and, therefore, works to offset the metabolic acidosis (see Figure 7–3).

As shown in Figure 7–10, when the pH, HCO_3^-, and P_{CO_2} all intersect in the yellow-colored area of the P_{CO_2}/HCO_3^-/pH nomogram, **metabolic acidosis with partial respiratory compensation** is present. In other words, the Pa_{CO_2} has decreased below the normal range, but the pH is still below normal. For example, when the P_{CO_2} is 25 torr, at a time when the pH is 7.30 and the HCO_3^- is 12 mEq/L, metabolic acidosis with partial respiratory compensation is confirmed (see Figure 7–10).

Metabolic acidosis with complete respiratory compensation is present when the P_{CO_2} decreases enough to move the acidic pH back to the normal range (7.35 or higher), which, in this case, would be below 20 torr (see Figure 7–10).

Combined Metabolic and Respiratory Acidosis

When the pH, HCO_3^-, and P_{CO_2} readings all intersect in the orange-colored area of the P_{CO_2}/HCO_3^-/pH nomogram, both **metabolic and respiratory acidosis** are present (Figure 7–11 on page 334). For example, if the reported P_{CO_2} is 70 torr, at a time when the pH is 7.10 and the HCO_3^- is 21 mEq/L, both metabolic and respiratory acidosis are present (see Figure 7–11). Both metabolic and respiratory acidosis are commonly seen in patients with acute ventilatory failure, which causes the blood P_{CO_2} to increase (respiratory acidosis) and the P_{O_2} to decrease (metabolic acidosis—caused by lactic acids).

Figure 7–10

When the pH, HCO_3^-, and P_{CO_2} all intersect in the yellow-colored area of the P_{CO_2}/HCO_3^-/pH nomogram, metabolic acidosis with partial respiratory compensation is present. For example, when the P_{CO_2} is 25 torr, at a time when the pH is 7.30 and the HCO_3^- is 12 mEq/L, metabolic acidosis with partial respiratory compensation is confirmed.

© Cengage Learning 2013

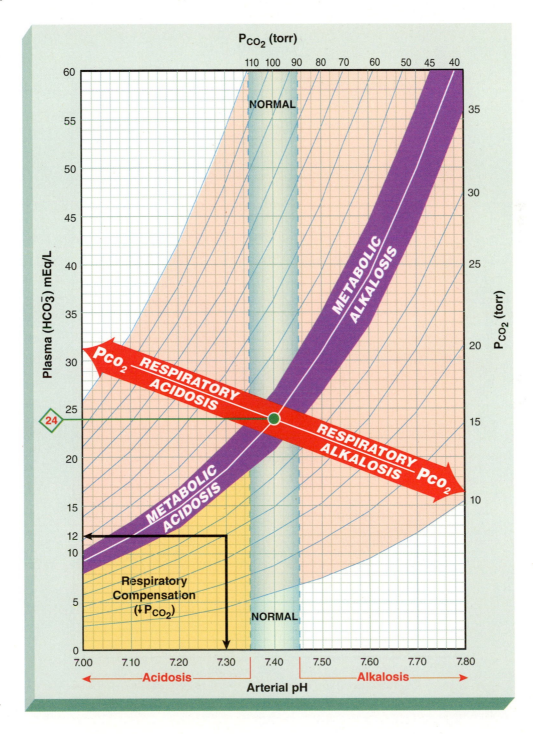

Figure 7–11

When the pH, HCO_3^-, and P_{CO_2} readings all intersect in the orange-colored area of the $P_{CO_2}/HCO_3^-/pH$ nomogram, combined metabolic and respiratory acidosis are present. For example, if the reported P_{CO_2} is 70 torr, at a time when the pH is 7.10 and the HCO_3^- is 21 mEq/L, combined metabolic and respiratory acidosis are present.

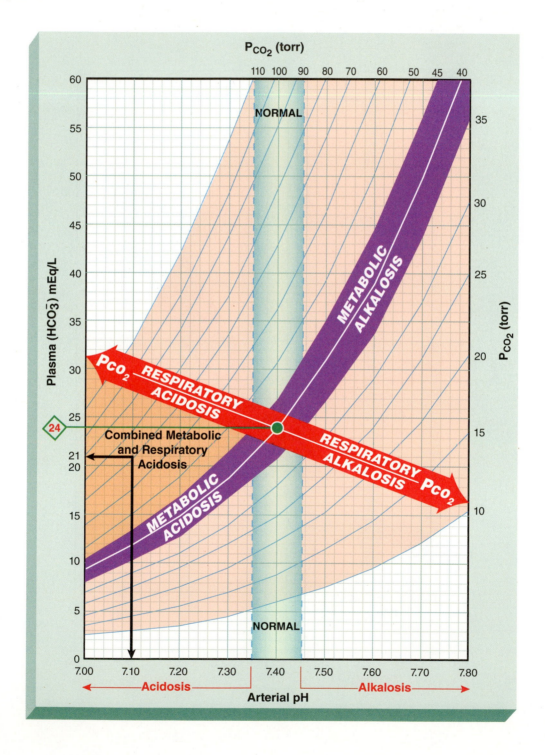

Clinical Connection—7-8

Case Study—Combined Metabolic and Respiratory Acidosis

Combined metabolic and respiratory acidosis is commonly seen in the patient who is in severe acute ventilatory failure—that is, when the pH is low, the Pa_{CO_2} is high, and the HCO_3^- and Pa_{O_2} are severely low. In these cases, not only is the patient suffering from the acidosis, caused by a sudden rise in the Pa_{CO_2} level, but also by an additional amount of H^+ ions caused by the anaerobic metabolism—which produces lactic acids as a by-product—that occurs when a low arterial oxygen level is present. For example, consider the following case scenario.

CASE: A 17-year-old male presents in the emergency room in severe respiratory distress. The patient is well known to the hospital staff. He has a long history of asthma and has been hospitalized for exacerbation of asthma three different times over the past four years. In fact, during his last hospital stay, he was on a mechanical ventilator for 48 hours. On this day, the patient appears semi-conscious and cyanotic. Palpation of the chest is unremarkable. On auscultation, loud bilateral wheezes and diminished heart sounds are noted. On a 2-liter nasal cannula, the arterial blood gases (ABGs) and vital signs are as follows:

ABGs		Vital Signs	
pH:	6.97	Blood pressure:	175/90
Pa_{CO_2}:	103	Heart rate:	110
HCO_3^-:	23	Respiratory rate: 8	
Pa_{O_2}:	33 (Sa_{O_2} 36%)	Temperature:	98.6°F

The clinical interpretation of the preceding ABG is **combined metabolic and respiratory acidosis** (acute ventilatory failure)—with **severe hypoxemia** (see Figure 7–11).

There are two sources responsible for the patient's acidosis—the lactic acid (caused by the low oxygen) and the acids produced by the high Pa_{CO_2} level (caused by the acute ventilatory failure). In this case, the patient needs to be immediately intubated, placed on a mechanical ventilator, and started on a regimen of first-line defense broncho-dilator therapy and oxygen therapy. Time is critical! While the mechanical ventilator is being set up, the respiratory therapist should aggressively ventilate the patient with 100 percent oxygen via a bag and mask.

Overall, the respiratory therapist has two primary goals: to appropriately ventilate the patient to decrease the high Pa_{CO_2} level back to the normal range (35 to 45 torr), to offset the acids produced by the Pa_{CO_2}, and to aggressively oxygenate the patient, to offset the lactic acid produced by the anaerobic metabolism. Once the excess acids are eliminated, the patient's pH should rapidly return to normal.

The respiratory therapist should always be on the lookout for lactic acidosis when the Pa_{O_2} is severely low.

Clinical Connection—7-9

Case Study—The Application of the P_{CO_2}/HCO_3^-/pH Nomogram to a Patient with Both Respiratory and Metabolic Acidosis

In the **Clinical Application Section—Case 2** (page 344), the respiratory therapist is called to help care for a 67-year-old man in cardiac arrest. This case illustrates how the P_{CO_2}/HCO_3^-/pH nomogram can be used to confirm that the patient has a combined respiratory and metabolic acidosis and prevent the unnecessary administration of sodium bicarbonate during an emergency situation.

Metabolic Alkalosis

The presence of other bases, not related to a decreased P_{CO_2} level or renal activity, can also be identified on the P_{CO_2}/HCO_3^-/pH nomogram. Clinically, this condition is called **metabolic alkalosis**. Metabolic alkalosis is present when the P_{CO_2} reading is within the normal range (35 to 45 torr), but not within the red normal blood buffer line when compared to the reported pH and HCO_3^- levels. This is because the pH and HCO_3^- readings are both higher than expected for a normal P_{CO_2} level.

When the reported pH and HCO_3^- levels are both higher than expected for a normal P_{CO_2} level, the P_{CO_2} reading will move up into the purple-colored bar titled "Metabolic Alkalosis" in Figure 7–12. In other words, the pH, HCO_3^-, and P_{CO_2} readings will all intersect within the purple-colored "Metabolic Alkalosis" bar. For example, when the reported P_{CO_2} is 40 torr (normal), at a time when the pH is 7.50 and the HCO_3^- is 31 mEq/L, metabolic alkalosis is confirmed (see Figure 7–12). Table 7–5 provides common causes of metabolic alkalosis.

Table 7–5	
Common Causes of Metabolic Alkalosis	
Hypokalemia	The depletion of total body potassium can occur from (1) several days of intravenous therapy without adequate replacement of potassium, (2) diuretic therapy, and (3) diarrhea. Whenever the potassium level is low, the kidneys attempt to conserve potassium by excreting hydrogen ions. This mechanism causes the blood base to increase. In addition, as the potassium level in the blood decreases, intracellular potassium moves into the extracellular space in an effort to offset the reduced potassium level in the blood serum. As the potassium (K^+) cation leaves the cell, however, a hydrogen cation (H^+) enters the cell. This mechanism causes the blood serum to become more alkalotic. Patients with hypokalemia frequently demonstrate the clinical triad of (1) metabolic alkalosis, (2) muscular weakness, and (3) cardiac dysrhythmia.
Hypochloremia	When the chloride ion (Cl^-) concentration decreases, bicarbonate ions increase in an attempt to maintain a normal cation balance in the blood serum. As the bicarbonate ion increases, the patient's blood serum becomes alkalotic. The kidneys, moreover, usually excrete potassium ions when chloride ions are unavailable, which, as described above, will also contribute to the patient's metabolic alkalosis.
Gastric suction or vomiting	Excessive gastric suction or vomiting causes a loss of hydrochloric acid (HCl) and results in an increase in blood base, that is, metabolic alkalosis.
Excessive administration of corticosteroids	Large doses of sodium-retaining corticosteroids can cause the kidneys to accelerate the excretion of hydrogen ions and potassium. Excessive excretion of either one or both of these ions will cause metabolic alkalosis.
Excessive administration of sodium bicarbonate	If an excessive amount of sodium bicarbonate is administered, metabolic alkalosis will occur. This used to occur frequently during cardiopulmonary resuscitation.
Diuretic therapy	Diuretic therapy can cause increased Cl^- and H^+ excretion and HCO_3^- retention. This condition can lead to metabolic alkalosis.
Hypovolemia	A low blood volume can lead to increased H^+ excretion and metabolic alkalosis.

Figure 7–12

When the reported pH and HCO_3^- levels are both higher than expected for a normal P_{CO_2} level, the P_{CO_2} reading will move up into the purple-colored bar titled "Metabolic Alkalosis." For example, when the reported P_{CO_2} is 40 torr (normal), at a time when the pH is 7.50 and the HCO_3^- is 31 mEq/L, metabolic alkalosis is confirmed.

© Cengage Learning 2013

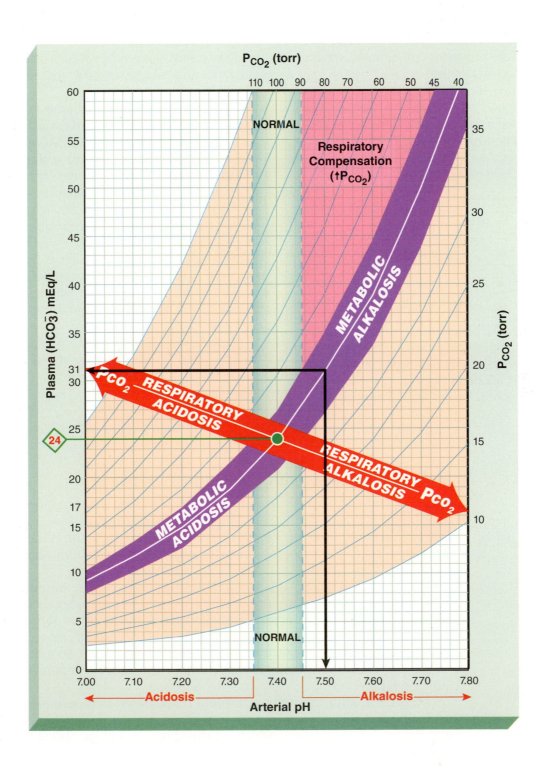

Clinical Connection—7-10

Case Study—Metabolic Alkalosis

Metabolic alkalosis is seen more often than metabolic acidosis. Although it is not as directly life threatening as metabolic acidosis, metabolic alkalosis is potentially dangerous. For example, consider the following case scenario.

   CASE: A post-op 64-year-old female is receiving intravenous therapy over a 3-day period with an inadequate potassium (K^+) replacement. Her K^+ level is 2.8 mEq/L. An electrocardiogram reveals premature atrial and ventricular contractions. Room air arterial blood gases (ABGs) and vital signs are as follows:

ABGs		Vital Signs	
pH:	7.55	Blood pressure:	110/65
Pa_{CO_2}:	43	Heart rate:	84
HCO_3^-:	36	Respiratory rate:	12
Pa_{O_2}:	96	Temperature:	98.6°F

The clinical interpretation of the preceding ABG is **metabolic alkalosis** (see Figure 7–12). A lower than normal level of potassium—called

hypokalemia—is a common cause of metabolic alkalosis and cardiac arrhythmias. Cardiac arrhythmias associated with hypokalemia include premature atrial and ventricular contractions, atrial and ventricular tachycardia, and ventricular fibrillation.

   Potassium plays an important role in normal cardiac function and skeletal and smooth muscle contraction. The normal range for serum potassium levels is 3.5 to 5 mEq/L—in this case, the patient's K^+ was 2.8 mEq/L. Shortly after the attending physician corrected the patient's potassium level, both the ABG values and cardiac function returned to normal. Hypokalemia and metabolic alkalosis are common causes of muscle weakness and difficult weaning from mechanical ventilation. The student should recall that alkalosis (increased pH) shifts the oxyhemoglobin curve to the left, making it more difficult for the hemoglobin to release oxygen to the tissues.

   Other causes of metabolic alkalosis include hypochloremia, gastric suction or vomiting, excessive administration of corticosteroids and sodium bicarbonate, diuretic therapy, and hypovolemia.

Metabolic Alkalosis with Respiratory Compensation

Under normal conditions, the immediate compensatory response to metabolic alkalosis is a decreased ventilatory rate (respiratory compensation). This action causes the Pa_{CO_2} to rise. As the P_{CO_2} increases, the H^+ concentration increases and, therefore, works to offset the metabolic alkalosis (see Figure 7–2).

   As shown in Figure 7–13, when the pH, HCO_3^-, and P_{CO_2} all intersect in the pink-colored area of the P_{CO_2}/HCO_3^-/pH nomogram, metabolic alkalosis with partial respiratory compensation is present. In other words, the Pa_{CO_2} has increased above the normal range, but the pH is still above normal. For example, when the P_{CO_2} is 60 torr, at a time when the pH is 7.50 and the HCO_3^- is 46 mEq/L, metabolic alkalosis with partial respiratory compensation is present (see Figure 7–13).

   Metabolic alkalosis with complete respiratory compensation is present when the Pa_{CO_2} increases enough to move the alkalotic pH back to the normal range (7.45 or lower), which, in this case, would be above 65 to 68 torr (see Figure 7–13).

Figure 7–13

When the pH, HCO_3^-, and P_{CO_2} all intersect in the pink-colored area of the P_{CO_2}/HCO_3^-/pH nomogram, metabolic alkalosis with partial respiratory compensation is present. For example, when the P_{CO_2} is 60 torr, at a time when the pH is 7.50 and the HCO_3^- is 46 mEq/L, metabolic alkalosis with partial respiratory compensation is present.

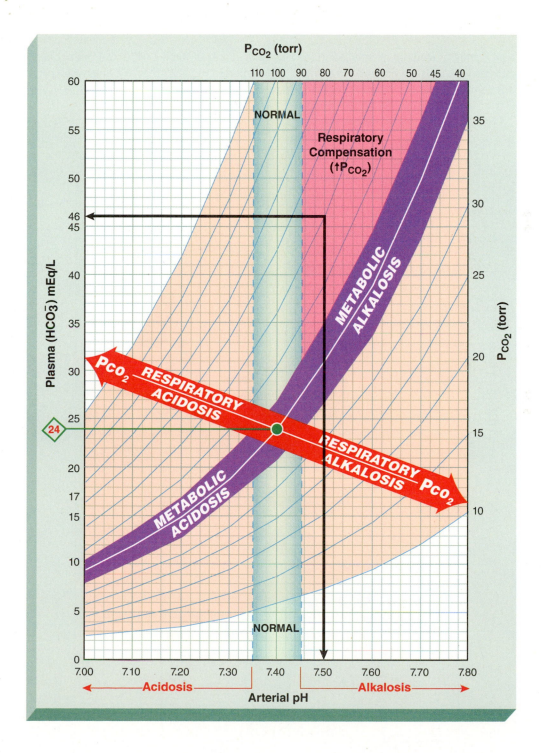

Combined Metabolic and Respiratory Alkalosis

When the pH, HCO_3^-, and P_{CO_2} readings all intersect in the blue-colored area of the $P_{CO_2}/HCO_3^-/pH$ nomogram, both **metabolic and respiratory alkalosis** are present (Figure 7–14). For example, if the reported P_{CO_2} is 25 torr, at a time when pH is 7.62 and the HCO_3^- is 25 mEq/L, both metabolic and respiratory alkalosis are present (see Figure 7–14).

Figure 7–14

When the pH, HCO_3^-, and P_{CO_2} readings all intersect in the blue-colored area of the $P_{CO_2}/HCO_3^-/pH$ nomogram, combined metabolic and respiratory alkalosis are present. For example, if the reported P_{CO_2} is 25 torr, at a time when pH is 7.62 and the HCO_3^- is 25 mEq/L, combined metabolic and respiratory alkalosis are present.

© Cengage Learning 2013

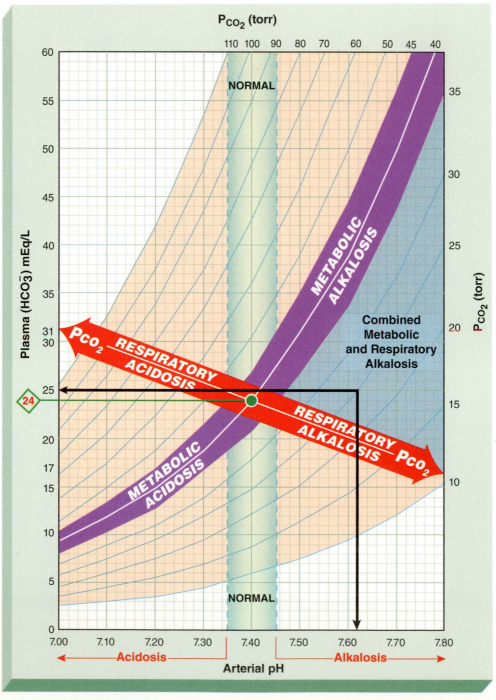

Clinical Connection—7-11

Case Study—Combined Metabolic and Respiratory Alkalosis

Combined metabolic and respiratory alkalosis can develop when an acute decrease in Pa_{CO_2}—regardless of the reason—is accompanied by any condition that causes metabolic alkalosis—for example, hypokalemia, hypochloremia, excessive gastric suction or vomiting, excessive administration of corticosteroids or sodium bicarbonate, diuretic therapy, or hypovolemia. For example, consider the following case scenario.

CASE: This 61-year-old female automobile accident victim is in the intensive care unit on a mechanical ventilator to allow time for her extensive multiple double rib fractures to heal. At this time, the mechanical ventilator is set as follows: rate—12 breaths per minute, tidal volume—0.85 liter, and oxygen concentration ($F_{I_{O_2}}$)—0.30. The morning chest radiograph reveals that her lungs are clear. For unrelated respiratory problems, she is receiving diuretic therapy, corticosteroids, and potassium to treat her hypokalemia. The patient's arterial blood gases (ABGs) and vital signs are shown in the table at next column:

ABGs		Vital Signs	
pH:	7.66	Blood pressure:	125/65
Pa_{CO_2}:	29	Heart rate:	80
HCO_3^-:	32	Respiratory rate: 12 (per ventilator)	
Pa_{O_2}:	92	Temperature:	98.6°F

The clinical interpretation of the preceidng ABG is **combined metabolic and respiratory alkalosis** (acute alveolar hyperventilation) (see discussion for Figure 7–14). The excessive HCO_3^- level is likely caused by the diuretic therapy, corticosteroids, and hypokalemia. The reduced Pa_{CO_2} is caused by overly aggressive mechanical alveolar ventilation—in this case, evidenced by a Pa_{CO_2} of 29 torr.

The attending physician should be notified to correct the metabolic alkalosis problems caused by the diuretic therapy, corticosteroids, and hypokalemia. The respiratory therapist's role would be to adjust the ventilator to increase the Pa_{CO_2} back to the patient's normal range (35 to 45 torr). This can easily be accomplished by either decreasing the tidal volume or decreasing the respiratory rate on the ventilator.

Base Excess/Deficit

The P_{CO_2}/HCO_3^-/pH nomogram also serves as an excellent tool to calculate the patient's total **base excess/deficit**. By knowing the base excess/deficit, nonrespiratory acid–base imbalances can be quantified. The base excess/deficit is reported in milliequivalents per liter (mEq/L) of base above or below the normal buffer base line of the P_{CO_2}/HCO_3^-/pH nomogram.

For example, if the pH is 7.25, and the HCO_3^- is 17 mEq/L, at a time when the Pa_{CO_2} is 40 torr, the P_{CO_2}/HCO_3^-/pH nomogram will confirm the presence of metabolic acidosis and a base excess of –7 mEq/L (more properly called a base deficit of 7 mEq/L) (see Figure 7–9). Metabolic acidosis may be treated by the careful intravenous infusion of sodium bicarbonate ($NaHCO_3$).

In contrast, if the pH is 7.50, and the HCO_3^- is 31 mEq/L, at a time when the Pa_{CO_2} is 40 torr, the P_{CO_2}/HCO_3^-/pH nomogram will verify the presence of metabolic alkalosis and a base excess of 7 mEq/L (see Figure 7–12). Metabolic alkalosis is treated by correcting the underlying electrolyte problem (e.g., hypokalemia or hypochloremia) or administering ammonium chloride (NH_4Cl).

Example of Clinical Use of P_{CO_2}/HCO_3^-/pH Nomogram

It has been shown that the P_{CO_2}/HCO_3^-/pH nomogram is an excellent clinical tool to confirm the presence of (1) respiratory acid–base imbalances, (2) metabolic acid–base imbalances, or (3) a combination of a respiratory and metabolic acid–base imbalances. The clinical application cases at the end of this chapter further demonstrate the clinical usefulness of the P_{CO_2}/HCO_3^-/pH nomogram.[4]

Chapter Summary

To fully master the clinical application of acid–base balance and the interpretation of arterial blood gases, the respiratory therapist must have a fundamental understanding of the following:

1. Acid–base balance and regulation, including the three major buffer systems.

2. The P_{CO_2}/HCO_3^-/pH relationship in respiratory acid–base imbalances, including acute ventilatory failure, chronic ventilatory failure and renal compensation, common causes of acute ventilatory failure, acute alveolar hyperventilation, chronic alveolar hyperventilation and renal compensation, and common causes of acute alveolar hyperventilation.

3. The P_{CO_2}/HCO_3^-/pH relationship in metabolic acid–base imbalances, including metabolic acidosis, common causes of metabolic acidosis, metabolic acidosis with respiratory compensation, both metabolic and respiratory acidosis, metabolic alkalosis, common causes of metabolic alkalosis, metabolic alkalosis with respiratory compensation, and both metabolic and respiratory alkalosis.

4. An understanding of base excess/deficit.

Clinical connections associated with these topics include (1) the P_{CO_2}/HCO_3^-/pH relationship—rule of thumb, and (2) case study examples for the following arterial blood gas findings:

- Acute ventilatory failure (acute respiratory acidosis).
- Chronic ventilatory failure (compensated respiratory acidosis).
- Acute alveolar hyperventilation (acute respiratory alkalosis).
- Chronic alveolar hyperventilation (compensated respiratory alkalosis).
- The application of the P_{CO_2}/HCO_3^-/pH nomogram to a victim of carbon monoxide poisoning.
- Metabolic acidosis.
- Combined metabolic and respiratory acidosis.
- The application of the P_{CO_2}/HCO_3^-/pH nomogram to a patient with both respiratory and metabolic acidosis.
- Metabolic alkalosis.
- Combined metabolic and respiratory alkalosis.

---

[4] See Appendix VI for a pocket-size P_{CO_2}/HCO_3^-/pH nomogram card that can be cut out, laminated, and used as a handy arterial blood gas reference tool in the clinical setting.

1 Clinical Application Case

A 36-year-old man, who had been working on his car in the garage while the motor was running, suddenly experienced confusion, disorientation, and nausea. A few minutes later he started to vomit. He called out to his wife, who was nearby. Moments later he collapsed and lost consciousness. His wife called 911. Eleven minutes later, the emergency medical team (EMT) arrived, quickly assessed the patient's condition, placed a non-rebreathing oxygen mask on the patient's face, and then transported him to the ambulance. En route to the hospital, the EMT reported that the patient continued to vomit intermittently. Because of this, the patient was frequently suctioned orally to prevent aspiration.

In the emergency department, the patient's skin was cherry red. Although he was still unconscious, he was breathing on his own through a non-rebreathing oxygen mask. A medical student assigned to the emergency department stated that it appeared that the patient was being over oxygenated—because his skin appeared cherry red—and that perhaps the oxygen mask should be removed. The respiratory therapist working with the patient strongly disagreed.

The patient's vital signs were blood pressure—165/105 mm Hg, heart rate—122 beats/min, and respirations—36 breaths/min. His arterial blood gas values on the non-rebreathing oxygen mask were pH—7.55, Pa_{CO_2}—25 torr, HCO_3^-—21 mEq/L, and Pa_{O_2}—539 torr. His carboxyhemoglobin level (CO_{Hb}) was 47 percent.

The patient was transferred to the intensive care unit, where he continued to be monitored closely. Although the patient never required mechanical ventilation, he continued to receive high concentrations of oxygen for the first 48 hours. By the end of the third day he was breathing room air and was conscious and able to talk with his family and the medical staff. His vital signs were blood pressure—117/77 mm Hg, heart rate—68 beats/min, and respirations—12 breaths/min. His arterial blood gas values were pH—7.4, Pa_{CO_2}—40 torr, HCO_3^-—24 mEq/L, and Pa_{O_2}—97 torr. His carboxyhemoglobin level (CO_{Hb}) was 3 percent. The patient was discharged on the fourth day.

Discussion

This case illustrates how clinical signs and symptoms can sometimes be very misleading and how the P_{CO_2}/HCO_3^-/pH nomogram can be used to determine the cause of certain findings on arterial blood gas analysis. Even though the patient's was very high (because of the non-rebreathing oxygen mask), the CO_{Hb} level of 47 percent had seriously impaired the patient's hemoglobin's ability to carry oxygen. In addition, any oxygen that was being carried by the hemoglobin was unable to detach itself easily from the hemoglobin. This was because CO_{Hb} causes the oxygen dissociation curve to shift to the left (refer to Figure 6–4).

Thus, despite the fact that the patient's Pa_{O_2} was very high (539 torr) in the emergency department, the patient's oxygen delivery system—and tissue oxygenation—was in fact very low and seriously compromised. The "cherry red" skin color noted by the medical student was a classic sign of carbon monoxide poisoning and not a sign of good skin color and oxygenation. The increased blood pressure, heart rate, and respiratory rate seen in the emergency department were compensatory mechanisms activated to counteract the decreased arterial oxygenation, that is, these mechanisms increased the total oxygen delivery (refer to D_{O_2} in Table 6–10).

Because it was reported that the patient had vomited excessively prior to the arterial blood gas sample being obtained in the emergency department, it was not readily apparent whether the high pH was a result of the low caused by the acute alveolar hyperventilation (which was caused by the low oxygen delivery) or a combination of both the acute alveolar hyperventilation and low and the loss of stomach acids (caused by the vomiting). The answer to this question can be obtained by using the P_{CO_2}/HCO_3^-/pH nomogram. In this case, when the pH, Pa_{CO_2}, and HCO_3^- values are applied to the P_{CO_2}/HCO_3^-/pH nomogram, it can be seen that the elevated pH was due solely to the decreased level, because all three variables cross through the normal buffer line (see Figure 7–7).[5]

---

[5] See Appendix VI for a credit-card size P_{CO_2}/HCO_3^-/pH nomogram that can be copied and laminated for use as a handy clinical reference tool.

Clinical Application Case

During a routine physical examination, a 67-year-old man had a cardiac arrest while performing a stress test in the pulmonary rehabilitation department. The patient had a long history of chronic bronchitis and emphysema. Although the patient had been in reasonably good health for the past 3 years, he had recently complained to his family physician of shortness of breath and heart palpitations. His physician ordered a full diagnostic evaluation of the patient, which included a complete pulmonary function study and stress test.

During the interview, the patient reported that he had not performed any form of exercise in years. In fact, he jokingly stated that whenever he would start to feel as if he should start to exercise, he would quickly sit down and the feeling would go away. The patient was about 35 pounds overweight and, during the stress test, appeared moderately ashen and diaphoretic. When the patient collapsed, a "Code Blue" was called and cardiopulmonary resuscitation was started immediately. When the Code Blue Team arrived, the patient had an oral airway in place and was being manually ventilated, with room air only, using a face mask and bag.

An intravenous infusion was started and the patient's heart activity was monitored with an electrocardiogram (ECG). An arterial blood gas sample was obtained and showed a pH of 7.10, Pa_{CO_2}—70 torr, HCO_3^-—21 mEq/L, Pa_{O_2}—38 torr, and Sa_{O_2}—50 percent. Upon seeing these results, the physician evaluated the patient's chest and breath sounds. It was quickly established that the patient's head was not hyperextended appropriately (which, as a result, impeded air flow through the oral and laryngeal airways). The patient's breath sounds were very diminished, and it was also noted that the patient's chest did not rise appropriately during each manual resuscitation. The patient was immediately intubated and manually ventilated with a bag and mask with an inspired oxygen concentration $F_{I_{O_2}}$ of 1.0. Despite the fact that the patient's pH was only 7.10 at this time, no sodium bicarbonate was administered.

Immediately after the patient was intubated, breath sounds could be heard bilaterally. Additionally, the patient's chest could be seen to move upward during each manual ventilation, and his skin started to turn pink. Another arterial blood sample was then drawn. While waiting for the arterial blood gas analysis results, epinephrine and norepinephrine were administered. Moments later, normal ventricular activity was seen. The arterial blood gas values from the second sample were pH—7.44, Pa_{CO_2}—35 torr, HCO_3^-—24 mEq/L, Pa_{O_2}—360 torr, and Sa_{O_2}—98 percent. Thirty minutes later, the patient was breathing spontaneously on an $F_{I_{O_2}}$ of 0.4, and he was conscious and alert. Two hours later, it was determined that the patient would not require mechanical ventilation and he was extubated. The patient was discharged from the hospital on the fourth day.

Discussion

This case illustrates how the $P_{CO_2}/HCO_3^-/pH$ nomogram can be used to confirm both a respiratory and metabolic acidosis and prevent the unnecessary administration of sodium bicarbonate during an emergency situation. As a result of the cardiopulmonary arrest, the patient's Pa_{CO_2} rapidly increased while, at the same time, his pH and Pa_{O_2} decreased. Because the patient's head was not positioned correctly, the lungs were not ventilated adequately. As a result, the Pa_{CO_2}, pH, and Pa_{O_2} continued to deteriorate. Fortunately, this was discovered when the first arterial blood gas values were seen.

The fact that the initial pH (7.10) and HCO_3^- (21 mEq/L) were both lower than expected for an acute increase in the Pa_{CO_2} (70 torr) suggested that there were additional acids present in the patient's blood (i.e., acids other than those produced by the increased Pa_{CO_2}). According to the $P_{CO_2}/HCO_3^-/pH$ nomogram, an acute increase in the patient's Pa_{CO_2} to 70 torr should have caused the pH to fall to about 7.22 and the HCO_3^- level should have increased to about 28 mEq/L (see Figure 7–5). In this case, both the pH and HCO_3^- were lower than expected. According to the $P_{CO_2}/HCO_3^-/pH$ nomogram, the patient had both a respiratory and metabolic acidosis (see Figure 7–11). In this case, the most likely cause of the metabolic acidosis was the low Pa_{O_2} (38 torr), which produces lactic acids (see Table 7–4).

The fact that the $P_{CO_2}/HCO_3^-/pH$ nomogram confirmed that the cause of the patient's lower than expected pH and HCO_3^- levels were solely due to the poor ventilation eliminated the need to administer sodium bicarbonate. In other words, because the patient's head was not positioned correctly, the patient's lungs were not being ventilated. This condition, in turn, caused the patient's Pa_{CO_2} to increase (which caused the pH to fall) and the Pa_{O_2} to decrease (which produced lactic acids and caused the pH to fall even further). In this case, therefore, the treatment of choice was to correct the cause of the respiratory and metabolic acidosis. Because the cause of the respiratory and metabolic acidosis was inadequate ventilation, the treatment of choice was aggressive ventilation.

Finally, as shown by the second arterial blood gas analysis, the arterial blood gases were rapidly corrected after intubation. In fact, the patient's Pa_{O_2} was overcorrected (360 torr). The patient's inspired oxygen concentration FI_{O_2} was subsequently reduced. If sodium bicarbonate had been administered to correct the patient's pH of 7.10 before the patient was appropriately ventilated, the pH and HCO_3^- readings would have been higher than normal after his Pa_{CO_2} was ventilated down from 70 torr to his normal level of about 40 torr.

Review Questions

1. During acute alveolar hypoventilation, the blood
   1. H_2CO_3 increases
   2. pH increases
   3. HCO_3^- increases
   4. P_{CO_2} increases
      A. 2 only
      B. 4 only
      C. 2 and 3 only
      D. 1, 3, and 4 only

2. The bulk of the CO_2 produced in the cells is transported to the lungs as
   A. H_2CO_3
   B. HCO_3^-
   C. CO_2 and H_2O
   D. Carbonic anhydrase

3. During acute alveolar hyperventilation, the blood
   1. P_{CO_2} increases
   2. H_2CO_3 decreases
   3. HCO_3^- increases
   4. pH decreases
      A. 2 only
      B. 4 only
      C. 1 and 3 only
      D. 2 and 4 only

4. In chronic hypoventilation, renal compensation has likely occurred when the
   1. HCO_3^- is higher than expected for a particular P_{CO_2}
   2. pH is lower than expected for a particular P_{CO_2}
   3. HCO_3^- is lower than expected for a particular P_{CO_2}
   4. pH is higher than expected for a particular P_{CO_2}
      A. 1 only
      B. 2 only
      C. 1 and 4 only
      D. 3 and 4 only

5. When metabolic acidosis is present, the patient's blood
   1. HCO_3^- is higher than expected for a particular P_{CO_2}
   2. pH is lower than expected for a particular P_{CO_2}
   3. HCO_3^- is lower than expected for a particular P_{CO_2}
   4. pH is higher than expected for a particular P_{CO_2}
      A. 1 only
      B. 2 only
      C. 3 and 4 only
      D. 2 and 3 only

6. Ketoacidosis can develop from
   1. an inadequate oxygen level
   2. renal failure
   3. an inadequate serum insulin level
   4. anaerobic metabolism
   5. an inadequate serum glucose level
      A. 1 only
      B. 2 and 3 only
      C. 4 and 5 only
      D. 3 and 5 only

7. Metabolic alkalosis can develop from
   1. hyperchloremia
   2. hypokalemia
   3. hypochloremia
   4. hyperkalemia
      A. 1 only
      B. 4 only
      C. 1 and 3 only
      D. 2 and 3 only

8. Which of the following HCO_3^- to H_2CO_3 ratios represent(s) an acidic pH?
   1. 18:1
   2. 28:1
   3. 12:1
   4. 22:1
      A. 1 only
      B. 2 only
      C. 3 only
      D. 1 and 3 only

9. If a patient has a level of 70 torr, what is the H_2CO_3 concentration?
      A. 1.3 mEq/L
      B. 1.5 mEq/L
      C. 1.7 mEq/L
      D. 2.1 mEq/L

10. The value of the pK in the Henderson-Hasselbalch equation is
      A. 1.0
      B. 6.1
      C. 7.4
      D. 20.1

11. Metabolic acidosis caused by a decreased HCO_3^- is often called
    A. hyperchloremic metabolic acidosis
    B. ketoacidosis
    C. hypokalemia
    D. lactic acidosis

12. Metabolic acidosis caused by fixed acids is present when the anion gap is greater than
    A. 9 mEq/L
    B. 14 mEq/L
    C. 20 mEq/L
    D. 25 mEq/L

13. What is the anion gap in the patient with the following clinical data?
    Na^+ 128 mEq/L
    Cl^- 97 mEq/L
    HCO_3^- 22 mEq/L

    _____

14. According to the P_{CO_2}/HCO_3^-/pH nomogram shown in Figure 7–15 on page 348, if the P_{CO_2} reported is 55 torr, at a time when the pH is 7.14 and the HCO_3^- is 18 mEq/L, what acid–base balance disturbance would be present?

    _____

15. According to the P_{CO_2}/HCO_3^-/pH nomogram shown in Figure 7–15, if the P_{CO_2} reported is 20 torr, at a time when the pH is 7.51 and the HCO_3^- is 16 mEq/L, what acid–base balance disturbance is present?

    _____

Clinical Application Questions

Case 1

1. In the emergency department, even though the patient's Pa_{CO_2} was very high (539 torr), the CO_{Hb} level of 47 percent (enhanced _____; impaired _____) the hemoglobin's ability to carry oxygen.

2. CO_{Hb} causes the oxygen dissociation curve to shift to the

    _____.

3. A classic sign of carbon monoxide (CO) poisoning is a skin color that is described as _____.

4. The increased blood pressure, heart rate, and respiratory rate seen in the emergency department were compensatory mechanisms activated to counteract the decreased arterial oxygenation. These mechanisms

    _____

Figure 7–15

Nomogram of P_{CO_2}/HCO$_3^-$/pH relationship.

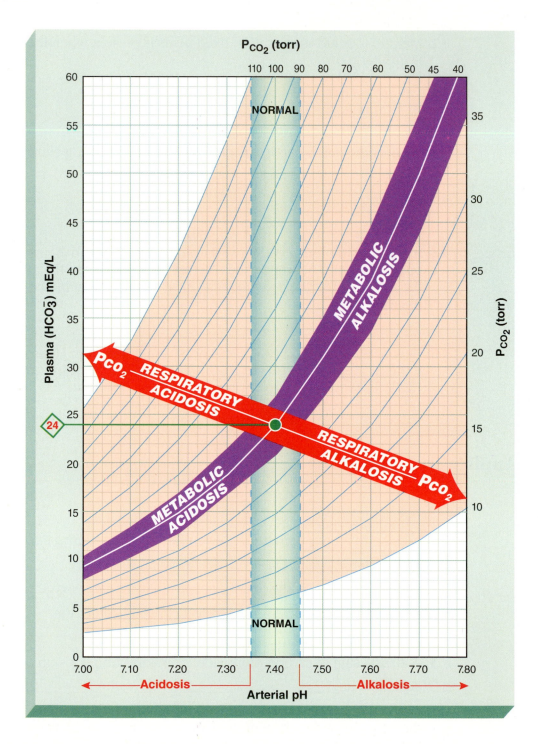

5. Initially, it was not clear why the patient's pH was so high. What were the two possible causes for the elevated pH?

A. _____

B. _____

6. The P_{CO_2}/HCO_3^-/pH nomogram verified that the sole cause of the elevated pH was due to the

_____.

Case 2

1. The fact that the initial pH (7.10) and HCO_3^- (21 mEq/L) were both lower than expected for an acute increase in the Pa_{CO_2} (70 torr) suggested that there were additional _____ present in the patient's blood.

2. In this case, the most likely cause of the metabolic acidosis was the

_____.

3. What was the treatment of choice in this case?

_____

4. If sodium bicarbonate had initially been administered to correct the patient's low pH level, the pH and HCO_3^- readings would have been _____ than normal after the had been lowered to the patient's normal level.

Chapter 8

Ventilation-Perfusion Relationships

Objectives

By the end of this chapter, the student should be able to:

1. Define *ventilation-perfusion ratio.*
2. Describe the overall ventilation-perfusion ratio in the normal upright lung.
3. Explain how the ventilation-perfusion ratio progressively changes from the upper to the lower lung regions in the normal upright lung.
4. Describe how an increased and decreased ventilation-perfusion ratio affects *alveolar gases.*
5. Describe the clinical connection associated with an increased ventilation-perfusion ratio caused by an excessive amount of blood loss.
6. Describe the clinical connection associated with a decreased ventilation-perfusion ratio caused by an upper airway obstruction.

7. Describe how the ventilation-perfusion ratio affects *end-capillary gases* and the *pH level*.
8. Define
   —Respiratory quotient
   —Respiratory exchange ratio
9. Describe the clinical connection associated with capnography.
10. Identify respiratory disorders that *increase* the ventilation-perfusion ratio.
11. Identify respiratory disorders that *decrease* the ventilation-perfusion ratio.
12. Complete the review questions at the end of this chapter.

Ventilation-Perfusion Ratio

Ideally, each alveolus in the lungs should receive the same amount of ventilation and pulmonary capillary blood flow. In reality, however, this is not the case. Overall, alveolar ventilation is normally about 4 L/min and pulmonary capillary blood flow is about 5 L/min, making the average overall ratio of ventilation to blood flow 4:5, or 0.8. This relationship is called the **ventilation-perfusion ratio** ($\dot{V}/\dot{Q}$ ratio) (Figure 8–1 on page 352).

Although the overall $\dot{V}/\dot{Q}$ ratio is about 0.8, the ratio varies markedly throughout the lung. In the normal individual in the upright position, the alveoli in the upper portions of the lungs (apices) receive a moderate amount of ventilation and little blood flow. As a result, the $\dot{V}/\dot{Q}$ ratio in the upper lung region is higher than 0.8.

In the lower regions of the lung, however, alveolar ventilation is moderately increased and blood flow is greatly increased, because blood flow is gravity dependent. As a result, the $\dot{V}/\dot{Q}$ ratio is lower than 0.8. Thus, the $\dot{V}/\dot{Q}$ ratio progressively decreases from top to bottom in the upright lung, and the average $\dot{V}/\dot{Q}$ ratio is about 0.8 (Figure 8–2 on page 353).

Figure 8–1

The normal ventilation-perfusion ratio ($\dot{V}/\dot{Q}$ ratio) is about 0.8.

© Cengage Learning 2013

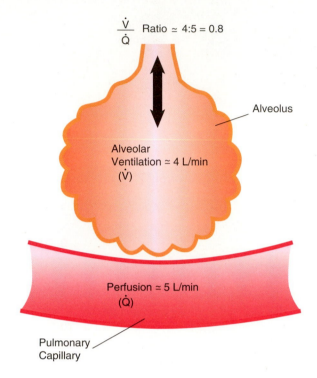

$\dfrac{\dot{V}}{\dot{Q}}$ Ratio $\simeq$ 4:5 = 0.8

Alveolus

Alveolar
Ventilation $\simeq$ 4 L/min
($\dot{V}$)

Perfusion $\simeq$ 5 L/min
($\dot{Q}$)

Pulmonary
Capillary

How the Ventilation-Perfusion Ratio Affects the Alveolar Gases

The $\dot{V}/\dot{Q}$ ratio profoundly affects the oxygen and carbon dioxide pressures in the alveoli ($P_{A_{O_2}}$ and $P_{A_{CO_2}}$). Although the normal $P_{A_{O_2}}$ and $P_{A_{CO_2}}$ are typically about 100 and 40 torr, respectively, this is not the case throughout most of the alveolar units. These figures merely represent an average.

The $P_{A_{O_2}}$ is determined by the balance between (1) the amount of oxygen entering the alveoli and (2) its removal by capillary blood flow. The $P_{A_{CO_2}}$ on the other hand, is determined by the balance between (1) the amount of carbon dioxide that diffuses into the alveoli from the capillary blood and (2) its removal from the alveoli by means of ventilation. Changing $\dot{V}/\dot{Q}$ ratios alter the $P_{A_{O_2}}$ and $P_{A_{CO_2}}$ levels for the reasons discussed in the following subsections.

Increased $\dot{V}/\dot{Q}$ Ratio

An increased $\dot{V}/\dot{Q}$ ratio can develop from either (1) an increase in ventilation or (2) a decrease in perfusion. When the $\dot{V}/\dot{Q}$ ratio increases, the $P_{A_{O_2}}$ rises and the $P_{A_{CO_2}}$ falls. The $P_{A_{CO_2}}$ decreases because it is washed out of the alveoli faster than it is replaced by the venous blood. The $P_{A_{O_2}}$ increases because it does not diffuse into the blood[1] as fast as it enters (or is ventilated into) the alveolus (Figure 8–3 on page 354). The $P_{A_{O_2}}$ also increases because the $P_{A_{CO_2}}$ decreases and, therefore, allows the $P_{A_{O_2}}$ to move closer to the partial pressure of atmospheric oxygen, which is about 159 torr at sea level (refer to Table 4–1). This $\dot{V}/\dot{Q}$ relationship is present in the upper segments of the upright lung (see Figure 8–2).

---

[1] Refer to how oxygen can be classified as either perfusion or diffusion limited in Chapter 4.

In the upright lung, the V̇/Q̇ ratio progressively decreases from the apex to the base. Note, however, that although the V̇/Q̇ ratio in the lung bases is lower than V̇/Q̇ ratio in the lung apices, the absolute amounts of ventilation and perfusion are greatest in the lung bases of the upright lung.

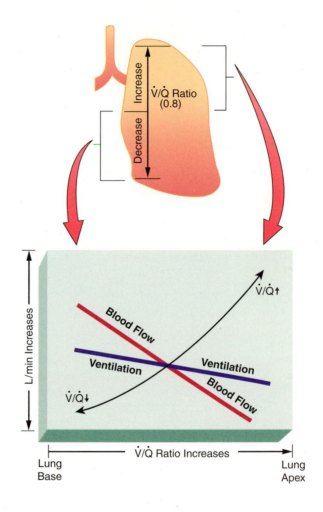

Clinical Connection—8-1

Case Study—An Increased Ventilation-Perfusion Ratio Caused by an Excessive Amount of Blood Loss

In the **Clinical Application Section—Case 1** (page 362), the respiratory therapist is called to help care for a 34-year-old male construction worker who was impaled by a steel enforement rod. This case nicely illustrates how an increased ventilation-perfusion ratio can develop as a result of an excessive amount of blood lost. Note the following paradox in this case: Even though the patient's $P_{A_{O_2}}$ and Pa_{O_2} are higher than normal—because of the increased ventilation-perfusion ratio—the actual amount of oxygen being transported to the patient's tissue cells is lower than normal because of the decreased blood flow.

Figure 8–3

When the $\dot{V}/\dot{Q}$ ratio is high, the alveolar oxygen pressure ($P_{A_{O_2}}$) increases and the alveolar carbon dioxide pressure ($P_{A_{CO_2}}$) decreases.

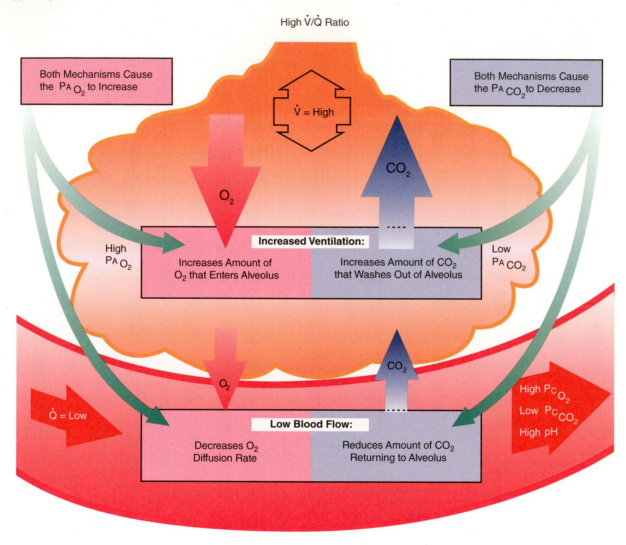

Decreased $\dot{V}/\dot{Q}$ Ratio

A decreased $\dot{V}/\dot{Q}$ ratio can develop from either a decrease in ventilation or an increase in perfusion. When the $\dot{V}/\dot{Q}$ ratio decreases, the $P_{A_{O_2}}$ falls and the $P_{A_{CO_2}}$ rises. The $P_{A_{O_2}}$ decreases because oxygen moves out of the alveolus and into the pulmonary capillary blood faster than it is replenished by ventilation. The $P_{A_{CO_2}}$ increases because it moves out of the capillary blood and into the alveolus faster than it is washed out of the alveolus (Figure 8–4). This $\dot{V}/\dot{Q}$ is present in the lower segments of the upright lung (see Figure 8–2).

Figure 8–4

When the $\dot{V}/\dot{Q}$ ratio is low, the alveolar oxygen pressure ($P_{A_{O_2}}$) decreases and the alveolar carbon dioxide pressure ($P_{A_{CO_2}}$) increases.

© Cengage Learning 2013

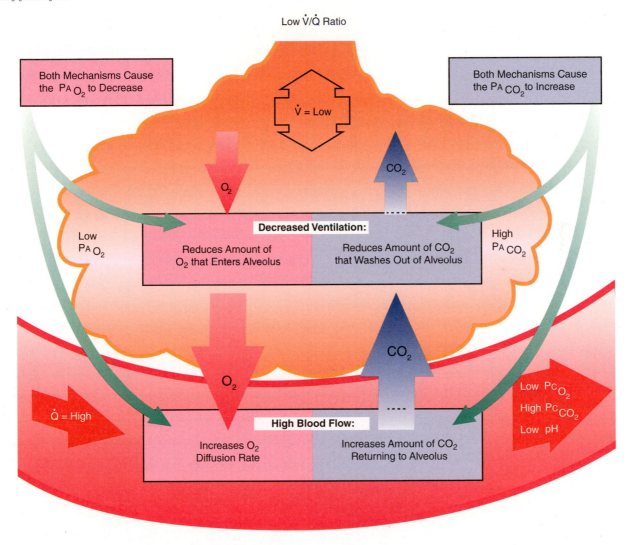

Clinical Connection—8-2

Case Study—A Decreased Ventilation-Perfusion Ratio Caused by an Upper Airway Obstruction

In the **Clinical Application Section—Case 2** (page 363), the respiratory therapist is called to help care for a 4-year-old boy who presented in the emergency department in severe respiratory distress. The boy had inhaled and lodged a quarter in his upper airway. This case nicely illustrates how an upper airway obstruction can cause a low ventilation-perfusion ratio. Note how quickly the patient's ventilation-perfusion ratio returns to normal after the quarter was successfully removed.

O₂–CO₂ Diagram

The effect of changing $\dot{V}/\dot{Q}$ ratios on the $P_{A_{O_2}}$ and $P_{A_{CO_2}}$ levels is summarized in the O₂–CO₂ diagram (Figure 8–5). The lines in the chart represent all the possible alveolar gas compositions as the $\dot{V}/\dot{Q}$ ratio decreases or increases. The O₂–CO₂ diagram (nomogram) shows that in the upper lung regions, the $\dot{V}/\dot{Q}$ ratio is high, the $P_{A_{O_2}}$ is increasing, and the $P_{A_{CO_2}}$ is decreasing. In contrast, the diagram shows that in the lower lung regions, the $\dot{V}/\dot{Q}$ ratio is low, the $P_{A_{O_2}}$ is decreasing, and the $P_{A_{CO_2}}$ is increasing.

How the Ventilation-Perfusion Ratio Affects the End-Capillary Gases

The oxygen and carbon dioxide pressures in the end-capillary blood ($P_{c_{O_2}}$ and $P_{c_{CO_2}}$) mirror the $P_{A_{O_2}}$ and $P_{A_{CO_2}}$ changes that occur in the lungs. Thus, as the $\dot{V}/\dot{Q}$ ratio progressively decreases from the top to the bottom of the upright lung, causing the $P_{A_{O_2}}$ to decrease and the $P_{A_{CO_2}}$ to increase, the $P_{c_{O_2}}$ and $P_{c_{CO_2}}$ also decrease and increase, respectively (see Figures 8–3 and 8–4).

Figure 8–5

The O₂–CO₂ diagram.

© Cengage Learning 2013

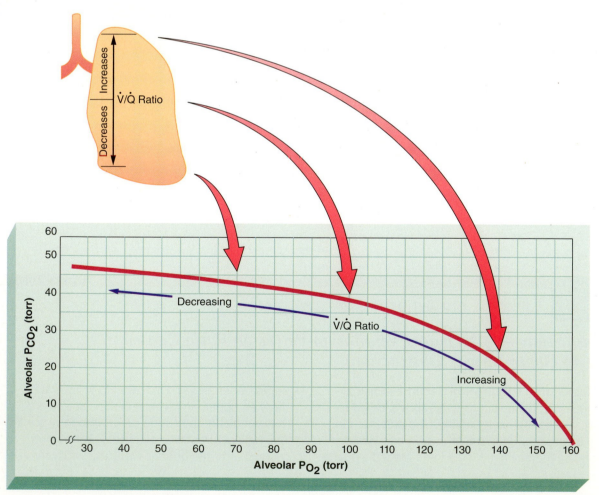

© Cengage Learning 2013

Figure 8–6

The mixing of pulmonary capillary blood gases (Pc_{O_2} and Pc_{CO_2}) from the upper and lower lung regions.

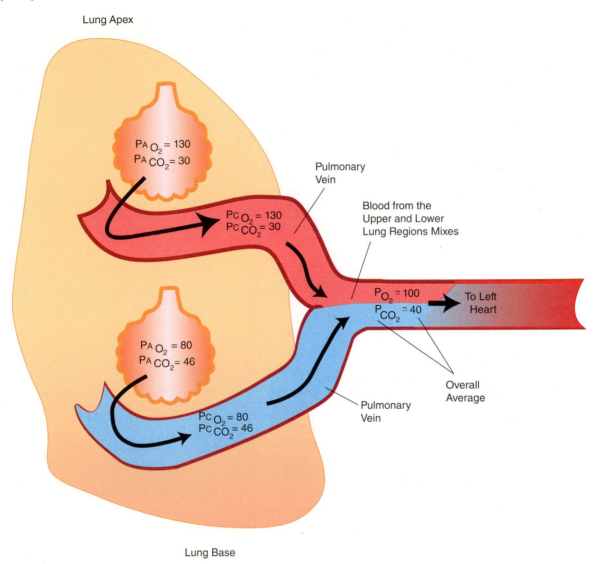

Lung Apex

$PA_{O_2} = 130$
$PA_{CO_2} = 30$

$Pc_{O_2} = 130$
$Pc_{CO_2} = 30$

Pulmonary Vein

Blood from the Upper and Lower Lung Regions Mixes

$P_{O_2} \simeq 100$
$P_{CO_2} \simeq 40$

To Left Heart

Overall Average

$PA_{O_2} = 80$
$PA_{CO_2} = 46$

$Pc_{O_2} = 80$
$Pc_{CO_2} = 46$

Pulmonary Vein

Lung Base

Downstream, in the pulmonary veins, the different Pc_{O_2} and Pc_{CO_2} levels are mixed and, under normal circumstances, produce a P_{O_2} of 100 torr and a Pc_{O_2} of 40 torr (Figure 8–6). The result of the Pc_{O_2} and Pc_{CO_2} mixture that occurs in the pulmonary veins is reflected downstream in the Pa_{O_2} and Pa_{CO_2} of an arterial blood gas sample (refer to Table 6–1).

Note also that as the PA_{CO_2} decreases from the bottom to the top of the lungs, the progressive reduction of the CO_2 level in the end-capillary blood causes the pH to become more alkaline. The overall pH in the pulmonary veins and, subsequently, in the arterial blood is normally about 7.35 to 7.45 (refer to Table 6–1).

Figure 8–7 on page 358 summarizes the important effects of changing $\dot{V}/\dot{Q}$ ratios.

Figure 8–7

How changes in the $\dot{V}/\dot{Q}$ ratio affect the $P_{A_{O_2}}$ and $P_{C_{O_2}}$, the $P_{A_{CO_2}}$ and $P_{C_{CO_2}}$, and the pH of pulmonary blood.

© Cengage Learning 2013

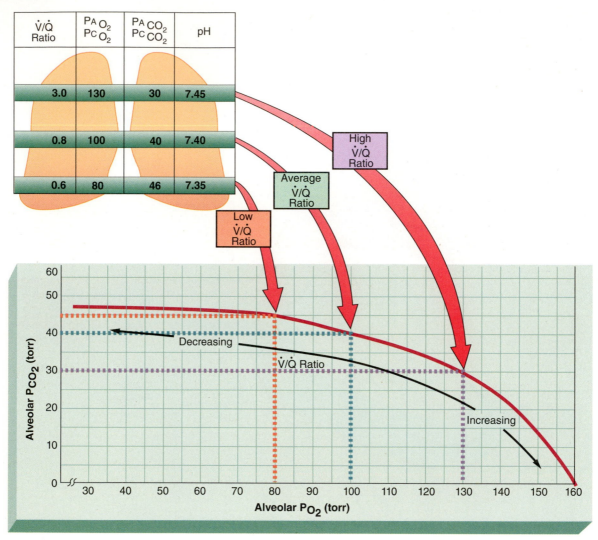

Respiratory Quotient

Gas exchange between the systemic capillaries and the cells is called **internal respiration**. Under normal circumstances, about 250 mL of oxygen are consumed by the tissues during 1 minute. In exchange, the cells produce about 200 mL of carbon dioxide. Clinically, the ratio between the volume of oxygen consumed ($\dot{V}_{O_2}$) and the volume of carbon dioxide produced ($\dot{V}_{CO_2}$) is called the **respiratory quotient** (RQ) and is expressed as follows:

$$RQ = \frac{\dot{V}_{CO_2}}{\dot{V}_{O_2}}$$

$$= \frac{200 \text{ mL CO}_2/\text{min}}{250 \text{ mL O}_2/\text{min}}$$

$$= 0.8$$

Respiratory Exchange Ratio

Gas exchange between the pulmonary capillaries and the alveoli is called **external respiration** because this gas exchange is between the body and the external environment. The quantity of oxygen and carbon dioxide exchanged during a period of 1 minute is called the **respiratory exchange ratio** (RR). Under normal conditions, the RR equals the RQ.

Clinical Connection—8-3

Capnography

Capnography is a rapid, continuous, noninvasive monitoring and graphic display of the patient's inhaled and exhaled carbon dioxide (CO_2) plotted against time. The gas sample is usually obtained by attaching an infrared CO_2 light sensor to the end of the patient's endotracheal tube or mask. The waveform produced is called a **capnogram** (Figure 8–8). The capnogram provides (1) a *direct* measurement of the partial pressure of CO_2 (P_{CO_2}), and/or the concentration of CO_2, that is eliminated by the lungs and (2) an *indirect* measurement of the partial pressure of the mixed venous blood CO_2 ($P\bar{v}_{CO_2}$), which is produced by the tissue cells and transport to the lungs for elimination.

The gas sample analyzed for the capnogram is called the **end-tidal CO_2 (ET_{CO_2})** or the **end-tidal partial pressure of carbon dioxide (PET_{CO_2})**—see Figure 8–8D. The normal ET_{CO_2} is 35 to 45 mm Hg, or about 5 percent. The normal ET_{CO_2} to Pa_{CO_2} gap is 2 to 3 torr. The respiratory therapist commonly uses capnography to collect important cardiopulmonary information—including the patient's ventilation-perfusion ($\dot{V}/\dot{Q}$) ratio, ventilatory pattern trends, verification of the endotracheal tube placement, the effectiveness of CPR, and CO_2 production. The following provides a brief overview and description of the kinds of fast and reliable information that can be obtained from capnography:

- **Ventilation-perfusion ($\dot{V}/\dot{Q}$) relationship.**
  A number of pulmonary conditions can alter the patient's $\dot{V}/\dot{Q}$ ratio. For example, pulmonary disorders that *decrease* the patient's $\dot{V}/\dot{Q}$ ratio—and, therefore, increase the ET_{CO_2} level on the capnogram—include chronic bronchitis, emphysema, and asthma. In fact, capnography

Figure 8–8

Capnogram waveform. **A** to **B** is post-inspiration (no CO_2 in inhaled gas). **B** is the beginning of alveolar exhalation (some CO_2). **B** to **C** is the exhalation upstroke where dead space gas mixes with alveolar gas (i.e., more CO_2). **C** to **D** is the continuation of exhalation with all alveolar gas (the plateau phase of the patient's exhaled CO_2 level). **D** is the end-expiration value (the peak CO_2 concentration)—this portion of the curve is commonly called the end-tidal CO_2 (ET_{CO_2} or PET_{CO_2}). Usually the end-tidal CO_2 value is used to follow the patient's ventilatory tends. The normal ET_{CO_2} to Pa_{CO_2} gap is 2 to 3 torr. **D** to **E** reflects the inspiration phase of respiration (zero C_2 being inhaled).

© Cengage Learning 2013

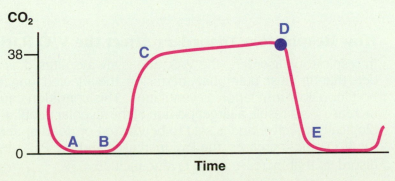

(continues)

Clinical Connection—8-3, continued

is an excellent way to monitor the effectiveness of bronchodilator therapy in the patient experiencing a severe asthmatic episode. This is because bronchospasm produces the classic "shark-fin" wave form on the capnogram as the patient struggles to exhale. The shark-fin-shaped appearance is a result of the slow and uneven alveolar CO_2 emptying that causes a right shift— a more horizontal sloping—of the B-C line on the capnogram. As the bronchospasm lessens in response to the bronchodilator therapy, the B-C line moves back to its normal (i.e., more vertical) upward slope—followed by the normal flat C-D plateau line (see Figure 8–8). Other causes of an increased ET_{CO_2} include hyperthermia (fever), sepsis, seizures, bicarbonate administration, and increased metabolic rates.

Pulmonary conditions that *increase* the patient's $\dot{V}/\dot{Q}$ ratio—and, therefore, decrease the ET_{CO_2} level on the capnogram—include cardiac arrest, pulmonary embolism, hypovolemia, congestive heart failure, hemorrhage, and pulmonary hypertension. Conditions that decrease or block blood flow through the lungs can greatly reduce the amount of CO_2 reaching the lungs, which in turn cause a rapid decrease in the ET_{CO_2} level.

- **Monitoring the patient's ventilation.** Capnography monitors the patient's ventilation, providing a breath-by-breath trend and an early warning system of an impending respiratory crisis. Such problems include:
  - Hyperventilation—ET_{CO_2} decreases
  - Hypoventilation—ET_{CO_2} increases

- **Confirming, maintaining, and assisting intubation.** Continuous end-tidal CO_2 levels can confirm a tracheal intubation. Zero ET_{CO_2} confirms that an endotracheal tube is incorrectly placed in the esophagus. In cases where it is difficult to visualize the vocal cords, a capnography sensor attached to the ET tube prior to intubation can assist in correctly placing the ET tube—that is, the capnogram shows a sudden rise in the ET_{CO_2} level.

- **Verifying the effectiveness of CPR.** Monitoring the ET_{CO_2} is a good way to assess the effectiveness of blood circulation during CPR. A rapid rise in the ET_{CO_2} level may also confirm the return of spontaneous circulation during periods of no chest compressions. Or, if the ET_{CO_2} suddenly drops after the CPR has been stopped, CPR may have to be restarted.

- **Monitoring sedated patients.** Capnography can be very helpful in monitoring any patient who is receiving pain management or sedation for signs of hypoventilation or apnea—that is, trends of increased ET_{CO_2} levels. A sudden drop in the ET_{CO_2} levels indicates the patient is beginning to arouse from sedation—that is, starting to breathe on his or her own—and will likely require more medication to prevent them from "bucking" the tube.

- **Monitoring hyperthermia.** When a patient spikes a fever, the metabolism increases and causes the ET_{CO_2} to rise. Early intervention in treating fevers can be life saving.

How Respiratory Disorders Affect the $\dot{V}/\dot{Q}$ Ratio

In respiratory disorders, the $\dot{V}/\dot{Q}$ ratio is always altered. For example, in disorders that diminish pulmonary perfusion, the affected lung area receives little or no blood flow in relation to ventilation. This condition causes the $\dot{V}/\dot{Q}$ ratio to increase. As a result, a larger portion of the alveolar ventilation will not be physiologically effective and is said to be **wasted** or **dead space ventilation**. When the $\dot{V}/\dot{Q}$ ratio increases, the $P_{A_{O_2}}$ increases and the $P_{A_{CO_2}}$ decreases. Pulmonary disorders that increase the $\dot{V}/\dot{Q}$ ratio include:

- Pulmonary emboli.
- Partial or complete obstruction in the pulmonary artery or some of the arterioles (e.g., atherosclerosis, collagen disease).
- Extrinsic pressure on the pulmonary vessels (e.g., pneumothorax, hydrothorax, presence of tumor).

- Destruction of the pulmonary vessels (e.g., emphysema).
- Decreased cardiac output.

In disorders that diminish pulmonary ventilation, the affected lung area receives little or no ventilation in relation to blood flow. This condition causes the $\dot{V}/\dot{Q}$ ratio to decrease. As a result, a larger portion of the pulmonary blood flow will not be physiologically effective in terms of gas exchange and is said to be **shunted blood**. When the $\dot{V}/\dot{Q}$ ratio decreases, the $P_{A_{O_2}}$ decreases and the $P_{A_{CO_2}}$ increases. Pulmonary disorders that decrease the $\dot{V}/\dot{Q}$ ratio include:

- Obstructive lung disorders (e.g., emphysema, bronchitis, asthma).
- Restrictive lung disorders (e.g., pneumonia, silicosis, pulmonary fibrosis).
- Hypoventilation from any cause.

Figure 8–9 summarizes the O_2–CO_2 effects of changing $\dot{V}/\dot{Q}$ ratios in response to respiratory disorders.

Figure 8–9

Alveolar O_2 and CO_2 pressure changes that occur as a result $\dot{V}/\dot{Q}$ of ratio changes caused by respiratory disorders: **A.** shunt unit; **B.** normal unit; **C.** dead space unit.

© Cengage Learning 2013

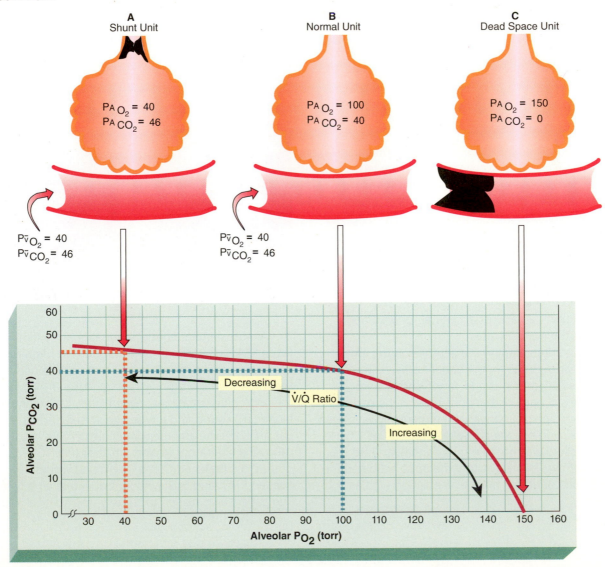

Chapter Summary

This chapter discusses how the ventilation-perfusion $\dot{V}/\dot{Q}$ ratio can profoundly affect alveolar oxygen ($P_{A_{O_2}}$) and carbon dioxide ($P_{A_{CO_2}}$) pressures. Essential components associated with this topic include (1) how the $\dot{V}/\dot{Q}$ ratio changes from the upper to lower lung regions in the normal upright lung and (2) how an increased and decreased $\dot{V}/\dot{Q}$ ratio affects the alveolar gases and end-capillary gases and pH level. Related topics include the respiratory quotient and respiratory exchange ratio and respiratory disorders that increase the $\dot{V}/\dot{Q}$ ratio (e.g., pulmonary emboli, decreased cardiac output) and decrease the $\dot{V}/\dot{Q}$ ratio (e.g., emphysema, bronchitis, pneumonia).

Clinical connections associated with these topics include (1) a case study illustrating an increased ventilation-perfusion ratio caused by an excessive amount of blood loss, (2) a case study describing a decreased ventilation-perfusion ratio caused by an upper airway obstruction, and (3) capnography.

1 Clinical Application Case

A 34-year-old male construction worker fell from a second-story platform and was impaled by a steel enforcement rod that was protruding vertically about 3 feet from a cement structure. The steel rod entered the side of his lower right abdomen and exited from the left side of the abdomen, about 2 cm below the twelfth rib (see the accompanying X-ray). Although the steel rod pierced the side of the descending aorta, no other major organs were seriously damaged.

The man was still conscious when workers cut through the steel rod to free him from the cement structure. While he was being cut free, an emergency medical team (EMT) inserted an intravenous infusion line, placed a non-rebreathing mask over his face, and worked to stop the bleeding as best they could. When the man was finally cut free, he was immediately transported to the trauma center. It was later estimated that he had lost about half of his blood volume at the accident site.

A full trauma team was assembled in the emergency department when the patient arrived. The patient was unconscious and very cyanotic. Even though he still had spontaneous breaths, he had an oral airway in place and was being manually ventilated with an inspired oxygen concentration ($F_{I_{O_2}}$) of 1.0. His blood pressure was 65/40 mm Hg and heart rate was 120 beats/min. The respiratory therapist intubated the patient and continued manual ventilation with an $F_{I_{O_2}}$ of 1.0.

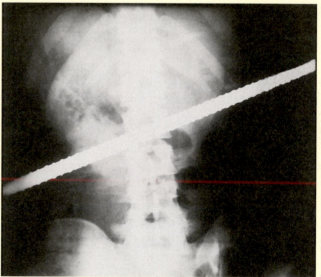

Courtesy: T. Des Jardins, WindMist LLC

Almost simultaneously, a portable X-ray film was taken STAT to aid the trauma surgeons in the removal of the steel rod. A blood specimen was obtained for the following laboratory assays: glucose, BUN (blood urea nitrogen), creatinine, electrolytes, CBC (complete blood cell) count, and a type and screen and blood gas analysis. The emergency department physician called the laboratory to alert lab staff that 10 units of un-cross-matched O negative blood would be needed STAT, and to stay 5 units ahead at all times. The patient was rushed to surgery. The surgical team learned during the operation that the patient's hematocrit was 15.3 percent and his hemoglobin level was 5.1 g%.

Four hours later, the patient was in stable condition in the surgical intensive care unit. The steel rod had been successfully removed, and his aorta was repaired. Although he was still listed in critical condition, his prognosis was described as good to excellent. At this time, however, the patient was still unconscious because of the drugs administered during surgery. He was on mechanical ventilation with the following settings: tidal volume 900 mL, respirations 12 breaths/min, FI_{O_2} 0.4, continuous positive airway pressure (CPAP) 5 cm H_2O, and a positive end-expiratory pressure (PEEP) of 5 cm H_2O.

His blood pressure was 126/79 mm Hg and heart rate was 78 beats/minute. Arterial blood gas values were pH—7.44, Pa_{CO_2}—36 torr, HCO_3^-—24 mEq/L, and Pa_{O_2}—136 torr. Oxygen saturation measured by pulse oximeter (Sp_{O_2}) was 98 percent. His hematocrit was 44 percent and hemoglobin level was 14.6 g%. The patient's recovery progressed very well. Two days later,

he was conscious and no longer on the ventilator. He was discharged 6 days later.

Discussion

This case illustrates an increased ventilation-perfusion ratio caused by an excessive amount of blood lost as a result of trauma (the penetrating steel rod). As the patient continued to lose blood, the blood flow through both of his lungs progressively decreased. As a result, alveolar ventilation progressively became greater than pulmonary blood flow. Thus, the patient's alveolar ventilation was becoming more and more "ineffective" physiologically. In other words, more and more of the patient's alveolar ventilation was becoming *wasted* or *dead space ventilation*. The paradox of this condition is that even though the patient's PA_{O_2} and Pa_{O_2} increased in response to an increased ventilation-perfusion ratio, the actual amount of oxygen being transported decreased because of the reduced blood flow (refer to Table 6–10). Fortunately, this pathologic process was reversed in surgery.

2	Clinical Application Case

A 4-year-old boy presented in the emergency department in severe respiratory distress. An hour earlier, the patient's mother had brought home some groceries in a large box. After removing the groceries, she noticed a silver quarter in the bottom of the box. She removed the quarter and placed it on the kitchen counter. She then gave the box to her 4-year-old son to play with. Thinking he was occupied for awhile, she went downstairs to the basement with her 10-year-old son to put a load of laundry in the washing machine. Moments later, they heard the youngest child cry.

Thinking that it was not anything serious, the mother asked the older boy to go get his brother. Seconds later, the older boy called to his mother that his brother looked blue and that he had vomited. The mother quickly went upstairs to the kitchen. She found her 4-year-old choking and expectorating frothy white sputum. She immediately knew what had

happened. The quarter was gone. Her 4-year-old had put the quarter in his mouth and had aspirated it.

Having been trained in cardiopulmonary resuscitation (CPR), she initiated the American Heart Association's Conscious-Obstructive CPR procedure. Her son's response, however, was not favorable. In fact, his choking appeared, and sounded, worse. Frothy white secretions continued to flow out of his mouth, and a loud, brassy-like sound could be heard each time he inhaled. His inspiratory efforts were clearly labored. Alarmed, the mother immediately drove her son to the emergency department a few miles away. The 10-year-old tried to comfort his brother as they drove to the hospital.

In the emergency department, the boy was conscious, crying, and in obvious respiratory distress. His skin was cyanotic and pale. He appeared very fatigued. Inspiratory stridor could be heard without the aid

(continues)

of stethoscope. He was sitting up on the side of the gurney, with his legs hanging over the edge, using his accessory muscles of inspiration. His vital signs were blood pressure—89/50 mm Hg, heart rate—105 beats/min, and respirations—6 breaths/min and labored. His breath sounds were very diminished. A portable chest X-ray film showed the quarter lodged about 2 cm above the vocal cords (see the accompanying X-ray). Oxygen saturation measured by pulse oximetry (SP_{O_2}) was 87 percent. The patient was immediately transferred to surgery and placed under general anethesia. The quarter was removed moments later without difficulty.

Discussion

This case illustrates a decreased $\dot{V}/\dot{Q}$ ratio caused by an upper airway obstruction. Although an arterial blood sample was not drawn in this case, one can easily predict what the values would have been by considering the following factors: As a result of the upper airway obstruction, the patient had a $\dot{V}/\dot{Q}$ low ratio in both lungs. In addition, in the emergency department the patient was becoming fatigued (his respiratory rate was 6 breaths/min), which further caused the $\dot{V}/\dot{Q}$ ratio to fall.

Thus, as the patient's $\dot{V}/\dot{Q}$ ratio progressively decreased, his PA_{O_2} decreased while, at the same time, his PA_{CO_2} increased. This condition, in turn, caused the

end-capillary oxygen pressure (Pc_{O_2}) and carbon dioxide pressure (Pc_{CO_2}) to decrease and increase, respectively. In addition, as the Pc_{CO_2} decreased, the pulmonary capillary blood pH also decreased (see Figures 8–4 and 8–7). If these arterial blood gas trends had continued, the patient would have died. Fortunately, when the quarter was successfully removed, the patient's $\dot{V}/\dot{Q}$ ratio quickly returned (increased) to normal. Today, the mother has the quarter on a charm bracelet.

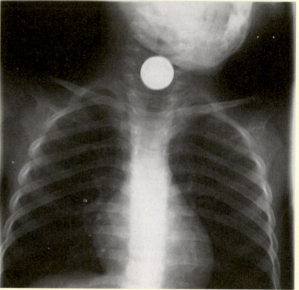

Courtesy T. Des Jardins, WindMist LLC

Review Questions

1. Overall, the normal $\dot{V}/\dot{Q}$ ratio is about
- A. 0.2
- B. 0.4
- C. 0.6
- D. 0.8

2. In the healthy individual in the upright position, the
1. $\dot{V}/\dot{Q}$ ratio is highest in the lower lung regions
2. PA_{O_2} is lowest in the upper lung regions
3. $\dot{V}/\dot{Q}$ ratio is lowest in the upper lung regions
4. PA_{CO_2} is highest in the lower lung regions

- A. 1 only
- B. 2 only
- C. 4 only
- D. 3 and 4 only

3. When the $\dot{V}/\dot{Q}$ ratio decreases, the
   1. $P_{A_{O_2}}$ falls
   2. $P_{C_{CO_2}}$ increases
   3. $P_{A_{CO_2}}$ rises
   4. $P_{C_{O_2}}$ decreases
      A. 1 only
      B. 3 only
      C. 2, 3, and 4 only
      D. 1, 2, 3, and 4

4. When alveolar ventilation is 7 L/min and the pulmonary blood flow is 9.5 L/min, the $\dot{V}/\dot{Q}$ ratio is about
   A. 0.4
   B. 0.5
   C. 0.6
   D. 0.7

5. If tissue cells consume 275 mL of O_2 per minute and produce 195 mL of CO_2 per minute, what is the RQ?
   A. 0.65
   B. 0.7
   C. 0.8
   D. 0.96

Clinical Application Questions

Case 1

1. As the patient continued to lose blood, his alveolar ventilation became more and more _____.

2. The patient's alveolar ventilation was _____ or _____ ventilation.

3. The paradox in this case was that even though the patient's $P_{A_{O_2}}$ and Pa_{O_2} increased in response to the increased ventilation-perfusion ratio, the actual amount of oxygen being transported (_____ decreased; _____ increased; _____ remained the same) because of the (_____ increased; _____ decreased) blood flow.

Case 2

1. As a result of the upper airway obstruction, the patient had a (_____low; _____high) ventilation-perfusion in both lungs.

2. The patient's fatigue and respiratory rate of 6 breaths/min further caused the ventilation-perfusion ratio to (_____rise; _____fall).

3. As a result of the upper airway obstruction and subsequent ventilation-perfusion ratio, the following values:
   A. $P_{A_{O_2}}$: _____ increased; _____ decreased; _____ remained the same
   B. $P_{A_{CO_2}}$: _____ increased; _____ decreased; _____ remained the same
   C. $P_{C_{O_2}}$: _____ increased; _____ decreased; _____ remained the same
   D. $P_{C_{CO_2}}$: _____ increased; _____ decreased; _____ remained the same
   E. pH: _____ increased; _____ decreased; _____ remained the same

Chapter 9

Control of Ventilation

Objectives

By the end of this chapter, the student should be able to:

1. Describe the function of the following respiratory neurons of the medullary respiratory centers:
   —The ventral respiratory group
   —The dorsal respiratory group
2. Describe the influence of the pontine respiratory centers on the medullary respiratory centers.
   —Pontine respiratory group
   —Apneustic center
3. Discuss the clinical connection associated with spinal cord trauma and diaphragmatic paralysis.
4. Describe the major areas of the body that influence breathing, and include:
   —Central chemoreceptors
   —Peripheral chemoreceptors
5. Discuss the clinical connection associated with altitude changes and the role of the peripheral chemoreceptors and central chemoreceptors in the stimulation of ventilation.
6. Describe the clinical connection associated with hydrogen ion (H^+) accumulation and its role in stimulating the peripheral chemoreceptors.
7. Describe the clinical connection associated with the hazards of oxygen therapy in patients with chronic hypercapnia and hypoxemia.
8. Describe other important factors that influence breathing, and include:
   —Hering-Breuer reflex
   —Deflation reflex
   —Irritant reflex
   —Juxtapulmonary-capillary receptors
   —Peripheral proprioceptor reflexes
   —Hypothalamic controls
   —Cortical controls
   —Aortic and carotid sinus baroreceptors
   —Miscellaneous factors
   - Sensory skin thermal receptors and superficial or deep receptors
     o Pain
     o Sudden cold stimulation
     o Stimulation of the pharynx or larynx
9. Describe the clinical connection associated with the unusual breathing reflexes.
10. Complete the review questions at the end of this chapter.

Introduction

The intrinsic rhythmicity of respiration is primarily controlled by specific neural areas located in the reticular substance of the medulla oblongata and pons of the brain. These neural areas possess monitoring, stimulating, and inhibiting properties that continually adjust the ventilatory patterns to meet specific metabolic needs. Also received and coordinated in these respiratory neural areas are the signals transmitted by the cerebral cortex during a variety of ventilatory maneuvers such as talking, singing, sniffing, coughing, or blowing into a woodwind instrument.

To fully understand the control of respiration, a basic knowledge of (1) the medullary respiratory centers, (2) the pontine respiratory centers and their influence on the medullary respiratory centers, and (3) factors that influence the rate and depth of breathing is necessary.

Control of Respiration

The Medullary Respiratory Centers

Although knowledge concerning this subject is incomplete, it is believed that two groups of interconnected respiratory neurons, located in the medulla oblongata, are responsible for coordinating the rhythmicity of respirations. These are the dorsal respiratory groups and the ventral respiratory groups (Figure 9–1). Collectively, these respiratory neurons are referred to as the medullary respiratory centers.

Ventral Respiratory Groups

The ventral respiratory groups (VRGs) are located bilaterally in two different areas of the medulla (see Figure 9–1). The VRGs consist of a complex network of neurons that run between the ventral brain stem of the spinal cord

---

Figure 9–1

Schematic of the respiratory components of the lower brainstem (pons and medulla oblongata). Pontine Respiratory Centers: PRG = pontine respiratory group; APC = apneustic center; DRG = dorsal respiratory group; VRG = ventral respiratory group; CC = central chemoreceptors.

© Cengage Learning 2013

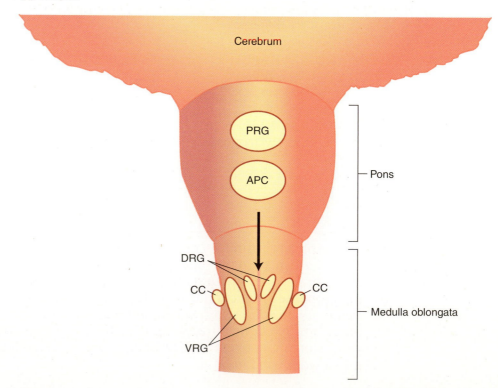

to the pons-medulla junction. The VGRs contain specialized neurons that fire during inspiration and another set of neurons that fire during expiration. When the inspiratory neurons are stimulated, a burst of electrical impulses travels along the phrenic nerve and the intercostal nerves—causing the diaphragm and external intercostal muscles to contract, respectively. This action, in turn, causes the thorax to expand and air flows into the lungs. When the VRGs' expiratory neurons fire, the inspiratory muscles relax, the lungs recoil, and expiration occurs passively. This inspiratory/expiratory cycle repeats continuously and produces a respiratory rate of about 12 to 15 breaths per minute.

Until recently, it was thought that the dorsal respiratory group neurons were primarily responsible for activating inspiration. It now appears, however, that not only are the VRG neurons responsible for triggering inspiration, but they also work to coordinate the rate, depth, and rhythm of breathing. In addition, it is now believed that the VRGs generate the gasping breaths commonly seen during periods of severe hypoxia—speculated by some to be the body's last-ditch effort to restore oxygen to the brain. Breathing completely stops when certain VRG neurons are suppressed—for example, by an overdose of morphine or alcohol.

Dorsal Respiratory Groups

The **dorsal respiratory groups (DRGs)** are located dorsally in the posterior region of the medulla oblongata near the root of cranial nerve IX. As mentioned earlier, it was once thought that the DRG neurons functioned as the primary inspiratory center—a task now known to be mainly performed by the VRGs. It is now known that the DRGs assimilate the various factors that influence breathing—for example, peripheral stretch receptors in the lungs, central chemoreceptors, and peripheral chemoreceptors (which will be described later in this chapter)—and relays this information to the VRGs. The VRGs, in turn, determine the rate, depth, and rhythm of breathing.

The Pontine Respiratory Centers—And Their Influence on the Medullary Respiratory Centers

The **pontine respiratory centers**, located in the pons, consist of two specialized group of neurons known as the **pontine respiratory group (PRG)**—formally called the *pneumotaxic center*—and the **apneustic center** (see Figure 9-1). Although these unique neural areas are known to exist, and can be made to operate under experimental conditions, their functional significance in humans is still not fully understood. It appears that the pontine respiratory centers function to some degree to modify and fine-tune the rhythmicity of breathing coordinated by the VRGs. For example, the neurons associated with the PRG are known to help smooth out the transition from inspiration and expiration—and the transition from expiration to inspiration. When the apneustic center is disrupted—for example, by a lesion—a prolonged or gasping type of inspiration occurs. This "breath-holding-like" phenomenon is called **apneustic breathing**. Under normal conditions, however, the apneustic center receives several different inhibitory signals, such as the lung inflation reflex (called the Hering-Breurer reflex), that suppress its function—thus, permitting expiration to occur.

Clinical Connection—9-1

Spinal Cord Trauma and Diaphragmatic Paralysis

Injury to the cervical (neck) area can have a profound effect on the patient's ability to move and breathe. The phrenic nerve for each hemidiaphragm emerges from the spinal cord at level C3 through C5 (Figure 9–2). Depending on the degree of involvement, injury to this region of the neck can damage the phrenic nerve and cause an *incomplete* or *complete* diaphragmatic paralysis. In addition, cervical neck injuries usually result in partial or full paralysis of the patient's legs and arms (quadreplegia). However, depending on the specific location and severity of the neck trauma, limited function may be retained.

Causes of phrenic nerve injuries include blunt trauma to the neck, brainstem stroke, and spinal cord tumor. Although most patients with an incomplete injury between C3 and C5 require mechanical ventilation, the majority of the cases can eventually be weaned successfully off the ventilator. On the other hand, a complete injury above the C3 and C5 level results in complete limb and diaphragmatic paralysis, ventilatory failure, and death, without immediate mechanical ventilation. In these cases, the respiratory therapist has an important role in managing the patient's overall ventilatory and bronchial hygiene care.

Figure 9–2

The phrenic nerve for each hemidiaphragm emerges from the spinal cord at level C3 through C5. Depending on the degree of involvement, injury to this region of the neck can damage the phrenic nerve and cause an incomplete or complete diaphragmatic paralysis.

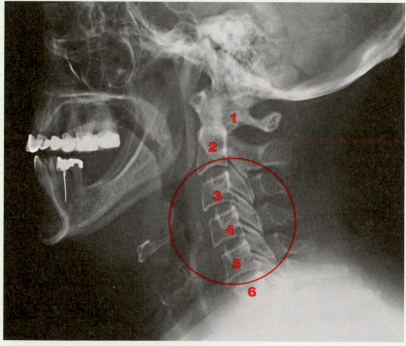

Courtesy T. Des Jardins, Windmist LLC

Factors That Influence the Rate and Depth of Breathing

From moment to moment, the medullary respiratory centers (VRG and DRG) activate specific ventilatory patterns based on information received from several areas throughout the body. The major known areas are the **central chemoreceptors** and the **peripheral chemoreceptors**. Other important factors that influence breathing originate from the (1) **Hering-Breuer reflex**, (2) **deflation reflex**, (3) **irritant reflex**, (4) **juxtapulmonary-capillary receptors**, (5) **peripheral proprioceptor reflexes**, (6) **hypothalamic controls**, (7) **cortical controls**, and (8) **aortic and carotid sinus baroreceptor reflexes**.

Central Chemoreceptors

The most powerful stimulus known to influence the medullary respiratory centers is an excess concentration of hydrogen ions [H^+] in the cerebrospinal fluid (CSF). The **central chemoreceptors**, which are located bilaterally and ventrally in the substance of the medulla, are responsible for monitoring the H^+ ion concentration of the CSF. In fact, a portion of the central chemoreceptors is actually in direct contact with the CSF. It is believed that the central chemoreceptors transmit signals to the respiratory components of the medulla by the following mechanism:

1. As the CO_2 level increases in the arterial blood (e.g., during hypoventilation), the CO_2 molecules diffuse across a semipermeable membrane, called the **blood-brain barrier**, which separates the blood from the CSF. The blood-brain barrier is very permeable to CO_2 molecules but relatively impermeable to H^+ and HCO_3^- ions.

2. As CO_2 moves into the CSF, it forms carbonic acid by means of the following reaction:

$$CO_2 + H_2O \leftrightarrows H_2CO_3 \leftrightarrows H^+ + HCO_3^-$$

3. Because the CSF lacks hemoglobin and carbonic anhydrase and has a relatively low bicarbonate and protein level, the overall buffering system in the CSF is very slow. Because of the inefficient CSF buffering system, the H^+ generated from the preceding reaction rapidly increases and, therefore, significantly reduces the pH in the CSF.

4. The liberated H^+ ions cause the central chemoreceptors to transmit signals to the respiratory component in the medulla, which, in turn, increases the alveolar ventilation.

5. The increased ventilation reduces the Pa_{CO_2} and, subsequently, the P_{CO_2} in the CSF. As the P_{CO_2} in the CSF decreases, the H^+ ion concentration of the CSF also falls. This action decreases the stimulation of the central chemoreceptors. Thus, the neural signals to the respiratory components in the medulla also diminish; this, in turn, causes alveolar ventilation to decrease.

6. In view of the preceding sequences, it should be understood that the central chemoreceptors regulate ventilation through the indirect effects of CO_2 on the pH of the CSF (Figure 9–3 on page 372).

Peripheral Chemoreceptors

The **peripheral chemoreceptors** are special oxygen-sensitive cells that react to the reductions of oxygen levels in the arterial blood. They are located high in the neck at the bifurcation of the internal and external carotid arteries and on the aortic arch (Figure 9–4 on page 373). They are close to, but distinct

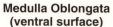

The relationship of the blood-brain barrier (BBB) to CO_2, HCO_3^-, and H^+. CO_2 readily crosses the BBB. H^+ and HCO_3^- do not readily cross the BBB. H^+ and HCO_3^- require the active transport system to cross the BBB. CSF = cerebrospinal fluid.

© Cengage Learning 2013

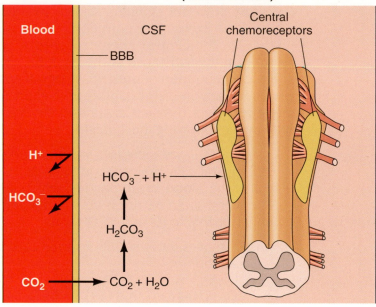

from, the *baroreceptors*. The peripheral chemoreceptors are also called the *carotid* and *aortic bodies.*

The carotid and aortic bodies are composed of epithelial-like cells and neuron terminals in intimate contact with the arterial blood. When activated by a low Pa_{O_2}, *afferent* (sensory) signals are transmitted to the respiratory components in the medulla by way of the glossopharyngeal nerve (ninth cranial nerve) from the carotid bodies and by way of the vagus nerve (tenth cranial nerve) from the aortic bodies. This action, in turn, causes *efferent* (motor) signals to be transmitted to the respiratory muscles, causing ventilation to increase (Figure 9–5 on page 374). Compared with the aortic bodies, the carotid bodies play a much greater role in initiating an increased ventilatory rate in response to reduced arterial oxygen levels.

As shown in Figure 9–6 on page 374, the peripheral chemoreceptors are not significantly activated until the oxygen content of the inspired air is low enough to reduce the Pa_{O_2} to 60 torr (Sa_{O_2} about 90 percent). Beyond this point, any further reduction in the Pa_{O_2} causes a marked increase in ventilation. *Suppression* of the peripheral chemoreceptors is seen, however, when the Pa_{O_2} falls below 30 torr.

In the patient with a low Pa_{O_2} and a chronically high Pa_{CO_2} level (e.g., end-stage emphysema), the peripheral chemoreceptors may be totally responsible for the control of ventilation. This is because a chronically high CO_2 concentration in the CSF inactivates the H^+ sensitivity of the central

Figure 9–4

Location of the carotid and aortic bodies (the peripheral chemoreceptors).

© Cengage Learning 2013

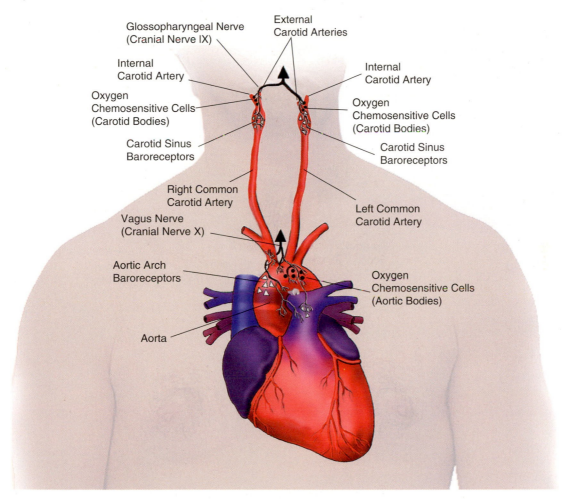

Glossopharyngeal Nerve (Cranial Nerve IX)

External Carotid Arteries

Internal Carotid Artery

Internal Carotid Artery

Oxygen Chemosensitive Cells (Carotid Bodies)

Oxygen Chemosensitive Cells (Carotid Bodies)

Carotid Sinus Baroreceptors

Carotid Sinus Baroreceptors

Right Common Carotid Artery

Left Common Carotid Artery

Vagus Nerve (Cranial Nerve X)

Aortic Arch Baroreceptors

Oxygen Chemosensitive Cells (Aortic Bodies)

Aorta

chemoreceptor—that is, HCO_3^- moves into the CSF via the active transport mechanism and combines with H^+, thus returning the pH to normal. A compensatory response to a chronically high CO_2 concentration, however, is the enhancement of the sensitivity of the peripheral chemoreceptors at higher CO_2 levels (Figure 9–7 on page 375).

Finally, it is important to understand that the peripheral chemoreceptors are specifically sensitive to the P_{O_2} of the blood and relatively insensitive to the oxygen content of the blood. The precise mechanism for this exclusive P_{O_2} sensitivity is not fully understood.

Clinically, this exclusive Pa_{O_2} sensitivity can be misleading. For example, there are certain conditions in which the Pa_{O_2} is normal (and, therefore, the peripheral chemoreceptors are not stimulated), yet the oxygen content of the blood is dangerously low. Such conditions include chronic anemia, carbon monoxide poisoning, and methemoglobinemia.

Figure 9–5

Schematic showing how a low Pa_{O_2} stimulates the respiratory components of the medulla to increase alveolar ventilation.

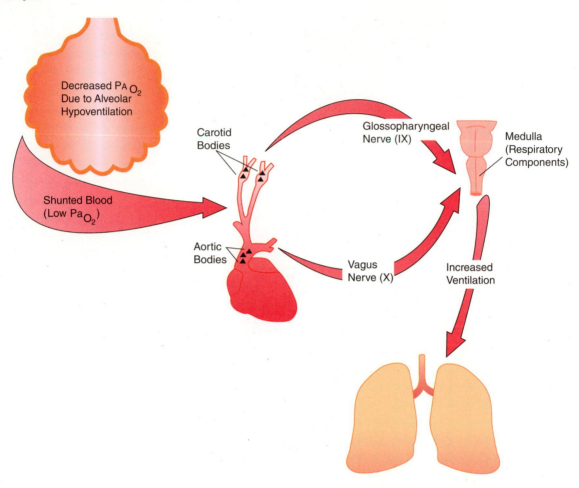

Figure 9–6

The effect of low Pa_{O_2} levels on ventilation.

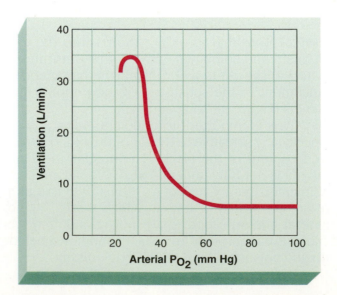

Figure 9–7

The effect of Pa_{O_2} on ventilation at three different Pa_{CO_2} values. Note that as the Pa_{CO_2} value increases, the sensitivity of the peripheral chemoreceptors increases.

© Cengage Learning 2013

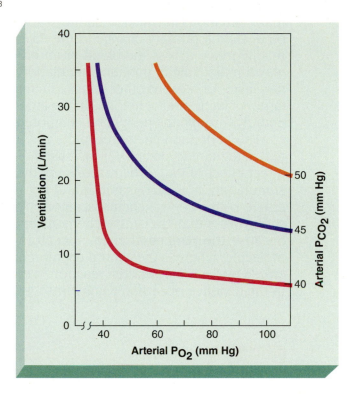

Clinical Connection—9-2

Altitude Changes—The Role of the Peripheral Chemoreceptors and Central Chemoreceptors in the Stimulation of Ventilation

In the **Clinical Application Section—Case 1** (page 383), the reader is provided with an overview of (1) why the respiratory rate is increased to a new baseline level when an individual, who normally resides at sea level, ascends to a high altitude for 2 weeks, and (2) why the respiratory rate continues to be higher than normal when the individual returns back to sea level. The following areas are discussed:

- How the oxygen peripheral chemoreceptors play an important—and overriding role—in

stimulating an increased ventilator rate at high altitudes.

- How the increased respiratory rate at a high altitude indirectly recalibrates the sensitivity of central chemoreceptors—to a lower Pa_{CO_2} (H^+) baseline level—during a 2-week period.

- How the central chemoreceptors continue to keep the respiratory rate higher than normal after the individual returns to sea level.

Other Factors That Stimulate the Peripheral Chemoreceptors

Although the peripheral chemoreceptors are primarily stimulated by a reduced Pa_{O_2} level, they are also activated by a decreased pH (increased H^+ level). This is an important feature of the peripheral chemoreceptors, because there are many situations in which a change in arterial H^+ ion levels can occur by means other than a primary change in the Pa_{O_2}. In fact, because the H^+ ions do not readily move across the blood-brain barrier, the peripheral chemoreceptors play a major role in initiating ventilation whenever the H^+ ion concentration increases for reasons other than an increased Pa_{CO_2}. For example, the accumulation of lactic acid or ketones in the blood stimulates hyperventilation almost entirely through the peripheral chemoreceptors (Figure 9–8).

The peripheral chemoreceptors are also stimulated by (1) hypoperfusion (e.g., stagnant hypoxia), (2) increased temperature, (3) nicotine, and (4) the direct effect of Pa_{CO_2}. The response of the peripheral chemoreceptors to Pa_{CO_2} stimulation, however, is minor and not nearly so great as the response generated by the central chemoreceptors. The peripheral chemoreceptors do respond faster than the central chemoreceptors to an increased Pa_{CO_2}. This occurs because the peripheral chemoreceptors are stimulated directly by the CO_2 molecule, whereas the central chemoreceptors are stimulated by the H^+ generated by the CO_2 hydration reaction in the CSF—a reaction that occurs slowly in the absence of carbonic anhydrase (see Figure 9–3).

Figure 9–8

The accumulation of lactic acids leads to an increased alveolar ventilation primarily through the stimulation of the peripheral chemoreceptors.

© Cengage Learning 2013

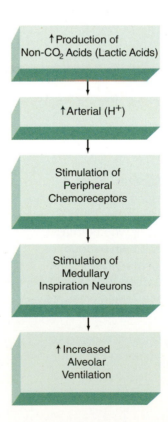

Other Responses Activated by the Peripheral Chemoreceptors

In addition to the increased ventilation activated by the peripheral chemoreceptors, other responses can occur as a result of peripheral chemoreceptor stimulation, including:

- Peripheral vasoconstriction.
- Increased pulmonary vascular resistance.
- Systemic arterial hypertension.
- Tachycardia.
- Increase in left ventricular performance.

Clinical Connection—9-3

Hydrogen Ion (H^+) Accumulation and Its Role in Stimulating the Peripheral Chemoreceptors

In the **Clinical Application Section—Case 2** (page 384), the respiratory therapist is called to assist in the care of a 44-year-old female unconscious as a result of a diabetic crisis. This case illustrates how clinical factors other than a decreased Pa_{O_2} can stimulate the oxygen peripheral chemoreceptors. Because the patient had not taken her insulin as prescribed, ketone acids had accumulated and caused the pH to fall. The excessive H^+ level stimulated the peripheral chemoreceptors and caused the patient's respiratory rate to increase. This case nicely shows (1) how the peripheral chemoreceptors can be stimulated by an excessive H^+ concentration, (2) how this action caused an increase the patient's respiratory rate, and (3) how the increased respiratory rate compensated for a low pH level by decreasing the Pa_{CO_2} level—another source of H^+.

Clinical Connection—9-4

The Hazards of Oxygen Therapy in Patients with Chronic Hypercapnia and Hypoxemia

In some patients with chronic hypercapnia (chronically higher than normal Pa_{CO_2} levels) and hypoxemia (e.g., COPD), the administration of too much oxygen may suppress the pheripheral oxygen chemoreceptors and depress ventilation. In other words, too much oxygen may cause acute ventilatory failure (acute respiratory acidosis) superimposed on the chonic ventilatory failure (compensated respiratory acidosis).

Clinically, oxygen-induced hypoventilation is commonly observed in the relaxed, unstimulated patient with chronic hyerapnia. Patients who are experiencing oxygen-induced hypoventilation are often described as sleepy, lethargic, and difficult to arouse, with slow and shallow breathing.

Although the precise mechanism responsible for this phenomenon is not known and continues to be the subject of much controversy and debate, the respiratory therapist must know that caution needs to be taken not to over-oxygenate patients with chronic ventilatory failure with hypoxemia (compensated respiratory acidosis).

Other Important Factors That Influence Breathing

Hering-Breuer Reflex

The Hering-Breuer reflex (also called the *inflation reflex*) is generated by stretch receptors, located in the visceral pleurae and in the walls of the bronchi and bronchioles, that become excited when the lungs overinflate. Signals from these receptors travel through the afferent fibers of the vagus nerve to the respiratory components in the medulla, causing inspiration to cease. In essence, the lungs themselves provide a feedback mechanism to terminate inspiration. Instead of a reflex to control ventilation, the Hering-Breuer reflex appears to be a protective mechanism that prevents pulmonary damage caused by excessive lung inflation. The significance of the Hering-Breuer reflex in the adult at normal tidal volumes is controversial; it appears to have more significance in the control of ventilation in the newborn.

Deflation Reflex

When the lungs are compressed or deflated, an increased rate of breathing results. The precise mechanism responsible for this reflex is not known. Some researchers believe that the increased rate of breathing may be due to the reduced stimulation of receptors serving the Hering-Breuer reflex rather than to the stimulation of specific deflation receptors. Others, however, think that the deflation reflex is not due to the absence of receptor stimulation of the Hering-Breuer reflex, because the reflex is still seen when the temperature of the bronchi and bronchioles is less than 8°C. The Hering-Breuer reflex is not active when the bronchi and bronchioles are below this temperature.

Irritant Reflex

When the lungs are exposed to noxious gases or accumulated mucus, the irritant receptors may also be stimulated. The irritant receptors are subepithelial mechanoreceptors located in the trachea, bronchi, and bronchioles. When the receptors are activated, a reflex vagal response causes the ventilatory rate to increase. Stimulation of the irritant receptors may also produce a reflex cough, sneeze, and bronchoconstriction.

Juxtapulmonary-Capillary Receptors

An extensive network of free nerve endings, called C-fibers, are located in the small conducting airways, blood vessels, and interstitial tissues between the pulmonary capillaries and alveolar walls. The C-fibers located near the alveolar capillaries are called juxtapulmonary-capillary receptors, or J-receptors. These receptors react to certain chemicals and to mechanical stimulation. For example, they are stimulated by alveolar inflamation, pulmonary capillary congestion and edema, humoral agents (e.g., serotonin, bradykinin), lung deflation, and emboli. When the J-receptors are stimulated, a reflex response triggers a rapid, shallow breathing pattern.

Peripheral Proprioceptor Reflexes

Peripheral proprioceptors are located in the muscles, tendons, joints, and pain receptors in muscles and skin. When stimulated, the proprioceptors send neural impulses to the medulla. The medulla, in turn, sends out an increased number of inspiratory signals. This may explain, in part, why moving an individual's limbs (e.g., during a drug overdose), or producing prolonged pain to the skin, stimulates ventilation. Sudden pain causes a short period of apnea, whereas prolonged pain causes the breathing rate to increase. The proprioceptors in the joints and tendons are also believed to play an important role in initiating and maintaining an increased respiratory rate during exercise. The more joints and tendons are involved, the greater the respiration rate.

Hypothalamic Controls

Strong emotions can activate sympathetic centers in the hypothalamus, which can alter respirations. For example, excitement causes the respiratory rate to increase. In addition, increased body temperature causes the respiration rate to increase, whereas decreased body temperature produces the opposite effect. For instance, a sudden cold stimulus (e.g., plunging into very cold water) can cause the cessation of breathing—or at the very least, a gasp.

Cortical Controls

Although the breathing pattern is normally controlled involuntarily by the medullary centers, one can also activate a conscious voluntary control over the rate and depth of breathing—or choose to hold the breath or take an extra deep breath.

Aortic and Carotid Sinus Baroreceptor Reflexes

The normal function of the aortic and carotid sinus baroreceptors, located near the aortic and carotid peripheral chemoreceptors (refer to Figure 5–12), is to initiate reflexes that cause a decreased heart and ventilatory rate in response to an elevated systemic blood pressure and an increased heart and ventilatory rate in response to a reduced systemic blood pressure.

To summarize, the *respiratory center* of the medulla oblongata coordinates both the involuntary and voluntary rhythm of breathing. The respiratory center (1) receives neural impulses from several different areas throughout the body, (2) evaluates and prioritizes these neural signals, and (3) based on the metabolic needs of the body, elicits neural impulses to the muscles of ventilation. Figure 9–9 on page 380 provides an overview of the complex functions of the medulla.

Miscellaneous Factors That May Influence Breathing

Finally, there are a number of known miscellaneous factors that may also influence breathing, including the following sensory impulses from thermal receptors on the skin and from superficial or deep pain receptors:

- **Pain.** A sudden painful stimulation causes a reflex apnea. However, a prolonged painful stimulus causes faster and deeper breathing.

The respiratory center coordinates signals from the higher brain region, great vessels, airways, lungs, and chest wall.
(+) = increased ventilatory rate; (–) = decreased ventilatory rate.

© Cengage Learning 2013

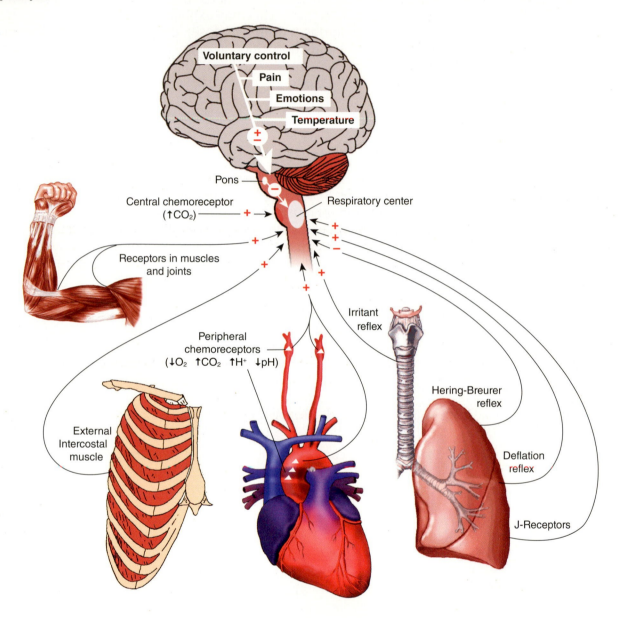

- **Sudden cold stimulation.** A sudden cold stimuli—such as a plunge into cold water—causes a reflex apnea.
- **Stimulation of the pharynx or larynx.** The stimulation of the pharynx or larynx by irritating chemicals or tactile stimulation causes a temporary apnea. This also includes the choking reflex, which is a valuable protective mechanism to prevent aspiration of food or liquids during swallowing.

Clinical Connection—9-5

Unusual Breathing Reflexes

Cough Reflex. Foreign matter in the trachea or large bronchi activates a cough reflex. The epiglottis and glottis reflexively close, and the expiratory muscles contract, causing the air pressure in the lungs to increase. This is followed by the sudden opening of the epiglottis and glottis, which results in an upward burst of gas that eliminates the offending foreign substance—the cough.

Sneeze Reflex. Similar to the cough reflex, a sneeze reflex is a forceful involuntary expulsion of air through the nose and mouth caused by an irritation to the mucous membranes of the nasal passageways. A sudden burst of air moves through the nose and mouth and forces the irritating substances (and mucus) out of the upper airway. It is estimated that the droplets from a sneeze can travel more than 100 miles per hour and travel up to 12 feet. What is called a **photo sneeze reflex** (also called a photic sneeze response, sun sneezing, and photogenic sneezing) is thought to be a genetic autosomal dominant trait, which is activated when an individual is suddenly exposed to bright light (Figure 9–10).

Hiccup. A hiccup is a characteristic sound that is generated by an involuntary contraction of the diaphragm, followed by the sudden closure of the glottis. Causes of hiccups include eating too much, drinking carbonated beverages, excessive consumption of alcohol, sudden temperature changes, and excitement or emotional stress. Although most episodes of hiccups do not last longer than a few minutes, recurrent and prolonged hiccup attacks sometimes occur. This problem is most often seen in men. Sedatives may be used in severe cases.

Yawn. A yawn is an involuntary act of opening the mouth wide and inhaling deeply. A yawn tends to occur when an individual is sleepy, drowsy, bored, or depressed. Yawning may be accompanied with upper body movements or the act of stretching to enhance chest expansion. Humans are not alone in the act of yawning. Dogs, cats, snakes, and even fish yawn. In spite of an extensive amount of research, the cause of yawning is not known. However, it is know that yawning is an involuntary movement that makes an individual's mouth open wide and breathe deeply. As the jaw drops, air flows into the lungs and the diaphragm moves downward. At the peak of the yawn, the lungs are stretched to capacity and the heart rate increases. Although many physiological aspects of a yawn have been well documented, researchers still cannot answer this fundamental question— Why do we yawn?

One common theory suggests that yawing serves to draw in more oxygen and to remove

Figure 9–10

Sneeze.

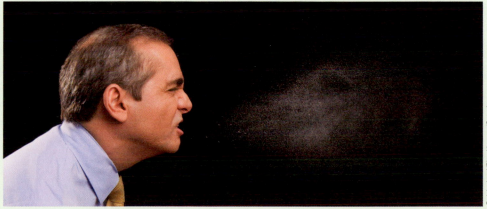

© John Lund/Blend Images/Getty Images

(continues)

Clinical Connection—9-5, continued

carbon dioxide. However, some researchers have tested this theory and found that administering oxygen to test subjects or decreasing their carbon dioxide did not prevent yawning. Some researchers suggest that yawning is contagious. Although this has not been scientifically confirmed, it is a good wager that a large number of students have had the inspiration to yawn after reading this clinical connection—correct?

Mammalian Diving Reflex. A fascinating, but poorly understood, physiological response called the *mammalian diving reflex* has been identified as the mechanism responsible for a number of remarkable recoveries of apparent cold water drowning victims—including some who have been submerged for more than 40 minutes! Even through drowning victims initially appear dead when pulled out of the cold water—that is, their breathing has stopped, their pupils are fixed and dilated, they appear cyanotic, and they have no pulse—cardiopulmonary resuscitation efforts are successful.

We do know that the diving reflex enhances breath holding in cold water. We also know that the diving reflex is an adaptation mechanism found in marine mammals (e.g., seals, otters, dolphins)—and, to a lesser extent, in humans. For example, the Weddell seals of Antarctica can hold their breath for up to 1 hour and can dive to depths of 500 meters. Although the diving reflex is weaker in human, it is known that when cold water—less than 20°C (68°F)—contacts the face or inside the nose, sensory neurons are stimulated that increase parasympathetic activity. The cold-water stimulation stops breathing, slows the heart rate, slows metabolism (decreasing oxygen and nutrient needs), and causes peripheral vasoconstriction—shunting blood to vital organs. The diving reflex is not observed during normal breath holding in air or during simulated dives in warm water. Apparently, the colder the water and the younger the victim, the better the chance of survival.

Clinical Connection—9-6

Second Wind

Second wind is a phenomenon associated with prolonged exercise—such as long-distance marathon running and bike racing—whereby the individual has a sudden transition from an ill-defined feeling of fatigue and shortness of breath to a more comfortable, less stressful feeling during the athletic event—oftentimes, with the strength to press on at—or greater than—their top performance. Today, the phrase "second wind" is commonly used as a metaphor for continuing on with renewed energy beyond the point of an individual's top performance—whether in other sports, a career or job performance, or life activities in general. Although the precise mechanism is still under debate, the stimulus for a second wind is thought to be associated with the following:

- **Lactic acid.** When individuals exercise for a long period of time, and push past the point of pain

and exhaustion, they may give their systemic vascular system enough time—that is, a warmup period—to find the correct balance between the supply of oxygen and the tissue cell metabolism, thereby offsetting the build up of lactic acid in the muscles.

- **Endorphins.** Endorphins are naturally occurring pain-reducing substances that are secreted by the anterior portion of the pituitary gland during stress and trauma. Endorphins act on certain parts of the brain to elicit a euphoria feeling, or what is commonly referred to as a "natural high."

- **Psychological.** The second wind may also be associated with a psychological factor—a by-product of the confidence and pride an individual may experience by exceeding his or her supposed limitation.

Chapter Summary

The respiratory neurons of the medulla oblongata coordinate both the involuntary and voluntary rhythm of breathing. The medullary *respiratory center* of the medulla receives neural impulses from several different areas throughout the body, evaluates and prioritizes the signals, and elicits neural impulses to the muscles of ventilation based on the metabolic need of the body.

To fully understand this subject, the respiratory therapist must have a basic knowledge of (1) the respiratory components of the medulla, including the ventral respiratory groups (VRGs) and the dorsal respiratory groups (DRGs); (2) the pontine respiratory centers and their influence on the medullary respiratory centers; and (3) the factors that influence the rate and depth of breathing—including the central chemoreceptors, peripheral chemoreceptors, Hering-Breuer reflex, deflation reflex, irritant reflex, juxtapulmonary-capillary receptors, peripheral proprioceptor reflexes, hypothalamic controls, cortical controls, and the aortic and carotid sinus baroreceptor reflexes. Miscellaneous factors that may also influence breathing include sudden and prolonged pain, sudden cold stimulation, and stimulation of the pharynx and larynx.

Clinical connections associated with these topics include (1) spinal cord trauma and diaphragmatic paralysis, (2) altitude changes and the role of the peripheral chemoreceptors and central chemoreceptors in the stimulation of ventilation, (3) hydrogen ion (H^+) accumulation and its role in stimulating the peripheral chemoreceptors, (4) the hazards of oxygen therapy in patients with chronic hypercapnia and hypoxemia, (5) unusual breathing reflexes, and (6) second wind.

1 Clinical Application Case

To facilitate the understanding of how the peripheral and central chemoreceptors control the ventilatory pattern, consider the following chain of events that develops when an individual who normally resides at sea level ascends to a high altitude (say, to the Colorado mountains to ski) for a period of 2 weeks.

Changes at High Altitudes

Stimulation of the Peripheral Chemoreceptors

1. As the individual ascends the mountain, the barometric pressure, and, therefore, the P_{O_2} of the atmosphere progressively decrease. (Remember that the oxygen percentage is still 21 percent.)

2. As the atmospheric P_{O_2} decreases, the individual's arterial oxygen pressure (Pa_{O_2}) also decreases.

3. As the individual continues to ascend the mountain, the Pa_{O_2} eventually falls low enough (to about 60 torr) to activate the peripheral chemoreceptors to stimulate the medulla to increase ventilation.

4. The increased ventilation initiated by the peripheral chemoreceptors causes a secondary decrease in the Pa_{CO_2}. In other words, the individual hyperventilates in response to the reduced Pa_{O_2} level.

5. Because the peripheral chemoreceptors do not acclimate to a decreased oxygen concentration, hyperventilation will continue for the entire time the individual remains at the high altitude.

Readjustment of the Central Chemoreceptors

In response to the hyperventilation that occurs while the individual is at the high altitude, the central chemoreceptors readjust to the lower CO_2 level because of the following chain of events:

1. As the individual hyperventilates to offset the low atmospheric P_{O_2}, the individual's Pa_{CO_2} level decreases.

(continues)

2. In response to the decreased Pa_{CO_2}, the CO_2 molecules in the CSF move into the blood until equilibrium occurs.

3. This reaction causes the pH of the CSF to increase.

4. Over the next 48 hours, however, HCO_3^- will also leave the CSF (via the active transport mechanism) to correct the pH back to normal.

In short, the individual's CSF readjusts to the low CO_2 level.

Changes After Leaving a High Altitude

Stimulation of the Central Chemoreceptors
Interestingly, even after the individual returns to a lower altitude, hyperventilation continues for a few days. The reason for this is as follows:

1. As the individual moves down the mountain, the barometric pressure steadily increases, and, therefore, the atmospheric P_{O_2} increases.

2. As the atmospheric P_{O_2} increases, the individual's Pa_{O_2} also increases and eventually ceases to stimulate the peripheral chemoreceptors.

3. As the stimulation of the peripheral chemoreceptors decreases, the individual's ventilatory rate decreases.

4. As the ventilatory rate declines, however, the individual's Pa_{CO_2} progressively increases.

5. As the Pa_{CO_2} increases, CO_2 molecules move across the blood-brain barrier into the CSF.

6. As CO_2 moves into the CSF, H^+ ions are formed, causing the pH of the CSF to decrease.

7. The H^+ ions liberated in the preceding reaction stimulate the central chemoreceptors to increase the individual's ventilatory rate.

8. Eventually, HCO_3^- ions move across the blood-brain barrier into the CSF to correct the pH back to normal. When this occurs, the individual's ventilatory pattern will be as it was before the trip to the mountains.

---

2   Clinical Application Case

A 44-year-old woman was found unconscious on her living room floor by her husband when he returned home from work. He immediately carried her to his car and drove her to the hospital. As he was driving, he called the hospital emergency department on his cell phone to alert the medical staff. He estimated that his time of arrival would be about 15 minutes. While on the phone, he also reported that his wife had a long history of diabetes. He stated that his wife had passed out three times in the past 2 years as a result of not taking her insulin as prescribed. The husband had no idea how long his wife had been unconscious before he found her.

Upon arrival, the patient was still unconscious and breathing very deeply and rapidly. The emergency department nurse placed an oxygen mask on the patient's face and started an intravenous infusion. A laboratory phlebotomist drew blood, and the respiratory therapist obtained an arterial blood sample from the patient's radial artery. The patient's vital signs were blood pressure—135/85 mm Hg, heart rate—97 beats/min, respirations—22 breaths/min, and temperature—37°C. The patient's respiratory pattern was charted by the respiratory therapist as Kussmaul's respiration. The patient's arterial blood gas values were pH—7.23, Pa_{CO_2}—24 torr, HCO_3^-—19 mEq/L, and Pa_{O_2}—405 torr. The respiratory therapist discontinued the patient's oxygen therapy. The second set of arterial blood gas values on room air were pH—7.23, Pa_{CO_2}—24 torr, HCO_3^-—19 mEq/L, and Pa_{O_2}—119 torr.

The laboratory report showed a blood glucose level of 837 mg/dL (normal, 70 to 150). The report also showed that her serum acetone level was 1:64 (normal, 0). The attending physician initiated insulin therapy. Two hours later, the patient was conscious and talking with her husband. Her vital signs were blood pressure—122/68 mm Hg, heart rate—75 beats/min, respirations—12 breaths/min, and temperature—37°C. Arterial blood gas values on room air at this time were pH—7.41, Pa_{CO_2}—39 torr, HCO_3^-—24 mEq/L, and Pa_{O_2}—95 torr. Her blood glucose level was 95 mg/dL, and her acetone level was zero. The patient was discharged the next day.

Discussion

This case illustrates how clinical factors other than an increased Pa_{CO_2} or decreased P_{O_2} can stimulate ventilation. Because the patient had not taken her insulin as prescribed, ketone acids (H^+) started to accumulate in her blood. As the ketone acid level increased, pH decreased. The excessive H^+ concentration stimulated the patient's peripheral chemoreceptors. Because the H^+ ion does not readily move across the blood-brain barrier, the peripheral chemoreceptors played a major role in causing the patient's ventilation to increase (see Figure 9–8).

In addition, note that as the patient's ventilation increased, her Pa_{CO_2} decreased (to 24 torr in the emergency department). The reduction in the Pa_{CO_2} was a compensatory mechanism—that is, the decreased Pa_{CO_2} worked to offset the acidic pH caused by the increased ketone acids. In other words, if the Pa_{CO_2} had been closer to normal level (around 40 torr) in the emergency department, the pH would have been lower than 7.23.

Note also that an increased respiratory rate does not necessarily mean that patient needs oxygen therapy. In this case, however, such therapy was appropriate (because of the patient's rapid breathing) until the cause of the rapid breathing was determined. When the results of the first arterial blood gas analysis were available (Pa_{O_2} was 405 torr), discontinuation of the oxygen therapy was the appropriate response.

Review Questions

1. The respiratory components of the medulla consist of which of the following?
1. Dorsal respiratory group
2. Apneustic center
3. Ventral respiratory group
4. Pneumotaxic center
   A. 1 only
   B. 2 only
   C. 1 and 3 only
   D. 2 and 4 only

2. Which of the following has the most powerful effect on the respiratory components of the medulla?
   A. Decreased O_2
   B. Increased H^+
   C. Decreased CO_2
   D. Increased pH

3. Which of the following may cause a temporary cessation in breathing?
1. Sudden pain
2. Stimulation of proprioceptor
3. Sudden cold
4. Inhalation of noxious gases
   A. 1 only
   B. 2 only
   C. 3 and 4 only
   D. 1 and 3 only

4. Which of the following will readily diffuse across the blood-brain barrier?
   1. CO_2
   2. H^+
   3. HCO_3^-
   4. H_2CO_3
      A. 1 only
      B. 2 only
      C. 3 only
      D. 2 and 4 only

5. When the systemic blood pressure increases, the aortic and carotid sinus baroreceptors initiate reflexes that cause a/an
   1. increased heart rate
   2. decreased ventilatory rate
   3. increased ventilatory rate
   4. decreased heart rate
      A. 1 only
      B. 2 only
      C. 3 only
      D. 2 and 4 only

6. The peripheral chemoreceptors are significantly activated when the P_{O_2} decreases to about
      A. 75 torr
      B. 70 torr
      C. 65 torr
      D. 60 torr

7. Stimulation of the peripheral chemoreceptors can cause which of the following?
   1. Tachycardia
   2. Decreased left ventricular performance
   3. Increased pulmonary vascular resistance
   4. Systemic arterial hypertension
      A. 1 only
      B. 2 only
      C. 4 only
      D. 1, 3, and 4 only

8. Suppression of the peripheral chemoreceptors begins when the P_{O_2} falls below
      A. 50 torr
      B. 40 torr
      C. 30 torr
      D. 20 torr

9. In addition to a low P_{O_2}, the peripheral chemoreceptors are also sensitive to a/an
   1. decreased H^+
   2. increased P_{CO_2}
   3. decreased pH
   4. increased temperature
      A. 2 only
      B. 3 only
      C. 1, 2, and 3 only
      D. 2, 3, and 4 only

10. Which of the following protects the lungs from excessive inflation?
    A. Juxtapulmonary-capillary receptors
    B. Hering-Breuer inflation reflex
    C. Deflation reflex
    D. Irritant reflex

Clinical Application Questions

Case 1

1. True _____ False _____ As an individual ascends a mountain, both the barometric pressure and atmospheric P_{O_2} decrease.

2. True _____ False _____ The oxygen percentage decreases as an individual ascends a mountain.

3. What stimulates the medulla to increase ventilation as an individual continues to ascend a mountain?

_____

4. As an individual continues to hyperventilate at high altitudes, the individual's Pa_{CO_2} (_____ increases; _____ decreases; _____ remains the same).

5. After an individual returns to a lower altitude, an increased ventilation continues for a few days. What causes the individual to maintain a higher than normal respiratory rate?

_____

Case 2

1. Because the patient had not taken her insulin as prescribed, what type of acid accumulated in her blood?

_____

2. What did the excess acid in the patient's blood stimulate that caused the patient's respiratory rate to increase?

_____

3. Do H^+ ions readily move across the blood-brain barrier?

Yes _____ No _____

4. Explain why the patient's increased ventilation was a compensatory mechanism to offset the acidic pH.

_____

_____

Chapter 10

Fetal Development and the Cardiopulmonary System

Objectives

By the end of this chapter, the student should be able to:

1. Describe the developmental events that occur during the following periods of fetal life:
   —Embryonic
   —Pseudoglandular
   —Canalicular
   —Terminal sac
2. Describe the clinical connection associated with the case study that illustrates the adverse effects of a premature birth on the cardiopulmonary system.
3. Describe how the following components relate to the placenta:
   —Umbilical arteries
   —Cotyledons
   —Fetal vessels
   —Chorionic villi
   —Intervillous space
   —Spiral arterioles
   —Umbilical vein
4. List the three major reasons oxygen transfers from maternal to fetal blood.
5. List the factors believed to cause the wide variance between the maternal and fetal P_{O_2} and P_{CO_2}.
6. Describe the clinical connection associated with the case study that illustrates the important role of the placenta as a lifeline between the mother and the baby during fetal life.
7. Describe how the following structures relate to the fetal circulation:
   —Umbilical vein
   —Liver
   —Ductus venosus
   —Inferior vena cava
   —Right atrium
   —Superior vena cava
   —Foramen ovale
   —Pulmonary veins
   —Left ventricle
   —Right ventricle
   —Ductus arteriosus
   —Common iliac arteries
   —External and internal iliacs
   —Umbilical arteries
8. Describe what happens to the following special structures of fetal circulation after birth:
   —Placenta
   —Umbilical arteries
   —Umbilical vein
   —Ductus venosus
   —Foramen ovale
   —Ductus arteriosus
9. Describe the clinical connection associated with amniocentesis.
10. Describe how the fetal lung fluid is removed from the lungs at birth.
11. List the number of alveoli present at birth and at 12 years of age.
12. Describe the clinical connection associated with the tests used to determine lung maturity in the fetus.
13. Describe the first breath, and include the pressure-volume changes of the lungs of the newborn during the first 2 weeks of life.
14. Identify the average newborn values for the following:
    —Lung compliance
    —Airway resistance
15. Describe how the following circulatory changes develop at birth:
    —Decrease in pulmonary vascular resistance
    —Closure of the foramen ovale
    —Constriction of the ductus arteriosus

(continues)

16. Describe the clinical connection associated with respiratory distress syndrome.

17. Describe the role of the following in the control of ventilation of the newborn:
—Peripheral chemoreceptors
—Central chemoreceptors
—Infant reflexes
  • Trigeminal
  • Irritant
  • Head paradoxical

18. List the normal values in the newborn for
—Lung volumes and capacities
—Respiratory rate
—Heart rate
—Blood pressure

19. Describe the clinical connection associated with the neonatal/pediatric respiratory care specialty.

20. Complete the review questions at the end of this chapter.

Fetal Lung Development

During fetal life, the development of the lungs is arbitrarily divided into four periods: *embryonic, pseudoglandular, canalicular,* and *terminal sac.*

Embryonic Period

The embryonic period encompasses the developmental events that occur during the first 5 weeks after fertilization. The lungs first appear as a small bud arising from the esophagus on the 24th day of embryonic life (Figure 10–1). On about the 28th day of gestation, this bud branches into the right and left lung buds. Between the 30th and 32nd day, primitive lobar bronchi begin to appear—two on the left lung bud and three on the right lung bud. By the end of the 5th week, cartilage can be seen in the trachea, and the main stem bronchi are surrounded by primitive cellular mesoderm, which gradually differentiates into bronchial smooth muscle, connective tissue, and cartilaginous plates.

Pseudoglandular Period

The pseudoglandular period includes the developmental processes that occur between the 5th and the 16th week of gestation. By the 6th week, all the segments are present and the subsegmental bronchi are also well represented. The subsegmental bronchi continue to undergo further branching, and by the 16th week all the subsegmental bronchi are present.

By the 10th week, ciliated columnar epithelial cells, a deeper basal layer of irregular cells, and a primitive basement membrane appear in the conducting airways. Goblet cells also begin to appear in the trachea and large bronchi. Between the 10th and 14th weeks, there is a sudden burst of bronchial branching. It is estimated that as many as 75 percent of the conducting airways develop at this time.

At 11 weeks of gestation, cartilage begins to appear in the lobar bronchi. Cartilaginous airways continue to form until about 24 weeks of gestation. By the 12th week, the bronchial mucous glands start to appear. Immature smooth-muscle cells are also noted at this time in the pulmonary arteries. As the tracheobronchial tree develops, new bronchial glands form until the 25th to 26th week of gestation. At birth, the concentration of bronchial glands is about 17 glands per square millimeter (mm^2). In the adult, the concentration drops to about 1 gland/mm^2, as a result of bronchial elongation and widening. By the 16th week, there are about 20 generations of bronchial airways.

© Cengage Learning 2013

Figure 10–1

Schematic of the developmental events that occur in the human lung during the embryonic and pseudoglandular periods (see text for explanation).

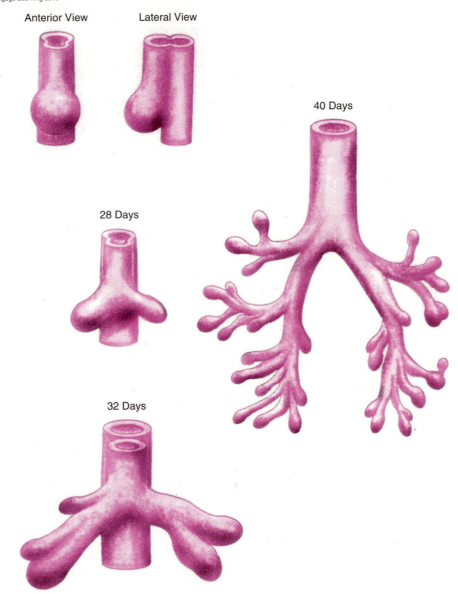

Anterior View   Lateral View

40 Days

28 Days

32 Days

Canalicular Period

The canalicular period includes the developmental events between the 17th and 24th week of gestation. During this time, the terminal bronchioles continue to proliferate and primitive respiratory bronchioles begin to appear. The lung mass becomes highly vascularized and the lung lobes are clearly recognizable. At about the 20th week of gestation, the lymphatic vessels begin to appear.

Terminal Sac Period

The terminal sac period begins at the 24th week of gestation and continues until term (between the 38th and 42nd week of gestation). The structures that appeared in the canalicular period continue to proliferate, and the entire

Clinical Connection—10-1

Case Study—Adverse Effects of a Premature Birth on the Cardiopulmonary System

In the **Clinical Application Section—Case 1** (page 405), the respiratory therapist is called to help care for a 1620-g (3-lb 9-oz) baby boy who was born 12 weeks early. This case illustrates the possible adverse effects of a premature birth on the infant's alveolar-capillary gas exchange units and pulmonary circulation.

acinus (respiratory bronchioles, alveolar ducts, alveolar sacs, and alveoli) develops. The type I and type II alveolar cells can be identified at this time, and pulmonary surfactant begins to appear.

Although pulmonary capillaries begin to appear at the 24th week, the air–blood interface between the alveoli and the pulmonary capillaries is poorly defined. Between the 26th and 28th weeks' gestation, the air–blood interface and the quantity of pulmonary surfactant begin to be sufficient enough to support life. By the 34th week, the respiratory acini are well developed. The smooth-muscle fibers in the conducting airways begin to appear during the last few weeks of gestation. These muscles continue to mature after birth.

Placenta

Following conception, the fertilized egg moves down the **uterine tube** (Fallopian tube) and implants into the wall of the uterus. The placenta develops at the point of implantation. Throughout fetal life, the placenta transfers maternal oxygen and nutrients to the fetus and transfers waste products out of the fetal circulation. When fully developed, the placenta appears as a reddish brown disk about 20 cm long and 2.5 cm thick. The placenta consists of about 15 to 20 segments called **cotyledons** (Figure 10–2). Each cotyledon is composed of **fetal vessels**, **chorionic villi**, and **intervillous spaces** (Figure 10–3 on page 394). The cotyledons provide an interface between the maternal and fetal circulation.

Deoxygenated blood is carried from the fetus to the placenta by way of two **umbilical arteries**, which are wrapped around the **umbilical vein** (see Figure 10–3). Normally, the P_{O_2} in the umbilical arteries is about 20 torr and the P_{CO_2} is about 55 torr. Once in the placenta, the umbilical arteries branch and supply each cotyledon. As the umbilical arteries enter the cotyledon, they again branch into the fetal vessels, which then loop around the internal portion of the fingerlike projections of the chorionic villi. Externally, the chorionic villi are surrounded by the intervillous space (see Figure 10–3).

Maternal blood from the uterine arteries enters the intervillous space through the **spiral arterioles**. The spiral arterioles continuously spurt jets of oxygenated blood and nutrients around the chorionic villi. Although the maternal blood P_{O_2} is usually normal during the last trimester of pregnancy (80 to 100 torr), the P_{CO_2} is frequently lower than expected (about 33 torr). This decrease in maternal P_{CO_2} is caused by the alveolar hyperventilation that develops as the growing infant restricts the mother's diaphragmatic excursion.

Figure 10–2

The placenta: **A.** fetal surface; **B.** maternal surface.

© Cengage Learning 2013

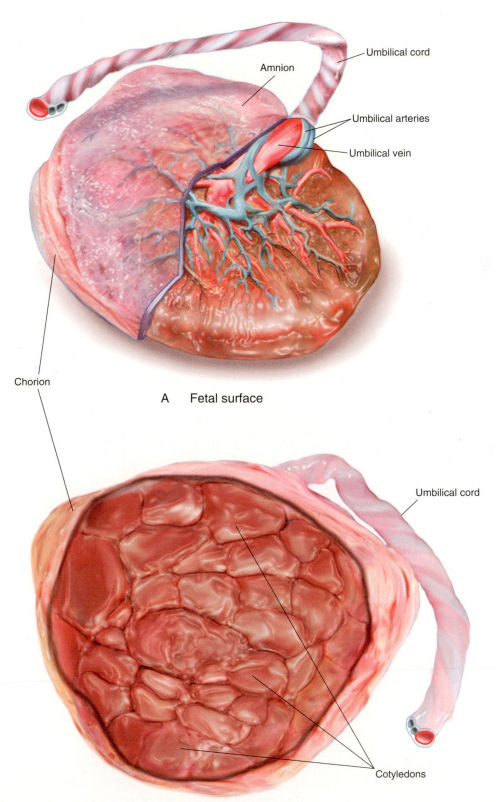

A   Fetal surface

B   Maternal surface

Figure 10–3

Anatomic structure of the placental cotyledon.

© Cengage Learning 2013

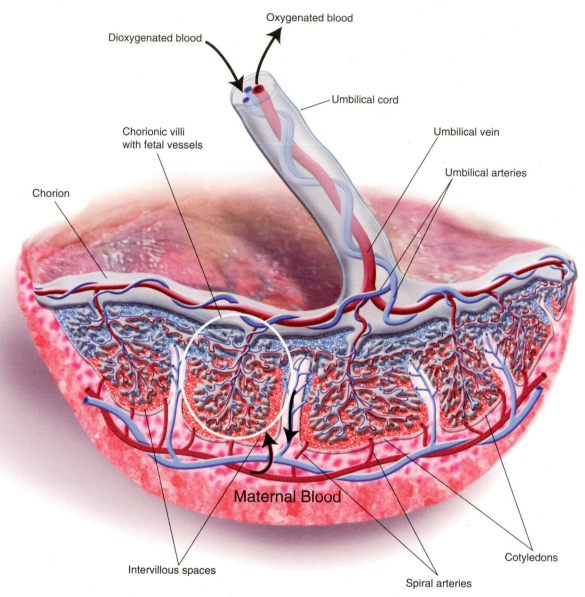

Once in the intervillous space, oxygen and nutrients in the maternal blood move through the tissues of the chorionic villi and enter the fetal blood. Oxygen transfers from the maternal to fetal blood because of the (1) maternal–fetal P_{O_2} gradient, (2) higher hemoglobin concentration in the fetal blood compared with that of maternal blood, and (3) greater affinity of fetal hemoglobin (Hb F) for oxygen than that of adult hemoglobin (Hb A). While the maternal oxygen and nutrients are moving into the fetal blood, carbon dioxide (P_{CO_2} of about 55 torr) and other waste products are moving out of the fetal blood and entering the maternal blood. The blood-to-blood barrier (chorionic villi) is about 3.5 μm thick.

Oxygenated fetal blood (actually a P_{O_2} of about 30 torr and a P_{CO_2} of about 40 torr) flows out of the chorionic villi via the fetal vessels and returns to

Clinical Connection—10-2

Case Study—The Placenta as an Important Lifeline Between Mother and Baby

In the **Clinical Application Section—Case 2** (page 406), the respiratory therapist is called to help care for a 1610-g (3-lb 7-oz) baby girl born 6 weeks early. The baby was delivered via a cesarean section shortly after the mother was diagnosed with having

abruptio placenta—the premature partial or total separation of the placenta from the uterus. This case illustrates the important role of the placenta as a lifeline between the mother and the baby during fetal life.

the fetus by way of the umbilical vein (see Figure 10–3). The wide variance between the maternal and fetal P_{O_2} and P_{CO_2} is thought to be caused by the following factors:

- The placenta itself is an actively metabolizing organ.
- The permeability of the placenta varies from region to region with respect to respiratory gases.
- There are fetal and maternal vascular shunts.

The fetal waste products in the maternal blood move out of the intervillous space by virtue of the arteriovenous pressure gradient. The pressure in the spiral arteries is about 75 mm Hg, and the pressure of the **venous orifices**, located adjacent to the spiral arteries, is about 8 mm Hg.

Fetal Circulation

The **umbilical vein** carries oxygenated blood and nutrients from the placenta to the fetus (Figure 10–4 on page 396). The umbilical vein enters the navel of the fetus and ascends anteriorly to the liver. About one-half of the blood enters the liver, and the rest flows through the **ductus venosus** and enters the **inferior vena cava**. This results in oxygenated fetal blood mixing with deoxygenated blood from the lower parts of the fetal body. The newly mixed fetal blood then travels up the inferior vena cava and enters the **right atrium**, where it again mingles with deoxygenated blood from the **superior vena cava**.

Once in the right atrium, most of the blood flows directly into the left atrium through the **foramen ovale**. While in the left atrium, the fetal blood again mingles with a small amount of deoxygenated blood from the pulmonary veins. The blood then enters the left ventricle and is pumped primarily to the heart and brain.

The rest of the blood in the right atrium moves into the right ventricle and is pumped into the pulmonary artery. Once in the pulmonary artery, most of the blood bypasses the lungs and flows directly into the aorta through the **ductus arteriosus**. A small amount of blood (about 15 percent) flows through the lungs and returns to the left atrium via the pulmonary veins. The Pa_{O_2} in the descending aorta is about 20 torr. Downstream, the **common iliac arteries** branch into the **external** and **internal iliacs**. The blood in the internal iliac branch passes into the umbilical arteries and again flows back to the placenta to pick up oxygen and to drop off waste products.

Figure 10–4

Fetal circulation.

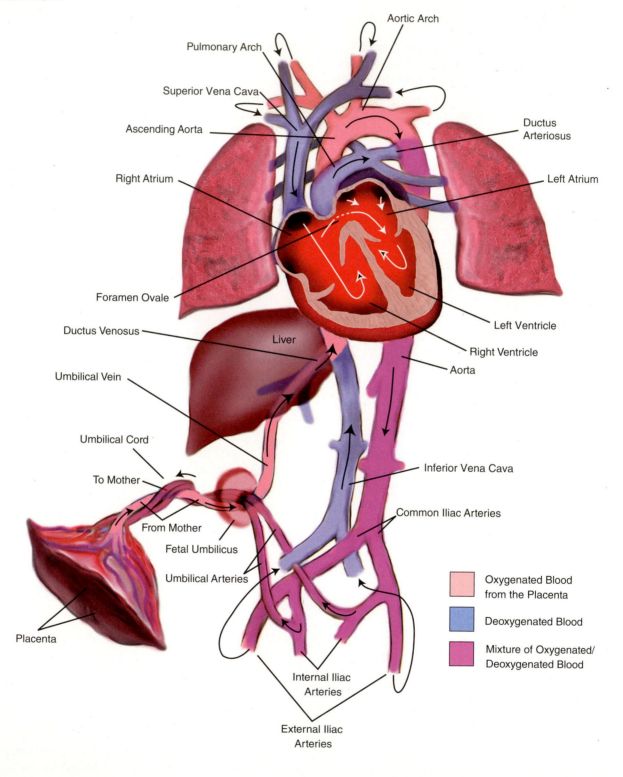

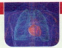

Clinical Connection—10-3

Amniocentesis

Amniocentesis is a procedure used to diagnose fetal abnormalities. As shown in Figure 10–5, an amniocentesis is performed by gently inserting a needle through the uterus and drawing out a small sample of amniotic fluid surrounding the fetus for laboratory analysis. The results from the fetal cells and other substances can reveal a number of important things about fetal development, including the lung maturity of the fetus, the bilirubin level (used to evaluate Rh incompatibility), the creatinine level (used to assess kidney function and maturity), the presence of any genetic disorders (assessed from cellular examinations), and evidence of *meconium* (first fetal stool—a thick and sticky, usually greenish to black material) in the amniotic fluid. Amniotic fluid stained with meconium indicates fetal asphyxia and possible meconium aspiration.

Figure 10–5

Amniocentesis.

© Cengage Learning 2013

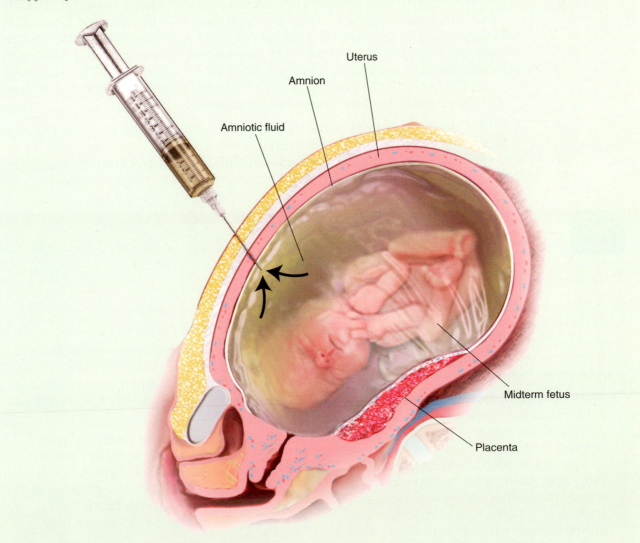

After birth—and once the lungs and the renal, digestive, and liver functions are established—the special structures of the fetal circulation are no longer required. These special structures go through the following changes:

- The placenta is expelled by the mother.
- The umbilical arteries atrophy and become the lateral umbilical ligaments.
- The umbilical vein becomes the round ligament (*ligamentum teres*) of the liver.
- The ductus venosus becomes the *ligamentum venosum*, which is a fibrous cord in the liver.
- The flap on the foramen ovale usually closes (as a result of the increased left atrium blood pressure) and becomes a depression in the interatrial septum called the *fossa ovalis*.
- The ductus arteriosus atrophies and becomes the *ligamentum arteriosum*.

Fetal Lung Fluids

It is estimated that at birth, the lungs are partially inflated with liquid approximately equal to the newborn's functional residual capacity. It was once thought that this liquid originated from the aspiration of amniotic fluid because the fetus normally demonstrates periods of rapid and irregular breathing during the last trimester of gestation. It is now known, however, that this is not the case. The fluid apparently originates from the alveolar cells during fetal development. At birth the fluid is removed from the lungs during the first 24 hours of life primarily by the following mechanisms:

- About one-third of the fluid is squeezed out of the lungs as the infant passes through the birth canal.
- About one-third of the fluid is absorbed by the pulmonary capillaries.
- About one-third of the fluid is removed by the lymphatic system.

 Clinical Connection—10-4

Tests Used to Determine Lung Maturity in the Fetus

There are several clinical tests available that can be used measure the lung maturity of the fetus. These include the **lecithin/sphingomyelin ratio**, the presence of **phosphatidylglycerol**, and more recently, the **surfactant/albumin ratio**.

1. The **lecithin/sphingomyelin ratio (L:S ratio)** is a common test of the fetal amniotic fluid to measure the maturity of the fetal lung. An amniotic fluid sample is collected—by means of a procedure called an *amniocentesis*—and processed. When the concentration of lecithin is two times greater than sphingomyelin—an L:S ratio of 2:1—the fetus lung development should be mature enough to produce sufficient pulmonary surfactant at birth. The L:S ratio is

relatively easy to measure and the validity and reliability of the test is good.

2. The test for **phosphatidylglycerol (PG)** is also useful to evaluate lung maturity. PG is a phospholipid found in pulmonary surfactant. The presence of PG in the amniotic fluid indicates a low risk of RDS.

3. The **surfactant/albumin ratio (S:A ratio)** is reported as milligrams of surfactant per gram of protein. An S:A ratio of less than 35 indicates immature lungs. An S:A ratio between 35 to 55 suggests uncertain lung maturity. An S:A ratio greater than 55 denotes lung maturity.

Number of Alveoli at Birth

About 24 million primitive alveoli are present at birth. This number, however, represents only about 10 percent of the adult gas exchange units. The number of alveoli continue to increase until about 12 years of age. Thus, it is important to note that respiratory problems during childhood can have a dramatic effect on the anatomy and physiology of the mature pulmonary system.

Birth

Moments after birth, an intriguing and dramatic sequence of anatomic and physiologic events occur. The function of the placenta is suddenly terminated, the lungs rapidly establish themselves as the organs of gas exchange, and all the features of adult circulation are set in place.

First Breath

At birth, the infant is bombarded by a variety of external sensory stimuli (e.g., thermal, tactile, visual). At the same time, the placenta ceases to function, causing the fetal blood P_{O_2} to decrease, the P_{CO_2} to increase, and the pH to decrease. Although the exact mechanism is unknown, the sensitivity of both the central and the peripheral chemoreceptors of the newborn increases dramatically at birth. In response to all these stimuli, the infant *inhales.*

To initiate the first breath, however, the infant must generate a remarkable negative intrapleural pressure to overcome the viscous fluid in the lungs. It is estimated that the intrapleural pressure must decrease to about –40 cm H_2O before any air enters the lungs. Intrapleural pressures as low as –100 cm H_2O have been reported. About 40 mL of air enter the lungs during the first breath. On exhalation, the infant expels about one-half of the volume obtained on the first breath, thus establishing the first portion of the residual volume. Figure 10–6 on page 400 illustrates the typical pressure-volume changes of the lungs that occur in the newborn during the first 2 weeks of life. The average *lung compliance* of the newborn is about 0.005 L/cm H_2O (5 mL/cm H_2O; the *airway resistance* is about 30 cm H_2O/L/sec.

Circulatory Changes at Birth

There are six fetal circulation structures that are no longer needed after birth—the **umbilical arteries, placenta, umbilical vein, ductus venosus, foramen ovale,** and **ductus arteriosus**. When the umbilical cord is clamped and cut, the two *umbilical arteries*, the *placenta*, and the *umbilical vein* no long function. The placenta is shed from the mother's uterus. The umbilical vein remaining in the infant's body eventually becomes the **round ligament** of the liver, and the ductus venousus becomes the **ligamentum venosum**.

In regard to the foramen ovale and ductus arteriosus, the following chain of events must occur—in this precise sequence—in order to stop their fetal circulation functions and, thereby, allow normal circulation to ensue:

1. As the infant inhales for the first time, the pulmonary vascular resistance falls dramatically. The major mechanisms that account for the decreased pulmonary vascular resistance are (a) the sudden increase in the alveolar P_{O_2}, which offsets the hypoxic vasoconstriction; (b) the removal of fluid from the lungs, reducing the external pressure on the pulmonary vessels,

Figure 10–6

The pressure-volume changes of the newborn's lungs during the first 2 weeks of life.

© Cengage Learning 2013

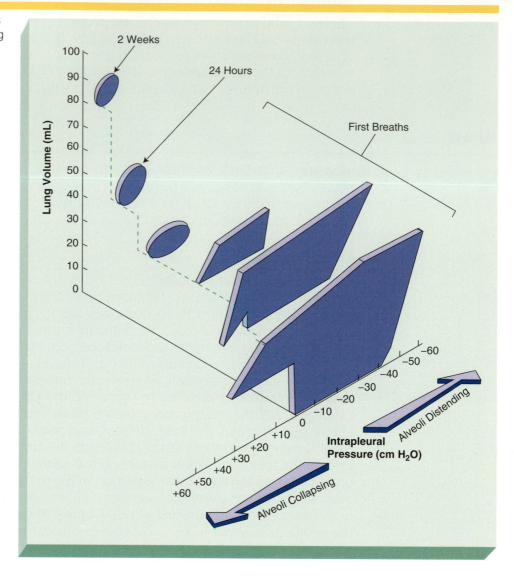

and (c) the mechanical increase in lung volume, which widens the caliber of the extra-alveolar vessels.

2. As the pulmonary vascular resistance decreases, a greater amount of blood flows through the lungs and, therefore, more blood returns to the left atrium. This causes the pressure in the left atrium to increase and the flap of the *foramen ovale* to close. The closure of the foramen ovale is further aided by the fall in pressure that occurs in the right atrium as the umbilical flow ceases. Complete structural closure, however, usually takes about 9 months or more. Eventually, the forman ovale becomes a small depression, called the **fossa ovalis**, in the wall of the right atrial septum.

3. A few minutes later, the smooth muscles of the *ductus arteriosus* constrict in response to the increased P_{O_2}. The newborn's P_{O_2} must increase to more than 45 to 50 torr in order for the ductus arteriosus to close. Under normal conditions, the ductus arteriosus eventually forms a fibrous cord called the **ligamentum arteriosum**.

Clinical Connection—10-5

Respiratory Distress Syndrome

Respiratory distress syndrome (RDS) is the most common cause of respiratory failure in the preterm baby. The *normal term* baby is between 38 and 42 weeks' gestation; a baby born before 38 weeks' gestation is called a *preterm baby* (premature). About 50 percent of the babies born between 26 and 28 weeks' gestation develop respiratory distress syndrome (RDS). About 25 percent of the babies born between 30 and 31 weeks' gestation develop RDS. These babies are born before their type II alveolar cells are mature enough to make an adequate amount of pulmonary surfactant. As a result, the baby's alveolar surface tension increases and causes the alveoli to collapse (atelectasis).

During the early stages of RDS, the treatment of choice is **continuous positive airway pressure (CPAP)**. The therapeutic benefits of CPAP include (1) the re-inflation of collapsed alveoli, (2) the decreased work of breathing, and (3) the return of the baby's oxygenation level to normal. The use of mechanical ventilation is avoided as long as possible. The administration of exogenous pulmonary surfactants may also be helpful to baby with RDS. Common exogenous preparations are **beractant** (Survanta®), **calfactant** (Infasurf®), and **poractant alfa** (Curosurf®).

4. If this P_{O_2} level is not reached, the ductus arteriosus will remain open, and the pulmonary vascular resistance will remain elevated, producing the syndrome known as **persistent pulmonary hypertension of the neonate (PPHN)** (previously known as persistent fetal circulation). Furthermore, should the neonate's P_{O_2} increase sufficiently to close the ductus arteriosus but then fall within the first 24 to 48 hours after birth, the ductus arteriosus will reopen. It is believed that other substances released at birth (such as bradykinin, serotonin, and prostaglandin inhibitors) contribute to the constriction of the ductus arteriosus.

Control of Ventilation in the Newborn

Within moments after birth, the newborn infant initiates the first breath. Although they are inhibited during fetal life, the peripheral and central chemoreceptors play a major role in activating the first breath. It is not precisely understood why these chemoreceptors are dormant during fetal life but suddenly activated at birth.

Peripheral Chemoreceptors

The exact role of the peripheral chemoreceptors in the newborn is not clearly defined. It is known, however, that in both preterm and term infants, hypoxia elicits a transient rise in ventilation, followed by a marked fall. The magnitude of the increase is similar whether the infant is in the rapid eye-movement (REM) state, quiet sleep state, or awake state. The late fall, however, is less marked or is absent when the infant is in the quiet sleep state. One to 2 weeks after birth, the infant demonstrates the adult response of sustained hyperventilation. The response to hypoxia is greater and more sustained in the term infant than in the preterm infant. Although it is known that the peripheral chemoreceptors of the adult are responsive to CO_2, little information is available about the peripheral chemoreceptors' sensitivity to changes in CO_2 and pH during the neonatal period.

Central Chemoreceptors

The central chemoreceptors of the newborn respond to the elevated CO_2 levels in a manner similar to that of the adult. The response to an increased CO_2 level is primarily an increased tidal volume, with little change in inspiratory time or ventilatory rate. The response of the central chemoreceptors may be more marked with increasing gestational age.

Infant Reflexes

Trigeminal Reflex

Stimulation of the newborn's trigeminal nerve (i.e., the face and nasal and nasopharyngeal mucosa) causes a decrease in the infant's respiration and heart rate. It has been reported that even gentle stimulation of the malar region in both preterm and term infants may cause significant respiratory slowing. Thus, various procedures (such as nasopharyngeal suctioning) may be hazardous to the newborn. Clinically, facial cooling has been used as a means of terminating paroxysms of supraventricular tachycardia in the newborn.

Irritant Reflex

Epithelial irritant receptors, located throughout the airways, respond to direct tactile stimulation, lung deflation, and irritant gases. This response is mediated by myelinated vagal fibers. Based on gestational age, these receptors elicit different responses. In preterm infants of less than 35 weeks' gestation, tracheal stimulation (e.g., endotracheal suctioning or intubation) is commonly followed by respiratory slowing or apnea. In the term infant, however, stimulation causes marked hyperventilation. The inhibitory response seen in the preterm infant may be due to vagal nerve immaturity (i.e., the vagal nerves are not adequately myelinated). Unmyelinated neurons are unable to transmit high-frequency discharges.

Head's Paradoxical Reflex

Head's paradoxical reflex is a deep inspiration that is elicited by lung inflation. In other words, the infant inhales and then tops the inspiration with a deep breath before exhalation occurs. This reflex is seen in the term infant and is thought to be mediated by the irritant receptors. The head paradoxical reflex may play a role in sighing, which is frequently seen in the newborn. This reflex is thought to be valuable in maintaining lung compliance by offsetting alveolar collapse.

Clinical Parameters in the Normal Newborn

Table 10–1 lists the average pulmonary function findings of the newborn. The vital signs of the normal newborn are listed in Table 10–2. Figure 10–7 illustrates graphically the average pH, Pa_{CO_2}, HCO_3^-, and Pa_{O_2} values of the normal infant over a period of 72 hours after birth.

Table 10–1

Approximate Lung Volumes (mL) and Capacities of the Normal Newborn

Tidal volume (V_T)	15	Vital capacity (VC)	115
Residual volume (RV)	40	Functional residual capacity (FRC)	80
Expiratory reserve volume (ERV)	40	Inspiratory capacity (IC)	75
Inspiratory reserve volume (IRV)	60	Total lung capacity (TLC)	155

© Cengage Learning 2013

Table 10–2

Vital Sign Ranges of the Normal Newborn

Respiratory rate (RR)	35–50/min
Heart rate (HR)	130–150/min
Blood pressure (BP)	60/40–70/45 mm Hg

© Cengage Learning 2013

Figure 10–7

The average pH, Pa_{CO_2}, HCO_3^-, and Pa_{O_2} values of the normal infant during the first 72 hours of life.

© Cengage Learning 2013

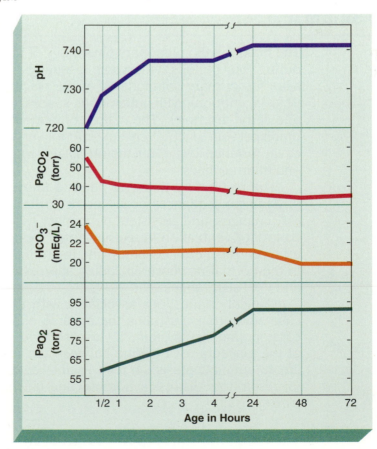

Clinical Connection—10-6

Neonatal/Pediatric Respiratory Care Specialty

The respiratory therapist can further broaden his or her career by pursuing additional education and training to become a credentialed **neonatal/pediatric respiratory care specialist**. The neonatal/pediatric specialist (NPS) works in children's hospitals, general hospitals, and neonatal intensive care units. The NPS is involved in treating and monitoring a variety of newborn breathing disorders. The NPS might monitor the breathing of premature babies, treat infants born with pulmonary disorders, or respond to the unique respiratory care needs of an infant in an emergency. Common respiratory disorders associated with the newborn infant include meconium aspiration syndrome, transient tachypnea of the newborn, respiratory distress syndrome, pulmonary air leak syndromes, respiratory syncytial virus infection, bronchopulmonary dysplasia, and congenital diaphragmatic hernia.

The **National Board for Respiratory Care Inc. (NBRC)** administers the credentialing examination for the neonatal/pediatric respiratory care specialty. The Neonatal/Respiratory Care Specialty Examination is designed to objectively measure essential knowledge, skills, and abilities required of respiratory therapists in the specialty area. Achievement of the **Certified Respiratory Therapist (CRT)** credential, plus one year of clinical experience in neonatal/pediatric respiratory care, or the **Registered Respiratory Therapist (RRT)** credential is required for admission to the Neonatal/Pediatric Specialty Examination (www.nbrc.org).

Chapter Summary

The major cardiopulmonary physiology of the fetus and the newborn develop during four periods: embryonic, pseudoglandular, canalicular, and terminal sac. The primary components of the placenta include the cotyledons, fetal vessels, chorionic villi, intervillous spaces, umbilical arteries, umbilical vein, and spiral arterioles. The major components of fetal circulation include the umbilical vein, ductus venosus, inferior vena cava, right atrium, superior vena cava, foramen ovale, ductus ateriosus, common iliac arteries, and external and internal iliacs.

The respiratory therapist needs a knowledge base of the anatomic and physiologic sequences occurring at birth, including the first breath, circulatory changes, and persistent pulmonary hypertension of the neonate (PPHN); control of ventilation in the newborn, including the peripheral chemoreceptors, central chemoreceptors, and infant reflexes; and the clinical parameters in the normal newborn, including approximate lung volumes and capacities and vital sign ranges.

Clinical connections associated with the preceding topics include (1) a case study that illustrates the adverse effects of a premature birth on the cardiopulmonary system, (2) a case study that illustrates the importance of the placenta as a lifeline between the mother and the baby during fetal life, (3) amniocentesis, (4) tests used to determine lung maturity in the fetus, (5) respiratory distress syndrome, and (6) the neonatal/pediatric respiratory care specialty.

1 Clinical Application Case

A 1620-g (3-lb 9-oz) boy was born 12 weeks early (at 28 weeks' gestation). His Apgar scores at delivery were 4 and 5.[1] The baby's skin was cyanotic, and he was in obvious respiratory distress. He demonstrated nasal flaring and intercostal retractions. A gruntlike sound could be heard without the aid of a stethoscope during each exhalation. The baby was transferred to the neonatal intensive care unit and placed on continuous positive airway pressure (CPAP) via nasal prongs at a pressure setting of 3 cm H_2O and an inspired oxygen concentration ($F_{I_{O_2}}$) of 0.4.

The baby's vital signs were respiratory rate—64 breaths/min, blood pressure—48/22 mm Hg, and apical heart rate—175 beats/min. On auscultation, bilateral crackles could be heard. A portable chest X-ray showed a "ground-glass" appearance and air bronchogram throughout both lung fields, consistent with respiratory distress syndrome (RDS). Umbilical arterial blood gas values were pH—7.53, Pa_{O_2}—28 torr, HCO_3^-—21 mEq/L, and P_{O_2}—41 torr. The neonatologist entered the following diagnosis in the infant's progress notes: "IRDS and PPHN" (persistent pulmonary hypertension of the neonate).

During the next 72 hours, the infant's clinical progress was stormy. Three hours after the baby was born, he was intubated and placed on a time-cycled, pressure-limited synchronized intermittent mandatory ventilation (SIMV) rate of 35 breaths/min, inspiratory time 0.5 second, peak inspiratory pressure (PIP) of 22 cm H_2O, an $F_{I_{O_2}}$ of 0.8, and positive end-expiratory pressure (PEEP) of 7 cm H_2O. The baby received Survanta® treatments (a synthetic pulmonary surfactant) through his endotracheal tube on day 2. On day 4, his clinical condition stabilized.

Although the baby was still intubated on day 5, he no longer required SIMV. The ventilator was set on the CPAP mode at a pressure setting of 3 cm H_2O with an $F_{I_{O_2}}$ of 0.4. The baby's vital signs were blood pressure—73/48 mm Hg, heart rate (apical)—122 beats/min, and respiratory rate—40 breaths/min. Normal vesicular breath sounds were heard over both lung fields. Chest X-ray showed substantial improvement throughout both lungs. The baby's umbilical arterial blood gas values were pH—7.41, Pa_{CO_2}—38 torr, HCO_3^-—24 mEq/L, and Pa_{O_2}—158 torr. The $F_{I_{O_2}}$ was decreased to 0.3. The neonatologist wrote the following assessment in the patient's chart: "IRDS has significantly improved and PPHN no longer appears to be present." The baby progressively improved and was discharged 3 days later.

Discussion

This case illustrates the possible adverse effects of a premature birth on the infant's alveolar-capillary gas exchange units and pulmonary circulation. During fetal development, the alveolar-capillary system and the quantity of pulmonary surfactant usually are not sufficient to support life until the 28th week of gestation or beyond. In this case, the baby was born at the very beginning of this time period. Thus, because of the immaturity of the baby's alveolar-capillary system, the ability of the type II cells to produce pulmonary surfactant was inadequate.

As a result of the insufficient amount of pulmonary surfactant, the pathologic processes of a common newborn respiratory disorder called respiratory distress syndrome (RDS) developed. The anatomic alterations of the lungs associated with RDS include interstitial and intra-alveolar edema and hemorrhage, alveolar consolidation, intra-alveolar hyaline membrane formation, and atelectasis. All of these pathologic processes cause the alveolar-capillary membrane's thickness to increase. As this condition progressively worsened, the diffusion of oxygen between the alveoli and the pulmonary capillary blood decreased, and the infant's lung compliance decreased. Clinically, the decreased diffusion of oxygen was manifested by cyanosis, increased respiration rate and heart rate, and decreased Pa_{O_2}. The decreased lung compliance was manifested by nasal flaring, intercostal retractions, exhalation grunting, bilateral crackles, and

---

[1] The Apgar score evaluates five factors: heart rate, respiratory effort, muscle tone, reflex irritability, and color. Each factor is rated 0, 1, or 2. The scoring system provides a clinical picture of the infant's condition following delivery. An Apgar score is taken at 1 minute after delivery. A second Apgar score is taken at 5 minutes after delivery to assess the infant's ability to recover from the stress of birth and adapt to extrauterine life. The baby is usually considered to be out of danger when the score is greater than 7.

(continues)

a ground-glass appearance and air bronchogram on the chest X-ray.

Finally, because the baby's Pa_{O_2} was less than 45 torr shortly after birth, the ductus arteriosus remained patent, producing the syndrome known as *persistent pulmonary hypertension of the neonate* (PPHN). As the infant's condition improved and his Pa_{O_2} increased, the ductus arteriosus closed and the signs and symptoms associated with PPHN disappeared. At the time of this writing, the baby was a perfectly normal 3-year-old boy who was attending half-day preschool sessions 5 days per week.

2 Clinical Application Case

While in her third trimester of pregnancy, a 28-year-old woman experienced vaginal bleeding, abdominal pain, uterine tenderness, and uterine contractions. Concerned, she alerted her husband, who immediately drove her to the hospital. In the emergency department, a provisional diagnosis of *abruptio placentae* (premature partial or total separation of the placenta from the uterus) was made. Because of the excessive hemorrhage, the medical staff felt that the abruptio placentae was extensive and that both the mother and the fetus were in a life-threatening situation. The patient received medication—STAT—for shock and blood replacement. She was then transferred to surgery and prepped for a cesarean section. Shortly after the delivery of the baby (and placenta), the bleeding stopped. The presence of a near-total abruptio placentae was confirmed during the surgery.

The initial assessment of the baby showed a premature female infant born 6 weeks early (at 34 weeks' gestation). She weighed only 1610 g (3 lb 7 oz). Her first Apgar score at delivery was 4. Her heart rate was less than 100 beats/min, respiratory rate was weak and irregular, skin color was blue, she demonstrated no grimace reflex when suctioned, and her muscle tone showed only moderate flexion. The baby was manually ventilated aggressively with an inspired oxygen concentration ($F_{I_{O_2}}$) of 1.0 and responded favorably within a few minutes. The second Apgar score was 8. Her heart rate was greater than 100 beats/min, she had a strong cry, her skin was pink, she demonstrated a grimace reflex when suctioned, and her muscle tone was improved.

The baby was transferred to the neonatal intensive care unit for close observation. Two hours later, the baby's vital signs were respiratory rate—44 breaths/min, blood pressure—66/42 mm Hg, and apical heart rate—135 beats/min. On auscultation, normal vesicular breath sounds were heard bilaterally. A portable chest X-ray was normal. The baby's umbilical arterial blood gas values were pH—7.33, Pa_{CO_2}—44 torr, HCO_3^-—23 mEq/L, and Pa_{O_2}—52 torr. Four days later, both the mother and the baby were discharged in good health.

Discussion

This case illustrates the important function of the placenta as a lifeline between the mother and the baby during fetal life. Because the placenta separated from the wall of the uterus, the maternal–placentae–fetal interface was seriously compromised. In short, the ability of the fetus to absorb oxygen, nutrients, and other substances and excrete carbon dioxide and other wastes was interrupted. Complete separation brings about immediate death of the fetus. Bleeding from the site of separation may cause abdominal pain, uterine tenderness, and uterine contraction. Bleeding may be concealed within the uterus or may be evident externally, sometimes as sudden massive hemorrhage (as in this case). In severe cases, shock and death can occur in minutes. A cesarean section must be performed immediately. Fortunately, in this case the mother and the baby were treated in a timely manner.

Review Questions

1. During the embryonic period, the lungs first appear at about the
   A. 10th day after fertilization
   B. 24th day after fertilization
   C. 6th week after fertilization
   D. 12th week after fertilization

2. The lungs are usually sufficiently mature to support life by the
   A. 24th week of gestation
   B. 28th week of gestation
   C. 32nd week of gestation
   D. 36th week of gestation

3. At birth, the number of alveoli represent about how much of the total adult gas exchange units?
   A. 10 percent
   B. 20 percent
   C. 30 percent
   D. 40 percent

4. The number of alveoli continues to increase until about
   A. 6 years of age
   B. 8 years of age
   C. 10 years of age
   D. 12 years of age

5. The average P_{O_2} in the umbilical arteries during fetal life is about
   A. 20 torr
   B. 40 torr
   C. 60 torr
   D. 80 torr

6. The average P_{O_2} in the umbilical vein during fetal life is about
   A. 20 torr
   B. 30 torr
   C. 40 torr
   D. 50 torr

7. The average P_{CO_2} in the umbilical arteries during fetal life is about
   A. 25 torr
   B. 35 torr
   C. 45 torr
   D. 55 torr

8. In the placenta, maternal blood is continuously pumped through the
   A. umbilical arteries
   B. chorionic villi
   C. fetal vessels
   D. intervillous space

9. In the fetal circulation, once blood enters the right atrium, most of the blood enters the left atrium by passing through the
   A. ductus arteriosus
   B. ductus venosus
   C. pulmonary arteries
   D. foramen ovale

10. Shortly after birth, the ductus arteriosus constricts in response to
    1. increased P_{O_2}
    2. decreased P_{CO_2}
    3. increased pH
    4. prostaglandins
       A. 1 only
       B. 2 only
       C. 3 and 4 only
       D. 1 and 4 only

Clinical Application Questions

Case 1

1. During fetal development, the alveolar-capillary system and the quantity of pulmonary surfactant usually are not sufficient to support life until the _____week of gestation.

2. As a result of the insufficient amount of pulmonary surfactant, the pathologic processes of a common newborn respiratory disease called _____ developed.

3. In this case, what are the major anatomic alterations of the lungs associated with the respiratory disease that developed in the infant?

   _____

   _____

   _____

   _____

   _____

   _____

4. Describe the pathophysiology that develops as the conditions listed in question 3 worsen.

   _____

   _____

   _____

5. Describe how the following conditions are manifested in the clinical setting:

Decreased pulmonary diffusion: _____

_____

_____

Decreased lung compliance: _____

_____

_____

6. Why did PPHN develop in the infant in this case? How did this condition improve?

_____

_____

_____

Case 2

1. Describe why the maternal–placentae–fetal interface was seriously compromised in this case. _____

_____

_____

2. Describe what condition(s) bleeding from the site of maternal–placenta separation may cause to the mother _____

_____

3. What may develop when the maternal–placenta separation is severe? What procedure must be performed immediately? _____

_____

Chapter 11

Aging and the Cardiopulmonary System

Objectives

By the end of this chapter, the student should be able to:

1. Describe the effects of aging on the following components of the *respiratory system:*
   —Static mechanical properties
   - Elastic recoil of the lungs
   - Lung compliance
   - Thoracic compliance
   —Lung volumes and capacities
   —Dynamic maneuvers of ventilation
   —Pulmonary diffusing capacity
   —Alveolar dead space ventilation
   —Pulmonary gas exchange
   —Arterial blood gases
   —Arterial-venous oxygen content difference
   —Hemoglobin concentration
   —Control of ventilation
   —Defense mechanisms
   —Exercise tolerance
   —Pulmonary diseases in the elderly
2. Describe the clinical connection associated with exercise and aging.
3. Describe the effects of aging on the following components of the *cardiovascular system:*
   —Structure of the heart
   —Work of the heart
   —Heart rate
   —Stroke volume
   —Cardiac output
   —Peripheral vascular resistance
   —Blood pressure
   —Aerobic capacity
4. Complete the review questions at the end of this chapter.

Introduction

The aging process is normal, progressive, and physiologically irreversible. Aging occurs despite optimal nutrition, genetic background, environmental surroundings, and activity patterns. The biological aging process, however, may demonstrate altered rates of progression in response to an individual's genetic background and daily living habits.

In 2011, the baby boomers—those born between 1946 and 1964—started to turn 65 years old. Presently, there are about 40 million people in the United States who are 65 and older—this number is projected to reach close to 90 million by 2050. Figure 11–1 on page 412 illustrates the actual and projected population of persons age 55 years and older for four different age groups from 1900 to 2040.

It is also projected that the number of annual short-stay hospital days of persons 65 years and older will increase from about 100,000 in 1980 to

Figure 11–1

The actual and projected population of adults age 55 years and older for four different age groups (1900 to 2040).

© Cengage Learning 2013

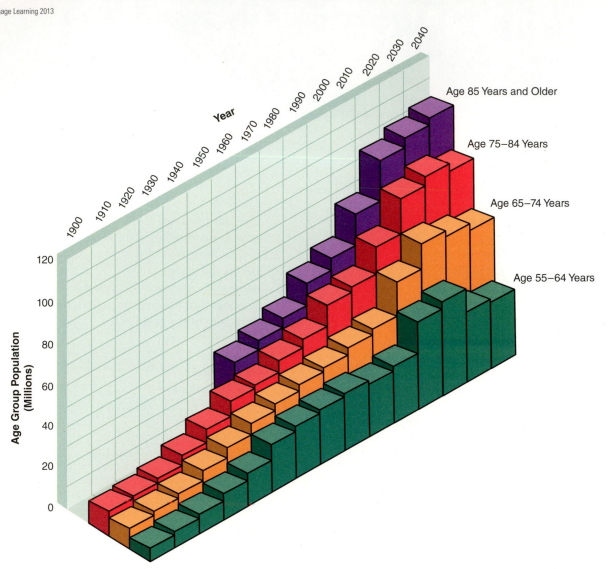

about 300,000 by the year 2050 (Figure 11–2). Because the mortality and morbidity rates rise sharply after age 65, the large size of this population will undoubtedly pose a tremendous challenge to the health care industry. A basic understanding of how the aging process affects the cardiopulmonary system is critical for the respiratory therapist.

The Effects of Aging on the Respiratory System

The growth and development of the lungs is essentially complete by about 20 years of age. Most of the pulmonary function indices reach their maximum levels between 20 and 25 years of age and then progressively decline. The precise effects of aging on the respiratory system are difficult to determine because the changes associated with time are often indistinguishable from those caused by disease. For example, factors such as long-term exposure

© Cengage Learning 2013

Figure 11–2

The actual and projected annual short-stay hospital days for adults age 65 years and older (1980 to 2050).

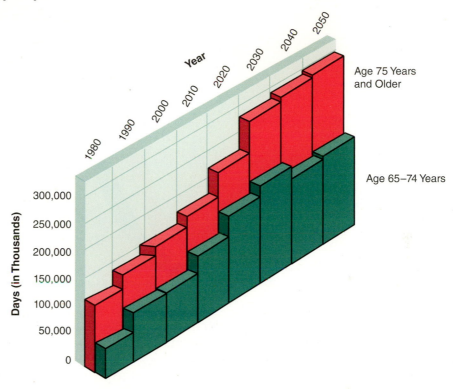

to environmental pollutants, recurring pulmonary infections, smoking, and some working conditions can cause alterations in the respiratory system that are not easily differentiated from changes due to aging alone. Despite these difficulties, the conclusions reached here appear to be well founded.

Static Mechanical Properties

The **functional residual capacity** is the volume remaining in the lungs when the elastic recoil of the lungs exactly balances the natural tendency of the chest wall to expand. With aging, the elastic recoil of the lungs decreases, causing lung compliance to increase. This is illustrated graphically as a shift to the left (steeper slope) of the volume-pressure curve (Figure 11–3 on page 414). The decrease in lung elasticity develops because the alveoli progressively deteriorate and enlarge after age 30. Structurally, the alveolar changes resemble the air sac changes associated with emphysema—commonly referred to as **senile emphysema** or **senile hyperinflation of the lungs**.

Even though the potential for greater lung expansion exists as an individual ages, it cannot be realized because of the structural limitations that develop in the chest wall. With aging, the costal cartilages progressively calcify, causing the ribs to slant downward, and this structural change causes the thorax to become less compliant. Because of these anatomic changes, the transpulmonary pressure difference, which is responsible for holding the airways open, is diminished with age.

Figure 11–3

Comparison of the pressure-volume curve of a 60-year-old adult with that of a 20-year-old adult.

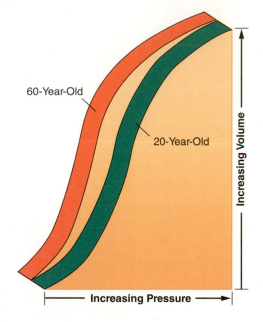

Finally, the reduction in chest wall compliance is slightly greater than the increase in lung compliance, resulting in an overall moderate decline in total compliance of the respiratory system. It is estimated that the work expenditure of a 60-year-old individual to overcome static mechanical forces during normal breathing is 20 percent greater than that of a 20-year-old. The decreased compliance of the respiratory system associated with age is offset by increased respiratory frequency, rather than by increased tidal volume during exertion.

Lung Volumes and Capacities

Figure 11–4 shows the changes that occur in the lung volumes and capacities with aging. Although studies differ, it is generally agreed that the total lung capacity (TLC) essentially remains the same throughout life. Should the TLC decrease, however, it is probably due to the decreased height that typically occurs with age.

It is well documented that the residual volume (RV) increases with age. This is primarily due to age-related alveolar enlargement and to small airway closure. As the RV increases, the RV/TLC ratio also increases. The RV/TLC ratio increases from approximately 20 percent at age 20 to about 35 percent at age 60. This increase occurs predominantly after age 40. Moreover, as the RV increases, the expiratory reserve volume (ERV) decreases. Most studies show that the functional residual capacity (FRC) increases with age, but not as much as the RV and the RV/TLC. Because the FRC typically increases with age, the inspiratory capacity (IC) decreases.

Because the vital capacity (VC) is equal to the TLC minus the RV, the VC inevitably decreases as the RV increases. It is estimated that in men, the VC decreases about 25 mL/year. In women, the VC decreases about 20 mL/year. In general, the VC decreases about 40 to 50 percent by age 70.

Figure 11–4

Schematic of the changes that occur in lung volumes and capacities with aging.

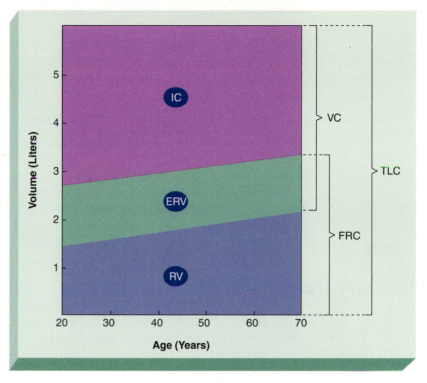

Dynamic Maneuvers of Ventilation

Because of the loss of lung elasticity associated with aging, there is inevitably a marked effect on the dynamics of ventilation. In fact, one of the most prominent physiologic changes associated with age is the reduced efficiency in forced air expulsion. This normal deterioration is reflected by a progressive decrease in the following dynamic lung functions:

- Forced vital capacity (FVC).
- Peak expiratory flow rate (PEFR).
- Forced expiratory flow$_{25-75\%}$ (FEF$_{25-75\%}$).
- Forced expiratory volume in 1 second (FEV$_1$).
- Forced expiratory volume in 1 second/forced vital capacity ratio (FEV$_1$/ FVC ratio).
- Maximum voluntary ventilation (MVV).

It is estimated that these dynamic lung functions decrease approximately 20 to 30 percent throughout the average adult's life. For example, it is reported that the FEV$_1$ decreases about 30 mL/year in men and about 20 mL/year in women after about age 20. Initially, the yearly decline in FEV$_1$ is relatively small, but accelerates with age. The FVC decreases about 15 to 30 mL/year in men and 15 to 25 mL/year in women. Precisely what causes the flow rates to decline is still being debated. However, because gas flow is dependent on the applied pressure and the airway resistance, changes in either or both of these factors could be responsible for the reduction of gas flow rates seen in the elderly.

Pulmonary Diffusing Capacity

The pulmonary diffusing capacity ($D_{L_{CO}}$) progressively decreases after about 20 years of age. It is estimated that the $D_{L_{CO}}$ falls about 20 percent over the course of adult life. In men, it is reported that $D_{L_{CO}}$ declines at a rate of about 2 mL/min/mm Hg; in women, the decline is about 1.5 mL/min/mm Hg. This decline results from decreased alveolar surface area caused by alveolar destruction, increased alveolar wall thickness, and decreased pulmonary capillary blood flow, all of which are known to occur with aging.

Alveolar Dead Space Ventilation

Alveolar dead space ventilation increases with advancing age. This is due, in part, to the decreased cardiac index associated with aging and the structural alterations of the pulmonary capillaries that occur as a result of normal alveolar deterioration. In other words, the natural loss of lung elasticity results in an increase in lung compliance, which, in turn, leads to an increase in dead space ventilation. It is estimated that the alveolar dead space ventilation increases about 1 mL/year throughout adult life.

Pulmonary Gas Exchange

The alveolar-arterial oxygen tension difference $P_{(A-a)O_2}$ progressively increases with age. Factors that may increase the $P_{(A-a)O_2}$ include the physiologic shunt, the mismatching of ventilation and perfusion, and a decreased diffusing capacity.

Arterial Blood Gases

In the normal adult, the Pa_{O_2} should be greater than 90 torr up to 45 years of age. After 45 years of age, the Pa_{O_2} generally declines. The minimum low Pa_{O_2}, however, should be greater than 75 torr—regardless of age. Contrary to earlier beliefs, it is now documented that the Pa_{O_2} progressively decreases between the ages of 45 and 75 years, and then often increases slightly and levels off.

The Pa_{CO_2} remains constant throughout life. A possible explanation for this is the greater diffusion ability of carbon dioxide through the alveolar-capillary barrier. Because the Pa_{CO_2} remains the same in the healthy older adult, the pH and HCO_3^- levels also remain constant.

Arterial-Venous Oxygen Content Difference

The maximum arterial-venous oxygen content difference $C(a - \bar{v})_{O_2}$ tends to decrease with age. Contributory factors include (1) decline in physical fitness, (2) less efficient peripheral blood distribution, and (3) reduction in tissue enzyme activity.

Hemoglobin Concentration

Anemia is a common finding in the elderly. Several factors predispose the elderly to anemia. Red bone marrow has a tendency to be replaced by fatty marrow, especially in the long bones. Gastrointestinal atrophy, which is commonly associated with advancing age, may slow the absorption of iron or vitamin B_{12}. Gastrointestinal bleeding is also more prevalent in the elderly. Perhaps the most important reasons for anemia in the elderly are sociologic rather than medical—for example, insufficient income to purchase food or decreased interest in cooking and eating adequate meals.

Control of Ventilation

Ventilatory rate and heart rate responses to hypoxia and hypercapnia diminish with age. This is due to a reduced sensitivity and responsiveness of the peripheral and central chemoreceptors and the slowing of central nervous system pathways with age. In addition, age slows the neural output to respiratory muscles and the lower chest wall and reduces lung mechanical efficiency. It is estimated that the ventilatory response to hypoxia is decreased more than 50 percent in the healthy male over 65 years of age; the ventilatory response to hypercapnia is decreased by more than 40 percent. These reductions increase the risk of pulmonary diseases (e.g., pneumonia, chronic obstructive pulmonary disease, and obstructive sleep apnea)

Defense Mechanisms

The rate of the mucociliary transport system declines with age. In addition, there is a decreased cough reflex in more than 70 percent of the elderly population. The decreased cough reflex is caused, in part, by the increased prevalence of medication use (e.g., sedatives) and neurologic diseases associated with the elderly. In addition, dysphagia (impaired esophageal motility), which is commonly seen in the elderly, increases the risk for aspiration and pneumonia.

Exercise Tolerance

In healthy individuals of any age, respiratory function does not limit exercise tolerance. The oxygen transport system is more critically dependent on the cardiovascular system than on respiratory function. The maximal oxygen uptake ($\dot{V}_{O_2max}$), which is the parameter most commonly used to evaluate an individual's aerobic exercise tolerance, peaks at age 20 and progressively and linearly decreases with age. Although there is considerable variation among individuals, it is estimated that from 20 to 60 years of age, a person's maximal oxygen uptake decreases by approximately 35 percent. Evidence indicates, however, that regular physical conditioning throughout life increases oxygen uptake and, therefore, enhances the capacity for exertion during work and recreation.

Pulmonary Diseases in the Elderly

Although the occurrence of pulmonary diseases increases with age, it is difficult to determine the precise relationship aging has to pulmonary disease. This is because aging is also associated with the presence of chronic diseases (e.g., lung cancer, bronchitis, emphysema). It is known, however, that the incidence of serious infectious pulmonary diseases is significantly greater in the elderly. Although the incidence of pneumonia and influenza has decreased dramatically in recent years, pneumonia and influenza are still a major causes of death in the elderly. Evidence suggests that this is partly due to the impaired defense mechanisms in the elderly.

Clinical Connection—11-1

Exercise and Aging

A regular exercise program throughout life can prevent, reduce, or delay some of the common effects associated with aging. There are four main types of exercises that seniors can benefit from:

- **Aerobic activities**—for example, walking, riding a bike, and swimming. These endurance exercises improve the health of the heart and circulatory systems.

- **Muscle strengthening**—for example, free weights or strengthening machines. These

activities build muscle tissue and reduce age-relate muscle loss.

- **Stretching exercises**—for example, leg, arm, and back stretching activities help to keep the body limber and flexible.

- **Balance exercises**—help to reduce chances of falling.

The accompanying chart provides an overview of the some of the well-documented health benefits of exercise.

Exercise vs. Aging		
	Effects of Aging	**Effects of Exercise**
Heart and Circulation		
Resting heart rate	Increase	Decrease
Maximum heart rate	Decrease	Slows the decrease
Maximum pumping capacity	Decrease	Increase
Heart muscle stiffness	Increase	Decrease
Blood vessel stiffness	Increase	Decrease
Blood pressure	Increase	Decrease
Risk of heart attack and stroke	Increase	Decrease
Blood		
Number of red blood cells	Decrease	No change
Blood viscosity	Increase	Decrease
Lungs		
Maximum oxygen uptake	Decrease	No change
Intestines		
Speed of emptying	Decrease	Increase
Bones		
Calcium content and strength	Decrease	Increase
Muscles		
Muscle mass and strength	Decrease	Increase

Clinical Connection—11-1, continued

Exercise vs. Aging

	Effects of Aging	Effects of Exercise
Metabolism		
Metabolic rate	Decrease	Increase
Body fat	Increase	Decrease
Blood sugar	Increase	Decrease
Insulin levels	Increase	Decrease
LDL ("bad") cholesterol	Increase	Decrease
HDL ("good") cholesterol	Decrease	Increase
Sex hormone levels	Decrease	Slows decrease
Nervous System		
Quality of sleep	Decrease	Increase
Risk of depression	Increase	Decrease
Memory lapse	Increase	Decrease

The Effects of Aging on the Cardiovascular System

A variety of adverse changes develop in the cardiovascular system with age. In fact, the major causes of death in the aging population are diseases of the cardiovascular system. The major changes in the cardiovascular system that develop as a function of age are discussed next.

Structure of the Heart

Between 30 and 80 years of age, the thickness of the left ventricular wall increases by about 25 percent. Cardiac hypertrophy, however, is not considered a primary change associated with aging. In the ventricles, the muscle fiber size progressively increases. Fibrosis develops in the lining of the chambers, and fatty infiltration occurs in the wall of the chambers. The amount of connective tissue increases, causing the heart to become less elastic. Thus, the compliance of the heart is reduced and the heart functions less efficiently as a pump. The heart valves thicken from calcification and fibrosis. This structural change causes the valves to become more rigid and less effective. As the valves become more rigid and distorted, the blood flow may be impeded and systolic murmurs may develop.

Work of the Heart

The work of the heart, which is defined as Stroke volume × Mean systolic blood pressure, decreases approximately 1 percent per year (Figure 11–5 on page 420).

Figure 11–5

Schematic of the effects of aging on the work of the heart. LVSWI = left ventricular stroke work index.

© Cengage Learning 2013

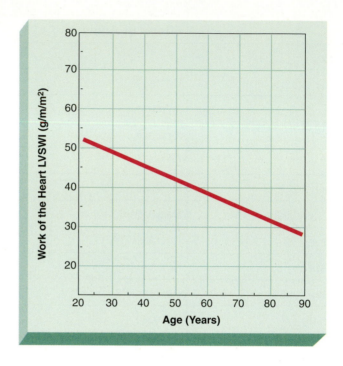

Heart Rate

Although the effects of age on the resting heart rate are debated, it is known that the increase in heart rate in response to stress is less in the elderly. The maximum heart rate can be estimated by the following formula:

Maximum heart rate = 220 − Age

Thus, the maximum heart rate for a 60-year-old is about 160 (220 − 60 = 160) beats/min. (Recent research has shown that some older subjects can achieve higher heart rates than those predicted by this method.) The reasons for the decreased maximum heart rate are unclear (Figure 11–6). It may be because of the diminished myocardial oxygen supply associated with advanced age. Another possibility is the decreased compliance of the heart in the elderly. The increase in heart rate in response to stress may be impaired because of increased connective tissue in the sinoatrial and atrioventricular junction and in the bundle branches. The number of catecholamine receptors on the muscle fibers may also be reduced.

With aging, moreover, it not only takes more time for the heart to accelerate, but it also takes more time to return to normal after a stressful event. Because of this, the expected increase in pulse rate in response to certain clinical situations (e.g., anxiety, pain, hemorrhage, and infectious processes) is often not as evident in the elderly.

Stroke Volume

The stroke volume diminishes with age. The precise reason for the reduction in the stroke volume is unknown. It is suggested, however, that it may be a reflection of poor myocardial perfusion, decreased cardiac compliance,

Figure 11–6

Schematic of the effects of aging on the maximum heart rate.

© Cengage Learning 2013

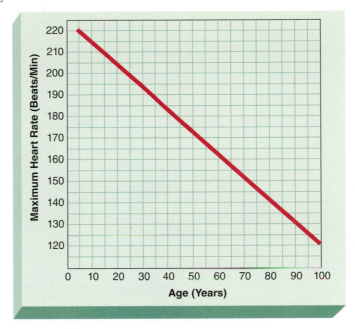

and poor contractility. As the stroke volume declines, the *stroke volume index* (Stroke volume ÷ Body surface area) also decreases.

Cardiac Output

As the stroke volume diminishes, the cardiac output inevitably declines (Cardiac output = Stroke volume × Heart rate). After age 20, the cardiac output decreases in a linear fashion about 1 percent per year (Figure 11–7 on page 422). Between the ages of 30 and 80, the cardiac output decreases about 40 percent in both men and women. As the cardiac output declines, the *cardiac index* (Cardiac output ÷ Body surface area) also decreases.

Peripheral Vascular Resistance

It is well documented that the elasticity of the major blood vessels decreases with advancing age. Both the arteries and veins undergo age-related changes. The intima thickens and the media becomes more fibrotic (refer to Figure 1–33). Collagen and extracellular materials accumulate in both the intima and media. As the peripheral vascular system becomes stiffer, its ability to accept the cardiac stroke volume declines. This age-related development increases the *resting pulse pressure* and the *systolic blood pressure*. It is estimated that the *total* peripheral vascular resistance increases about 1 percent per year (Figure 11–8 on page 422).

As the peripheral vascular resistance increases, the perfusion of the body organs decreases. This progressive decline in organ perfusion partly explains the many organ debilities seen in elderly people. As the vascular system becomes stiffer with age, its tolerance to change diminishes. For example, a sudden move from the horizontal to the vertical position may cause a marked drop in systemic blood pressure, causing dizziness, confusion, weakness,

Schematic of the effects of aging on cardiac output.

© Cengage Learning 2013

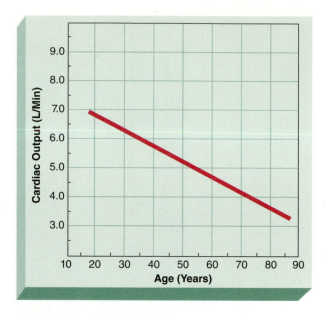

Schematic of the effects of aging on total peripheral vascular resistance.

© Cengage Learning 2013

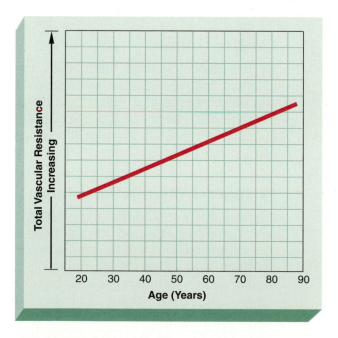

and fainting. Arterial stiffening also makes the baroreceptors, located in the carotid sinuses and aortic arch, sluggish and less able to moderate blood pressure changes.

Blood Pressure

As described previously, factors associated with aging that increase blood pressure are increasing stiffness of large arteries and increasing total peripheral resistance. Other factors, such as obesity, sodium intake, and stress, can also elevate blood pressure.

Aerobic Capacity

Aerobic capacity decreases about 50 percent between 20 and 80 years of age. This is primarily due to the reduction in muscle mass and strength associated with aging. Other possible causes include the inadequate distribution of blood flow to working muscles and the decreased ability of the tissue cells to extract oxygen.

Chapter Summary

A fundamental knowledge base of the effects of aging on the cardiopulmonary system is an important part of respiratory care. The major components are the influence of aging on the respiratory system, including the static mechanical properties of the lungs, lung volumes and capacities, dynamic maneuvers of ventilation, pulmonary diffusing capacity, and alveolar dead space ventilation, as well as pulmonary gas exchange, arterial blood gases, arterial-venous oxygen content difference, hemoglobin concentration, control of ventilation, defense mechanisms, exercise tolerance, and presence of pulmonary diseases. The knowledge base should also include the effects of aging on the cardiovascular system, including the structure of the heart, work of the heart, heart rate, stroke volume, cardiac output, peripheral vascular resistance, blood pressure, and aerobic capacity.

Review Questions

1. As an individual ages, the
   A. residual volume decreases
   B. expiratory reserve volume increases
   C. functional residual capacity decreases
   D. vital capacity decreases

2. Most of the lung function indices reach their maximum levels between
   A. 5–10 years of age
   B. 10–15 years of age
   C. 15–20 years of age
   D. 20–25 years of age

3. With advancing age, the
   1. lung compliance decreases
   2. chest wall compliance increases
   3. lung compliance increases
   4. chest wall compliance decreases
      A. 2 only
      B. 3 only
      C. 1 and 2 only
      D. 3 and 4 only

4. As an individual ages, the
1. forced vital capacity increases
2. peak expiratory flow rate decreases
3. forced expiratory volume in 1 second increases
4. maximum voluntary ventilation increases
   A. 1 only
   B. 2 only
   C. 2 and 4 only
   D. 3 and 4 only

5. With advancing age, the
1. Pa_{CO_2} increases
2. Pa_{O_2} decreases
3. $P_{(A-a)O_2}$ decreases
4. $C(a - \bar{v})_{O_2}$ decreases
   A. 1 only
   B. 2 only
   C. 3 and 4 only
   D. 2 and 4 only

6. The maximum heart rate of a 45-year-old person is
   A. 155 beats/min
   B. 165 beats/min
   C. 175 beats/min
   D. 185 beats/min

7. Over the course of life, the diffusion capacity decreases by about
   A. 5 percent
   B. 10 percent
   C. 15 percent
   D. 20 percent

8. Between 30 and 80 years of age, the cardiac output decreases by about
   A. 10 percent
   B. 20 percent
   C. 30 percent
   D. 40 percent

9. With advancing age, the
1. blood pressure increases
2. stroke volume decreases
3. cardiac output increases
4. heart work decreases
   A. 1 only
   B. 2 only
   C. 3 and 4 only
   D. 1, 2, and 4 only

10. Between 20 and 60 years of age, the RV/TLC ratio
   A. increases from 20 to 25 percent
   B. increases from 20 to 30 percent
   C. increases from 20 to 35 percent
   D. increases from 20 to 40 percent

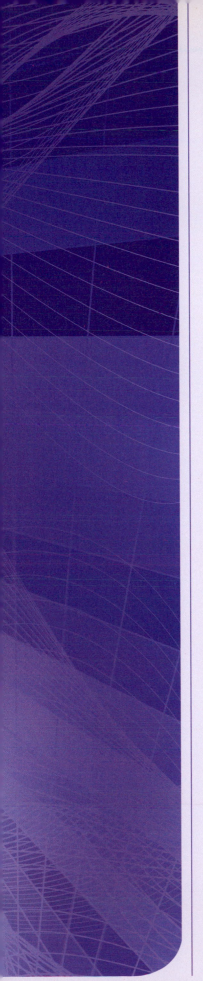

Section Two

Advanced Cardiopulmonary Concepts and Related Areas—The Essentials

Chapter 12

Electrophysiology of the Heart

Objectives

By the end of this chapter, the student should be able to:

1. Describe the electrophysiology of the heart, including:
—Action potential
- Phase 0
- Phase 1
- Phase 2
- Phase 3
- Phase 4

2. Describe the properties of the cardiac muscle, including:
—Automaticity
—Excitability
—Conductivity
—Contractility

3. Explain the following refractory periods of the heart:
—Absolute refractory period
—Relative refractory period
—Nonrefractory period

4. Identify the major components of the conductive system of the heart, including:
—Sinoatrial node
—Atrioventricular junction
—Bundle of His
—Right and left bundle branches
—Purkinje fibers

5. Describe the clinical connection associated with synchronized cardioversion and unsynchronized cardioversion.

6. Describe the cardiac effects of the
—Sympathetic nervous system
—Parasympathetic nervous system

7. Complete the review questions at the end of this chapter.

Introduction

The heart contracts by generating and propagating **action potentials**, which are electrical currents that travel across the cell membranes of the heart. The electrical events of an action potential are identical in skeletal muscles, cardiac muscle, and neurons. In neurons, however, a transmitted action potential is called a **nerve impulse**. When the heart is relaxed (i.e., not generating an action potential), the cardiac muscle fibers are in what is called their **polarized** or **resting state**. During this period, there is an electrical charge difference across the fibers of the heart cells. This electrical difference between the electrolytes inside the cell membranes and the electrolytes outside of the cell membranes is called the **resting membrane potential (RMP)**.

The primary electrolytes responsible for the electrical difference across the RMP are **potassium (K⁺)**, **sodium (Na⁺)**, and **calcium (Ca²⁺)**. Similar to all the cells in the body, the concentration of K^+ is greatest inside the cardiac cell—about 151 mEq/L—and the concentration of K^+ outside the cardiac cell is about 4 mEq/L. For Na^+ and Ca^{2+}, the opposite is true. The concentration of Na^+ outside the cardiac cell is about 144 mEq/L and about 7 mEq/L inside the cell; the concentration of Ca^{2+} is about 5 mEq/L outside the cell and less than 1 mEq/L inside the cell.

When the cardiac cell is in its resting or polarized state, the inside of the cell is negatively charged with the K^+ cation, and the outside of the cell is positively charged with the Na^+ cation. The way in which this relationship (i.e., negative inside the cell and positive outside of the cell) develops with two cations (positive ions) is as follows: in the polarized state, the Na^+/K^+ pump establishes (1) an increased Na^+ concentration outside of the cell and (2) an increased K^+ concentration inside of the cell. Both ions then diffuse along their concentration gradients; that is, K^+ diffuses out of the cell while, at the same time, Na^+ diffuses into the cell. For every 50 to 75 K^+ ions that diffuse out of the cell, only 1 Na^+ diffuses into the cell. This exchange ratio results in a deficiency of positive cations inside the cell; that is, an electrical difference (RMP) between the electrolytes inside the cell and the electrolytes outside the cell is generated (Figure 12–1).

The potential force of the RMP is measured in millivolts (mV) (1 mV = 0.001 V). The RMP of the myocardial cells is about −90 mV. The cornerstone to the understanding of the electrophysiology of the heart is the five electrophysiologic phases of the action potential. An electrocardiogram (ECG) is used to record the five phases of the action potential. A variety of heart abnormalities can disrupt any of these five electrophysiologic phases and, therefore, disrupt and alter the configuration of a normal ECG tracing.

Figure 12–1

The polarized state. For each Na^+ ion that diffuses into the cell, about 75 K^+ ions diffuse out of the cell. The result is a deficiency of positive cations inside the cell; this is a cell with a negative charge.

© Cengage Learning 2013

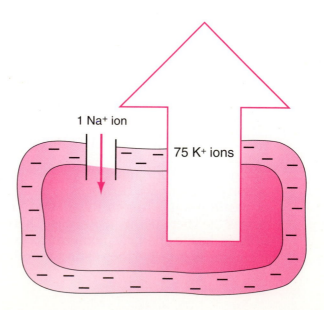

The Five Phases of the Action Potential

Depolarization

Depolarization is the trigger for myocardial contraction.

Phase 0: Rapid depolarization (early phase). Under normal conditions, the ventricular muscle fibers are activated between 60 and 100 times/min by an electrical impulse initiated by the sinoatrial (SA) node. This action changes the RMP and allows a rapid inward flow of Na^+ into the cell through specific Na^+ channels. This process causes the inside of the cell to become positively charged. The voltage inside the cell at the end of depolarization is about +30 mV. This electrophysiologic event produces a rapid up-stroke in the action potential (see Figure 12–2).

Repolarization

Repolarization is the process by which the cells of the heart return to their resting state.

Figure 12–2

The action potential and the Na^+, K^+, and Ca^{2+} changes during phases 0, 1, 2, 3, and 4.

© Cengage Learning 2013

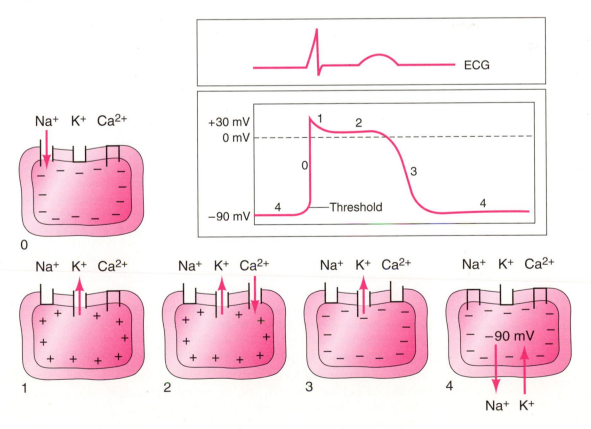

Phase 1: Initial repolarization. Immediately after phase 0, the channels for K^+ open and permit K^+ to flow out of the cell, an action that produces an early, but incomplete, repolarization (repolarization is slowed by the phase 2 influx of Ca^{2+} ions). Phase 1 is illustrated as a short downward stroke in the action potential curve just before the plateau (see Figure 12–2).

Phase 2: Plateau state. During this period, there is slow inward flow of Ca^{2+}, which, in turn, significantly slows the outward flow of K^+. The plateau phase prolongs the contraction of the myocardial cells (see Figure 12–2).

Phase 3: Final rapid repolarization. During this period, the inward flow of Ca^{2+} stops, the outward flow of K^+ is again accelerated, and the rate of repolarization accelerates (see Figure 12–2).

Phase 4: Resting or polarized state. During this period, the voltage-sensitive ion channels return to their pre-depolarization permeability. The excess Na^+ inside the cell (that occurred during depolarization) and the loss of K^+ (that occurred during repolarization) are returned to normal by the Na^+ and K^+ ion pumps. An additional Na^+ and Ca^{2+} pump removes the excess of Ca^{2+} from the cell (see Figure 12–2).

Properties of the Cardiac Muscle

The heart is composed of two types of cardiac cells: contractile muscle fibers and specialized "pacemaker cells" called autorhythmic cells. The myocardial contractile fiber cells make up the bulk of the musculature of the myocardium and are responsible for the pumping activity of the heart. Approximately 1 percent of the heart is composed of the autorhythmic cells, the majority of which are located in the SA node. These cells have the unique ability to initiate an action potential spontaneously, which, in turn, triggers the myocardial fibers to contract. The cardiac cells of the heart have four specific properties: automaticity, excitability, conductivity, and contractility.

- Automaticity is the unique ability of the cells in the SA node (pacemaker cells) to generate an action potential without being stimulated. This occurs because the cell membranes of the pacemaker cells permit Na^+ to leak into the cell during phase 4. As Na^+ enters the cell, the RMP slowly increases. When the threshold potential (TP) of the pacemaker cells is reached (between −40 and −60 mV), the cells of the SA node rapidly depolarize (Figure 12–3). Under normal conditions, the unique automaticity of the pacemaker cells stimulates the action potential of the heart's conductive system (i.e., atria, atrioventricular [AV] junction, bundle branches, Purkinje fibers, ventricles) at regular and usually predictable intervals (Figure 12–4).

- Excitability (irritability) is the ability of a cell to reach its threshold potential and respond to a stimulus or irritation. The lower the stimulus needed to activate a cell, the more excitable the cell; conversely, the greater the stimulus needed, the less excitable the cell. The presence of ischemia and hypoxia cause the myocardial cell to become more excitable.

Figure 12–3

Schematic comparing action potential of pacemaker and nonpacemaker (working) myocardial cells.

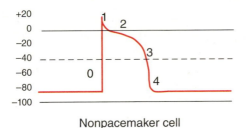

Nonpacemaker cell

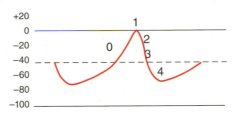

Pacemaker cell

Figure 12–4

Conductive system of the heart.

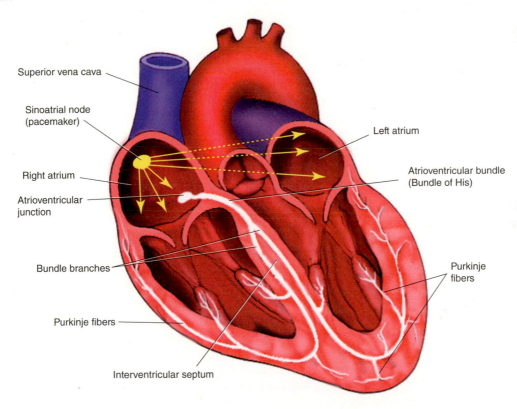

- **Conductivity** is the unique ability of the heart cells to transmit electrical current from cell to cell throughout the entire conductive system.
- **Contractility** is the ability of cardiac muscle fibers to shorten and contract in response to an electrical stimulus.

Refractory Periods

Additional properties of the myocardial contractile fibers and autorhythmic cells are refractory periods, which entail (1) the ionic composition of the cells during different phases of the action potential and (2) the ability of the cells to accept a stimulus.

The **absolute refractory period** is the time in which the cells cannot respond to a stimulus. The ionic composition of the cells is not in place to receive a stimulus. Phases 0, 1, 2, and about half of phase 3 represent the absolute refractory period (see Figure 12–2).

The **relative refractory period** is the time in which repolarization is almost complete and where a strong stimulus may cause depolarization of some of the cells. Some cells may respond normally, some in an abnormal way, and some not at all. The second half of phase 3 represents the relative refractory period of the action potential (see Figure 12–2).

The **nonrefractory period** occurs when all the cells are in their resting or polarized state. The cells are ready to respond to a stimulus in a normal fashion. Phase 4 represents the nonrefractory period (see Figure 12–2).

The duration of each refractory period may vary in response to use of medications or recreational drugs, or presence of disease, electrolyte imbalance, myocardial ischemia, or myocardial injury.

The Conductive System

As shown in Figure 12–4, the components of the conductive system include the **sinoatrial node** (SA node), **atrioventricular junction** (AV junction), **bundle of His**, the **right** and **left bundle branches**, and the **Purkinje fibers**. The electrical cycle of the heart begins with the SA node, or pacemaker. The SA node initiates the cardiac contraction by producing an electrical impulse that travels through the right and left atria. In the right atrium, the electrical impulse is conducted through the **anterior internodal tract**, **middle internodal tract**, and **posterior internodal tract**. All three internodal pathways become one at the AV junction. The **Bachmann's bundle** conducts electrical impulses from the SA node directly to the left atrium. The electrical impulse generated by the SA node cause the right and left atria to contract simultaneously. This action, in turn, forces the blood in the atria to move into the ventricles.

The AV junction is located just behind the tricuspid in the lower portion of the right interatrial septum. The AV junction relays the electrical impulse from the atria to the ventricles via the bundle of His (also called the AV bundle). The bundle of His enters the intraventricular septum and divides into the left and right bundle branches. At the heart's apex, the Purkinje fibers spread throughout the posterior portion of the ventricle and head back toward the base of the heart. In the normal heart, the total time required for an electrical impulse to travel from the SA node to the end of the Purkinje fibers is about 0.22 second. In other words, the entire heart depolarizes in about 0.22 second.

Autonomic Nervous System

Even though the conductive system of the heart has its own intrinsic pacemaker, the autonomic nervous system plays an important role in the rate of impulse formation, conduction, and contraction strength. The regulation of the heart is controlled by neural fibers from both the sympathetic and parasympathetic nervous systems.

Sympathetic neural fibers innervate the atria and ventricles of the heart. When stimulated, the sympathetic fibers cause an *increase* in the heart rate, AV conduction, cardiac contractility, and excitability. **Parasympathetic** neural

Clinical Connection—12-1

Synchronized Cardioversion Defibrillation versus Unsynchronized Cardioversion Defibrillation

Synchronized cardioversion defibrillation is a low-energy shock that is synchronized with the peak of the QRS complex (ventricular depolarization). When the "sync" option is engaged on a defibrillator and the shock button is pushed, there will be a delay in the shock until the defibrillator reads and synchronizes the shock with the patient's ECG rhythm—the peak of the R-wave in the patient's QRS complex. A synchronized cardioversion avoids shocking the patient's heart during the repolarization phase. Common indications for synchronized cardioversion include unstable atrial fibrillation, atrial flutter, atrial tachycardia, and supraventricular tachycardia.

Unsynchronized cardioversion defibrillation is a high-energy shock that is delivered as soon as the shock button is pushed on the defibrillator. The electrical current may fall randomly anywhere within the cardiac cycle—the QRS complex. An unsynchronized cardioversion is used when there is no coordinated electrical heart activity—a pulseless ventricular tachycardia or ventricular fibrillation—or when the defibrillator fails to synchronize with the electrical activity of the heart in an unstable patient.

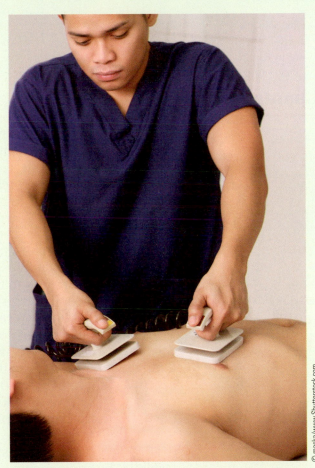

© maska/www.Shutterstock.com.

fibers, via the vagus nerve, innervate the SA node, atrial muscle fibers, and the AV junction. The parasympathetic system has little or no influence on the ventricular musculature. Stimulation of the parasympathetic system causes a *decrease* in heart rate, AV conduction, contractility, and excitability.

Under normal circumstances, the heart action is maintained in a state of balanced control because of the opposing effects of the sympathetic and parasympathetic systems. However, a variety of dysrhythmias can develop when the autonomic nervous system is influenced by medications or abnormal conditions. When the sympathetic nervous system is stimulated by a drug (e.g., epinephrine), the heart rate will increase. On the other hand, when a drug (i.e., propranol) blocks the sympathetic nervous system, the parasympathetic nervous system takes control and the heart rate decreases. Table 12–1 on page 434 summarizes cardiac response to autonomic nervous system changes.

Table 12–1			
Cardiac Response to Autonomic Nervous System Changes			
Sympathetic Stimulation	**Sympathetic Block**	**Parasympathetic Stimulation**	**Parasympathetic Block**
↑ Heart rate	↓ Heart rate	↓ Heart rate	↑ Heart rate

© Cengage Learning 2013

Chapter Summary

Cardiac contractions are a function of action potentials (electrical currents) that sweep across the cell membranes of the heart. Each action potential consists of five phases: phases 0, 1, 2, 3, and 4. Phase 0 represents depolarization, and phases 1, 2, 3, and 4 represent different stages of repolarization. The cardiac cells of the heart have four specific properties: automaticity, excitability, conductivity, and contractility. Automaticity is the unique ability of the cells in the sinoatrial (SA) node (pacemaker cells) to generate an action potential without being stimulated. Excitability (irritability) is the ability of a cell to reach its threshold potential and respond to a stimulus or irritation. Conductivity is the ability of the heart cells to transmit electrical current from cell to cell throughout the entire conductive system. Contractility is the ability of cardiac muscle fibers to shorten and contract in response to an electrical stimulus.

An additional property of the myocardial contractile fibers and autorhythmic cells is refractory periods, which include (1) the ionic composition of the cells during different phases of the action potential and (2) the ability of the cells to accept a stimulus. The absolute refractory period is the phase in which the cells cannot respond to a stimulus. The relative refractory period is the time in which repolarization is partially complete and a strong stimulus may cause depolarization of some of the cell. The nonrefractory period is when all the cells are in their resting or polarized state and are ready to respond to a stimulus in a normal fashion. The components of the conductive system are the sinoatrial node (SA node), atrioventricular junction (AV junction), bundle of His, the right and left bundle branches, and the Purkinje fibers. Finally, although the conductive system of the heart has its own intrinsic pacemaker, the autonomic nervous system plays an important role in the rate of impulse formation, conduction, and contraction strength. The regulation of the heart is controlled by neural fibers from both the sympathetic and parasympathetic nervous systems. A clinical connections associated with the preceding topics includes Synchronized Cardioversion Defibrillation versus Unsynchronized Cardioversion Defibrillation.

Review Questions

1. Which of the following is the rapid upstroke in the action potential?
    A. Phase 0
    B. Phase 1
    C. Phase 2
    D. Phase 3

2. When does the inward flow of Ca^{2+} into the heart stop?
  A. Phase 1
  B. Phase 2
  C. Phase 3
  D. Phase 4

3. Which of the following is the plateau stage of the action potential?
  A. Phase 0
  B. Phase 1
  C. Phase 2
  D. Phase 3

4. The sinoatrial node is also called the
  A. pacemaker
  B. action potential
  C. resting membrane potential
  D. relative refractory period

5. Which of the following slows the heart rate and AV conduction?
  A. Resting membrane potential
  B. Parasympathetic nervous system
  C. Pacemaker
  D. Phase 0

6. When can a strong stimulus cause an unwanted depolarization of the heart?
  A. Absolute refractory period
  B. Relative refractory period
  C. Nonrefractory period
  D. Phase 0

7. Which of the following is called the resting state?
  A. Phase 1
  B. Phase 2
  C. Phase 3
  D. Phase 4

8. Which of the following means the ability to transmit electrical current from one cell to another?
  A. Conductivity
  B. Excitability
  C. Contractility
  D. Automatcity

9. An electrical difference across the fibers of the heart is called the
  A. absolute refractory period
  B. resting membrane potential
  C. action potential
  D. depolarization

10. The entire sequence of electrical changes during depolarization and repolarization is called
  A. nonrefractory period
  B. conductivity
  C. contractility
  D. action potential

Chapter 13

The Standard 12-ECG Lead System

Objectives

By the end of this chapter, the student should be able to:

1. Describe the components of the standard limb leads, including:
   —Standard limb leads
   - Bipolar leads
     o Lead I
     o Lead II
     o Lead III
   - Unipolar leads
     o aVR
     o aVL
     o aVF
   —Axes
   —Einthoven's triangle

2. Describe how an electrical impulse of the heart is recorded when it
   —Moves toward a positive electrode
   —Moves away from a positive electrode (toward a negative electrode)
   —Moves perpendicular to a positive and negative electrode

3. Identify how the following limb leads monitor the frontal plane of the heart:
   —Left lateral leads
   —Inferior leads

4. Describe the clinical connection associated with electrocardiograms (ECGs)—the role of the respiratory therapist.

5. Describe the components of the precordial (chest) leads, including:
   —V1
   —V2
   —V3
   —V4
   —V5
   —V6

6. Identify how the following precordial leads monitor the horizontal plane of the heart:
   —Anterior leads
   —Lateral leads

7. Describe the modified chest lead.

8. Describe the normal electrocardiogram (ECG) configurations and their expected measurements, including:
   —The components of the ECG paper
   —P wave
   —PR interval
   —QRS complex
   —ST segment
   —T wave
   —U wave
   —QT interval

9. Complete the review questions at the end of this chapter.

Introduction

The electrocardiogram (ECG) is a graphic representation of the electrical activity of the heart's conductive system recorded over a period of time. Under normal conditions, ECG tracings have very predictable directions, durations, and amplitudes. Because of this fact, the various components of the ECG tracing can be identified, assessed, and interpreted as to normal or abnormal function. The ECG is also used to monitor the heart's response to therapeutic interventions. Because the ECG is such a useful tool in the clinical setting, the respiratory therapist must have a basic and appropriate understanding of ECG analysis. The essential knowledge components required for a systematic 12-ECG interpretation are discussed.

The Standard 12-ECG Lead System

The standard 12-ECG system consists of four limb electrodes and six chest electrodes. Collectively, the electrodes (or leads) view the electrical activity of the heart from 12 different positions—6 *standard limb leads* and 6 *precordial (chest) leads* (Table 13–1). Each lead (1) views the electrical activity of the heart from a different angle, (2) has a positive and negative component, and (3) monitors specific portions of the heart from the point of view of the positive electrode in that lead.

Standard Limb Leads

As shown in Figure 13–1, the *standard limb leads* are leads I, II, III, aVR, aVL, and aVF. They are called the limb leads because they are derived from electrodes attached to the arms and legs. Leads I, II, and III are bipolar leads, which means they use two electrodes to monitor the heart, one positive and one negative. As illustrated in Figure 13–2 on page 440, an imaginary line can be drawn between the positive and negative electrodes for leads I, II, and III.

Table 13–1		
ECG Lead Systems		
Standard Limb Leads		**Precordial (Chest) Leads**
Bipolar Leads	**Unipolar Leads**	**Unipolar Leads**
Lead I	aVR	V1
Lead II	aVL	V2
Lead III	aVF	V3
		V4
		V5
		V6

© Cengage Learning 2013

© Cengage Learning 2013

Figure 13–1

The standard limb leads—leads I, II, III, aVR, aVL, and aVF. Each of the standard limb electrodes can function as either a positive or negative electrode.

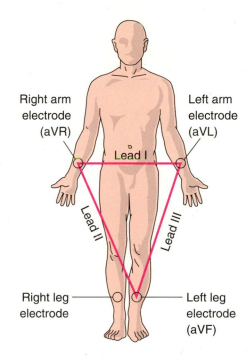

Lead	Right arm	Right leg	Left leg	Left arm
I	−			+
II	−		+	
III			+	−
aVR	+	−	−	−
aVL	−	−	−	+
aVF	−	−	+	−

These lines represent the **axis** of each lead. The triangle formed around the heart by the three axes is called *Einthoven's triangle*.

Electrical impulses that travel more toward the positive electrode (relative to the axis of the lead) are recorded as positive deflections in that lead (see lead I, Figure 13–3A on page 440). When an electrical current travels perpendicular to the lead axis, an equiphasic (half up and half down deflection) or a straight line is recorded (see lead II, Figure 13–3B). Electrical impulses that move away from the positive electrode (or more toward the negative electrode) are recorded as negative deflections in that lead (see lead III, Figure 13–3C). In the normal

Figure 13–2

Leads I, II, and III axes form Einthoven's triangle.

© Cengage Learning 2013

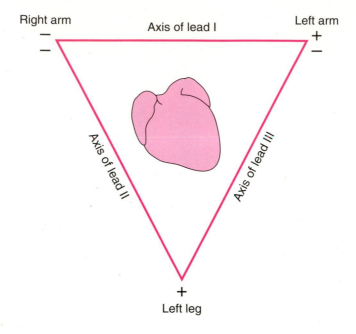

Figure 13–3

Einthoven's triangle around the heart. The arrow represents an electrical impulse moving across the surface of the heart. **A.** In lead I, the impulse is moving toward the positive electrode and is recorded as a positive deflection. **B.** In lead II, the impulse is moving perpendicular to the lead axis, and an equiphasic or straight line is recorded. **C.** In lead III, the impulse is moving toward the negative electrode and is recorded as a negative deflection.

© Cengage Learning 2013

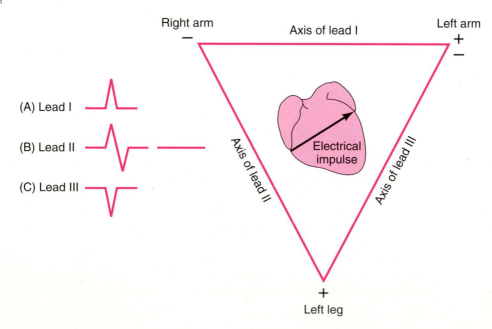

Figure 13–4

In the normal heart, the dominant electrical current in the heart flows from the base to the apex in a right-to-left direction.

© Cengage Learning 2013

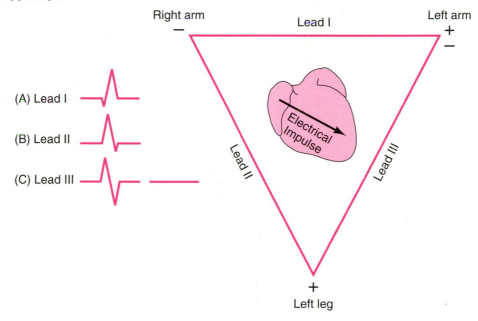

heart, the largest electrical impulse travels from the base of the heart to the apex, in a right to left direction (Figure 13–4).

The aVR, aVL, and aVF leads are **unipolar leads** (see Figure 13–1). Unipolar leads monitor the electrical activity of the heart between the positive electrode (i.e., aVR, aVL, aVF) and the zero electrical reference point at the center of the heart. In essence, the center of the heart functions as a negative electrode. Thus, the axis for these leads is drawn from the electrode and the center of the heart. When the negative electrodes are eliminated in the aVR, aVL, and aVF, the amplitude of the ECG recordings is augmented by 50 percent. This is the reason for the letter *a*, which stands for augmentation; the *V* represents voltage. The letters *R*, *L*, and *F* represent where the positive electrode is placed.

Collectively, the limb leads monitor the electrical activity of the heart in the **frontal plane**, which is the electrical activity that flows over the anterior surface of the heart; from the **base to the apex of the heart**, in a **right to left** direction. Leads I and aVL are called **left lateral leads**, because they monitor the left lateral side of the heart. Leads II, III, and aVF view the lower surfaces of the heart and are called **inferior leads**. The aVR lead does not contribute much information for the 12-ECG interpretation and because of this fact, it is generally ignored. Figure 13–5 on page 442 summarizes the frontal plane and the limb leads.

Precordial (Chest) Leads

Figure 13–6 on page 442 shows the chest position of the *precordial leads*, which are also unipolar leads (i.e., the center of the heart functions as the

Figure 13–5

The frontal plane and the limb leads.

© Cengage Learning 2013

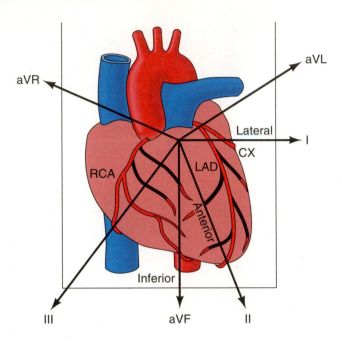

Figure 13–6

A. The position of the electrodes on the rib thorax; **B.** the precordial leads as they reflect the surface of the myocardium.

© Cengage Learning 2013

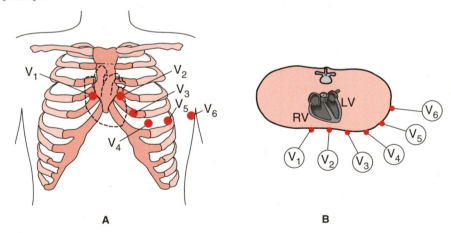

negative reference point, similar to the aVR, aVL, and aVF leads). Figure 13–7 shows the axes of the six precordial leads. The precordial leads monitor the heart from the horizontal plane, which means they record electrical activity that transverses the heart. Leads V1 and V2 monitor the right ventricle, V3 and V4 monitor the ventricular septum, and V5 and V6 view the left ventricle. Leads V1, V2, V3, and V4 are also called anterior leads, and leads V5 and V6 are also called lateral leads. Figure 13–8 summarizes the horizontal plane and its leads.

Figure 13–7

The axes of the six precordial leads.

© Cengage Learning 2013

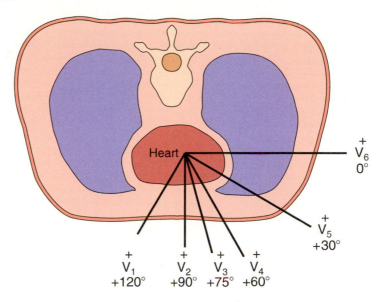

Figure 13–8

The horizontal plane and its leads.

© Cengage Learning 2013

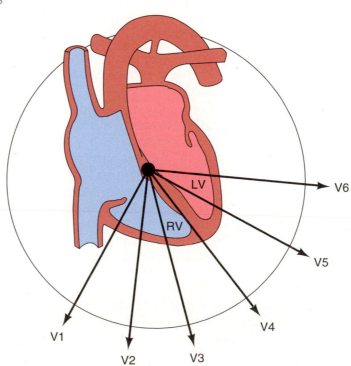

Figure 13–9

The position of the electrodes for the monitoring system MCL₁.

© Cengage Learning 2013

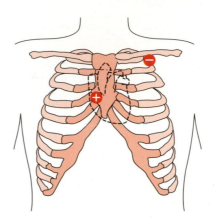

Modified Chest Lead

The *modified chest lead* (MCL₁) is a bipolar chest lead similar to the precordial lead V1. The positive electrode is placed on the chest (in the same position as V1) and the negative electrode is placed on the left arm or left shoulder area (Figure 13–9). The MCL₁ may be helpful in visualizing some waveforms.

Normal ECG Configurations and Their Expected Measurements (Lead II)

The ECG Paper

All ECG systems use the same standard paper and run at the same speed of 25 mm/sec (Figure 13–10). From left to right, each **small square** has a duration of 0.04 second. Each **large square**, delineated by the darker lines, has five small squares, and a duration of 0.20 second. The paper on all ECG monitors runs at a speed of 5 large squares per second, or 300 large squares per minute (5 large squares × 60 seconds = 300 squares/min). The vertical portion of each small square also represents an **amplitude** (or voltage) of **0.1 millivolt** (mV), and **1 millimeter** (1 mm) in distance. Prior to each test, the ECG monitor is standardized so that 1 mV is equal to 10 mm (10 small vertical squares). As shown in Figure 13–11, most ECG paper has small vertical line marks in the margins every 15 large squares, or every 3 seconds (0.20 × 15 = 3 seconds). Fundamental to the evaluation and interpretation of ECG recordings is the ability to measure the duration and amplitude of the waveforms.

The electrical activity of the heart is monitored and recorded on the ECG paper. As illustrated in Figure 13–12 on page 446, the normal ECG configurations are composed of **waves**, **complexes**, **segments**, and **intervals** recorded as voltage (on a vertical axis) against time (on a horizontal axis). A single *waveform* begins and ends at the baseline. When the waveform continues past the baseline, it changes into another waveform. Two or more waveforms

Figure 13–10

The ECG monitoring paper, with the blocks enlarged to illustrate the minimum units of measurement. The smallest of the blocks has three values (see solid red block): 0.04 second in duration (horizontal measurement), 0.1 mV in amplitude (vertical measurement), and 1 mm in height (also a vertical measurement). Five horizontal blocks would measure 0.20 second. Five blocks on the vertical would measure 5 mm and/or 0.5 mV. Note the darker lines that delineate five of the smallest blocks.

© Cengage Learning 2013

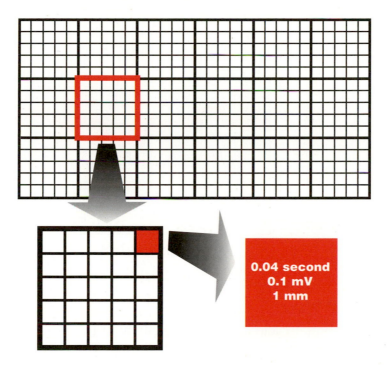

Figure 13–11

ECG monitoring paper showing markers indicating 3- and 6-second intervals. There are 15 blocks in 3 seconds and 30 blocks in 6 seconds.

© Cengage Learning 2013

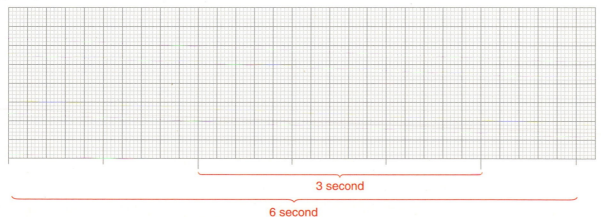

together are a *complex*. A flat, straight, or isoelectric line is called a *segment*. A waveform, or complex, connected to a segment is called an *interval*. All ECG tracings above the baseline are described as **positive** deflections. Waveforms below the baseline are **negative** deflections.

Figure 13–12

The normal ECG configurations.

© Cengage Learning 2013

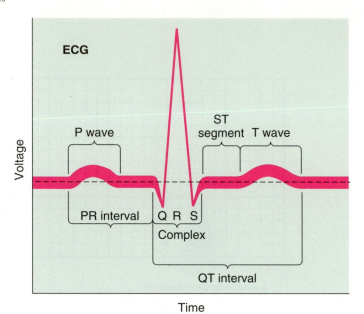

The P Wave

The normal cycle of electrical activity in the heart begins with atrial depolarization and is recorded as the *P wave*. The shape of the P wave is usually symmetrical and upright. The P wave is followed by a short pause, while the electrical current passes through the AV node. This is seen on the ECG tracing as a flat, or isoelectric, line (a segment) after the P wave. The normal duration of the P wave is 0.08 to 0.11 second (2 to $2\frac{1}{2}$ small horizontal squares). The normal amplitude of the P wave is 0.2 and 0.3 mV (2 to 3 small vertical squares) (Figure 13–13).

An increased duration or amplitude of the P wave indicates the presence of atrial abnormalities, such as hypertension, valvular disease, or congenital heart defect. Repolarization of the atria is usually not recorded on an ECG tracing, because atrial repolarization normally occurs when the ventricles are depolarizing, which is a greater electrical activity. When depolarization of the atria occurs from outside the SA node, the P wave configuration appears different than an SA node-induced P wave. The rhythm of the SA wave will also be disrupted and reset. When the atria depolarize in response to a stimulus outside the SA node, the wave is called a *P prime (P') wave*.

The PR Interval

The *PR interval* starts at the beginning of the P wave and ends at the beginning of the QRS complex. The normal duration of the PR interval is 0.12 to 0.20 second (3 to 5 small horizontal squares). The PR interval represents the total atrial (supraventricular) electrical activity prior to the activation of the bundle of His, ventricular branches, and Purkinje fiber system (see Figure 13–13).

Figure 13–13

The durations of the normal ECG configurations.

© Cengage Learning 2013

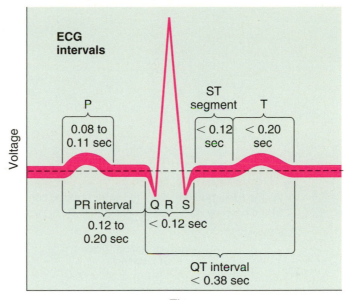

The QRS Complex

The *QRS complex* represents ventricular depolarization. Because the muscle mass of the ventricles is greater than that of the atria, the amplitude of the QRS complex is higher than the P wave. The QRS complex consists of three separate waveforms: **Q wave**, **R wave**, and **S wave**. The first negative deflection (below the baseline) after the P wave is the *Q wave* (Figure 13–14A on page 448). The next tall positive deflection (above the baseline) is the *R wave* (Figure 13–14B). The *S wave* is the small negative deflection (below the baseline) that follows the R wave (Figure 13–14C).

Relative to the ECG lead, the QRS complex may not have a Q wave or an S wave. Under normal conditions, the duration of the QRS complex is less than 0.12 second ($2\frac{1}{2}$ little squares) (see Figure 13–13). Abnormal ventricular-induced QRS complex waves are longer than 0.12 second. Other characteristics of an abnormal QRS complex include premature ventricular contractions (PVCs), increased amplitude, and T waves of opposite polarity.

The ST Segment

The *ST segment* represents the time between ventricular depolarization and repolarization (see Figure 13–13). The ST segment begins at the end of the QRS complex (called the J point) and ends at the beginning of the T wave. Normally, the ST segment measures 0.12 second or less. The ST segment may be elevated or depressed due to myocardial injury, ischemia, and certain cardiac medications. A flat, horizontal ST segment above or below the baseline is highly suggestive of ischemia. Figure 13–15 on page 448 shows four different ST segment variations.

Figure 13–14

A. Q waveform of the QRS complex; **B.** R waveform of the QRS complex; **C.** S waveform of the QRS complex.

© Cengage Learning 2013

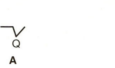

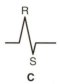

A

B

C

Figure 13–15

A. The ST segment highlighted within cardiac complex. **B.** Note the variations in ST segments in at the baseline. **C.** 3-mm ST segment ↑. **D.** 3-mm ST segment ↓.

© Cengage Learning 2013

Ventricular Repolarization
ST Segment

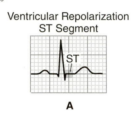

A

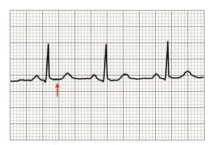

B

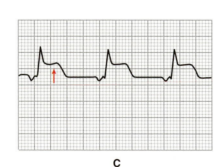

C

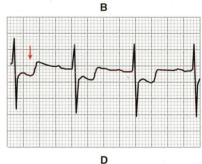

D

The T Wave

The *T wave* represents ventricular repolarization, rest, and recovery (see Figure 13–13). Normally, the T wave has a positive deflection of about 0.5 mV, although it may have a negative deflection. It may, however, be of such low amplitude that it is difficult to read. The duration of the T wave normally measures 0.20 second or less.

At the beginning of the T wave, the ventricles are in their effective refractory period. At about the peak of the T wave, the ventricles are in their relative refractory period and, thus, are vulnerable to stimulation (see Figure 13–13). T waves are sensitive indicators for the presence of a number of abnormalities, including acid–base imbalances, hyperventilation, hyperkalemia, ischemia, and the use of various drugs. Figure 13–16 shows common T wave variations.

© Cengage Learning 2013

Figure 13–16

A. The T wave representing ventricular depolarization; **B.** measuring the T wave with ST segment elevation; **C.** measuring an inverted T wave with ST segment depression.

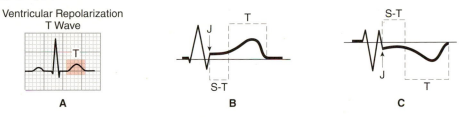

Figure 13–17

The U wave highlighted (arrow) within the cardiac complex. U waves plot only with other U waves, just as P waves plot with P waves, and QRS plots with the QRS complex.

© Cengage Learning 2013

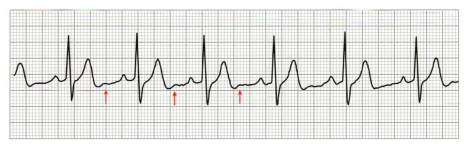

The U Wave

The *U wave* follows the T wave and has the same polarity (deflection) as the T wave (Figure 13–17). Its origin and mechanism are not known. Because of its low voltage, the U wave usually is flat and not seen; however, it often becomes prominent in the presence of certain electrolyte disturbances, certain medications, and heart disease.

The QT Interval

The *QT interval* is measured from the beginning of the QRS complex to the end of the T wave (see Figure 13–13). The QT interval represents total ventricular activity, that is, ventricular depolarization (QRS) and repolarization (ST segment and the T wave). The normal QT interval measures about 0.38 second, and varies in males and females and with age. As a general rule, the QT interval should be about 40 percent of the measured RR interval.

Finally, note that the QT interval varies indirectly to the heart rate; that is, the faster the heart rate, the shorter the QT interval time. This is because when the heart rate is fast, repolarization is also faster. The QT interval time is longer with slower heart rates. The QT interval often varies with use of certain cardiac drugs that alter the heart's action potential and refractory times.

Chapter Summary

The electrocardiogram (ECG) is a graphic representation of the electrical activity of the heart's conductive system monitored and recorded over a period of time. The essential knowledge components for the standard 12-ECG system include (1) the standard limb leads—leads I, II, III, aVR, aVL, and aVF; (2) how an electrical impulse of the ventricle is recorded; (3) the precordial (chest) leads—V_1, V_2, V_3, V_4, V_5, and V_6; and (4) the normal ECG configurations. Table 13–2 summarizes the normal ECG configurations and corresponding activity of the heart. The clinical connection associated with these topics includes the electrocardiogram—the role of the respiratory therapist.

Table 13–2	
Summary of Normal ECG Configurations and Heart Activity	

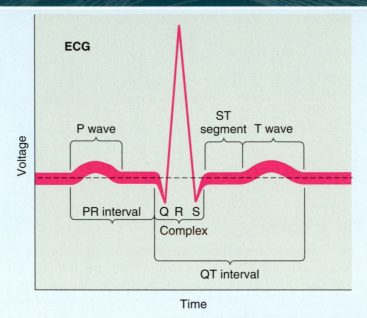

ECG Configuration	Heart Activity
P wave	Atrial depolarization
PR interval	Total atrial electrical activity prior to activation of the bundle of His, ventricular branches, and Purkinje fiber system
QRS complex	Ventricular depolarization
ST segment	Time between ventricular depolarization and repolarization
T wave	Ventricular repolarization
U wave	Usually is flat or not seen. Often prominent in the presence of certain electrolyte disturbances, certain medications, and heart disease
QT interval	Total ventricular activity (QRS complex, ST segment, and T wave)

Clinical Connection—13-1

Electrocardiograms (ECGs)—The Role of the Respiratory Therapist

In many hospitals throughout the United States, the respiratory therapist is the person who obtains the ECG—which places the respiratory therapist at the patient's bedside at a prime time to both witness and respond to life-threatening arrhythmias. This is why the respiratory practitioner must have a good ECG knowledge base; the therapist must also be able to interpret ECG results correctly. Without a doubt, the early recognition—and intervention—of a serious cardiac problem can minimize heart damage. Oftentimes, the respiratory therapist serves as the first link in care for the patient experiencing a cardiac arrest and is a vital part of the health care team once the patient has stabilized. In addition, a fundamental knowledge base and understanding of ECG changes can further enhance the respiratory therapist's patient assessment and treatment plans. Chapter 14 provides the reader the essential information required to interpret the most commonly seen cardiac arrhythmias.

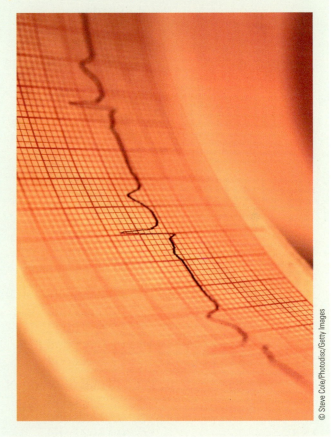

© Steve Cole/Photodisc/Getty Images

Review Questions

1. Which of the following is (are) unipolar leads?
   1. aVL
   2. Lead II
   3. V6
   4. Lead III
   5. aVR
      A. 3 only
      B. 1 and 5 only
      C. 2 and 4 only
      D. 1, 3, and 5 only

2. The imaginary line that can be drawn between the positive and negative electrodes in leads I, II, and III is called the
   A. axis
   B. vector
   C. equiphasic line
   D. baseline

3. Which of the following monitor the electrical activity of the heart in the frontal plane?
  1. aVL
  2. Lead II
  3. aVR
  4. Lead III
  5. aVF
      A. 1 and 3 only
      B. 1, 4, and 5 only
      C. 2, 3, 4, and 5 only
      D. 1, 2, 3, 4, and 5

4. Which of the following monitor the left ventricle?
  1. V1
  2. V2
  3. V3
  4. V5
  5. V6
      A. 1 only
      B. 5 only
      C. 2 and 3 only
      D. 4 and 5 only

5. The small squares on the standard ECG paper represent
      A. 0.02 second
      B. 0.04 second
      C. 0.06 second
      D. 0.08 second

6. The normal duration of the P wave is no longer than
      A. 0.80 second
      B. 0.11 second
      C. 0.15 second
      D. 0.20 second

7. The normal duration of the PR interval is no longer than
      A. 0.12 second
      B. 0.15 second
      C. 0.20 second
      D. 0.50 second

8. The normal duration of the QRS complex is less than
      A. 0.01 second
      B. 0.05 second
      C. 0.12 second
      D. 0.15 second

9. The normal duration of the ST segment is
      A. 0.12 second or less
      B. 0.15 second or less
      C. 0.20 second or less
      D. 0.50 second or less

10. The normal duration of the T wave is
      A. 0.05 second or less
      B. 0.10 second or less
      C. 0.15 second or less
      D. 0.20 second or less

Objectives

By the end of this chapter, the student should be able to:

1. Describe the systematic approach to ECG interpretation, including:
   —General inspection
   —Analysis of ventricular activity
   —Analysis of atrial activity
   —Assessment of atrioventricular relationship
2. Describe the P wave, PR interval, QRS complex, QRS rate, and QRS rhythm in the normal sinus rhythm.
3. Describe the P wave, PR interval, QRS complex, QRS rate, and QRS rhythm in the following abnormal sinus mechanisms:
   —Sinus bradycardia
   —Sinus tachycardia
   —Sinus arrhythmia
   —Sinus block
   —Sinus arrest
4. Describe the clinical connection associated with the treatment protocol of bradycardia.
5. Describe the P wave, PR interval, QRS complex, QRS rate, and QRS rhythm in the following abnormal atrial mechanisms:
   —Premature atrial complex
   —Atrial bigeminy
   —Atrial tachycardia
   —Atrial flutter
   —Atrial fibrillation
6. Describe the P wave, PR interval, QRS complex, QRS rate, and QRS rhythm for the following abnormal ventricular mechanisms:
   —Premature ventricular contraction

   • Uniform PVCs
   • Multiform PVCs
   • Paired PVCs
   • Bigeminal PVCs
   • Trigeminal PVCs
   —Ventricular tachycardia
   —Ventricular flutter
   —Ventricular fibrillation
   —Asystole
7. Describe the clinical connections associated with treatment protocol for a pulseless arrest.
8. Describe the clinical connection associated with the treatment protocol for ventricular fibrillation and pulseless ventricular tachycardia.
9. Describe the clinical connection associated with the treatment protocol for asystole and pulseless electrical activity.
10. Describe the P wave, PR interval, QRS complex, QRS rate, and QRS rhythm in the following atrioventricular (AV) defects:
    —Sinus rhythm with first-degree AV block
    —Sinus rhythm with second-degree AV block
    —Complete AV block
11. Complete the review questions at the end of the chapter.

How to Analyze the Waveforms

There are many correct ways in which to approach electrocardiograph (ECG) interpretation. Fundamental to all good methods is a consistent, systematic approach. Some practitioners, for example, begin by looking at the P waves and then move on to the QRS complexes, whereas others start by looking at the QRS complexes and then the P waves. Both approaches are correct. The key is to be systematic and consistent. Table 14–1 provides an overview of the steps involved in a good systematic approach to ECG analysis. A short discussion of this approach follows.

Step 1: Does the General Appearance of the ECG Tracing Appear Normal or Abnormal?

Closely scan the ECG tracing and identify each of the wave components. Note any specific wave abnormalities. Are there any abnormalities—in terms of appearance or duration—in the P waves, QRS complexes, ST segments, or T waves? Do the complexes appear consistent from one beat to the next? Does the rate appear too slow or too fast? Does the rhythm appear regular or irregular? Are there any extra beats or pauses? It is often helpful to circle any possible abnormalities during step 1. This initial process helps to pinpoint problem areas that can be inspected more carefully during the steps discussed next.

Table 14–1

Systematic Approach to ECG Interpretation

Step 1: General inspection

Step 2: Analysis of ventricular activity (QRS complexes)
- Rate
- Rhythm
- Shape

Step 3: Analysis of atrial activity
- Rate
- Rhythm
- Shape

Step 4: Assessment of atrioventricular relationship
- Conduction ratio
- Discharge sequence (P:QRS or QRS:P)
- PR interval

Step 5: ECG interpretation
- Normal sinus rhythm
- Cardiac dysrhythmias

© Cengage Learning 2013

Step 2: Does the Ventricular Activity (QRS Complexes) Appear Normal or Abnormal?

Rate

When the ventricular heart rate is **regular**, the rate can be determined by counting the number of large squares between two consecutive QRS complexes and then dividing 300 by the number of large squares. For example, if there are three large squares between two QRS complexes, then the ventricular rate would be 100/min (300 ÷ 3 = 100) (Figure 14–1). Table 14–2 shows the estimated heart rate for different numbers of large squares between two QRS complexes. Appendix VII provides a more complete presentation of the estimated heart rate for different numbers of large squares between two QRS complexes.

When the ventricular heart rate is **irregular**, the rate can be calculated by using the vertical 3-second marks in the upper margins of the ECG paper. This is done by counting the number of QRS complexes in a 6-second interval (two 3-second marks), then multiplying this number by 10. For example, if seven

---

Figure 14–1

ECG recording with markers denoting the number of large squares (blocks) between the QRS complexes (RR interval). Because there are three such blocks between QRS complexes, dividing 3 into 300 provides the estimated rate of 100 per minute.

© Cengage Learning 2013

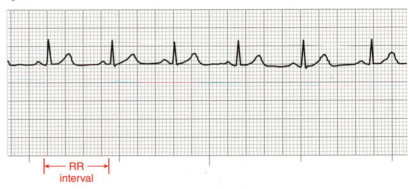

├── RR ──┤
interval

Table 14–2

Calculating Heart Rate by Counting the Number of Large ECG Squares

Distance between Two QRS Complexes (number of large squares)	Estimated Heart Rate (per min)
1	300
2	150
3	100
4	75
5	60
6	50

© Cengage Learning 2013

QRS complexes are present in two 3-second intervals (6 seconds), then the ventricular rate is about 70 beats/min (bpm) (7 × 10 = 70). Normal *adult* heart rate is between 60 and 100 bpm. A heart rate of less than 60 bpm is classified as bradycardia. A heart rate greater than 100 bpm is called tachycardia.

Rhythm

The ventricular rhythm is determined by comparing the shortest RR intervals with the longest RR intervals. When the time variation between the shortest RR interval and the longest RR interval is greater than 0.12 second, the rhythm is *irregular*; a variation of 0.12 or less is a *regular* rhythm.

Shape

Finally, determine if the shape of the QRS complexes is identical from one complex to another. Are the QRS complexes of the expected polarity, considering the monitoring lead? The shape as well as the duration of the QRS complex help to determine the origin of the ventricular depolarization. The normal QRS duration is 0.10 second (2.5 little squares) or less. A QRS complex that is narrow and lasts 0.10 second or less represents a supraventricular origin (i.e., sinoatrial [SA] node or atrial source) and normal intraventricular conduction. When the QRS complex is greater than 0.10 second and the shape is distorted (e.g., increased amplitude, opposite polarity, slurred), then an abnormal electrical source (ectopic focus) is likely to be present within the ventricle.

Step 3: Does the Atrial Activity Appear Normal or Abnormal?

Similar to the assessment of the QRS complexes, the rate, rhythm, and shape of the atrial activity (P waves) are evaluated. The rate of the atrial activity is calculated in the same way as the QRS complexes (see Table 14–2). Normally, the P wave rate and the QRS rate are the same. The atrial rhythm is calculated in the same way as the QRS rhythm, except that in this case PP intervals are used. The shape of the P waves is then evaluated. Abnormalities may include P waves that are not of expected polarity, atrial flutter, fibrillation, or P prime (P′) waves (i.e., waves initiated outside the SA node).

Step 4: Does the Atrioventricular (AV) Relationship Appear to be Normal?

Is the AV conduction ratio 1:1? In other words, is a P wave followed by a QRS complex? When the AV conduction ratio is greater than 1:1 (e.g., 2:1, 3:1), not all the atrial impulses are being conducted to the ventricles. For example, an AV conduction ratio of 2:1 or 3:1 indicates that every second or third atrial impulse is being blocked. In some cases, the AV conduction is completely blocked and the P waves and QRS complexes are totally unrelated. The best method to determine the AV conduction ratio is to ask these two questions:

1. Is each P wave followed by a QRS complex?

2. Is each QRS complex preceded by a single P wave?

When the answer to each of these questions is no, evaluate the rhythm to determine if a pattern exists. An excellent method to determine this is to measure the PR intervals to see if the intervals are fixed or variable. The PR

ECG tracing of a normal sinus rhythm.

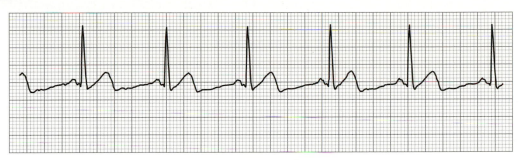

interval is measured from the beginning of the P wave to the start of the QRS complex. The PR interval represents the time between the start of atrial depolarization to the beginning of ventricular depolarization. During a normal sinus rhythm, the PR interval is constant from one beat to the next and is no longer than 0.20 second. A PR interval greater than 0.20 second represents an abnormal delay in AV conduction.

Step 5: What Is the ECG Interpretation?

Normal Sinus Rhythm

If there are no variations from the normal sinus rhythm (NSR)—the gold standard by which most ECG dysrhythmias are measured, compared, and analyzed—then the ECG tracing is normal. When the ECG tracing varies from the normal sinus rhythm, however, the interpretation must incorporate all the information that describes the abnormal electrical activity of the heart. Thus, in view of these facts, the recognition of the normal sinus rhythm is an essential prerequisite to the interpretation of abnormal ECG tracings. The following summarizes the ECG characteristics of the normal sinus rhythm, as viewed from lead II:

- **P wave:** The P waves are positive (upright) and uniform. A QRS complex follows every P wave.
- **PR interval:** The duration of the PR interval is between 0.12 and 0.20 second and is constant from beat to beat.
- **QRS complex:** The duration of the QRS complex is 0.12 second or less. A P wave precedes every QRS complex.
- **QRS rate:** Between 60 and 100 bpm.
- **QRS rhythm:** Regular.

Figure 14–2 shows an ECG tracing of a normal sinus rhythm.

Common Cardiac Dysrhythmias

The most common cardiac dysrhythmias can be subdivided into the following four major categories: sinus mechanisms, atrial mechanisms, ventricular mechanisms, and AV conduction defects. Table 14–3 on page 458 provides an overview of the major dysrhythmias found under each of these categories.

Table 14–3			
Common Cardiac Dysrhythmias			
Sinus Mechanisms	Atrial Mechanisms	Ventricular Mechanisms	AV Conduction Defects

Sinus bradycardia
Sinus tachycardia
Sinus arrhythmia
Sinus block
Sinus arrest
	Premature atrial complex (PAC)
	Atrial bigeminy
	Atrial tachycardia
	Atrial flutter
	Atrial fibrillation
		Premature ventricular complex (PVC)
		  Uniform PVCs
		  Multiform PVCs
		  Paired PVCs
		  Bigeminal PVCs
		  Trigeminal PVCs
		Ventricular tachycardia
		Ventricular flutter
		Ventricular fibrillation
		Asystole
			Sinus rhythm with first-degree AV block
			Sinus rhythm with second-degree AV block
			Complete AV block

© Cengage Learning 2013

The Sinus Mechanisms

Sinus Bradycardia

Bradycardia means "slow heart." In *sinus bradycardia*, the heart rate is less than 60 bpm. The ECG characteristics of sinus bradycardia in lead II are as follows:

- **P wave:** The P waves are positive and uniform. Each P wave is followed by a QRS complex.
- **PR interval:** The PR interval has a normal duration between 0.12 and 0.20 second and is constant from beat to beat.
- **QRS complex:** The QRS complex duration is 0.12 second or less. P wave precedes every QRS complex.
- **QRS rate:** Less than 60 bpm.
- **QRS rhythm:** Regular.

Figure 14–3 shows an ECG tracing of sinus bradycardia. Figure 14–4 shows the presence of sinus bradycardia in two leads in a healthy adult.

Sinus bradycardia is often normal in athletes who have increased their cardiac stroke volume through physical conditioning. Common pathologic causes of sinus bradycardia include a weakened or damaged SA node, severe or chronic hypoxemia, increased intracranial pressure, obstructive sleep apnea, and use of certain drugs (most notably beta-blocking agents). Sinus bradycardia may lead to a decreased cardiac output and lowered blood pressure. In severe cases, sinus bradycardia may lead to a decreased perfusion and tissue hypoxia. The individual may have a weak or absent pulse, poor capillary refill, cold and clammy skin, and a depressed sensorium.

Figure 14–3

An ECG tracing showing one (+) P wave to the left of each QRS complex; the PR interval is consistent, and the heart rate is less than 60 bpm. These computations represent a sinus bradycardia.

© Cengage Learning 2013

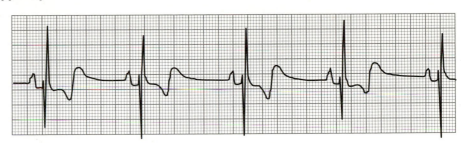

Figure 14–4

An ECG tracing showing sinus bradycardia in two leads from a physically fit adult.

© Cengage Learning 2013

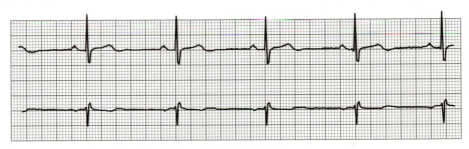

Sinus Tachycardia

Tachycardia means "fast heart." In *sinus tachycardia*, the heart rate is between 100 and 160 bpm, and the rhythm is regular. The ECG characteristics of sinus tachycardia in lead II are as follows:

- **P wave:** The P waves are positive and uniform. Each P wave is followed by a QRS complex.
- **PR interval:** The PR interval has a normal duration between 0.12 and 0.20 second and is constant from beat to beat.

Clinical Connection—14-1

Bradycardia: ACLS Treatment Protocol*

Atropine: The first drug of choice for symptomatic bradycardia.

Dopamine: Second-line drug for symptomatic bradycardia when atropine is not effective.

Epinephrine: Can be used as an equal alternative to dopamine when atropine is not effective.

* Advanced Cardiac Life Support (http://acls-algorithms.com)

Figure 14–5

An ECG tracing from an exercising adult. Note there is a single (+) P wave to the left of each QRS complex; the rate is 150 bpm.

© Cengage Learning 2013

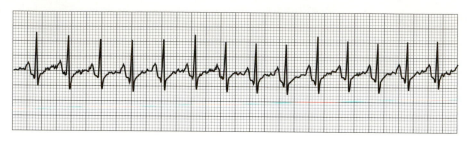

- **QRS complex:** The QRS complex duration is 0.12 second or less. A P wave precedes every QRS complex.
- **QRS rate:** Between 100 and 160 bpm.
- **QRS rhythm:** Regular.

Figure 14–5 shows an ECG tracing of sinus tachycardia.

In adults, sinus tachycardia is the normal physiologic response to exercise, emotions, fever, pain, fear, anger, and anxiety. Sinus tachycardia is also caused by physiologic stress such as hypoxemia, hypovolemia, severe anemia, hyperthermia, massive hemorrhage, hyperthyroidism, and any condition that leads to an increased sympathetic stimulation. Pathologic conditions associated with sinus tachycardia include congestive heart failure, cardiogenic shock, myocardial ischemia, heart valve disorders, pulmonary embolism, hypertension, and infarction.

Sinus Arrhythmia

In *sinus arrhythmia*, the heart rate varies by more than 10 percent. The P-QRS-T pattern is normal, but the interval between groups of complexes (e.g., the PP or RR intervals) vary. The ECG characteristics in sinus arrhythmia in lead II are as follows:

- **P wave:** The P waves are positive and uniform. Each P wave is followed by a QRS complex.
- **PR interval:** The PR interval has a normal duration between 0.12 and 0.20 second and is constant from beat to beat.
- **QRS complex:** The QRS complex duration is 0.12 second or less. A P wave precedes every QRS complex.
- **QRS rate:** Varies by more than 10 percent.
- **QRS rhythm:** Irregular.

Figure 14–6 shows an ECG tracing of a sinus arrhythmia.

A sinus arrhythmia is normal in children and young adults. The patient's pulse will often increase during inspiration and decrease during expiration. No treatment is required unless there is a significant alteration in the patient's arterial blood pressure.

Sinus (SA) Block

In a *sinus (SA) block*, also called a *sinus exit block*, the SA node initiates an impulse but the electrical current through the atria is blocked. Thus, the atria—and the ventricles—do not depolarize or contract, resulting in no P wave or

Figure 14–6

An ECG tracing of sinus arrhythmia 54 to 71 bpm..

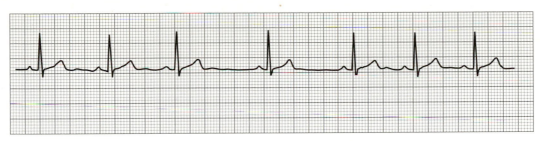

QRS complex. The next P-QRS-T complex, however, appears at the precise time it would normally appear if the sinus block had not occurred. In other words, the ECG shows that the heart has skipped a beat. The ECG characteristics for sinus block in lead II are as follows:

- **P wave:** The P waves are positive and uniform; however, an entire P-QRS-T complex is missing.
- **PR interval:** The PR interval has a normal duration between 0.12 and 0.20 second and is constant from beat to beat, except for the pause when an entire cycle is missing. The PR interval may be slightly shorter after the pause.
- **QRS complex:** Except for the missing cycle, the QRS complex duration is 0.12 second or less, and a P wave precedes every QRS complex.
- **QRS rate:** The rate may vary according to the number and position of missing P-QRS-T cycles.
- **QRS rhythm:** The rhythm may be regular or irregular according to the number and position of missing P-QRS-T cycles.

Figure 14–7 shows an ECG tracing of a sinus block.

Sinus Arrest

Sinus arrest (SA node arrest) is the sudden failure of the SA node to initiate an impulse (i.e., no P wave). It is common to see two, three, or four P-QRS-T complexes missing following a normal P-QRS-T complex. This period of inactivity is then followed by a normal sinus rhythm. Generally, there is no pattern of frequency of occurrence; that is, the individual may demonstrate one or two periods of sinus arrests, and then demonstrate a normal sinus rhythm for

Figure 14–7

An ECG tracing showing SA block.

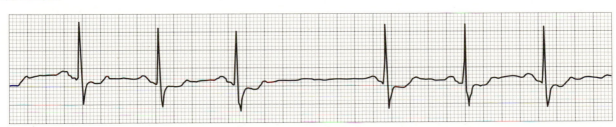

An ECG tracing from an 82-year-old patient showing sinus arrest. The patient required insertion of an electronic pacemaker.

© Cengage Learning 2013

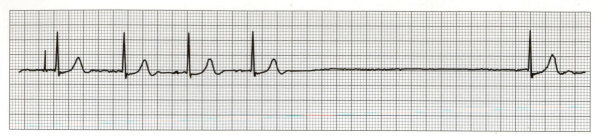

minutes, or even hours, before another sinus arrest appears. When the sinus arrest is excessively long, the AV node usually takes over and initiates a new (but slower) rhythm called an *escape rate*. The ECG characteristics for sinus arrest in lead II are as follows:

- **P wave:** No P wave.
- **PR interval:** The PR interval has a normal duration between 0.12 and 0.20 second and is constant from beat to beat.
- **QRS complex:** The QRS complex duration is 0.10 second or less. After a sinus arrest, however, the QRS duration may be greater than 0.12 second when the escape rhythm is initiated by the AV node.
- **QRS rate:** Normal sinus rhythm during nonsinus arrest periods.
- **QRS rhythm:** The QRS complexes before and after the sinus arrest are regular. The escape rate may be regular or irregular.

Figure 14–8 shows an ECG tracing of a sinus arrest.

The Atrial Mechanisms

Premature Atrial Complex

A *premature atrial complex* (PAC) results when abnormal electrical activity in the atria causes the atria to depolarize before the SA node fires. An electrical current that originates outside the SA node is called an **ectopic focus**. An ectopic focus in the atria results in a **P prime** (P′) on the ECG tracing. The P′ is usually easy to identify. It will be early or premature and it will usually vary in size and shape from the normal sinus P wave. PACs also disrupt the sinus rate and rhythm. When the sinus node regains control, the rate and rhythm will return to normal. The QRS configuration is usually normal. The ECG characteristics of a PAC in lead II are as follows:

- **P wave:** The P′ wave will appear different than a normal SA node-induced P wave. The P′ may be hidden, or partially hidden, in the preceding T wave. P′ waves hidden in the T wave often distort or increase the amplitude of the T wave. A PAC may not successfully move into the ventricles if the AV node or bundle branches are in their complete refractory period. This is called a *blocked* or *nonconducted* PAC.
- **PR interval:** The P′R interval may be normal or prolonged, depending on the timing of the PAC. Most often, however, the P′R interval is different from the normal SA node rhythm.

- **QRS complex:** Except for the abnormal cycle generated by the P' wave, the QRS complex duration is 0.12 second or less, and a normal P wave precedes every QRS complex.
- **QRS rate:** Varies.
- **QRS rhythm:** Irregular.

Figure 14–9 shows an ECG tracing of a sinus rhythm with PAC. Figure 14–10 is an ECG tracing illustrating a sinus rhythm with two nonconducted PACs.

Depending on their severity and frequency, PACs may be of no clinical significance, or they may result in harmful atrial arrhythmias. Causes of PACs include hypoxemia, impending heart failure, right coronary artery disease, excessive use of digitalis, pericarditis, ingestion of stimulants or caffeine, and recreational drug abuse. PACs are commonly seen in patients with chronic obstructive pulmonary disease (COPD) when the disease is accompanied by increased pulmonary vascular resistance. PACs are also frequently seen in females during the third trimester of pregnancy because of the increased workload of the mother's heart, which develops primarily because (1) the mother's blood volume increases by as much as 50 percent during the third trimester and (2) the additional perfusion of the fetus and placenta causes the peripheral vascular resistance to increase.

Figure 14–9

An ECG tracing showing one (+) P wave to the left of each of the first three sinus beats, a sinus rhythm at 96 bpm. The next QRS complex is similar to the sinus QRSs but is premature and has a (+) P' superimposed on the previous T wave. The sinus P waves do not plot through the event. The PACs recur (arrow) each time, disturbing sinus rhythm. The ECG interpretation would be sinus rhythm at 96 bpm with frequent PACs.

© Cengage Learning 2013

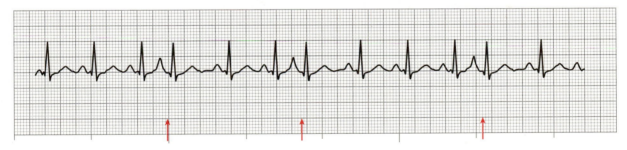

Figure 14–10

An ECG tracing showing one (+) P wave to the left of each of the first two sinus beats, a sinus rhythm. A sudden pause occurs in the cadence of the sinus mechanism. Look back at the last T wave and note the increased amplitude. The height of the T wave is a combination of P wave and T wave amplitudes. The sinus P waves do not plot through the event, and the cadence of the sinus rhythm resumes at about 75 bpm. The ECG interpretation would be sinus rhythm at 75 bpm with frequent, nonconducted PACs.

© Cengage Learning 2013

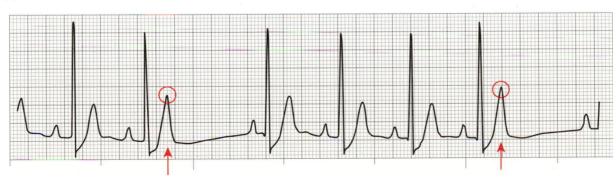

An ECG tracing showing a sinus mechanism with one (+) P for each QRS. However, not all the P waves are similar. In fact, there appear to be premature QRS complexes, each with a premature P' wave, creating a pattern; every other beat is an ectopic. When every other beat is an ectopic, this is *bigeminy*. In this case, the ectopic has its origin in the atria. Thus, the ECG interpretation would be sinus rhythm at 86 bpm with *atrial bigeminy*.

© Cengage Learning 2013

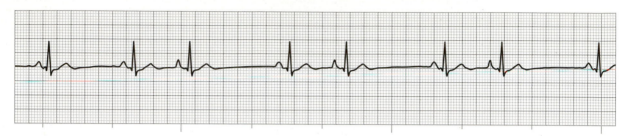

Atrial Bigeminy

Atrial bigeminy are said to be present when every other beat is an ectopicatrial beat—a PAC. In other words, the ECG tracing shows a PAC, a normal sinus beat, a PAC, a normal sinus beat, and so on (Figure 14–11). Atrial bigeminy are often one of the first signs of congestive heart failure. Patients with atrial bigeminy should be assessed for peripheral edema, sudden weight gain, and adventitious breath sounds.

Atrial Tachycardia

Atrial tachycardia is present when an atrial ectopic focus depolarizes the atria at a rate of 130 to 250 bpm. Generally, the AV node delays many of the atrial ectopic beats and the resulting ventricular rate is usually normal. The ventricular rhythm may be regular or irregular. When atrial tachycardia appears suddenly and then disappears moments later, it is referred to as paroxysmal atrial tachycardia. The ECG characteristics of atrial tachycardia in lead II are as follows:

- **P' wave:** Starts abruptly, at rates of 130 to 250 bpm. The P' wave may or may not be seen. Visible P' waves differ in configuration from the normal sinus P wave. At more rapid rates, the P' is hidden in the preceding T wave and cannot be seen as a separate entity.
- **P'R interval:** The PR interval has a normal duration between 0.12 and 0.20 second and is constant from beat to beat. The P'R interval is difficult to measure at rapid rates.
- **QRS complex:** The QRS complex duration is 0.12 second or less. A P wave usually precedes every QRS complex, although a 2:1 AV conduction ratio is often seen. The QRS complexes during atrial tachycardia may be normal or abnormal, depending on the degree of ventricular refractoriness and AV conduction time.
- **QRS rate:** Very regular.
- **QRS rhythm:** Atrial tachycardia begins suddenly and is very regular.

Figure 14–12 shows an example of atrial tachycardia. Figure 14–13 shows an example of paroxysmal atrial tachycardia.

Atrial tachycardia is associated with conditions that stimulate the sympathetic nervous system, such as anxiety, excessive ingestion of caffeine or alcohol, and smoking. Unlike sinus tachycardia, which generally goes unnoticed

Figure 14–12

An example of the onset of atrial tachycardia. In the beginning, the tracing shows a sinus rhythm at 100 bpm. A PAC (arrow) begins the sudden change in rate at 188 bpm.

© Cengage Learning 2013

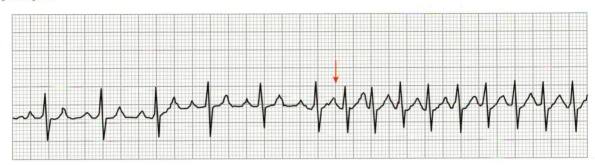

Figure 14–13

An ECG tracing showing a narrow QRS complex of similar configuration throughout. Plotting out the P waves, the atrial rate is 86 bpm for the first two complexes. The rate changes suddenly. Note the PAC (arrow) at the beginning of the tachycardia. The rate here is 136 bpm, and T waves are distorted and lumpy, indicating the atrial ectopics. The rate changes again, beginning with a pause and reverting to a sinus rhythm. The visible sudden onset and end of the tachycardia is called *paroxysm*. The identification is sinus at 86 → atrial tachycardia (PAT) at 136 per minute → sinus at 86 per minute. The sinus P waves do not plot through this event.

© Cengage Learning 2013

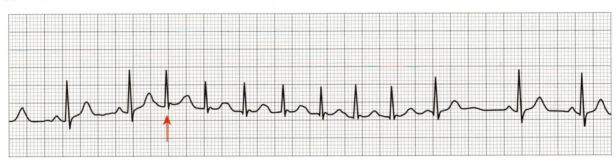

by the patient, the patient "feels" the sudden onset of atrial tachycardia. Young adults sometimes have sudden periods of paroxysmal atrial tachycardia. Atrial tachycardia is also associated with the early stages of menopause.

Atrial Flutter

A consequence of PACs is the development of *atrial flutter*. In atrial flutter, the normal P wave is absent and replaced by two or more regular sawtooth-like waves, called *flutter* or *ff waves*. The QRS complex is normal and the ventricular rate may be regular or irregular, depending on the relationship of the atrial to ventricular beats. Figure 14–14 on page 466 shows an atrial flutter with a regular rhythm and with a 4:1 conduction ratio (i.e., four atrial beats for every ventricular beat). Usually, the atrial rate is constant between 200 and 300 bpm, whereas the ventricular rate is in the normal range. The ECG characteristics of atrial flutter in lead II are as follows:

- **ff waves:** Atrial depolarization is regular. Commonly has a sawtooth-like or sharktooth-like appearance.
- **P'R interval:** The P'R interval of the ff waves is typically 0.24 to 0.40 second and consistent with the QRS complex.

Figure 14–14

Atrial flutter with a 4:1 conduction ratio.

© Cengage Learning 2013

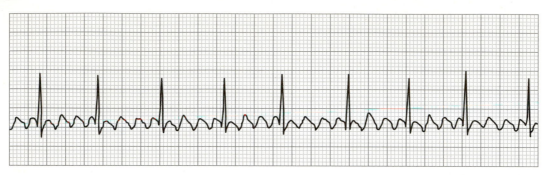

Figure 14–15

A. ECG showing new-onset atrial flutter in a patient; **B.** a continuous ECG tracing from a patient with recurrent atrial flutter. The patient was taking lanoxin 0.25 mg daily for 37 days.

© Cengage Learning 2013

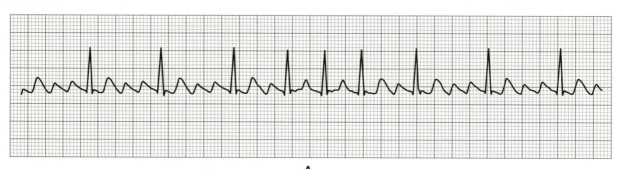

A

B

- **QRS complex:** The QRS complex duration is usually 0.12 second or less. Depending on the degree of ventricular refractoriness, the QRS may be greater than 0.12 second. When this is the case, the ff waves distort the QRS complexes and T waves.
- **QRS rate:** The QRS rate is a function of the degree of ventricular refractoriness and of the AV conduction time.
- **QRS rhythm:** Depending on AV conduction, the QRS rhythm may be regular or irregular.

Figure 14–15 shows three different examples of atrial flutter.

Atrial flutter is frequently seen in patients over 40 years of age with COPD (e.g., emphysema, chronic bronchitis), chronic heart disease (e.g., congestive heart failure, valvular heart disease), chronic hypertension, myocardial ischemia, myocardial infarction, hypoxemia, quinidine excess, pulmonary embolus, and hepatic disease.

Atrial Fibrillation

Another consequence of PACs is the development of *atrial fibrillation*, which is a chaotic, disorganized, and ineffective state occurring within the atria. During atrial fibrillation, the AV node is bombarded by hundreds of atrial ectopic impulses at various rates and amplitudes. Atrial fibrillation is usually easy to identify and is often referred to as *coarse fibrillation*. Unlike atrial flutter, atrial fibrillation is commonly seen in the clinical setting. The atrial rate cannot be measured because it often reaches rates between 300 and 600 bpm. The atrial P' waves are called *fib* or *ff* waves. Atrial fibrillation may reduce the cardiac output by as much as 20 percent because of the atrial quivering and loss of atrial filling (the so-called atrial kick). The characteristics of atrial fibrillation seen on ECG are:

- **ff waves:** Atrial depolarization is chaotic and irregular.
- **PR interval:** There are no PR intervals.
- **QRS complex:** The QRS complex duration is usually 0.12 second or less. The ff waves often distort the QRS complexes and T waves.
- **QRS rate:** The QRS rate is a function of the degree of ventricular refractoriness and conduction time.
- **QRS rhythm:** Depending on AV conduction, the QRS rhythm may be regular or irregular.

Figure 14–16 shows an example of atrial fibrillation with an irregular QRS rhythm.

Atrial fibrillation is associated with COPD, valvular heart disease, congestive heart failure, ischemic heart disease, and hypertensive heart disorders. Paroxysmal atrial fibrillation may also occur as a result of emotional stress, excessive alcohol consumption, and excessive straining and vomiting.

Figure 14–16

ECG tracing showing narrow QRS complex with an irregular rhythm. The chaotic pattern between the QRS complexes is the atrial fibrillation. This coarse pattern is easily seen.

© Cengage Learning 2013

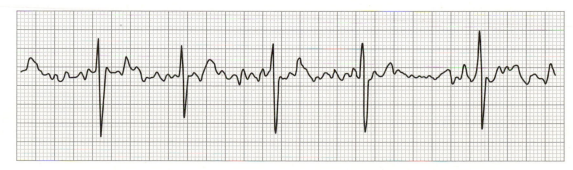

The Ventricular Mechanisms

Premature Ventricular Contraction

A *premature ventricular contraction* (PVC) is the result of abnormal electrical activity arising within the ventricles. The QRS complex is not preceded by a P wave; rather it is wide, bizarre, and unlike the normal QRS complex. The QRS has an increased amplitude with a T wave of opposite polarity; that is, a positive QRS complex is followed by a negative T wave. The characteristics of a PVC seen on ECG are:

- **P wave:** There is no P wave before a PVC. The P waves of the dominant rhythm are normal.
- **PR interval:** There is no PR interval before a PVC. The PR interval of the dominant rhythm is normal.
- **QRS complex:** The QRS complex is wide (long duration), bizarre, and unlike the normal QRS complex. The QRS of the PVC usually has an increased amplitude with a T wave of opposite polarity. The QRS-T may also present with diminished amplitude and be narrow (short duration).
- **QRS rate:** The QRS rate is that of the underlying rhythm.
- **QRS rhythm:** The rhythm is that of the underlying rhythm, and PVCs disturb the regularity.

Figure 14–17 shows an ECG tracing with a PVC.

PVCs may occur in various forms, including **uniform PVCs**, **multiform PVCs**, **paired PVCs**, **bigeminal PVCs**, and **trigeminal PVCs**. *Uniform PVCs* (also called unifocal) orginate from one focus. All the PVCs on an ECG tracing are similar in appearance, size, and amplitude (see Figure 14–17). *Multiform PVCs* (also called multifocal) originate from more than one focus. When this occurs, the PVCs take on different shapes and amplitudes (Figure 14–18). *Paired PVCs* (also called couplets) are two closely coupled PVCs in a row. Paired PVCs are dangerous because the second PVC can occur when the ventricle is refractory and may cause ventricular fibrillation (Figure 14–19). Ventricular *bigeminy* is a PVC every other beat (i.e., a normal sinus beat, PVC, sinus beat, PVC, etc.) (Figure 14–20). Ventricular *bigeminy* is often seen in patients receiving digitalis. *Trigeminy* occurs when every third beat is a PVC (see Figure 14–21 on page 470).

Figure 14–17

An ECG tracing of rhythm and two premature ventricular complexes (PVCs). Note the difference in morphology in the QRS complexes: the QRS of the premature complex is different from the dominant QRSs because it does not use the ventricular conduction pathways. The premature ventricular QRS is opposite from its T wave. The sinus P waves plot through the events because sinus cadence is undisturbed. The PVCs are similar to each other and are *uniform* in appearance. The ECG interpretation would be sinus rhythm at 86 bpm with frequent, uniform PVCs.

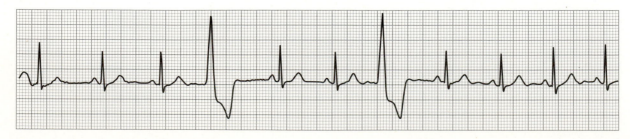

Note the difference between the PVCs. The ECG interpretation would be sinus rhythm about 78 bpm with frequent, *multiformed* PVCs.

© Cengage Learning 2013

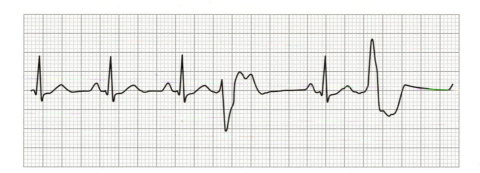

An ECG tracing showing sinus rhythm with frequent, uniform PVCs and two examples of *paired* PVCs or *couplets*. Couplets indicate the beginning of reentry and are regarded as dangerous.

© Cengage Learning 2013

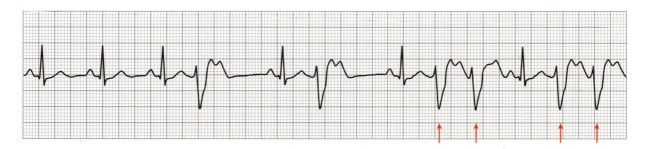

ECG tracing illustrating ventricular *bigeminy* (every other complex is a PVC).

© Cengage Learning 2013

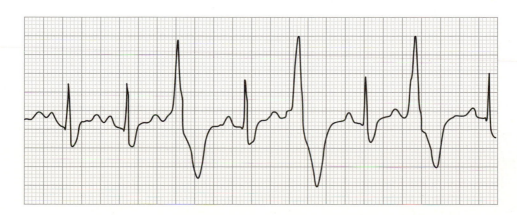

Figure 14–21

ECG tracing illustrating *trigeminy* (every third complex is a PVC).

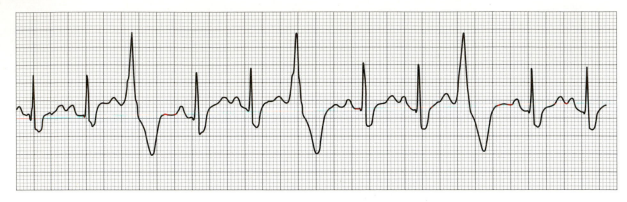

Common causes of PVCs include intrinsic myocardial disease, electrolyte disturbances (e.g., hypokalemia), hypoxemia, acidemia, hypertension, hypovolemia, stress, and congestive heart failure. PVCs may also develop as a result of use of caffeine or certain medications such as digitalis, isoproterenol, dopamine, and epinephrine. PVCs may also be a sign of theophylline, alpha-agonist, or beta-agonist toxicity.

Ventricular Tachycardia

Three or more PVCs occurring in a row represent *ventricular tachycardia*. The QRS complex is wide and bizarre in appearance, making it difficult or impossible to identify the P and T waves. The rate is regular, or slightly irregular, between 100 and 170 bpm. Ventricular tachycardia is often initiated by a PVC that is significantly premature, although it may occur suddenly after a normal sinus rhythm. When ventricular tachycardia appears suddenly and then disappears moments later, it is referred to as **paroxysmal** or **intermittent** ventricular

---

Clinical Connection—14-2

Pulseless Arrest: ACLS Treatment Protocol*

The **pulseless arrest algorithm** is the most important algorithm in the ACLS Protocol. The following four dysrhythmias produce a pulseless arrest:

- Ventricular tachycardia (VT).

- Ventricular fibrillation (VF).

- Asystole.

- Pulseless electrical activity (PEA).

The ACLS provides the following two pathways in the pulseless arrest algorithm: (1) VF/VT pathway and (2) asystole/PEA pathway. See Clinical Connection 14–3: Ventricular Fibrillation and Pulseless Ventricular Tachycardia and Clinical Connection 14–4: Asystole and Pulseless Activity later in this chapter for these two treatment protocol pathways.

---

* Advanced Cardiac Life Support (http://acls-algorithms.com)

An ECG tracing from a 55-year-old patient with ventricular tachycardia. The patient responded to antiarrhythmic medication and was reportedly successfully reperfused.

© Cengage Learning 2013

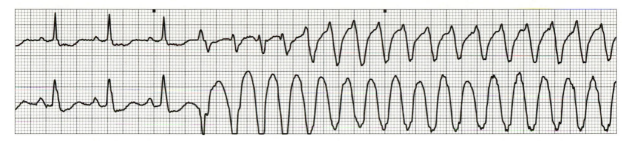

tachycardia. When the ECG tracing shows only ventricular tachycardia, it is called *sustained ventricular tachycardia* or *V-tach*. The blood pressure level is often decreased during ventricular tachycardia. The characteristics of ventricular tachycardia seen on ECG are:

- **P wave:** The P wave usually cannot be identified during ventricular tachycardia.
- **PR interval:** The PR interval cannot be measured.
- **QRS complex:** The QRS duration is usually greater than 0.12 second and bizarre in appearance. The T wave usually cannot be identified.
- **QRS rate:** Between 100 and 170 bpm. Three or more consecutive PVCs constitute ventricular tachycardia.
- **QRS rhythm:** Regular or slightly irregular.

Figure 14–22 shows an ECG tracing of ventricular tachycardia.

Ventricular Flutter

In ventricular flutter, the ECG shows poorly defined QRS complexes. The rhythm is regular or slightly irregular, and the rate is 250 to 350 bpm. Ventricular flutter is rarely seen in the clinical setting because it usually deteriorates quickly into ventricular fibrillation. There is usually no discernible peripheral pulse. The characteristics of ventricular flutter seen on ECG are:

- **P wave:** The P wave is usually not distinguishable.
- **PR interval:** The PR interval is not measurable.
- **QRS complex:** The QRS duration is usually greater than 0.12 second and bizarre in appearance. The T wave is usually not separated from the QRS complex.
- **QRS rate:** Between 250 and 350 bpm.
- **QRS rhythm:** Regular or slightly irregular.

Figure 14–23 on page 472 shows an ECG tracing of ventricular flutter.

Ventricular Fibrillation

Ventricular fibrillation is characterized by multiple and chaotic electrical activities of the ventricles. The ventricles literally quiver out of control with no beat-producing rhythm. Ventricular fibrillation is a terminal rhythm. It may

Figure 14-23

An ECG tracing showing a sinus beat followed by an R-on-T PVC, which caused ventricular flutter as confirmed on a 12-lead ECG.

© Cengage Learning 2013

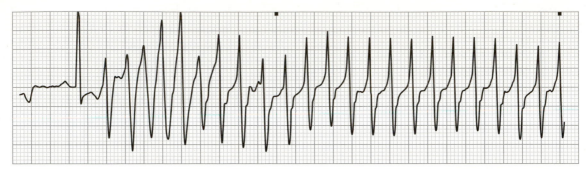

follow PVCs, ventricular tachycardia, and ventricular flutter. During ventricular fibrillation, there is no cardiac output or blood pressure and, without treatment (defibrillation), the patient will die in minutes. The characteristics of ventricular fibrillation seen on ECG are:

- **P wave:** The P waves cannot be identified.
- **PR interval:** The PR interval is not measurable.
- **QRS complex:** The QRS complex cannot be identified.
- **QRS rate:** A rate cannot be calculated.
- **QRS rhythm:** The rhythm is chaotic because of multiple, disorganized ventricular contractions.

Figure 14–24 shows three different examples of ventricular fibrillation.

Clinical Connection—14-3

Ventricular Fibrillation and Pulseless Ventricular Tachycardia: ACLS Treatment Protocol*

Defibrillation: Today, most defibrillators are biphasic. Biphasic means the electrical current moves from one paddle to the other—and then back in the other direction. A biphasic defibrillator requires less energy (compared to a monophasic defibrillator) to restore a normal heart rhythm and is believed to cause fewer skin burns and cellular heart damage. When a biphasic defibrillator is used in the treatment of VF or PVT, a dose of 120 to 200 Joules is used for the shock.

Vasopressors: Vasopressor agents are used to produce vasoconstriction and to increase blood pressure. **Epinephrine** is primarily used for its vasoconstrictive effects. During CPR, epinephrine is commonly used to help increase blood flow to the brain and heart. Vasopressin is also used for its vasoconstrictive effects and has been shown to have effects similar to those of epinephrine

Antiarrhythmic drugs: Amiodarone, Lidocaine, and **magnesium** are used for their antiarrhythmic effects. Amiodarone is used for a wide variety of atrial and ventricular tachy-arrhythmias and for rate control of rapid atrial arrhythmias. Lidocaine can be given via tracheal tube for stable ventricular tachycardia. Magnesium is used for ventricular fibrillation.

* Advanced Cardiac Life Support (http://acls-algorithms.com)

Figure 14–24

ECG tracings from three patients with ventricular fibrillation.

© Cengage Learning 2013

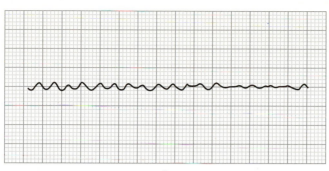

A

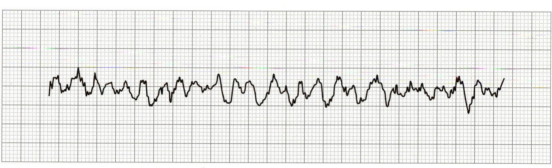

B

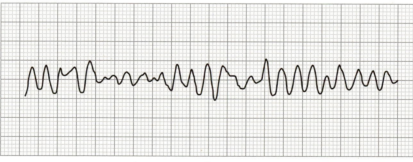

C

Asystole (Cardiac Standstill)

Asystole is the complete absence of electrical and mechanical activity. As a result, the cardiac output stops and the blood pressure falls to about 5 to 7 mm Hg. The ECG tracing appears as a flat line and indicates severe damage to the heart's electrical conduction system (Figure 14–25 on page 474). Occasionally, periods of disorganized electrical and mechanical activity may be generated during long periods of asystole; this is referred to as an *agonal rhythm* or a *dying heart*.

Figure 14–25

ECG tracings from the same patient: **A.** an apparent asystole or fine ventricular fibrillation; **B.** ventricular fibrillation confirmed on lead I.

© Cengage Learning 2013

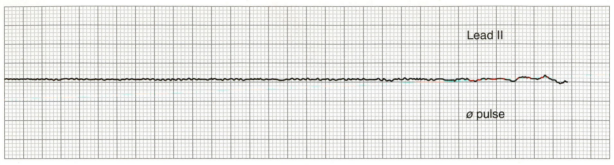

Lead II

ø pulse

A

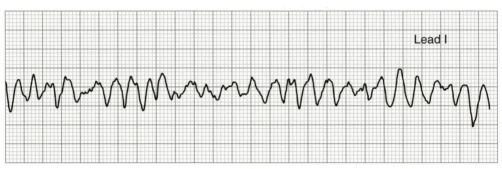

Lead I

B

Clinical Connection—14-4

Asystole and Pulseless Electrical Activity: ACLS Treatment Protocol*

Asystole is defined as a cardiac arrest rhythm in which there is no discernible electrical activity on the ECG Monitor. Asystole is sometimes referred to as a "flat line." Treatment Protocol is:

Epinephrine: Used for cardiac arrests—ventricular fibrillation, pulseless ventricular tachycardia, asystole, and pulseless electrical activity.

Vasopressin: Used as an alternative pressor to epinephrine.

Note: Atropine has been removed from the algorithm per 2010 ACLS Guidelines.

* Advanced Cardiac Life Support (http://acls-algorithms.com)

Figure 14–26

An ECG tracing illustrating a sinus rhythm at 60 bpm with a consistently prolonged PR interval that is greater than 0.20 second. Note that the PR segment is greater than 0.12 second. The ECG interpretation would be sinus rhythm at 60 bpm with first-degree AV block.

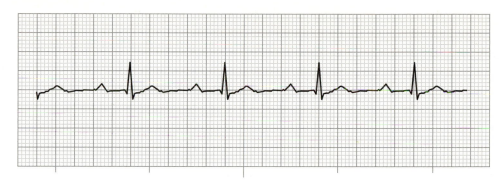

AV Conduction Defects

Sinus Rhythm with First-Degree AV Block

When the atrial impulse is delayed as it moves through the AV node, the PR interval increases. When the PR interval is consistently greater than 0.20 second, a *first-degree AV block* is said to exist. The ECG characteristics of first-degree AV block in lead II are:

- **P wave:** The P waves are positive and uniform. Each P wave is followed by a QRS complex.
- **PR interval:** The PR interval is consistently greater than 0.20 second from beat to beat.
- **QRS complex:** The duration of the QRS complex is 0.12 second or less. Each QRS complex is preceded by a P wave.
- **QRS rate:** The rate is usually based on the normal sinus rhythm and is constant between 60 and 100 bpm.
- **QRS rhythm:** The rhythm is dependent on the sinus rhythm. When a sinus arrhythmia is present, the rhythm will vary accordingly.

Figure 14–26 shows a first-degree AV block. Note that the only variation from a normal sinus rhythm is the prolonged PR interval.

Causes of first-degree AV block include right coronary artery disease, endocarditis, myocarditis, electrolyte disturbances, and aging.

Sinus Rhythm with Second-Degree AV Block: The Wenckebach Phenomenon

The **Wenckebach phenomenon** is a progressive delay in the conduction of the atrial impulse through the AV junction until, eventually, an atrial impulse is completely blocked from the ventricles. In other words, in a sinus rhythm, progressive lengthening of the PR segment occurs until a P wave is not conducted. This is because the progressive prolongation of the PR interval ultimately causes the P wave to occur during the refractory period of the

Figure 14–27

An ECG tracing showing progressive prolongation of the PR interval until the sinus P wave does not conduct into the ventricles. There is no ventricular depolarization, hence the missed QRS. The PR after the dropped beat is consistent with each instance. The ECG interpretation would be sinus rhythm at 86 bpm with second-degree AV block, Wenckebach, probably type I (QRS 0.08 second) inverted T waves, and ventricular rate 57 to 75 bpm.

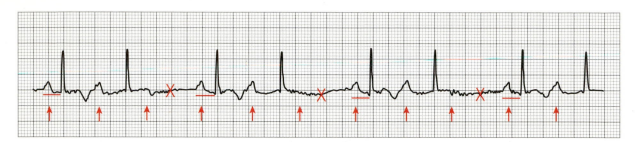

ventricles, resulting in a missed QRS complex. The next P wave occurs right on time. The first PR interval immediately after the missed QRS complex is the first PR interval of the next Wenckebach cycle. The Wenckebach phenomenon may repeat itself with variations in the number of conducted beats. The characteristics of the Wenckebach phenomenon seen on ECG are:

- Progressive prolongation of the PR interval.
- The complex Wenckebach cycle begins and ends with a P wave.
- There is one more P wave than QRS complexes in a cycle.
- Irregular or decreasing RR intervals.

Figure 14–27 shows an ECG tracing of the Wenckebach phenomenon.

Complete AV Block

When the pathology of the AV junction is severe, all the sinus impulses may be blocked. When a **complete AV block** is present, the *bundle of His* takes control of the ventricular rhythm at a rate of 40 to 60 bpm. This mechanism is referred to as the *escape junctional pacemaker*. The ventricular rhythm is regular. The sinus rhythm continues at its normal rate (60 to 100 bpm), completely independent of the ventricular rhythm. The sinus rhythm is regular.

When the complete AV block is caused by pathology below the bundle of His, the ventricular rhythm is controlled by what is called a ventricular escape mechanism. The rate of the ventricular escape mechanism is between 20 and 40 bpm. Similar to complete AV block above the bundle of His, the atrial and ventricular rates will be independent of each other and regular in rhythm.

To summarize, in complete AV block, the atrial rate is faster and completely independent of the ventricular rate. There is no relationship between the P and QRS complexes, and there are no PR intervals. The atria remain under the control of the SA node, and the ventricles are under the control of the bundle of His or of a ventricular escape mechanism. The ECG characteristics of complete AV block in lead II are as follows:

- **P wave:** The P waves are positive and uniform. There is no relationship between the P waves and the QRS complexes. The atrial rate is faster than the ventricular escape rate.

Figure 14–28

An ECG illustrating complete AV block, probably at the level of the AV node because the QRS is 0.06 second. The atrial rate is faster than the QRS rate, and the P waves and QRS complexes are independent of each other. There are no consistent PR intervals. The ECG interpretation would be sinus rhythm at 50 bpm with complete AV block, a junctional rhythm with a ventricular rate at 40 bpm.

© Cengage Learning 2013

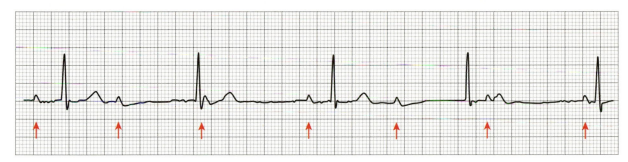

- **PR interval:** There are no measurable PR intervals because there is no relationship between the P waves and QRS complexes.
- **QRS complex:** The duration of the QRS complex may be normal or greater than 0.12 second. When the pathology is above the bundle of His, the QRS complex is usually normal (<0.12 second). When the pathology is below the bundle of His, the duration of the QRS complexes will be greater than 0.12 second.
- **QRS rate:** The atrial rate is faster and completely independent of the ventricular rate. A junctional escape pacemaker produces a rate between 40 and 60 bpm. A ventricular escape pacemaker produces a rate between 20 and 40 bpm.
- **QRS rhythm:** Both a junctional escape pacemaker and a ventricular escape pacemaker produce a regular rhythm.

Figure 14–28 shows an ECG tracing with complete AV block.

Chapter Summary

A consistent, systematic approach is fundamental to all good methods of ECG interpretation. This chapter presented a five-step systematic approach to ECG interpretation. *Step 1* is the *general inspection*, which requires the examiner to closely scan the ECG tracing to determine if the general appearance of the ECG tracing looks normal or abnormal. *Step 2* is the *analysis of ventricular activity* for rate, rhythm, and shape. *Step 3* is the *analysis of atrial activity* for rate, rhythm, and shape. *Step 4* is the *assessment of the atrioventricular relationship*, which includes the conduction ratio, discharge sequence, and PR interval. *Step 5* is the *ECG interpretation*, which determines if there is a normal sinus rhythm or cardiac dysrhythmias present.

The common cardiac dysrhythmias are the *sinus mechanisms*, which include sinus bradycardia, sinus tachycardia, sinus arrhythmia, sinus block, and sinus arrest; the *atrial mechanisms*, which include premature atrial complex, atrial bigeminy, atrial tachycardia, atrial flutter, and atrial fibrillation; *ventricular mechanisms*, which include premature ventricular complex (PVC), uniform PVCs, multiform PVCs, paired PVCs, bigeminal PVCs, trigeminal PVCs, ventricular tachycardia, ventricular flutter, ventricular fibrillation, and asystole; and *AV conduction defects*, which include sinus rhythm with first-degree AV block, sinus rhythm with second-degree AV block, and complete AV block.

Clinical connections associated with this chapter include the treatment protocol for bradycardia, pulse arrest, ventricular fibrillation and pulseless ventricular tachycardia, and asystole and pulseless electrical activity.

Review Questions

1.
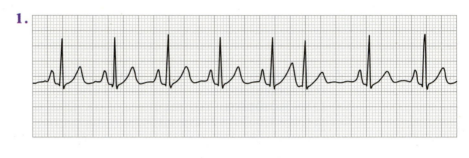

QRS duration: _____ QT duration: _____

Ventricular rate and rhythm: _____

Atrial rate and rhythm: _____

PR interval: _____

Interpretation: _____

2.
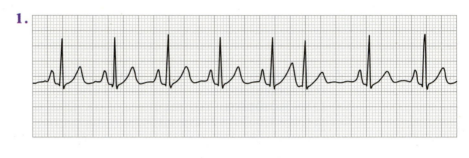

QRS duration: _____ QT duration: _____

Ventricular rate and rhythm: _____

Atrial rate and rhythm: _____

PR interval: _____

Interpretation: _____

3.

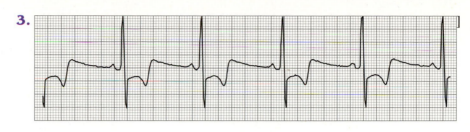

QRS duration: _____ QT duration: _____

Ventricular rate and rhythm: _____

Atrial rate and rhythm: _____

PR interval: _____

Interpretation: _____

4.

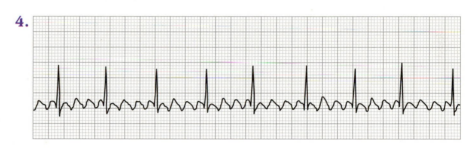

QRS duration: _____ QT duration: _____

Ventricular rate and rhythm: _____

Atrial rate and rhythm: _____

PR interval: _____

Interpretation: _____

5.

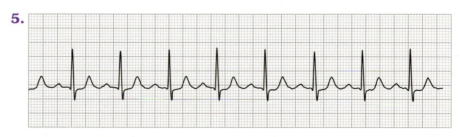

QRS duration: _____ QT duration: _____

Ventricular rate and rhythm: _____

Atrial rate and rhythm: _____

PR interval: _____

Interpretation: _____

6.

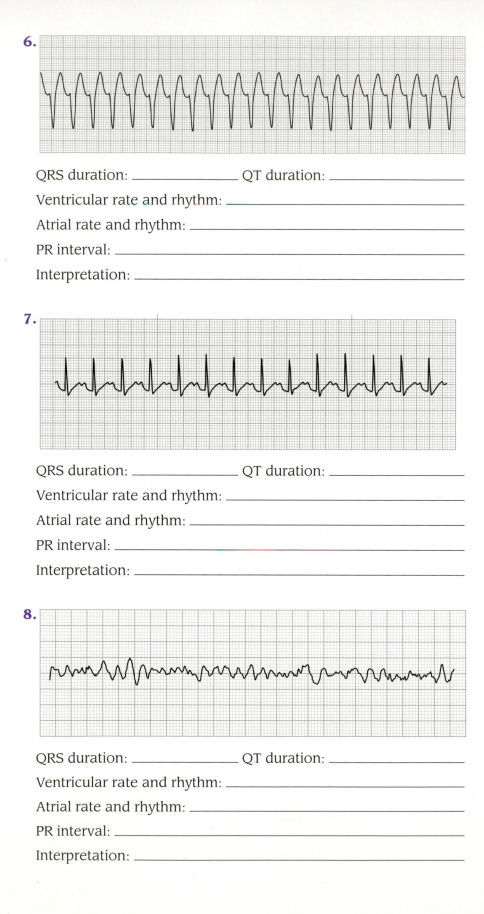

QRS duration: _____ QT duration: _____

Ventricular rate and rhythm: _____

Atrial rate and rhythm: _____

PR interval: _____

Interpretation: _____

7.

QRS duration: _____ QT duration: _____

Ventricular rate and rhythm: _____

Atrial rate and rhythm: _____

PR interval: _____

Interpretation: _____

8.

QRS duration: _____ QT duration: _____

Ventricular rate and rhythm: _____

Atrial rate and rhythm: _____

PR interval: _____

Interpretation: _____

9.

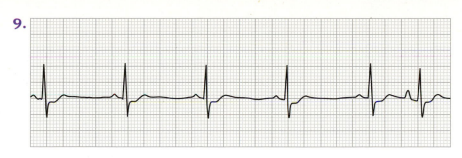

QRS duration: _____ QT duration: _____

Ventricular rate and rhythm: _____

Atrial rate and rhythm: _____

PR interval: _____

Interpretation: _____

10.

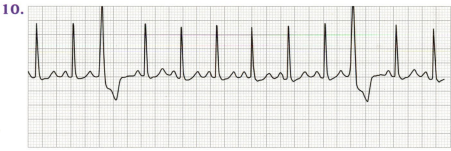

QRS duration: _____ QT duration: _____

Ventricular rate and rhythm: _____

Atrial rate and rhythm: _____

PR interval: _____

Interpretation: _____

Chapter 15

Hemodynamic Measurements

Objectives

By the end of this chapter, the student should be able to:

1. List the abbreviations and normal ranges of the following hemodynamic values *directly* measured by means of the pulmonary artery catheter:
   —Central venous pressure
   —Right atrial pressure
   —Mean pulmonary artery pressure
   —Pulmonary capillary wedge pressure
   —Cardiac output
2. Describe the clinical connection associated with the adverse effects of an elevated afterload on a patient's hemodynamic parameters.
3. Describe the clinical connection associated with the use of best PEEP in adjusting a patient's hemodynamic profile.
4. List the abbreviations and normal ranges of the following *computed* hemodynamic values:
   —Stroke volume
   —Stroke volume index
   —Cardiac index
   —Right ventricular stroke work index
   —Left ventricular stroke work index
   —Pulmonary vascular resistance
   —Systemic vascular resistance
5. List factors that increase and decrease the following:
   —Stroke volume
   —Stroke volume index
   —Cardiac output
   —Cardiac index
   —Right ventricular stroke work index
   —Left ventricular stroke work index
6. Describe the clinical connection that outline the hemodynamic changes associated with the following:
   —Cor pulmonale
   —Congestive heart failure
   —COPD
   —Lung collapse
   —Hypovolemia
   —Pulmonary embolism
7. List the factors that increase and decrease the *pulmonary vascular resistance*.
8. List the factors that increase and decrease the *systemic vascular resistance*.
9. Complete the review questions at the end of this chapter.

Hemodynamic Measurements Directly Obtained by Means of the Pulmonary Artery Catheter

The term **hemodynamics** is defined as the study of the forces that influence the circulation of blood. With the advent of the pulmonary artery catheter (Figure 15–1 on page 484), the hemodynamic status of the critically ill patient can be accurately determined at the bedside.[1] The pulmonary artery catheter

---

[1] See Appendix V for a representative example of a cardiopulmonary profile sheet used to monitor the hemodynamic status of the critically ill patient.

Clinical Connection—15-1

Case Study—The Adverse Effects of an Elevated Afterload on a Patient's Hemodynamic Parameters

In the **Clinical Application Section—Case 1** (page 494), the respiratory therapist is called to help care for a 71-year-old woman with sudden chest pain. This case illustrates how an elevated afterload can cause harmful changes in a patient's hemodynamic profile. For example, the patient's early hemodynamic profile shows a very high SVR and PCWP and a low CI,[2] which verifies the elevated afterload. The case further shows how the administration of nitroprusside can be used to correct an elevated afterload, and return the SVR, PCWP, and CI values back to normal.

[2] SVR = systemic vascular resistance; PCWP = pulmonary capillary wedge pressure; CI = cardiac index.

Figure 15–1

Insertion of the pulmonary catheter. The insertion site of the pulmonary catheter may be the basilic, brachial, femoral, subclavian, or internal jugular veins. The latter two are the most common insertion sites. As the catheter advances, pressure readings and waveforms are monitored to determine the catheter's position as it moves through the right atrium (RA), right ventricle (RV), pulmonary artery (PA), and finally into a pulmonary capillary wedge pressure (PCWP) position. Immediately after a PCWP reading, the balloon is deflated to allow blood to flow past the tip of the catheter. When the balloon is deflated, the catheter continuously monitors the pulmonary artery pressure.

© Cengage Learning 2013

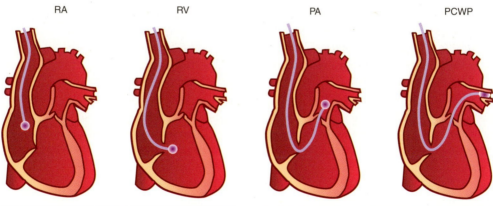

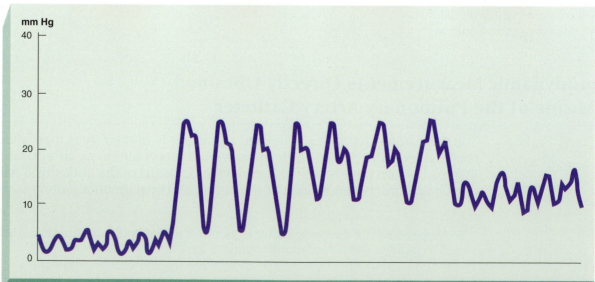

Table 15–1

Hemodynamic Values Directly Obtained by Means of the Pulmonary Artery Catheter

Hemodynamic Value	Abbreviation	Normal Range
Central venous pressure	CVP	0–8 mm Hg
Right atrial pressure	RAP	0–8 mm Hg
Mean pulmonary artery pressure	$\overline{\text{PAP}}$	9–18 mm Hg
Pulmonary capillary wedge pressure (also pulmonary artery wedge; pulmonary artery occlusion)	PCWP PAW PAO	4–12 mm Hg
Cardiac output	CO	4–8 L/min

© Cengage Learning 2013

has enabled the respiratory therapist to measure several hemodynamic parameters directly. These direct measurements, in turn, can be used to compute other important hemodynamic values. Table 15–1 lists the major hemodynamic values that can be measured directly.

Hemodynamic Values Computed from Direct Measurements

Table 15–2 lists the major hemodynamic values that can be calculated from the direct measurements listed in Table 15–1. Today, such calculations are obtained either from a programmed calculator or by using the specific hemodynamic formula and a simple handheld calculator. Note, moreover, that because the hemodynamic parameters vary with the size of an individual, some hemodynamic values are "indexed" by body surface area (BSA). Clinically, the BSA is obtained from a height–weight nomogram (see Appendix IV). The normal adult BSA is 1.5 to 2 m^2.

Table 15–2

Computed Hemodynamic Values

Hemodynamic Value	Abbreviation	Normal Range
Stroke volume	SV	60–130 mL
Stroke volume index	SVI	30–65 mL/beat/m^2
Cardiac index	CI	2.5–4.2 L/min/m^2
Right ventricular stroke work index	RVSWI	7–12 g m/m^2
Left ventricular stroke work index	LVSWI	40–60 g m/m^2
Pulmonary vascular resistance	PVR	20–120 dynes $\times$ sec $\times$ cm^{-5}
Systemic vascular resistance	SVR	800–1500 dynes $\times$ sec $\times$ cm^{-5}

© Cengage Learning 2013

Clinical Connection—15-2

Case Study—The Use of Best PEEP in Adjusting a Patient's Hemodynamic Profile

In the **Clinical Application Section—Case 2** (page 495), the respiratory therapist is called to help care for a 35-year-old man who was found unconscious, face down, in about 4 inches of water at a local beach. This case illustrates how the use of best level of **positive end-expiratory-pressure** (**PEEP**)—commonly referred to as **best PEEP**—was the PEEP level that caused the least reduction of cardiac output and produced the maximum total oxygen delivery.

Stroke Volume

The stroke volume (SV) is the volume of blood ejected by the ventricles with each contraction. The preload, afterload, and myocardial contractility are the major determinants of stroke volume. Stroke volume is derived by dividing the cardiac output (CO) by the heart rate (HR).

$$SV = \frac{CO}{HR}$$

For example, if an individual has a cardiac output of 4.5 L/min (4500 mL/min) and a heart rate of 75 beats/min, the stroke volume would be calculated as follows:

$$SV = \frac{CO}{HR}$$

$$= \frac{4500 \text{ mL/min}}{75 \text{ beats/min}}$$

$$= 60 \text{ mL/beat}$$

Table 15–3 lists factors that increase and decrease the stroke volume.

Clinical Connection—15-3

Cor Pulmonale—Hemodynamic Changes

Cor pulmonale is the enlargement of the *right* ventricle caused by primary lung disease. Cor pulmonale eventually results in the inability of the right ventricle to pump blood effectively to the lungs (also called right-heart failure). When the right ventricle starts to fail, blood returning to the heart backs up and pools throughout the peripheral vascular system—for example, in the liver, legs, neck veins, ankles, feet, and hands. Hemodynamic changes associated with cor pulmonale are shown in the table below.

Hemodynamic Indices											
CVP	RAP	$\overline{PAP}$	PCWP	CO	SV	SVI	CI	RVSWI	LVSWI	PVR	SVR
↑↑	↑↑	↓	↓	O	O	O	O	O	O	O	O

O = unchanged

Table 15–3

Factors Increasing and Decreasing Stroke Volume (SV), Stroke Volume Index (SVI), Cardiac Output (CO), Cardiac Index (CI), Right Ventricular Stroke Work Index (RVSWI), and Left Ventricular Stroke Work Index (LVSWI)

Increases	Decreases
Positive Inotropic Drugs (Increased Contractility)	**Negative Inotropic Drugs (Decreased Contractility)**
Dobutamine	Propranolol
Epinephrine	Timolol
Dopamine	Metoprolol
Isoproterenol	Atenolol
Digitalis	Nadolol
Amrinone	
	Abnormal Conditions
Abnormal Conditions	Septic shock (late stages)
Septic shock (early stages)	Congestive heart failure
Hyperthermia	Hypovolemia
Hypervolemia	Pulmonary emboli
Decreased vascular resistance	Increased vascular resistance
	Myocardial infarction
	Hyperinflation of Lungs
	Mechanical ventilation
	Continuous positive airway pressure (CPAP)
	Positive end-expiratory pressure (PEEP)

© Cengage Learning 2013

Stroke Volume Index

The stroke volume index (SVI) (also known as stroke index) is derived by dividing the stroke volume (SV) by the body surface area (BSA).

$$SVI = \frac{SV}{BSA}$$

For example, if a patient has a stroke volume of 60 mL and a body surface area of 2 m², the stroke volume index would be determined as follows:

$$SVI = \frac{SV}{BSA}$$

$$= \frac{60 \text{ mL/beat}}{2 \text{ m}^2}$$

$$= 30 \text{ mL/beat/m}^2$$

Assuming that the heart rate remains the same, as the stroke volume index increases or decreases, the cardiac index also increases or decreases.

Clinical Connection—15-4

Congestive Heart Failure—Hemodynamic Changes

Congestive heart failure (CHF) (also called left-heart failure) is the inability of the *left* ventricle to pump blood effectively. When a patient has CHF, the right ventricle continues to pump blood to the lungs, but the left ventricle does not adequately pump the returning blood from the lungs into the systemic circulation.

As a result, the vascular system in the lungs becomes engorged with blood, the pulmonary capillary blood pressure increases, and fluid leaks out of the capillaries into the alveoli—causing the condition known as **pulmonary edema**. Hemodynamic changes associated with CHF are shown in the table below

Hemodynamic Indices											
CVP	RAP	$\overline{PAP}$	PCWP	CO	SV	SVI	CI	RVSWI	LVSWI	PVR	SVR
O	↑	↑	↑↑	↓	↓	↓	↓	↑	↓	↑	↓

O = unchanged

The stroke volume index reflects the (1) contractility of the heart, (2) overall blood volume status, and (3) amount of venous return. Table 15–3 lists factors that increase and decrease the stroke volume index.

Cardiac Index

The cardiac index (CI) is calculated by dividing the cardiac output (CO) by the body's surface area (BSA).

$$CI = \frac{CO}{BSA}$$

Clinical Connection—15-5

COPD—Hemodynamic Changes

Respiratory disorders classifed as **chronic obstructive pulmonary disorders (COPD)** are chronic bronchitis, emphysema, cystic fibrosis, and

bronchiectasis. Hemodynamic changes associated with COPD are shown in the table below.

Hemodynamic Indices											
CVP	RAP	$\overline{PAP}$	PCWP	CO	SV	SVI	CI	RVSWI	LVSWI	PVR	SVR
↑	↑	↑↑	O	O	O	O	O	↑	O	↑	O

O = unchanged

For example, if a patient has a cardiac output of 5 L/min and a body surface area of 2 m², the cardiac index is computed as follows:

$$CI = \frac{CO}{BSA}$$

$$= \frac{5 \text{ L/min}}{2 \text{ m}^2}$$

$$= 2.5 \text{ L/min/m}^2$$

See Table 15–3 for a list of factors that increase and decrease the cardiac index.

Right Ventricular Stroke Work Index

The right ventricular stroke work index (RVSWI) measures the amount of work required by the right ventricle to pump blood. The RVSWI is a reflection of the contractility of the right ventricle. In the presence of normal right ventricular contractility, increases in afterload (e.g., caused by pulmonary vascular constriction) cause the RVSWI to increase, until a plateau is reached. When the contractility of the right ventricle is diminished by the presence of disease, the RVSWI does not increase appropriately. The RVSWI is derived from the following formula:

$$RVSWI = SVI \times (\overline{PAP} - CVP) \times 0.0136 \text{ g/mL}$$

where SVI is stroke volume index, $\overline{PAP}$ is mean pulmonary artery pressure, CVP is central venous pressure, and the density of mercury factor 0.0136 g/mL is needed to convert the equation to the proper units of measurement—that is, gram meters/square meter (g m/m²).

For example, if a patient has an SVI of 35 mL, a $\overline{PAP}$ of 20 mm Hg, and a CVP of 5 mm Hg, the patient's RVSWI is calculated as follows:

$$RVSWI = SVI \times (\overline{PAP} - CVP) \times 0.0136 \text{ g/mL}$$

$$= 35 \text{ mL/beat/m}^2 \times (20 \text{ mm Hg} - 5 \text{ mm Hg}) \times 0.0136 \text{ g/mL}$$

$$= 35 \text{ mL/beat/m}^2 \times 15 \text{ mm Hg} \times 0.0136 \text{ g/mL}$$

$$= 7.14 \text{ g m/m}^2$$

Factors that increase and decrease the RVSWI index are listed in Table 15–3.

Left Ventricular Stroke Work Index

The left ventricular stroke work index (LVSWI) measures the amount of work required by the left ventricle to pump blood. The LVSWI is a reflection of the contractility of the left ventricle. In the presence of normal left ventricular contractility, increases in afterload (e.g., caused by systemic vascular constriction) cause the LVSWI to increase until a plateau is reached. When the contractility of the left ventricle is diminished by the presence of disease, the LVSWI does not increase appropriately. The following formula is used for determining this hemodynamic variable:

$$LVSWI = SVI \times (MAP - PCWP) \times 0.0136 \text{ g/mL}$$

Clinical Connection—15-6

Lung Collapse—Hemodynamic Changes

Respiratory disorders that cause the lung to collapse include flail chest, pneumothorax, and hemothorax.

Hemodynamic changes associated with lung collapse are shown in the table below.

Hemodynamic Indices											
CVP	RAP	$\overline{\text{PAP}}$	PCWP	CO	SV	SVI	CI	RVSWI	LVSWI	PVR	SVR
↑	↑	↑	↓	↓	↓	↓	↓	↑	↓	↑	↓

O = unchanged

where SVI is stroke volume index, MAP is mean arterial pressure, PCWP is pulmonary capillary wedge pressure, and the density of mercury factor 0.0136 g/mL is needed to convert the equation to the proper units of measurement—that is, g m/m².

For example, if a patient has an SVI of 30 mL, an MAP of 100 mm Hg, and a PCWP of 5 mm Hg, then:

$$\text{LVSWI} = \text{SVI} \times (\text{MAP} - \text{PCWP}) \times 0.0136 \text{ g/mL}$$

$$= 30 \text{ mL/beat/m}^2 \times (100 \text{ mm Hg} - 5 \text{ mm Hg}) \times 0.0136 \text{ g/mL}$$

$$= 30 \text{ mL/beat/m}^2 \times (95 \text{ mm Hg}) \times 0.0136 \text{ g/mL}$$

$$= 38.76 \text{ g m/m}^2$$

Table 15–3 lists factors that increase and decrease the LVSWI.

Clinical Connection—15-7

Hypovolemia—Hemodynamic Changes

Hypovolemia is a blood disorder consisting of a decrease in the volume of circulating blood. Common causes include dehydration, bleeding, vomiting, severe burns, and drugs such as

diuretics or vasodilators used to treat hypertensive individuals. Hemodynamic changes associated with hypovolemia are shown in the table below.

Hemodynamic Indices											
CVP	RAP	$\overline{\text{PAP}}$	PCWP	CO	SV	SVI	CI	RVSWI	LVSWI	PVR	SVR
↓↓	↓	↓	↓	↓	↓	↓	↓	↓	↓	O	↑

O = unchanged

Vascular Resistance

As blood flows through the pulmonary and the systemic vascular system, there is resistance to flow. The pulmonary system is a *low-resistance* system, whereas the systemic vascular system is a *high-resistance* system.

Pulmonary Vascular Resistance

The pulmonary vascular resistance (PVR) measurement reflects the afterload of the right ventricle. It is calculated by the following formula:

$$PVR = \frac{\overline{PAP} - PCWP}{CO} \times 80$$

where $\overline{PAP}$ is the mean pulmonary artery pressure, PCWP is the pulmonary capillary wedge pressure, CO is the cardiac output, and 80 is a conversion factor for adjusting to the correct units of measurement (dyne $\times$ sec $\times$ cm^{-5}).

For example, to determine the PVR of a patient who has a $\overline{PAP}$ of 15 mm Hg, a PCWP of 5 mm Hg, and a CO of 5 L/min:

$$PVR = \frac{\overline{PAP} - PCWP}{CO} \times 80$$
$$= \frac{15 \text{ mm Hg} - 5 \text{ mm Hg}}{5 \text{ L/min}} \times 80$$
$$= \frac{10 \text{ mm Hg}}{5 \text{ L/min}} \times 80$$
$$= 160 \text{ dynes} \times \text{sec} \times \text{cm}^{-5}$$

Table 15–4 on page 492 lists factors that increase the pulmonary vascular resistance. Factors that decrease the pulmonary vascular resistance are listed in Table 15–5 on page 492.

Systemic or Peripheral Vascular Resistance

The systemic or peripheral vascular resistance (SVR) measurement reflects the afterload of the left ventricle. It is calculated by the following formula:

$$SVR = \frac{MAP - CVP}{CO} \times 80$$

Clinical Connection—15-8

Pulmonary Embolism—Hemodynamic Changes

A **pulmonary embolism** is the blockage of a pulmonary artery by fat, air tumor, or thrombus that usually arises from a peripheral vein (most frequently one of the deep veins of the legs). Hemodynamic changes associated with pulmonary embolism are shown in the table below.

Hemodynamic Indices											
CVP	RAP	$\overline{PAP}$	PCWP	CO	SV	SVI	CI	RVSWI	LVSWI	PVR	SVR
↑	↑	↑↑	↓	↓	↓	↓	↓	↑	↓	↑	O

O = unchanged

Table 15–4

Factors That Increase Pulmonary Vascular Resistance (PVR)

Chemical Stimuli
Decreased alveolar oxygenation
  (alveolar hypoxia)
Decreased pH (acidemia)
Increased P_{CO_2} (hypercapnia)

Pharmacologic Agents
Epinephrine
Norepinephrine
Dobutamine
Dopamine
Phenylephrine

Hyperinflation of Lungs
Mechanical ventilation
  Continuous positive airway pressure (CPAP)
  Positive end-expiratory pressure (PEEP)

Pathologic Factors
Vascular blockage
  Pulmonary emboli
  Air bubble
  Tumor mass

Vascular wall disease
  Sclerosis
  Endarteritis
  Polyarteritis
  Scleroderma

Vascular destruction
  Emphysema
  Pulmonary interstitial fibrosis

Vascular compression
  Pneumothorax
  Hemothorax
  Tumor

Humoral Substances
Histamine
Angiotensin
Fibrinopeptides
Prostaglandin $F_{2\alpha}$
Serotonin

© Cengage Learning 2013

Table 15–5

Factors That Decrease Pulmonary Vascular Resistance (PVR)

Pharmacologic Agents	Humoral Substances
Oxygen	Acetylcholine
Isoproterenol	Bradykinin
Aminophylline	Prostaglandin E
Calcium-channel blocking agents	Prostacyclin (prostaglandin I_2)

© Cengage Learning 2013

where MAP is the mean arterial pressure, CVP is the central venous pressure, CO is the cardiac output, and 80 is a conversion factor for adjusting to the correct units of measurement (dyne $\times$ sec $\times$ cm^{-5}). (Note: The right atrial pressure [RAP] can be used in place of the CVP value.)

Table 15–6

Factors That Increase and Decrease Systemic Vascular Resistance (SVR)

Increases SVR	Decreases SVR
Vasoconstricting Agents	**Vasodilating Agents**
Dopamine	Nitroglycerin
Norepinephrine	Nitroprusside
Epinephrine	Morphine
Phenylephrine	Inamrinone
	Hydralazine
Abnormal Conditions	Methyldopa
Hypovolemia	Diazoxide
Septic shock (late stages)	Phentolamine
$\downarrow P_{CO_2}$	
	Abnormal Conditions
	Septic shock (early stages)
	$\uparrow P_{CO_2}$

$\uparrow$ increased, $\downarrow$ decreased

© Cengage Learning 2013

For example, if a patient has an MAP of 80 mm Hg, a CVP of 5 mm Hg, and a CO of 5 L/min, then:

$$SVR = \frac{MAP - CVP}{CO} \times 80$$

$$= \frac{80 \text{ mm Hg} - 5 \text{ mm Hg}}{5 \text{ L/min}} \times 80$$

$$= \frac{75 \text{ mm Hg} \times 80}{5 \text{ L/min}}$$

$$= 1200 \text{ dynes} \times \sec \times cm^{-5}$$

Table 15–6 lists factors that increase and decrease the systemic vascular resistance.

Chapter Summary

The hemodynamic status of the critically ill patient can be directly measured at the bedside using a pulmonary catheter. Direct hemodynamic measurements include the central venous pressure (CVP), right atrial pressure (RAP), mean pulmonary artery pressure (PAP), pulmonary capillary wedge pressure (PCWP), and cardiac output (CO). The direct hemodynamic measurements, in turn, can be used to compute the following hemodynamic values: stroke volume (SV), stroke volume index (SVI), cardiac index (CI), right ventricular stroke work index (RVSI), left ventricular stroke work index (LVSWI), pulmonary vascular resistance (PVR), and systemic vascular resistance (SVR). Currently, these calculations are obtained either from a programmed calculator or by using the hemodynamic formula and a handheld calculator.

Clinical connections associated with the preceding topics include (1) a case study that illustrates the adverse effects of an elevated afterload on a patient's hemodynamic parameters, (2) a case study that illustrates the use of best PEEP in adjusting a patient's hemodynamic profile, (3) cor pulmonale hemodynamic changes, (4) congestive heart failure hemodynamic changes, (5) COPD hemodynamic changes, (6) lung collapse hemodynamic changes, (7) hypovolemia hemodynamic changes, and (8) pulmonary embolism hemodynamic changes.

1 Clinical Application Case

A 71-year-old woman reported sudden chest pain to her husband while working in her garden. Moments later she collapsed; her husband called 911 immediately. Upon arrival, the paramedics charted these vital signs: blood pressure—64/35 mm Hg, heart rate—32 beats/min, and respiratory rate—4 breaths/min and shallow. Cardiopulmonary resuscitation (CPR) was initiated, and the patient was transferred to the hospital. En route to the hospital, an intravenous line was inserted, and a bolus of epinephrine was administered.

In the emergency department, the patient's vital signs were blood pressure—78/50 mm Hg, heart rate—42 beats/min, and spontaneous respiratory rate—16 breaths/min. Dopamine was administered, and the heart rate increased to 60 beats/min. Despite the improved heart rate, however, the patient's blood pressure remained low, and her skin was cold and clammy. After administration of 3 L/min oxygen via nasal cannula, the patient's arterial blood gas values were pH—7.54, Pa_{CO_2}—25 torr, HCO_3^-—22 mEq/L, Pa_{O_2}—62 torr.

Her electrocardiogram (ECG) showed a complete heart block.[3] The patient was immediately transferred to the coronary care unit (CCU). At the bedside, a transvenous cardiac pacing wire was placed under fluoroscopy, and the ventricles were paced at a rate of 80 beats/min. A pulmonary catheter was then inserted (see Figure 15–1), and a hemodynamic profile was obtained (see Hemodynamic Profile No. 1).

After evaluating the first hemodynamic profile, the physician made the diagnosis of cardiogenic shock and prescribed nitroprusside for the patient. One hour later, while on an inspired oxygen concentration ($F_{I_{O_2}}$) of 0.5, the patient's arterial blood gas values were pH—7.43, Pa_{CO_2}—33 torr, HCO_3^-—24 mEq/L, and Pa_{O_2}—108 torr. Urine output was 35 mL/hr. The patient's skin was warm and dry, and respiratory rate 12 breaths/min. At this time, a second hemodynamic profile was obtained (see Hemodynamic Profile No. 2).

---

[3] The ventricles were contracting independently from the sinus atrial node rhythm (Figure 14–28).

Discussion

This case illustrates the adverse "ripple" effects of an elevated afterload (Chapter 5) on a patient's hemodynamic parameters. The very high SVR and PCWP and low CI in Hemodynamic Profile No. 1 showed that the patient's afterload was elevated. Although dopamine is a good agent to increase the patient's CI (cardiac index), in larger doses it causes the SVR (systemic vascular resistance) to increase. Because the SVR was already high, nitroprusside (a vasodilator) was used to reduce the patient's afterload.

Hemodynamic Profile		
Parameter*	Profile No. 1	Profile No. 2
BP	88/54	91/55
HR	80 paced	80 paced
CVP	9	9
RAP	10	10
$\overline{PAP}$	18	16
PCWP	21	13
CI	1.1	1.8
SVR	2295	1670
Urine output (mL/hr)	0	35

*BP = blood pressure; HR = heart rate; CVP = central venous pressure; RAP = right atrial pressure; $\overline{PAP}$ = mean pulmonary artery pressure; PCWP = pulmonary capillary wedge pressure; CI = cardiac index; SVR = systemic vascular resistance. Normal ranges are given in Tables 15–1 and 15–2.

After the administration of the nitroprusside, the patient's blood pressure essentially remained the same in the second hemodynamic profile, while her PCWP, CI, SVR, and urine output all improved significantly. In short, as the patient's SVR decreased in response to the nitroprusside, the left ventricular afterload also decreased. This action, in turn, allowed blood to be more readily ejected from the left ventricle. A cardiac pacemaker was permanently implanted and the patient progressively improved. The patient was discharged after 7 days.

| 2 | Clinical Application Case |

A 35-year-old man was found unconscious, face down, in about 4 inches of water at a local beach. He had fallen asleep on the beach at low tide while intoxicated. His pulse was weak, and he was not breathing. Someone called 911, and the lifeguard started cardiopulmonary resuscitation (CPR). When the paramedics arrived, CPR was continued with an inspired oxygen concentration ($F_{I_{O_2}}$) of 1.0, and the patient was transferred to the local hospital.

In the emergency department, the patient was semiconscious. Although he demonstrated a spontaneous respiratory rate of 8 breaths/min, his breathing was labored and shallow. His pulse rate was 115 beats/min and blood pressure was 95/60 mm Hg. Chest X-ray showed a normal-size heart, but patches of alveolar infiltrates (white areas) were visible throughout both lung fields. The laboratory report showed that the patient's alcohol level was 0.53, complete blood cell (CBC) count was normal, and hemoglobin level was normal, at 15 g% (refer to Chapter 6). On an $F_{I_{O_2}}$ of 1.0, his arterial blood gas values were pH—7.27, Pa_{CO_2}—62 torr, HCO_3^-—26 mEq/L, and Pa_{O_2}—38 torr.

The patient was intubated and transferred to the intensive care unit. At the time of intubation, sand and seaweed were suctioned from the patient's trachea. A pulmonary artery catheter and arterial line were inserted (see Figure 15–1). The patient was placed on a mechanical ventilator with the following settings: tidal volume—750 mL, respiration rate—12 breath/min, $F_{I_{O_2}}$—1.0, and positive end-expiratory pressure (PEEP)—5 cm H_2O. The patient's arterial blood gas values on these settings were pH—7.47, Pa_{CO_2}—28 torr, HCO_3^-—22 mEq/L, Pa_{O_2}—57 torr, and Sa_{O_2}—91 percent. At this time, a hemodynamic profile and arterial blood sample were obtained (see Hemodynamic Profile No. 1).

After reviewing the clinical data in the first hemodynamic profile, the physician had the respiratory therapist decrease the patient's tidal volume to 650 mL to increase the patient's Pa_{CO_2}, which had been reduced too much by the first ventilator settings (the decreased Pa_{CO_2} was the cause of elevated pH). Because the patient's Pa_{O_2} was still very low on an $F_{I_{O_2}}$ of 1.0, the PEEP was increased to 10 cm H_2O. A second arterial blood gas analysis showed the following values: pH—7.42, Pa_{CO_2}—36 torr, HCO_3^-—23 mEq/L, Pa_{O_2}—61 torr, and Sa_{O_2}—90 percent. A second hemodynamic profile was then obtained (see Hemodynamic Profile No. 2).

After reviewing the patient's second arterial blood gas analysis and second hemodynamic profile, the physician had the respiratory therapist decrease the PEEP back to 5 cm H_2O. Fifteen minutes later, a third arterial blood gas analysis showed a pH of 7.42, Pa_{CO_2}—36 torr, HCO_3^-—23 mEq/L, Pa_{O_2}—59 torr, and Sa_{O_2}—90 percent. A third hemodynamic profile was then obtained (see Hemodynamic Profile No. 3). Despite the fact that the patient's Pa_{O_2} was less than satisfactory at this time, the physician asked the respiratory therapist to maintain the preceding treatment parameters.

Discussion

This case illustrates that the best level of PEEP (commonly referred to as "best PEEP") was the PEEP level that produced the least depression of cardiac output and the maximum total oxygen delivery. Inspection of the three hemodynamic profiles shows that 5 cm H_2O was the most effective by these criteria.[4] Despite the fact that the patient's clinical course was stormy, he was eventually weaned from the ventilator 16 days after his admission. Although he did regain consciousness, he was amnesic. He was also diagnosed to have moderate to severe mental and neuromuscular disorders. He was transferred to the rehabilitation unit where, at the time of this writing, progress was reported as slow.

---

[4] Chapter 6 shows how the patient's oxygen delivery for each level of PEEP can be calculated by using the total oxygen delivery (D_{O_2}) formula. It is strongly recommended that the reader calculate and compare the D_{O_2} when the patient was on 5 cm H_2O PEEP versus 10 cm H_2O PEEP. The D_{O_2} formula will show that even though the patient's Pa_{O_2} was less than desirable at 5 cm H_2O of PEEP, the cardiac output (and, therefore, the total oxygen delivery) was greater.

Hemodynamic Profile

Parameter*	Profile No. 1 PEEP 5 cm H_2O	Profile No. 2 PEEP 10 cm H_2O	Profile No. 3 PEEP 5 cm H_2O
BP	90/60	95/68	91/62
HR	107	105	98
CI	1.9	1.5	1.9
CO	3.83	3.1	3.82
SVI	36	31	37
SVR	1490	170	1493

*BP = blood pressure; HR = heart rate; CI = cardiac index; CO = cardiac output; SVI = stroke volume index; SVR = systemic vascular resistance.

Review Questions

Directions: On the line next to the hemodynamic parameters in Column A, match the normal range from Column B. Items in Column B may be used once, more than once, or not at all.

COLUMN A
Hemodynamic Parameters

1. _____ Mean pulmonary artery pressure

2. _____ Pulmonary vascular resistance

3. _____ Cardiac output

4. _____ Left ventricular stroke work index

5. _____ Central venous pressure

6. _____ Stroke volume index

7. _____ Pulmonary capillary wedge pressure

8. _____ Systemic vascular resistance

9. _____ Right atrial pressure

10. _____ Cardiac index

COLUMN B
Normal Range

a. 4–8 L/min

b. 800–1500 dynes $\times$ sec $\times$ cm^{-5}

c. 60–130 mL

d. 2–8 mm Hg

e. 20–120 dynes $\times$ sec $\times$ cm^{-5}

f. 9–18 mm Hg

g. 30–65 mL/beat/m^2

h. 80 mm Hg

i. 2.5–4.2 L/min/m^2

j. 4–12 mm Hg

k. 40–60 g m/m^2

l. 7–12 g m/m^2

11. Which of the following increases an individual's cardiac output?
1. Epinephrine
2. Hypovolemia
3. Mechanical ventilation
4. Hyperthermia
   A. 1 only
   B. 2 only
   C. 3 only
   D. 1 and 4 only

12. Pulmonary vascular resistance increases in response to
1. acidemia
2. oxygen
3. mechanical ventilation
4. epinephrine
   A. 2 only
   B. 3 only
   C. 1 and 3 only
   D. 1, 3, and 4 only

13. An individual's systemic vascular resistance increases in response to
1. morphine
2. hypovolemia
3. increased P_{CO_2}
4. epinephrine
   A. 1 only
   B. 2 only
   C. 3 only
   D. 2 and 4 only

14. Which of the following decreases an individual's stroke volume index?
1. Dobutamine
2. Mechanical ventilation
3. Propranolol
4. Congestive heart failure
   A. 2 only
   B. 4 only
   C. 1 and 3 only
   D. 2, 3, and 4 only

15. An individual's pulmonary vascular resistance decreases in response to
1. bradykinin
2. emphysema
3. norepinephrine
4. hypercapnia
   A. 1 only
   B. 2 only
   C. 3 and 4 only
   D. 2 and 3 only

Clinical Application Questions

Case 1

1. Although dopamine is a good agent to increase the patient's CI, in larger doses it cause _____

_____

2. Why was nitroprusside administered in this case?

_____

_____

3. Why did the patient's PCWP, CI, SVR, and urine output all improve after the administration of nitroprusside?

_____

_____

Case 2

1. Why was a PEEP of 5 cm H_2O the "best PEEP" in this case?

_____

_____

2. Using the total oxygen delivery formula (D_{O_2}) (discussed in Chapter 6), calculate and compare the D_{O_2} when the patient was receiving 5 cm H_2O PEEP compared with 10 cm H_2O PEEP.

_____

_____

Chapter 16

Renal Failure and Its Effects on the Cardiopulmonary System

Objectives

By the end of this chapter, the student should be able to:

1. Describe how the following relate to the kidney:
   —Hilum
   —Ureters
   —Cortex
   —Medulla
   —Renal pelvis
   —Major calyces
   —Minor calyces
   —Renal papillae
   —Renal pyramid
   —Nephrons
2. Describe how the following relate to the nephron:
   —Glomerulus
   —Proximal tubule
   —Loop of Henle
   —Distal tubule
   —Bowman's capsule
   —Renal corpuscle
   —Proximal convoluted tubule
   —Descending limb of the loop of Henle
   —Ascending limb of the loop of Henle
   —Distal convoluted tubule
   —Collecting duct
3. Describe how the following blood vessels relate to the nephron:
   —Renal arteries
   —Interlobar arteries
   —Arcuate arteries
   —Interlobular arteries
   —Afferent arterioles
   —Efferent arterioles
   —Peritubular capillaries
   —Interlobular veins
   —Arcuate vein
   —Interlobar vein
   —Renal vein
4. Describe the role of the following in the formation of urine:
   —Glomerular filtration
   —Tubular reabsorption
   —Tubular secretion
5. Describe the role of the following in the control of urine concentration and volume:
   —Countercurrent mechanism
   —Selective permeability
6. Describe the role of the kidneys in regulating the following:
   —Sodium
   —Potassium
   —Calcium, magnesium, and phosphate
   —Acid–base balance
7. Describe the role of the following in controlling the blood volume:
   —Capillary fluid shift system
   —The renal system
8. Describe the clinical connection associated with the adverse effects of poor blood circulation on kidney and lung function.
9. Identify common causes of renal disorders, including the following:
   —Congenital disorders
   —Infections
   —Obstructive disorders
   —Inflammation and immune responses
   —Neoplasms
10. Identify causes of the following types of renal disorders:
    —Prerenal conditions
    —Renal conditions
    —Postrenal conditions

(continues)

11. Describe how mechanical ventilation alters urinary output.
12. Describe the clinical connection associated with a prerenal abnormality caused by second- and third-degree burns.
13. Describe cardiopulmonary problems that can develop with renal failure, including the following:
    —Hypertension and edema
    —Metabolic acidosis
    —Electrolyte abnormalities
      • Chloride
      • Potassium
    —Anemia
    —Bleeding
    —Cardiovascular problems
14. Complete the review questions at the end of this chapter.

The composition of blood is largely determined by what the kidneys retain and excrete. The kidneys filter dissolved particles from the blood and selectively reabsorb the substances that are needed to maintain the normal composition of body fluids. When the renal system fails, a variety of indirect cardiopulmonary problems develop, including hypertension, congestive heart failure, pulmonary edema, anemia, and changes in acid–base balance. Because of this fact, a basic understanding of the cause, classification, and clinical manifestations of renal failure is essential in respiratory care.

The Kidneys

The kidneys are two bean-shaped organs located against the posterior wall of the abdominal cavity, one on each side of the vertebral column (Figure 16–1). In the adult, each kidney is about 12 cm long, 6 cm wide, and 3 cm thick. Medially, in the central concave portion of each kidney there is a longitudinal fissure called the **hilum**. The renal artery, renal vein, and nerves enter and leave kidneys through the hilum. The **ureters**, which transport urine from the kidneys to the bladder, also exit the kidneys through the hilum.

As shown in Figure 16–2 on page 502, the **cortex**, which is the outer one-third of the kidney, is a dark brownish red layer. The middle two-thirds of the kidney, the **medulla**, can be seen as a light-colored layer. Within the kidney, the ureter expands to form a funnel-shaped structure called the **renal pelvis**. The renal pelvis subdivides into two or three tubes called **major calyces** (singular, **calyx**), which in turn divide into several smaller tubes called **minor calyces**. A series of small structures called **renal papillae** (or *papillary ducts*) extends from the calyx toward the cortex of the kidney to form a triangular-shaped structure called the **renal pyramid**. The peripheral portions of the papillary ducts serve as collecting ducts for the waste products selectively filtered and excreted by the **nephrons**.

The Nephrons

The nephrons are the functional units of the kidneys (Figure 16–3 on page 503). Each kidney contains about 1 million nephrons. Each nephron consists of a **glomerulus**, **proximal tubule**, **loop of Henle**, and **distal tubule**. The distal tubules empty into the collecting ducts. Although the collecting ducts technically are not part of the renal pyramid, they are considered a functional part of the nephron because of their role in urine concentration, ion salvaging, and acid–base balance.

Figure 16–1

The organs of the urinary system. Urine is formed by the kidneys and flows through the ureters to the bladder, where it is eliminated via the urethra.

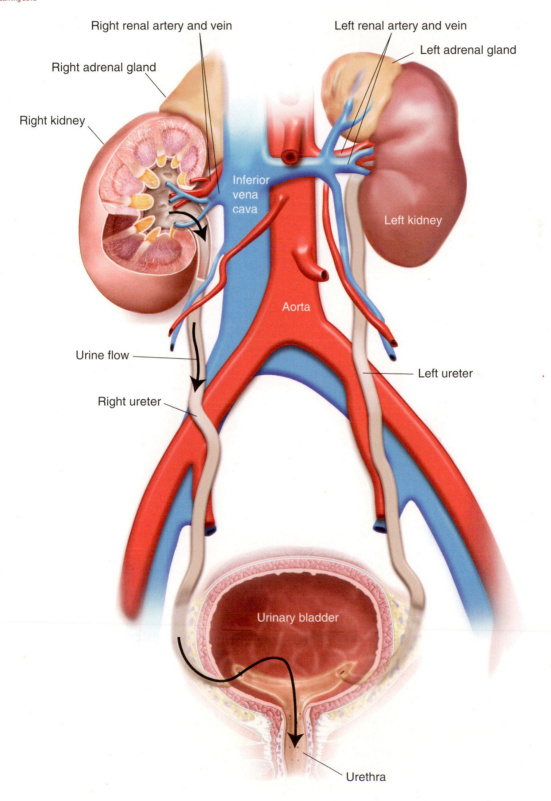

Figure 16–2

Cross-section of the kidney.

© Cengage Learning 2013

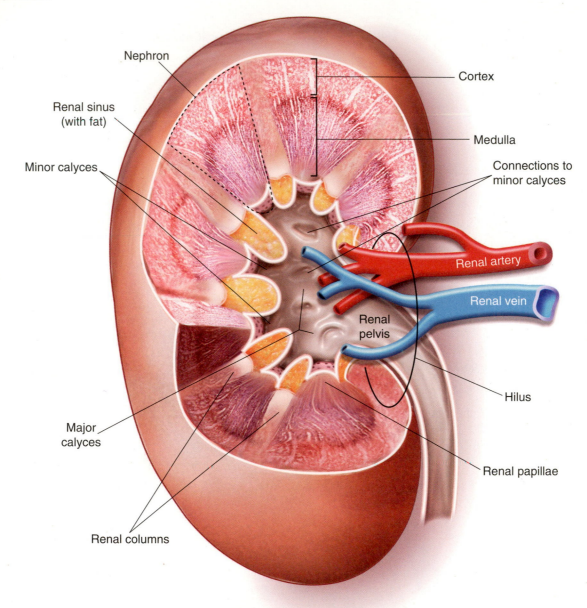

The glomerulus consists of a network of interconnected capillaries encased in a thin-walled, saclike structure called **Bowman's capsule**. The glomerulus and Bowman's capsule constitute what is known as a **renal corpuscle**. Urine formation begins with the filtration of fluid and low-molecular-weight particles from the glomerular capillaries into Bowman's capsule. The substances that are filtered pass into the **proximal convoluted tubule**, which lies in the cortex.

The proximal tubule dips into the medulla to form the *descending* limb of the loop of Henle. The tubule then bends into a U-shaped structure to form the loop of Henle. As the tubule straightens, it ascends back toward the cortex

Figure 16–3

The nephron.

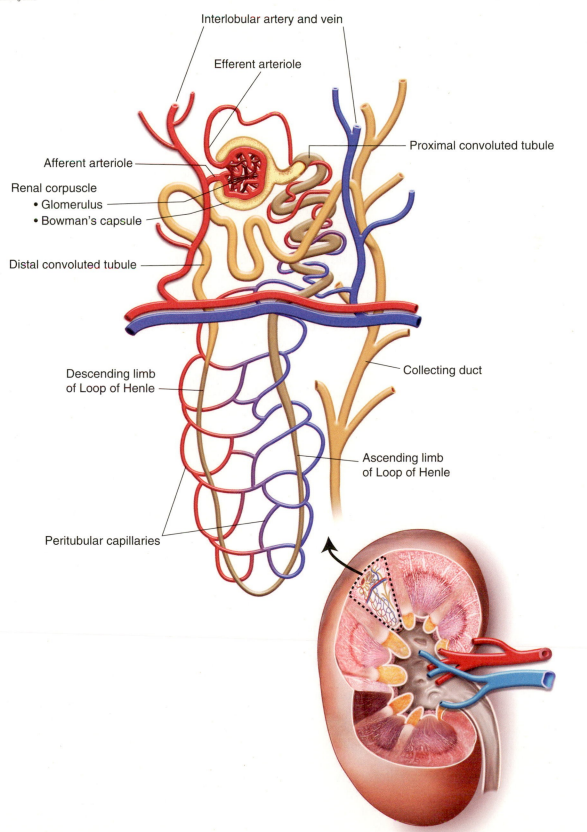

as the *ascending* limb of the loop of Henle. The tubule again becomes convoluted as it enters the cortex. This portion of the nephron is called the distal convoluted tubule (see Figure 16–3). The distal convoluted tubule empties into the collecting duct. The collecting duct then passes through the renal pyramid to empty into the minor and major calyces, which in turn drain into the renal pelvis (see Figure 16–2). From the renal pelvis, the mixture of waste products (collectively referred to as urine) drains into the ureter, where it is carried by peristalsis to the urinary bladder. The urine is stored in the urinary bladder until it is discharged from the body through the urethra (see Figure 16–3).

Blood Vessels of the Kidneys

As shown in Figure 16–4, the right and left renal arteries carry blood to the kidneys. Shortly after passing through the hilum of the kidney, the renal artery divides into several branches called the interlobar arteries. At the base of the renal pyramids, the interlobar arteries become the arcuate arteries. Divisions of the arcuate arteries form a series of interlobular arteries, which enter the cortex and branch into the afferent arterioles.

The afferent arterioles deliver blood to the capillary cluster that forms the glomerulus. After passing through the glomerulus, the blood leaves by way of the efferent arterioles. The efferent arterioles then branch into a complex network of capillaries called the peritubular capillaries, which surround the various portions of the renal tubules of the nephron (see Figure 16–3).

The peritubular capillaries reunite to form the interlobular veins, followed by the arcuate vein, the interlobar vein, and the renal vein. The renal vein eventually joins the inferior vena cava as it courses through the abdominal cavity.

Urine Formation

The formation of urine involves glomerular filtration, tubular reabsorption, and tubular secretion.

Glomerular Filtration

Urine formation begins in the renal corpuscle. Water and dissolved substances such as electrolytes are forced out of the glomerular capillaries by means of the blood pressure (*hydrostatic pressure*). The filtration of substances through the capillary membrane of the glomerulus is similar to the filtration in other capillaries throughout the body. The permeability of the glomerular capillary, however, is much greater than that of the capillaries in other tissues. As the filtrate leaves the glomerular capillaries, it is received in Bowman's capsule.

The rate of filtration is directly proportional to the hydrostatic pressure of the blood. The hydrostatic pressure in the glomerular capillary is about 55 mm Hg. This pressure, however, is partially offset by the hydrostatic pressure in Bowman's capsule of about 15 mm Hg. The osmotic pressure of the plasma is another important factor that offsets glomerular filtration. In other words, in the capillaries the hydrostatic pressure acting to move water and dissolved particles outward is opposed by the inward osmotic pressure generated by the presence of protein in the plasma. Under normal conditions, the osmotic

Figure 16–4

A. Illustration of the blood vessels of the kidney. **B.** Renal arteriogram: 1—interlobar artery; 2—tip of catheter in renal artery; 3—renal artery; 4—intestine. It is not unusual to have portions of the intestine overlying the kidney on renal arteriogram studies.

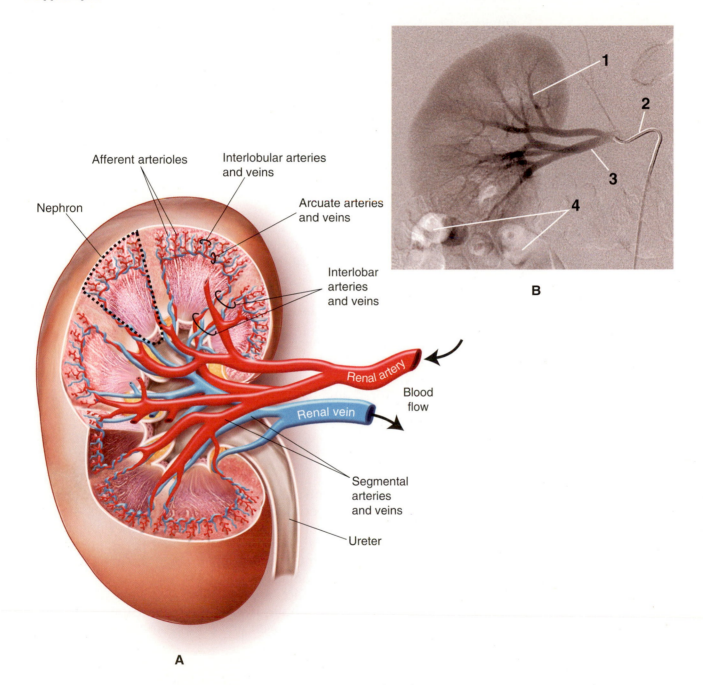

pressure is about 30 mm Hg. As shown in Table 16–1 on page 506, the net filtration pressure, which is the algebraic sum of the three relevant forces, is about 10 mm Hg. The glomeruli filter about 125 mL of fluid per minute (about 180 L/day). Of this 125 mL, however, only about 1 mL is excreted as urine. The average urine output is about 60 mL/hour, or 1440 mL/day.

Table 16–1	
Forces of Glomerular Filtration	
Factors	**Force**
Enhances Filtration	
Glomerular capillary blood pressure	+55 mm Hg
Opposes Filtration	
Fluid pressure in Bowman's capsule	−15 mm Hg
Osmotic force (caused by the protein concentration difference)	−30 mm Hg
Net Filtration Pressure	+10 mm Hg

© Cengage Learning 2013

Tubular Reabsorption

As the glomerular filtrate passes through the (1) proximal convoluted tubule, (2) loop of Henle, and (3) distal convoluted tubule, water, sodium, glucose, and other substances leave the tubule and enter the blood in the peritubular capillaries. Some substances, such as glucose and amino acids, are completely reabsorbed. About 99 percent of the filtered water and sodium is reabsorbed. About 50 percent of urea is reabsorbed and the electrolyte reabsorption is generally a function of need.

Although tubular reabsorption occurs throughout the entire renal tubule system, the bulk of it occurs in the proximal convoluted portion. Certain sections of the tubule, however, reabsorb specific substances, using particular modes of transport. For example, the proximal tubule reabsorbs glucose by means of *active transport*, whereas water reabsorption occurs throughout the renal tubule by *osmosis*.

Tubular Secretion

Tubular secretion is the mechanism by which various substances are transported from the plasma of the peritubular capillaries to the fluid of the renal tubule (the *opposite* direction of tubular reabsorption). In essence, this mechanism constitutes a second pathway through which fluid can gain entrance into the renal tubule (the first being *glomerular filtration*). The most important substances transported into the tubules by means of secretion are hydrogen (H^+) and potassium (K^+) ions. In fact, most of the hydrogen and potassium ions found in the urine enter the tubules by secretion. Thus, the mechanisms that control the rates of tubular hydrogen and potassium secretion regulate the level of these substances in the blood.

Urine Concentration and Volume

The composition and volume of extracellular fluids are controlled by the kidneys' ability to produce either a dilute or concentrated urine. The kidneys are able to do this by two mechanisms: the **countercurrent mechanism** and the **selective permeability of the collecting ducts**.

Countercurrent Mechanism

The countercurrent mechanism controls water reabsorption in the distal tubules and collecting ducts. It accomplishes this through the unique anatomic position of certain nephrons. About one in every five nephrons descends deep into the renal medulla. These nephrons are called **juxtamedullary nephrons**. The normal osmolality of the glomerular filtrate is approximately 300 mOsm/L.[1] The osmolality of the interstitial fluid increases from about 300 mOsm/L in the cortex to about 1200 mOsm/L as the juxtamedullary nephron descends into the renal medulla. This sets up a strong active transport of sodium out of the descending limb of the loop of Henle. The increased amount of sodium in the interstitial fluid, in turn, prevents water from returning to the peritubular capillaries surrounding the tubules.

Selective Permeability

As shown in Figure 16–5 on page 508, the permeability of the collecting ducts is regulated by the antidiuretic hormone (ADH), which is produced in the hypothalamus and is released by the pituitary gland. The hypothalamic cells manufacture ADH in response to input from numerous vascular baroreceptors, particularly a group found in the left atrium (see Figure 16–5). When the atrial blood volume and, therefore, pressure increase, the baroreceptors are activated to transmit neural impulses to the hypothalamus, causing the production of ADH to be inhibited. This causes tubules to be impermeable to water and the urine to be greater in volume and more dilute.

In contrast, decreased atrial pressure (*dehydration*) decreases the neural impulses originating from the baroreceptors and causes the production of ADH to increase. The result is the rapid movement of water out of these portions of the tubules of the nephron and into the interstitium of the medullary area by osmosis. This causes the urine volume to decrease and its concentration to increase.

The specific gravity (*osmolality*) of urine varies with its concentration of solutes. The urine produced by the healthy kidney has a specific gravity of about 1.003 to 1.030 under normal conditions. During periods of diminished renal function, the urine specific gravity may fall to levels of 1.008 to 1.012.

Regulation of Electrolyte Concentration

The kidneys play a major role in maintaining a normal cellular environment by regulating the concentration of various ions. Some of the more important ions regulated by the kidneys are sodium, potassium, calcium, magnesium, and phosphate.

Sodium Ions

Sodium ions (Na^+) account for more than 90 percent of the positively charged ions in the extracellular fluid. Because the sodium ions cause almost all of the osmotic pressure of the fluids, it follows that the sodium ion concentration

---

[1] Milliosmols (mOsm/L) = 1000 milliosmols = 1 osmol, which is the unit in which osmotic pressure is expressed. We speak of osmols or milliosmols per liter.

Figure 16–5

The pathway by which antidiuretic hormone (ADH) is controlled. When the baroreceptors in the left atrium sense an increased pressure (increased plasma volume), they send neural impulses to the hypothalamus, causing the production of ADH to decrease. In contrast, a decreased pressure (decreased plasma volume) causes the production of ADH to increase.

© Cengage Learning 2013

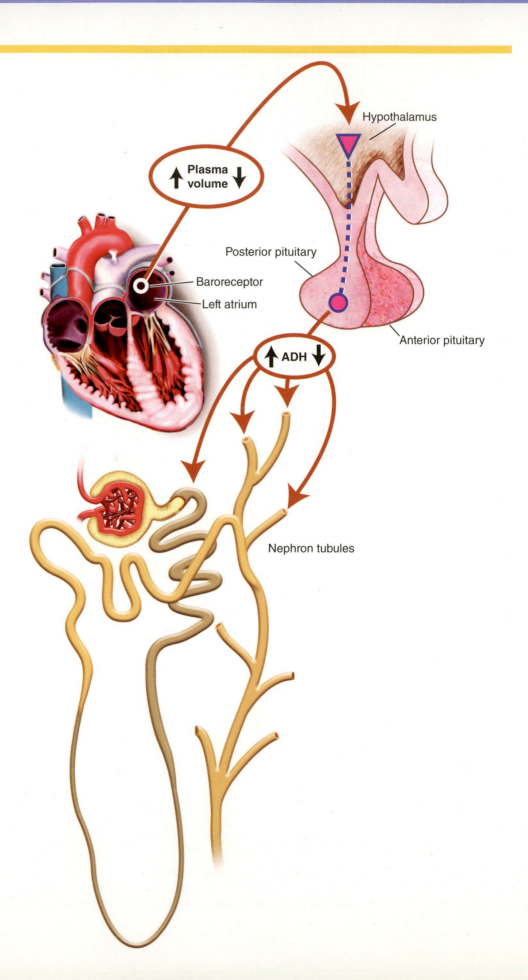

↑ Plasma volume ↓

Hypothalamus

Posterior pituitary

Baroreceptor

Left atrium

Anterior pituitary

↑ ADH ↓

Nephron tubules

directly affects the osmolality of the fluids. Thus, when the sodium concentration increases, there is a corresponding increase in the extracellular fluid osmolality. In contrast, the extracellular fluid osmolality decreases when there is a decreased sodium concentration.

The kidneys control the concentration of sodium primarily by regulating the amount of water in the body. When the sodium level becomes too high, the amount of water in the body increases by (1) secretion of ADH, which causes the kidney to retain water, and (2) stimulation of thirst, which causes the individual to drink liquids.

Potassium Ions

A balanced potassium (K^+) level is essential for normal nerve and muscle function. When the potassium level becomes too low, muscle weakness, diarrhea, metabolic alkalosis, and cardiac arrhythmias develop—such as premature atrial and ventricular contractions, atrial and ventricular tachycardia, and ventricular fibrillation.

An excessively high potassium concentration causes muscle weakness, metabolic acidosis, and life-threatening arrhythmias (e.g., widening of the QRS complex). In response to a high K^+ level, the kidneys work to return the concentration to normal by means of two negative feedback control mechanisms: (1) the direct effect the excess potassium has on the epithelial cells of the renal tubules to cause an increased transport of potassium out of the peritubular capillaries and into the tubules of the nephrons, where it is subsequently passed in the urine, and (2) the stimulating effect the elevated potassium level has on the adrenal cortex, causing it to release increased quantities of *aldosterone*. Aldosterone stimulates the tubular epithelial cells to transport potassium ions into the nephron tubules and, hence, into the urine. The extracellular potassium concentration is normally 3.5 to 5 mEq/L.

Calcium, Magnesium, and Phosphate Ions

The precise mechanisms by which calcium, magnesium, and phosphate concentrations are regulated by the kidneys are not well understood. It is known, however, that elevated levels of any one of these ions in the extracellular fluid cause the tubules to decrease reabsorption and to pass the substances into the urine. In contrast, when any one of these substances is low in concentration, the tubules rapidly reabsorb the substance until its concentration in the extracellular fluids returns to normal.

Role of the Kidneys in Acid–Base Balance

In addition to the natural acid–base buffers (refer to Chapter 7) of the body fluids (e.g., HCO_3^-, phosphate, and protein buffers), and the respiratory system's ability to regulate the elimination of CO_2, the renal system also plays an important role in maintaining a normal acid–base balance by its ability to regulate the excretion of hydrogen ions and the reabsorption of bicarbonate ions.

All the renal tubules are capable of secreting hydrogen ions. The rate of secretion is directly proportional to the hydrogen ion concentration in the blood. Thus, when the extracellular fluids become too acidic, the kidneys excrete hydrogen ions into the urine. In contrast, when the extracellular fluids

Figure 16–6

The effect of extracellular fluid pH on urine pH.

© Cengage Learning 2013

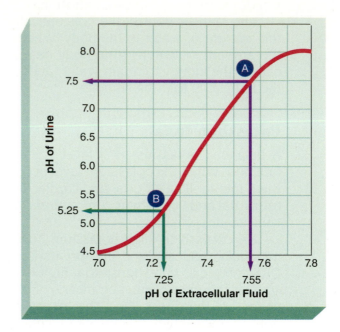

become too alkaline, the kidneys excrete basic substances (primarily sodium bicarbonate) into the urine.

This principle is illustrated in Figure 16–6, which shows that at point A, the pH of the extracellular fluid is 7.55. Because this is alkaline, the pH of the urine is also alkaline (pH 7.5), because the kidneys excrete alkaline substances from the body fluids. In contrast, the extracellular pH at point B is 7.25 and the pH of the urine is very acidic (pH 5.25), because of excretion of large quantities of acidic substances (primarily hydrogen ions) from the body fluids. In both of these examples, the excretion of either acidic or alkaline substances moves the pH toward normal.

Blood Volume

In the adult, the normal blood volume is about 5 L, and it rarely increases or decreases more than a few hundred milliliters from that value. The capillary fluid shifts and the renal system are the two major mechanisms responsible for this constancy of the blood volume.

Capillary Fluid Shift System

Under normal circumstances, the pressure in the systemic capillaries is about 17 mm Hg. When the pressure rises above this value, fluid begins to leak into the tissue spaces, causing the blood volume to decrease toward normal. In contrast, when the blood volume falls, the capillary pressure decreases and fluid is then absorbed from the interstitial spaces, causing the blood volume to move back toward normal. This mechanism, however, has its limitations, because the tissue spaces cannot expand indefinitely when the blood volume becomes too high, nor can the tissue spaces supply an inexhaustible amount of fluid when the blood volume is too low.

Clinical Connection—16-1

Case Study—The Adverse Effects of Poor Blood Circulation on Kidney and Lung Function

In the **Clinical Application Section—Case 1** (page 517), the respiratory therapist is called to help care for a 73-year-old woman who was admitted to the hospital for severe renal failure and left ventricular heart failure. This case illustrates how poor blood circulation adversely affects the patient's lung and kidney functions. The case further shows how all the clinical manifestations demonstrated in this case—for example, white fluffy patches on the chest X-ray and a shape reduction in urine output—can be traced back to the patient's left ventricular failure (a prerenal abnormality).

The Renal System

When the blood volume increases, the glomerular pressure in the kidney rises, causing the amount of the glomerular filtrate and the volume of the urine to increase. In addition, the pressure in the peritubular capillaries decreases fluid reabsorption from the tubules, which further increases the volume of urine.

Increased blood volume increases the glomerular pressure (normally 60 mm Hg) by means of two mechanisms: (1) the increased blood volume increases the blood flow through the afferent arterioles that lead into the kidneys and thus increases the intrarenal pressure and (2) the increased blood volume stretches the atria of the heart, which contain stretch receptors called **volume receptors**. When the volume receptors in the atria are stretched, a neural reflex is initiated which causes the renal afferent arterioles to dilate. This causes the blood flow into the kidneys to increase and thus increases the amount of urine formed. Furthermore, when the volume receptors are stretched, the secretion of ADH by the posterior pituitary gland is inhibited, which in turn increases the urine output.

Renal Failure

The renal system is subject to the same types of disorders as other organs. The more common causes of renal failure are (1) congenital disorders, (2) infections, (3) obstructive disorders, (4) inflammation and immune responses, and (5) neoplasms.

Common Causes of Renal Disorders

Congenital Disorders

Approximately 10 percent of infants are born with a potentially life-threatening malformation of the renal system. Such abnormalities include unilateral renal agenesis, renal dysplasia, and polycystic disease of the kidney.

Infections

Urinary tract infections are the second most common type of bacterial infections (after respiratory tract infections). Urinary tract infections are seen

Table 16–2
Factors That Obstruct Urinary Flow

Calculi (bladder or kidney stones)

Normal pregnancy

Prostatic hypertrophy

Infection and inflammation causing scar tissue

Neurologic disorders (e.g., spinal cord injury, diabetic neuropathy)

© Cengage Learning 2013

more often in women than men. Approximately 20 percent of all women will develop at least one urinary tract infection during their lifetime. These infections range from bacteriuria to severe kidney infections that cause irreversible damage to the kidneys.

Obstructive Disorders

Urinary obstruction can affect all age groups and can occur in any part of the urinary tract. About 90 percent of obstructions are located below the level of the glomerulus. Some factors that predispose individuals to urinary flow obstruction are listed in Table 16–2. Persons who have a urinary obstruction are prone to infections, a heightened susceptibility to calculus formation, and permanent kidney damage.

Inflammation and Immune Responses

Kidney inflammation is caused by altered immune responses, drugs and related chemicals, and radiation. Inflammation can cause significant alterations in the glomeruli, tubules, and interstitium. The various forms of glomerulonephritis are believed to be caused by natural immune responses.

Neoplasms

Cancer of the kidneys accounts for 1 to 2 percent of all cancers. Although cancer of the kidneys is relatively rare in the adult, one form of cancer—Wilms' tumor—accounts for about 70 percent of all cancers of early childhood.

Classification of Renal Disorders

Renal disorders are commonly classified according to the anatomic portion of the renal system responsible for the renal decline. The major classifications are (1) prerenal, (2) renal, and (3) postrenal.

Prerenal Conditions

Prerenal conditions consist of abnormalities that impair blood flow to the kidneys. Prerenal problems are the most common and generally are reversible if identified and treated early. Table 16–3 lists some common prerenal causes of renal failure.

Table 16–3

Prerenal Abnormalities

Hypovolemia
    Decrease of gastrointestinal tract fluid
    Hemorrhage
    Fluid sequestration (e.g., burns)

Septicemia

Heart failure

Renal artery atherosclerosis

© Cengage Learning 2013

Table 16–4

Renal Abnormalities

Renal ischemia

Injury to the glomerular membrane caused by nephrotoxic agents
    Aminoglycoside agents (e.g., gentamicin, kanamycin)
    Heavy metals (e.g., lead, mercury)
    Organic solvents (e.g., ethylene glycol)
    Radiopaque contrast media
    Sulfonamides

Acute tubular necrosis

Intratubular obstruction
    Uric acid crystals
    Hemolytic reactions (e.g., blood transfusion reactions)

Acute inflammatory conditions
    Acute pyelonephritis
    Necrotizing papillitis

© Cengage Learning 2013

Normally, about 20 to 25 percent of the cardiac output is filtered by the kidneys. When the volume of blood falls (e.g., in cardiac failure or hemorrhage), the blood flow to the kidneys may decrease sharply. Thus, one of the early clinical manifestations of prerenal failure is a sharp reduction in urine output.

Renal Conditions

Renal abnormalities involve conditions that obstruct flow through the kidneys. Table 16–4 lists the five categories of renal abnormalities.

Postrenal Conditions

An obstruction of the urinary tract at any point between the calyces and the urinary meatus is known as a postrenal obstruction. Table 16–5 on page 514 lists some abnormalities included in the postrenal category.

Table 16–5
Postrenal Abnormalities
Ureteral obstruction (e.g., calculi, tumors)
Bladder outlet obstruction (e.g., prostatic hypertrophy)

© Cengage Learning 2013

Clinical Connection—16-2

Case Study—A Prerenal Abnormality Caused by Second- and Third-Degree Burns

In the **Clinical Application Section—Case 2** (page 518), the respiratory therapist is called to help care for a 42-year-old male firefighter who was found unconscious in a smoke-filled room with second- and third-degree burns over portions of his left shoulder, left arm, and left hand and over the anterior portion of his chest and abdominal region. This case illustrates how the patient's burns caused fluid sequestration, which in turn caused hypovolemia—a prerenal abnormality.

Mechanical Ventilation as a Cause of Renal Failure

It is well documented that mechanical ventilation can alter urinary output. *Positive pressure ventilation* decreases urinary output, whereas *negative pressure ventilation* increases urinary output. It is believed that this is due in part to the blood pressure changes that occur in response to mechanical ventilation. In positive pressure ventilation, the venous return is often impeded, causing the blood volume and, therefore, the pressure in the atria to diminish. The reduced pressure stimulates the volume receptors in the atria to send more impulses to the pituitary gland, causing more ADH to be released. As the concentration of ADH increases, the amount of urine formed by the kidneys decreases.

Cardiopulmonary Disorders Caused by Renal Failure

In chronic renal failure, a variety of cardiopulmonary problems can develop. In acute renal failure, the body's ability to eliminate nitrogenous wastes, water, and electrolytes is impaired. As the renal system declines further, the blood urea nitrogen (BUN), creatinine, potassium, and phosphate levels rapidly increase, and metabolic acidosis develops. Water retention gives rise to peripheral edema and pulmonary congestion. During end-stage renal failure, virtually every portion of the body is affected. In terms of specific cardiopulmonary problems, the following problems can be expected in patients with renal failure.

Hypertension and Edema

When the renal function is impaired, the kidneys lose their ability to excrete sodium. Consequently, the ingestion of sodium leads to hypertension and edema.

Metabolic Acidosis

With the decline in renal function, the kidneys' ability to secrete hydrogen ions (H^+) and to conserve bicarbonate (HCO_3^-) progressively decreases. Furthermore, during the more advanced stages of renal failure, hyperkalemia is a frequent finding. Thus, because of the increased H^+ and K^+ ion levels and the loss of HCO_3^-, *metabolic acidosis* is an almost inevitable clinical manifestation in end stage renal failure (refer to Metabolic Acidosis, page 328).

Renal Acid–Base Disturbances Caused by Electrolyte Abnormalities

Chloride abnormalities can lead to acid–base disturbances through the renal system. For example, when the plasma chloride (Cl^-) level falls below normal, the amount of Cl^- available for glomerular filtration decreases. Under normal circumstances, when the positive sodium ion (Na^+) is reabsorbed by the tubules, the negative Cl^- ion must also be reabsorbed to maintain electrical neutrality. In the absence of adequate amounts of Cl^-, however, the electrical balance is maintained by the secretion of hydrogen ions (H^+). The loss of H^+ results in *hypochloremic alkalosis.* In contrast, when the plasma Cl^- level is higher than normal, the secretion of H^+ ions is reduced. This in turn causes a reduction in bicarbonate reabsorption and *hyperchloremic acidosis.*

Potassium abnormalities can also lead to acid–base disturbances through the renal system. For example, under normal conditions the potassium ion (K^+) behaves similarly to the H^+ ion in that it is secreted in the renal tubules in exchange for Na^+. In the absence of Na^+, neither K^+ nor H^+ can be secreted. When the K^+ level is higher than normal, however, the competition with H^+ for Na^+ exchange increases. When this happens, the amount of H^+ ions secreted is reduced, which in turn decreases the amount of HCO_3^- reabsorption. The end-product of this process is *hyperkalemic acidosis.* When the K^+ level is lower than normal, the competition with H^+ for Na^+ exchange decreases. Consequently, the amount of H^+ secreted is increased, which in turn increases the amount of HCO_3^- reabsorption. The end-product of this process is *hypokalemic alkalosis.*

Anemia

The kidneys are a primary source of the hormone *erythropoietin*, which stimulates the bone marrow to produce red blood cells (RBCs). When the renal system fails, the production of erythropoietin is often inadequate to stimulate the bone marrow to produce a sufficient amount of RBCs. In addition, the toxic wastes that accumulate as a result of renal failure also suppress the ability of bone marrow to produce RBCs. Both of these mechanisms contribute to the anemia seen in chronic renal failure.

Bleeding

Approximately 20 percent of persons with chronic renal failure have a tendency to bleed as a result of platelet abnormalities. Clinically, this is manifested by epistaxis (nosebleed), gastrointestinal bleeding, and bruising of the skin and subcutaneous tissues.

Cardiovascular Problems

Hypertension is often an early sign of renal failure. In severe cases, the increased extracellular fluid volume, caused by sodium and water retention, gives rise to edema, congestive heart failure, and pulmonary edema. Pericarditis is also seen in about 50 percent of persons with chronic renal failure. This condition develops as a result of the pericardium being exposed to the metabolic end-products associated with renal decline.

Chapter Summary

When the renal system fails, a number of indirect cardiopulmonary problems can develop, such as hypertension, congestive heart failure, pulmonary edema, anemia, and changes in acid–base balance. Because of this fact, a basic understanding of the cause, classification, and clinical manifestations of renal failure is essential to advanced respiratory care. The primary content areas are the kidneys, including the hilum, ureters, cortex, medulla, renal pelvis, major calyces, renal papillae, and renal pyramid; the nephrons, including the glomerulus, proximal tubule, loop of Henle, distal tubule, Bowman's capsule, renal corpuscle, proximal convoluted tubule, distal convoluted tubule, and collecting duct; and the blood vessels of the kidneys, including the renal arteries, interlobar arteries, arcuate arteries, interlobular arteries, afferent and efferent arterioles, peritubular capillaries, interlobular veins, arcuate vein, interlobar vein, and renal vein.

In addition, the respiratory therapist needs a strong knowledge base of urine formation, including glomerular filtration, tubular reabsorption, and tubular secretion; urine concentration and volume, including countercurrent mechanism and selective permeability of the collecting ducts; the regulation of electrolyte concentration, including sodium, potassium, calcium, magnesium, and phosphate ions; and the role of the kidneys in acid–base balance and blood volume, including the capillary fluid shift system and the renal system. Causes of renal failure include congenital disorders, infections, obstructive disorders, inflammation and immune responses, neoplasms (tumors), and mechanical ventilation. Finally, chronic renal failure may lead to a variety of cardiopulmonary problems, including hypertension and edema, metabolic acidosis, electrolyte abnormalities, anemia, bleeding, and cardiovascular disorders.

Clinical connections associated with these topics include (1) the adverse effects of poor blood circulation on kidney and lung function and (2) a prerenal abnormality caused by second- and third-degree burns.

A 73-year-old woman was admitted to the hospital for severe renal failure and left ventricular heart failure. An electrocardiogram (ECG) revealed a slow, irregular sinus rhythm with occasional premature ventricular contractions (PVCs). Her ankles, hands, and eyelids were swollen. Her skin was pale, damp, and cool. She had a spontaneous cough, productive of a small amount of white, frothy sputum. A chest X-ray showed white, fluffy patches that spread outward from the hilar areas to the peripheral borders of both lungs. Her left ventricle appeared moderately enlarged.

The patient's vital signs were blood pressure—183/97 mm Hg, heart rate—101 beats/min, respirations—18 breaths/min and deep, and temperature—37°C. The laboratory report showed that the patient's blood urea nitrogen (BUN), creatinine, potassium, and phosphate levels were all higher than normal. The patient had no urine output. On room air, her arterial blood gas values were pH—7.29, Pa_{CO_2}—32 torr, HCO_3^-—17 mEq/L, and Pa_{O_2}—64 torr. The respiratory therapist started the patient on 4 L/min of oxygen via a nasal cannula and drew a second arterial blood sample 25 minutes later. The results showed a pH of 7.28, Pa_{CO_2}—30, HCO_3^-—16, and Pa_{O_2}—86. No remarkable change was seen in the patient's vital signs.

Although the patient received aggressive medical treatment to correct her cardiac and renal problems, her pulmonary congestion did not significantly improve until she started to produce urine, 24 hours after admission. On day 4, the patient's condition was upgraded. Her skin color was normal, and her skin was warm and dry to the touch. She no longer had a productive cough. When the patient was asked to produce a strong cough, no sputum was produced.

Her peripheral edema was resolved and her vital signs were blood pressure—132/84 mm Hg, heart rate—74 beats/min, and respiratory rate—10 breaths/min. Her laboratory report showed no remarkable problems, and her ECG was normal. A second chest X-ray showed normal lungs and normal heart size. On room air, her arterial blood gas values were pH—7.39, Pa_{CO_2}—39 torr, HCO_3^-—24 mEq/L, and Pa_{O_2}—93 torr. The patient was discharged on day 5.

Discussion

This case illustrates the adverse effects of poor blood circulation on the function of the kidneys and lungs. Essentially, all of the clinical manifestations in this case can be traced back to the patient's left ventricular failure (a prerenal abnormality). As pointed out in this chapter, prerenal problems are the most common and are generally reversible if identified and treated early. One of the early clinical manifestations of prerenal failure is a sharp reduction in urine output. On admission, the patient had no urine output. With the decline in renal function, the kidney's ability to secrete hydrogen ions (H^+) and to conserve (HCO_3^-) progressively decreases. Furthermore, during the more advanced stages of renal failure, hyperkalemia (increased K^+) is a frequent finding. Thus, because of the increased H^+ and K^+ ion levels and the loss of HCO_3^-, *metabolic acidosis* is an inevitable clinical manifestation in severe renal failure.

Because of the left ventricular failure, fluid progressively accumulated in the patient's lungs and extremities. The fluid accumulation, in turn, increased the density of the alveolar-capillary membranes, causing the white fluffy patches visible on the patient's chest X-ray. In addition, as the fluid accumulation in her lungs worsened, the oxygen diffusion across the alveolar-capillary membrane decreased (refer to Figure 4–7). This pathologic process was verified by the Pa_{O_2} of 64 torr on admission. Moreover, because the blood flow through the pulmonary system was impeded (because of the left ventricular failure), blood accumulated throughout the patient's extremities, thus causing swelling in the ankles, hands, and eyelids. Fortunately, the patient received aggressive treatment in a timely manner to reverse all of these potentially fatal pathologic processes.

A 42-year-old male firefighter was found unconscious in a smoke-filled room on the fourth floor of a burning office building. He had second- and third-degree burns over portions of his left shoulder, left arm, and left hand and over the anterior portion of his chest and abdominal region. His pulse was rapid, and his respiratory rate was slow and gasping. He was quickly carried out of the building and placed in a waiting ambulance. It was later estimated that the patient had been unconscious in the smoke-filled room for more than 10 minutes. En route to the hospital, the patient was manually ventilated with 100 percent oxygen. An intravenous infusion was started, and Ringer's lactated solution was administered. The patient's clothing was cut away, and the burn wounds were covered to prevent shock, fluid loss, and heat loss.

When the patient arrived in the emergency department, the skin that was not burned appeared cherry red. His vital signs were blood pressure—96/55 mm Hg and heart rate—124 beats/min. He was still being manually ventilated with 100 percent oxygen. Bilateral bronchospasm and crackles were heard when his lungs were auscultated. The patient was then intubated. Black, frothy secretions were suctioned from his lungs. A chest X-ray showed white fluffy densities throughout both lung fields. Arterial blood gas values were pH—7.52, Pa_{CO_2}—28 torr, HCO_3^-—22 mEq/L, Pa_{O_2}—47 torr. His *carboxyhemoglobin* (CO_{Hb}) level was 47 percent. The emergency department physician felt the patient was hypovolemic and going into shock.

The patient was transferred to the intensive care unit and placed on a mechanical ventilator. His progress was stormy during the first 24 hours. The respiratory care team had to make several ventilator adjustments. The patient's hemodynamic profile was classified as critical (see Hemodynamic Profile No. 1). His cardiopulmonary status, however, was finally stabilized on the second day. At this time, the patient's ventilator settings were a ventilatory rate of 12 breaths/min, an inspired oxygen concentration (FI_{O_2}) of 1.0, and a positive end-expiratory pressure (PEEP) of +15 cm H_2O. Arterial blood gas values were pH—7.38, Pa_{CO_2}—37 torr, HCO_3^-—24 mEq/L, Pa_{O_2}—78 torr, and Sa_{O_2}—93 percent.

Hemodynamic Profile

Parameter*	Profile No. 1	Profile No. 2
BP	63/39 mm Hg	125/83 mm Hg
CVP	12 mm Hg	3 mm Hg
RAP	13 mm Hg	3 mm Hg
$\overline{PAP}$	25 mm Hg	14 mm Hg
CO	2.7 L/min	5.8 L/min
Urine Output	0 mL/hr	54 mL/hr

*BP = blood pressure; CVP = central venous pressure; RAP = right atrial pressure; $\overline{PAP}$ = mean pulmonary artery pressure; CO = cardiac output.

Two days later, the patient's cardiopulmonary status was upgraded to fair. His ventilator settings at this time were 6 breaths/min, FI_{O_2}—0.5, and PEEP—+8 cm H_2O. Arterial blood gas values were pH—7.41, Pa_{CO_2}—38 torr, HCO_3^-—24 mEq/L, Pa_{O_2}—84 torr, and Sa_{O_2}—93 percent. His carboxyhemoglobin (CO_{Hb}) level was 11 percent. His hemodynamic status had significantly improved, and he was producing urine (see Hemodynamic Profile No. 2). The patient progressively improved and was discharged 2 weeks later.

Discussion

Similar to case 1, this case illustrates a prerenal abnormality. The patient's burns caused fluid sequestration, which in turn lead to *hypovolemia* (see Table 16–3). As a result of the hypovolemia, the blood flow though the patient's kidneys decreased. Again, one of the early clinical manifestations of prerenal failure is a sharp reduction in urine output. Note the low cardiac output and no urine output charted on Hemodynamic Profile No.1. Fortunately, the patient responded favorably to therapy, and his hemodynamic status and urine output returned to normal (see Hemodynamic Profile No. 2).

Note also that the patient's pulmonary status, unrelated to the poor kidney function, was very serious on admission. The patient's pathologic lung changes in the distal airways and alveoli were most likely caused by the irritant and toxic gases and suspended soot particles associated with incomplete combustion and smoke. Many of the substances found in smoke are extremely caustic to the tracheobronchial tree and poisonous to the body. The injuries that develop from smoke inhalation include inflammation of the tracheobronchial tree, bronchospasm, excessive bronchial secretions and mucus plugging, decreased mucosal ciliary transport mechanism, atelectasis, alveolar edema, and frothy secretions. Evidence of this condition was documented by the white, fluffy densities found throughout both lung fields and the low Pa_{O_2} (47 torr) at admission. Finally, the patient's carbon monoxide level (CO_{Hb}—47 percent) was dangerously high in the emergency department. Although the patient initially responded slowly to respiratory care, the described pathologic processes were ultimately reversed, and the cardiopulmonary status was normal at the time of discharge.

Review Questions

1. The outer one-third of the kidney is called the
    A. medulla
    B. minor calyces
    C. renal pyramid
    D. cortex

2. Glomerular filtration is directly proportional to
    A. blood cell size
    B. hydrostatic pressure
    C. osmotic pressure
    D. the patient's fluid intake

3. Tubular reabsorption occurs primarily in the
    A. renal corpuscle
    B. proximal convoluted tubule
    C. loop of Henle
    D. distal convoluted tubule

4. The major substance(s) transported by means of tubular secretion is (are)
    1. H^+
    2. Cl^-
    3. K^+
    4. HCO_3^-
    5. Na^+
        A. 1 only
        B. 2 and 4 only
        C. 4 and 5 only
        D. 1 and 3 only

5. The urine produced by the healthy kidney has a specific gravity of about
    A. 1.000–1.001
    B. 1.006–1.020
    C. 1.003–1.030
    D. 1.060–1.080

6. Which of the following can be classified as a prerenal condition?
1. Heart failure
2. Intratubular obstruction
3. Bladder outlet obstruction
4. Hypovolemia
   A. 2 only
   B. 4 only
   C. 2 and 3 only
   D. 1 and 4 only

7. Which of the following are the functional units of the kidneys?
   A. Collecting ducts
   B. Major calyces
   C. Peritubular capillaries
   D. Nephrons

8. Which of the following empties urine into the bladder?
   A. Collecting ducts
   B. Ureters
   C. Distal convoluted tubules
   D. Urethra

9. Normally, the net glomerular filtration pressure is about
   A. 5 mm Hg
   B. 10 mm Hg
   C. 15 mm Hg
   D. 20 mm Hg

10. Which of the following is(are) part of the nephron?
1. Proximal convoluted tubules
2. Loop of Henle
3. Glomerulus
4. Distal convoluted tubules
   A. 3 only
   B. 2, 3, and 4 only
   C. 1, 2, and 3 only
   D. 1, 2, 3, and 4

Clinical Application Questions

Case 1

1. In this case, all of the clinical manifestations can be traced back to the

patient's _____

_____

_____.

2. What was the early clinical manifestation of prerenal failure presented?

_____

_____

_____.

3. Why did metabolic acidosis develop? _____

_____

_____.

4. What clinical manifestations developed as a result of left ventricular

failure? _____

_____

_____

_____.

Case 2

1. What was the cause of the prerenal abnormality in this case?

_____

_____

_____.

2. What lung injuries developed as a result of smoke inhalation?

_____

_____

_____.

3. What was the clinical evidence that the lung injuries listed in

question 2 were present? _____

_____

_____.

Chapter 17

Sleep Physiology and Its Relationship to the Cardiopulmonary System

Objectives

By the end of this chapter, the student should be able to:

1. Differentiate sleep from a coma.
2. Define polysomography.
3. Define a polysomnogram epoch.
4. Describe the purpose of the following monitors:
   —Electroencephalogram (EEG)
   —Electro-oculogram (EOG)
   —Electromyogram (EMG)
   —Oximeter
   —CO_2 analyzer
5. Differentiate among the following EEG waveforms:
   —Beta waves
   —Alpha waves
   —Theta waves
   —Delta waves
   —K complexes
   —Sleep spindles
   —Sawtooth waves
   —Vertex waves
6. Describe the clinical connection associated with the sleep disorder specialist—trends, education, and certification.
7. Identify the major epoch physiologic components associated with the following types of sleep:
   —Eyes open—wake (stage W)
   —Eyes closed—drowsy
   —Stage N1, non-REM sleep (light sleep)
   —Stage N2, non-REM sleep (light sleep)
   —Stage N3, non-REM deep sleep (slow-wave sleep; deep sleep)
   —REM sleep
8. Describe the clinical connection associated with the types of sleep studies.
9. Outline the normal sleep cycle.
10. Describe the following two most widely accepted theories regarding the purpose of sleep:
    —Restoration
    —Energy conservation
11. Describe circadian rhythms.
12. Describe the normal sleep patterns for the following groups:
    —Newborns and infants
    —Toddlers and preschoolers
    —Children and adolescents
    —Young adults and older adults
13. List factors that affect sleep initiation and maintenance
14. Describe the following common sleep disorders:
    —Insomnia
    —Hypersomnia
    —Narcolepsy
    —Sleep apnea
      • Obstructive sleep apnea (OSA)
      • Central sleep apnea (CSA)
      • Mixed sleep apnea
    —Periodic limb movement disorder (PLMD)
    —Restless legs syndrome (RLS)
15. Discuss the clinical connection associated with the clinical signs and symptoms of obstructive sleep apnea.
16. Describe the clinical connection associated with the therapeutic effects of continuous positive airway pressure (CPAP) in obstructive sleep apnea.
17. Discuss the clinical connection associated with the risk factors linked to obstructive sleep apnea.
18. Discuss the clinical connection associated with the risk factors linked to central sleep apnea.

(continues)

19. Describe the clinical connection associated with the management of sleep apnea.
20. Describe the clinical connection associated with the role of the respiratory therapist in caring for the obstructive sleep apnea patient.
21. Describe the physiologic changes that occur during sleep in the following:
—Autonomic nervous system
—Musculoskeletal system
—Thermal regulation
—Renal function
—Genital function
—Gastrointestinal function
—Endocrine function
—Cardiovascular function
—Sleep-related arrhymias
—Cerebral blood flow
—Respiratory physiology
22. Complete the review questions at the end of this chapter.

Introduction

Sleep is a naturally occurring state of partial unconsciousness, diminished activity of the skeletal muscles, and depressed metabolism from which a person can be awakened by stimulation. Because sleep is readily reversible, it is distinguished from a *coma,* which is a state of unconsciousness from which a person cannot be awakened—even by the most forceful stimuli. Interestingly, an individual's environmental monitoring often continues to function during sleep, as illustrated by the fact that a strong stimulus—like a baby's cry—can immediately awaken a parent. In fact, it is well documented that individuals who sleepwalk can actually navigate around objects or climb stairs while truly asleep.

All mammals and birds sleep. Body size appears to play an important role in determining the amount of sleep a species needs. In general, large mammals need less sleep than small mammals. For example, a giraffe or elephant sleeps about 3 to 4 hours a day, whereas a cat or ferret needs about 12 to 14 hours of sleep a day. Bats, opossums, and armadillos sleep 18 or more hours a day. The newborn requires about 17 hours of sleep a day, whereas the adult needs about 6 to 8 hours a day.

During the past several years, there has been a tremendous increase in the demand for sleep medicine diagnostic and therapeutic services—driven, in part, by (1) the heightened appreciation of sleep disorders in the general population and (2) the increased scientific research studies now available concerning sleep and sleep disorders. In response to the increased need for these services, many specialized sleep centers and laboratories are now available throughout the health care industry. These sleep centers offer **polysomography** (sleep studies) with qualified sleep technologists who provide many diagnostic and therapeutic services.

An **epoch** or **polysomnogram** is a recorded measurement of time during a sleep study of multiple physiologic variables that can be used to identify the different phases of sleep and, importantly, sleep disorders. For example, sleep-related disorders, such as *obstructive sleep apnea*, are now known to adversely affect the cardiopulmonary system in numerous ways, and the respiratory therapist commonly treats them.

The major physiologic variables provided during a polysomnogram include (1) an **electroencephalogram** (EEG), which measures the electrophysiologic changes in the brain; (2) an **electro-oculogram** (EOG), which monitors the movements of the eyes; and (3) an **electromyogram** (EMG), which measures muscle activity. Table 17–1 provides an overview of common EEG waveforms.

Table 17–1

Common EEG Waveforms

An **electroencephalogram** (EEG) measures the electrophysiologic changes in the brain. The EEG electrical activity is characterized by frequency in cycles per second or hertz (Hz), amplitude (voltage), and the direction of major defection (polarity). The following are the most common frequency ranges.

Beta Waves
(>13 Hz)

One of the four brain waves, characterized by relatively low voltage or amplitude and a frequency greater than 13 Hz. Beta waves are known as the "busy waves" of the brain. They are recorded when the patient is awake and alert with eyes open. They are also seen during Stage N1 sleep.

Alpha Waves
(8–13 Hz)

One of the four brain waves, characterized by a relatively high voltage or amplitude and a frequency of 8–13 Hz. Alpha waves are known as the "relaxed waves" of the brain. They are commonly recorded when the individual is awake, but in a drowsy state and when the eyes are closed. Alpha waves are commonly seen during Stage N1 sleep. Bursts of alpha waves are also seen during brief awakenings from sleep called arousals. Alpha waves may also be seen during REM sleep.

Theta Waves
(4–7 Hz)

One of the four types of brain waves, characterized by a relatively low frequency of 4–7 Hz and low amplitude of 10 microvolts (μV). Theta waves are known as the "drowsy waves" of the brain. They are seen when the individual is awake, but relaxed and sleepy. They are also recorded in Stage 1 sleep, REM sleep, and as background waves during Stage N2 sleep.

Delta Waves
(<4 Hz)

The slowest of the four types of brain waves. Delta waves are characterized by a frequency of less than 4 Hz and high amplitude (>75 μV) broad waves. Although delta EEG activity is usually defined as <4 Hz, in human sleep scoring, the slow-wave activity used for staging is defined as EEG activity < 2 Hz (> 0.5 second duration) and a peak-to-peak amplitude of >75 μV. Delta waves are called the "deep-sleep waves." They are associated with a dreamless state from which an individual is not easily aroused. Delta waves are seen primarily during Stage N3 sleep.

K Complexes

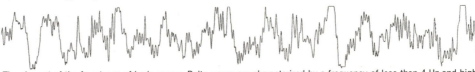

K complexes are intermittent high-amplitude, biphasic waves of at least 0.5 second duration that signal the start of Stage N2 sleep (green bars). A K complex consists of a sharp negative wave (upward deflection), followed immediately by a slower positive wave (downward deflection), that is >0.5 second. K complexes are usually seen during Stage N2 sleep. They are sometimes seen in Stage N3. Sleep spindles are often superimposed on K complexes.

Sleep Spindles

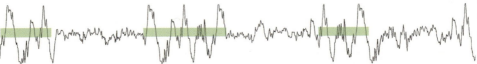

Sleep spindles are sudden bursts of EEG activity in the 12–14 Hz frequency (6 or more distinct waves) and duration of 0.5 to 1.5 seconds (pink bars). Sleep spindles mark the onset of Stage N2. They may be seen in Stage N3, but usually do not occur in REM sleep.

Sawtooth Waves

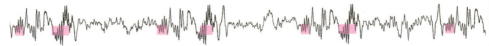

Sawtooth waves are notched-jagged waves of frequency in the theta range (3–7 Hz) (brown bars). They are commonly seen during REM sleep. Although sawtooth waves are not part of the criteria for REM sleep, their presence is a clue that REM sleep is present.

Vertex Waves

Vertex waves are sharp negative (upward deflection) EEG waves, often in conjunction with high amplitude and short (2–7 Hz) activity (yellow bar). The amplitude of many of the vertex sharp waves are greater than 20 μV and, occasionally, they may be as high as 200 μV. Vertex waves are usually seen at the end of Stage N1.

© Cengage Learning 2013

Figure 17–1

Eyes open—wake. As shown in the yellow bar, the EEG records beta waves with high-frequency, low-amplitude activity, and sawtooth waves. EOG is low frequency and variable, and the EMG activity is relatively high. The epoch appears similar to REM sleep.

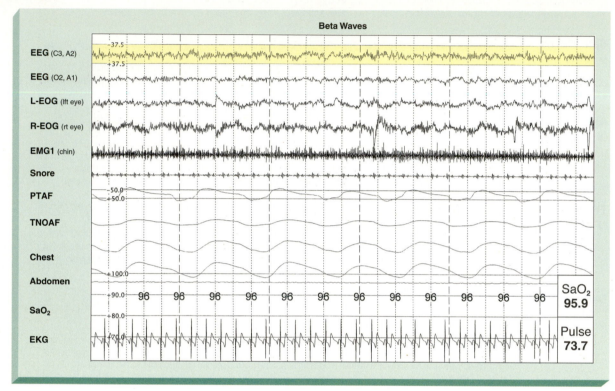

Other physiologic features typically monitored during a sleep study include (1) the presence or absence of snoring, (2) nasal and oral airflow, (3) chest movement, (4) abdomen movement, (5) Sa_{O_2}, and (6) an electrocardiogram (ECG). End-tidal CO_2 monitoring as a surrogate for airflow is used in sleep studies of neonates and infants and more and more often in adults. Thermistors, which sense change in temperature (exhaled air is warmer than inspired air), are also used for this purpose.

Figure 17–1 provides a representative sleep study epoch of a patient with "eyes open and awake." Most sleep study epochs are 30 seconds in duration. Thus, between 720 and 960 separate epoch recordings are generated over a 6- to 8-hour sleep study period.

Types of Sleep

Non-rapid-eye-movement sleep (non-REM sleep or NREM sleep) and rapid-eye-movement sleep (REM sleep) are the two major types of sleep. The following subsections provide a more in-depth discussion of the two major types of sleep and the physiologic changes commonly observed during a full sleep cycle.

Clinical Connection—17-1

The Sleep Disorder Specialist—Trends, Education, and Certification

The respiratory therapist can further broaden his or her career by pursuing additional education and training as a **sleep disorder specialist (SDS)** (Figure 17–2). The SDS performs sleep tests and works with physicians to provide a variety of information needed for the diagnosis of sleep disorders. For example, the SDS:

- Monitors of brain waves, eye movements, muscle activity, multiple breathing variables, and blood oxygen levels during sleep, using specialized recording equipment.

- Interprets the recording as it happens, and responds appropriately to emergencies.

- Instructs the patient in recording and maintaining a sleep diary of 7 to 14 days of wake/sleep cycles.

- Provides support services related to the treatment of sleep-related problems, including helping patients use devices for the treatment of breathing problems during sleep and helping individuals develop good sleep habits.

The **National Board for Respiratory Care Inc. (NBRC)** administers the credentialing examination for the sleep disorder specialist. The NBRC's Sleep Disorder Specialty examination program is designed for a respiratory therapist with an NBRC respiratory care credential and experience or education in the field of sleep medicine. The admission requirements are the following:

- Be a certified respiratory therapist (CRT) or registered respiratory therapist (RRT) having completed a Commission on Accreditation for Respiratory Care (CoARC) or Committee on Accreditation Allied Health Education Programs (CAAHEP) accredited respiratory therapist program, including a sleep add-on track.

Figure 17–2

A sleep disorder specialist.

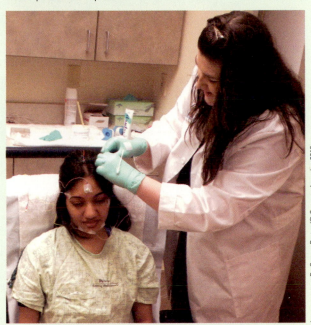

Image courtesy Dr. George Burton/© Cengage Learning 2013

- Be a CRT with 6 months of full-time[1] clinical experience following certification in a sleep diagnostics and treatment setting under medical supervision (MD, DO, or PhD).

- Be an RRT with 3 months of full-time clinical experience following certification in a sleep diagnostic and treatment setting under medical supervision.

---

[1] Full-time experience is defined as a minimum of 21 hours per week per calendar year in a sleep diagnostics and treatment setting under medical supervision following Certification acceptable to the Board. Clinical experience must be completed before the candidate applies for this examination (http://www.nbrc.org).

Eyes Open—Wake

The eyes open—wake state (stage W) appears very similar to REM sleep. The EEG shows beta waves with high frequency, low-amplitude activity, and sawtooth waves. The EOG is low frequency and variable, and the EMG activity is relatively high (see Figure 17–1).

Eyes closed—wake. As shown in the purple bar, the EEG records prominent alpha waves (>50 percent). The EOG tracing often shows slow, rolling eye movements, and the EMG activity is relatively high.

© Cengage Learning 2013

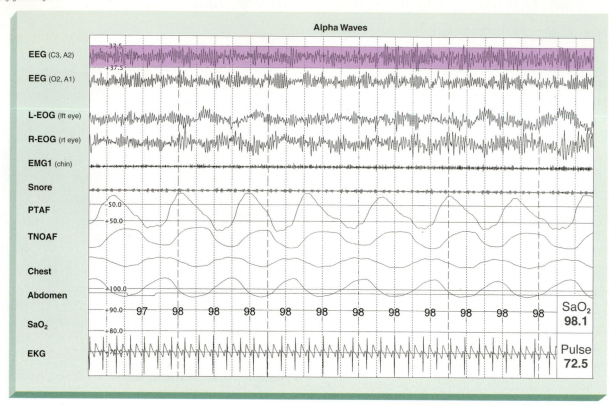

Eyes Closed—Wake

The EEG during the eyes closed—wake (drowsy) period is characterized by prominent alpha waves (>50 percent). The EOG tracing usually shows slow, rolling eye movements, and the EMG activity is relatively high (Figure 17–3).

Non-REM Sleep (N Sleep)

Non-REM sleep consists of three stages of sleep. In general, stage N1 and stage N2 are described as *light sleep stages*, and stage N3 is referred to as *slow-wave sleep* and *deep sleep*. Non-REM sleep accounts for about 75 to 80 percent of sleep time in the average adult. During the first 30 to 45 minutes of sleep, an individual passes through all three stages of non-REM sleep, progressively moving toward slow-wave sleep—stage N3. In the average young adult, stage N1 comprises about 3 to 8 percent of sleep time, stage N2 about 45 to 55 percent, and stage N3 makes up about 15 to 20 percent of total sleep time. The following is a general overview of the three stages of non-REM sleep.

Stage N1

Stage N1 is the transitional stage between drowsiness and sleep. The person feels sleepy and often experiences a drifting or floating sensation. The sleeper

Figure 17–4

Stage N1 non-REM sleep. EEG records low-voltage, mixed-frequency activity, with alpha waves (8–12 Hz, <50 percent) (purple bar) and theta waves (blue bar). Some beta waves (>13 Hz) (yellow bar) may also appear. Vertex waves commonly appear toward the end of stage N1 (orange bar). The EOG shows slow, rolling eye movements. The EMG reveals decreased activity and muscle relaxation. Respirations become regular, and the heart rate and blood pressure decrease slightly. Snoring may occur.

© Cengage Learning 2013

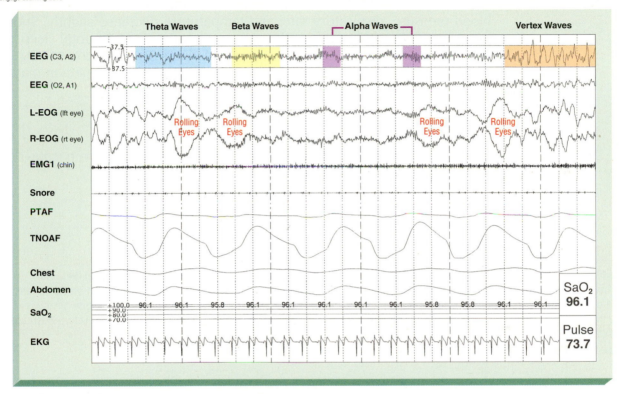

may experience sudden muscle contractions called **hypnic myoclonia**. These contractions are frequently preceded by a sensation of starting to fall. These sudden muscle movements are similar to the "jump" one elicits when startled. Under normal conditions, stage N1 lasts between 10 to 12 minutes and is very light sleep. A person can be easily awakened during this period.

As the person moves into stage N1, the EEG shows light sleep comprised of low-voltage, mixed-frequency activity, with **alpha waves** (8–12 Hz[2]; <50 percent) and **theta waves**. Alpha waves indicate that the brain is in a calm and relaxed state of wakefulness. Some **beta waves** (>13 Hz) may also appear. **Vertex waves** commonly appear toward the end of stage N1. The EOG shows slow, rolling eye movements. The EMG reveals decreased activity and muscle relaxation. Breathing become regular, and the heart rate and blood pressure decrease slightly ("nocturnal dipping"). Minute ventilation, cerebral blood flow, and muscle tone diminish. Snoring may occur. If awakened, persons may state that they were not asleep (Figure 17–4).

---

[2] Hz = cycles per second.

Stage N2

Stage N2 is still a relatively light sleep stage, although arousal is a bit more difficult. The EEG becomes more irregular and is comprised predominantly of **theta waves** (4–7 Hz), intermixed with sudden bursts of **sleep spindles** (12–18 Hz) and one or more **K complexes**. **Vertex waves** may also be seen during this stage. The EOG shows either slow eye movements or absence of slow eye movements. The EMG has low electrical activity. The heart rate, blood pressure, respiratory rate, and temperature decrease slightly. Snoring may occur. Stage N2 occupies the greatest proportion of the total sleep time and accounts for about 40 to 50 percent of sleep. The duration of stage N2 NREM sleep is between 10 and 15 minutes. If awakened, the person may say he or she was thinking or daydreaming (Figure 17–5).

Stage N3

Stage N3 sleep can be divided into the following two main categories: (1) slow-wave sleep and (2) deep sleep.

Figure 17–5

Stage N2 non-REM sleep. The EEG becomes more irregular and is comprised mostly of theta waves (4–7 Hz) (blue bar), intermixed with sudden bursts of sleep spindles (12–18 Hz) (pink bar), and one or more K complexes (green bars). Vertex waves may also be seen during this stage (yellow bar). The EOG shows either slow eye movements or absence of slow eye movements. The EMG has low electrical activity. The heart rate, blood pressure, respiratory rate, and temperature decrease slightly. Snoring may occur.

© Cengage Learning 2013

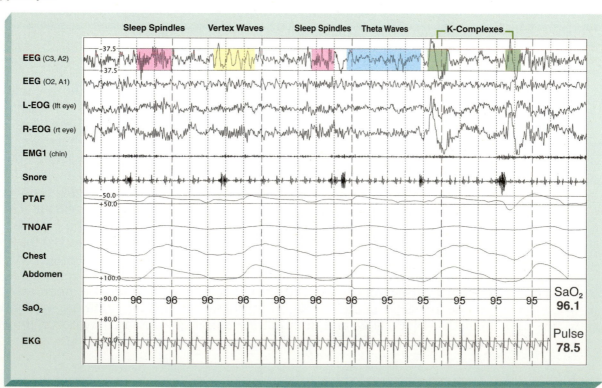

Stage N3—Slow-Wave Sleep. *Slow-wave sleep* is present when 20 to 50 percent of the EEG activity consists of high-amplitude (>75 µV), slow-frequency (2 Hz or slower) **delta waves**. Both **sleep spindles** and **K complexes** may be present during this period of stage N3. There is little or no eye movement on the EOG, and the EMG activity is low. The skeletal muscles are very relaxed, but tone is maintained. There is a continued decrease in the heart rate, blood pressure, respiratory rate, body temperature, and oxygen consumption. Snoring may occur. Dreaming may occur, but is less dramatic, more realistic, and may lack plot. The sleeper becomes more difficult to arouse. Stage N3 is usually reached about 20 to 25 minutes after the onset of stage N1 (Figure 17–6).

Stage N3—Deep Sleep. *Deep sleep* is present when more than 50 percent of the EEG activity consists of **delta waves** (amplitude >75 µV and frequency 2 Hz or less). The EOG shows no eye movements, and the EMG has little or no electrical activity. The sleeper is very relaxed and seldom moves. The vital signs reach their lowest, normal level. In fact, the sleeper's heart and

---

Figure 17–6

Stage N3 non-REM (slow-wave) sleep. EEG records 20 to 50 percent activity of high-amplitude (>75 µV), slow-frequency (2 Hz or slower) delta waves (orange bar). Sleep spindles (pink bar) and K complexes (green bar) may be present during stage N3. The EOG records little or no eye movement, and the EMG activity is low. There is a continued decrease in the heart rate, blood pressure, respiratory rate, body temperature, and oxygen consumption. Snoring may occur.

© Cengage Learning 2013

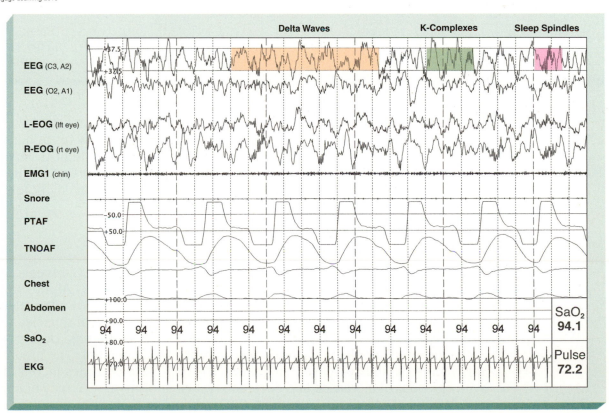

Figure 17-7

Stage N3 non-REM (deep) sleep. EEG records more than 50 percent activity of delta waves (amplitude >75 μV, frequency 2 Hz or less) (orange bar). The EOG shows no eye movements, and the EMG has little or no electrical activity. The sleeper's heart and respiratory rate are generally decreased 20 to 30 percent below normal waking-hour levels.

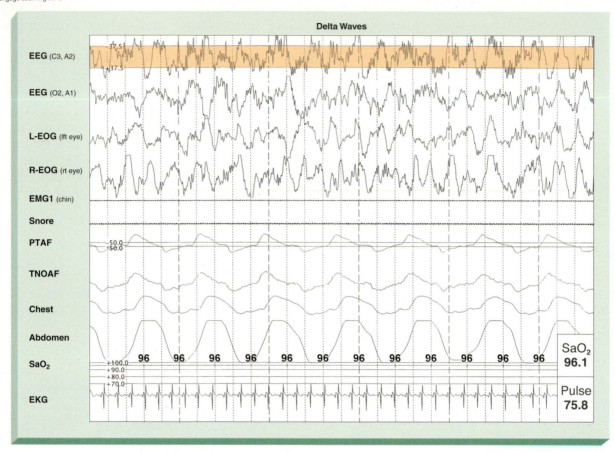

respiratory rate are generally decreased 20 to 30 percent below his or her normal waking-hour levels. Oxygen consumption is low. The patient is very difficult to awaken. This period of stage N3 is thought to be important for mental and physical restoration. This is the stage in which bed-wetting, night terrors, and sleepwalking are most likely to occur (Figure 17-7).

REM Sleep

REM sleep resembles the eyes open—wake state. The EEG reveals low-voltage, mixed EEG activity, and frequent sawtooth waves. Alpha waves may be present. The EOG shows REM. The EMG recording shows low electrical activity, and a temporary paralysis of most of the skeletal muscles (e.g., arms, legs) is present. Diaphragmatic muscle activity continues. During REM sleep, brain metabolism may increase as much as 20 percent. The breathing rate increases and decreases irregularly. The heart rate becomes inconsistent with episodes of increased and decreased rates. Snoring may or may not present. When the sleeper is very tired, the duration of each REM period is very

Figure 17–8

REM sleep. Resembles the eyes open—wake epoch. The EEG records low-voltage, mixed EEG activity and frequent sawtooth waves (brown bar). Alpha waves may be present (purple bar). The EOG records rapid eye movement (REM). The EMG records low electrical activity and documents a temporary paralysis of most of the skeletal muscles (e.g., arms, legs). The breathing rate increases and decreases irregularly. During REM sleep, the heart rate becomes inconsistent with episodes of increased and decreased rates. Snoring may or may not be present. REM is not as restful as NREM sleep. REM is also known as paradoxic sleep. Most dreams occur during REM sleep.

© Cengage Learning 2013

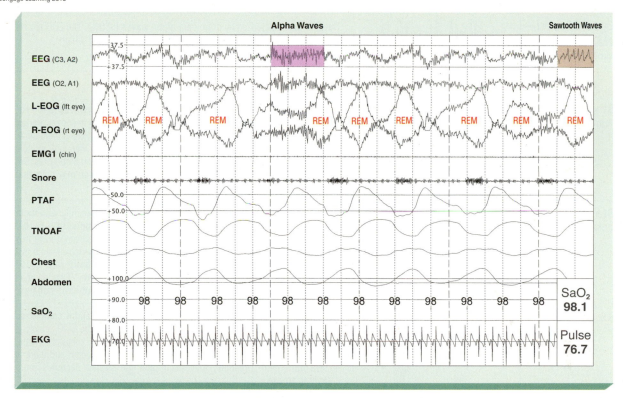

short or even absent. As the person becomes more rested through the sleep period, the length of the REM sleep periods increase.

About 25 percent of the sleep of the young normal adult consists of REM sleep. The first REM sleep period usually occurs about 70 to 90 minutes after one falls asleep and lasts 5 to 30 minutes. REM is not as restful as NREM sleep. In fact, REM sleep is also known as **paradoxic sleep**, because the EEG pattern is similar to the normal awake pattern. Most dreams occur during REM sleep. They are frequently remembered during the wakeful state and are often described as having vivid content, full color, sounds, implausible or bizarre settings, and a sense of paralysis (Figure 17–8).

Table 17–2 on page 534 summarizes the sleep stages, according to the current American Academy of Sleep Medicine standards.[3]

---

[3] *The AASM Manual for the Scoring of Sleep & Associated Events: Rules, Terminology, and Technical Specifications* (Copyright 2011 American Academy of Sleep Medicine, 2510 North Frontage Road, Darien, Il 60561, Telephone: 630-737-9700).

Table 17–2
Sleep Stages

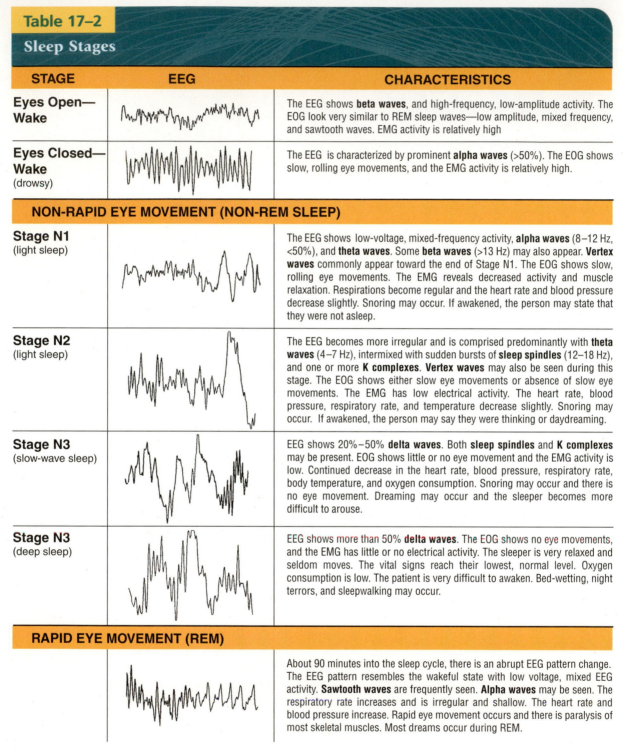

STAGE	EEG	CHARACTERISTICS
Eyes Open—Wake		The EEG shows **beta waves**, and high-frequency, low-amplitude activity. The EOG look very similar to REM sleep waves—low amplitude, mixed frequency, and sawtooth waves. EMG activity is relatively high
Eyes Closed—Wake (drowsy)		The EEG is characterized by prominent **alpha waves** (>50%). The EOG shows slow, rolling eye movements, and the EMG activity is relatively high.
NON-RAPID EYE MOVEMENT (NON-REM SLEEP)		
Stage N1 (light sleep)		The EEG shows low-voltage, mixed-frequency activity, **alpha waves** (8–12 Hz, <50%), and **theta waves**. Some **beta waves** (>13 Hz) may also appear. **Vertex waves** commonly appear toward the end of Stage N1. The EOG shows slow, rolling eye movements. The EMG reveals decreased activity and muscle relaxation. Respirations become regular and the heart rate and blood pressure decrease slightly. Snoring may occur. If awakened, the person may state that they were not asleep.
Stage N2 (light sleep)		The EEG becomes more irregular and is comprised predominantly with **theta waves** (4–7 Hz), intermixed with sudden bursts of **sleep spindles** (12–18 Hz), and one or more **K complexes**. **Vertex waves** may also be seen during this stage. The EOG shows either slow eye movements or absence of slow eye movements. The EMG has low electrical activity. The heart rate, blood pressure, respiratory rate, and temperature decrease slightly. Snoring may occur. If awakened, the person may say they were thinking or daydreaming.
Stage N3 (slow-wave sleep)		EEG shows 20%–50% **delta waves**. Both **sleep spindles** and **K complexes** may be present. EOG shows little or no eye movement and the EMG activity is low. Continued decrease in the heart rate, blood pressure, respiratory rate, body temperature, and oxygen consumption. Snoring may occur and there is no eye movement. Dreaming may occur and the sleeper becomes more difficult to arouse.
Stage N3 (deep sleep)		EEG shows more than 50% **delta waves**. The EOG shows no eye movements, and the EMG has little or no electrical activity. The sleeper is very relaxed and seldom moves. The vital signs reach their lowest, normal level. Oxygen consumption is low. The patient is very difficult to awaken. Bed-wetting, night terrors, and sleepwalking may occur.
RAPID EYE MOVEMENT (REM)		
		About 90 minutes into the sleep cycle, there is an abrupt EEG pattern change. The EEG pattern resembles the wakeful state with low voltage, mixed EEG activity. **Sawtooth waves** are frequently seen. **Alpha waves** may be seen. The respiratory rate increases and is irregular and shallow. The heart rate and blood pressure increase. Rapid eye movement occurs and there is paralysis of most skeletal muscles. Most dreams occur during REM.

Clinical Connection—17-2

Types of Sleep Studies

The majority of sleep studies are done in sleep disorders centers, which may be "facility-based" (associated with hospitals) or freestanding (Figure 17–9). In some settings, limited studies may be done in the home. In fully accredited sleep disorders centers, the following tests are commonly performed:

- **Nocturnal polysomnography** (nights)—**Polysomnography** (PSG), also known as a **sleep study**, is a study of sleep. The test result is called a **polysomnogram**, also abbreviated PSG. The results of the PSG are used as a diagnostic tool in sleep medicine. The PSG monitors many body functions including brain (EEG) activities, eye movements (EOG), muscle activity or skeletal muscle activation (EMG), respiratory airflow, pulse oximetry, expired CO_2, and heart rhythm (ECG) during sleep.

- **Multiple sleep latency testing** (MSLT) (days)—The MSLT is used to measure the time elapsed from the start of a daytime nap period to the first signs of sleep, called **sleep latency**. The test is based on the idea that the sleepier people are, the faster they will fall asleep. The MSLT can

be used (1) to test for **narcolepsy**, (2) to test for physical tiredness versus true excessive daytime sleepiness, and (3) to determine if treatments for breathing disorders are working. The primary purpose of MSLT is to serve as an objective measure of sleepiness. The test consists of four or five 20-minute nap opportunities that are scheduled about 2 hours apart. A MSLT is usually performed after an overnight sleep study. During the test, the patient's brain waves (EEG, muscle activity (EMG) and eye movements (EOG) are recorded.

- **Maintenance of wakefulness testing (MWT)** (nights or days, depending on work time being studied)—The MWT is used to evaluate how alert an individual is during the day. The MWT determines whether or not a patient is able to stay awake for a defined period of time. The test indicates how well an individual is able to function and remain alert during periods of quiet time and inactivity.

Figure 17–9

Nocturnal polysomnography (sleep study).

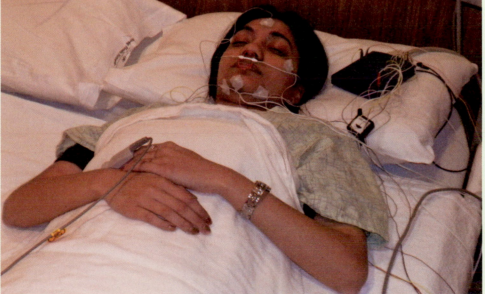

Image courtesy Dr. George Burton/ © Cengage Learning 2013

Normal Sleep Cycles

Under normal circumstances, most people require 10 to 30 minutes to fall asleep. The time needed to fall asleep is called **sleep latency**. A sleep latency period of less than 5 minutes indicates excessive sleepiness; a sleep latency period of longer than 30 minutes is associated with the lack of sleepiness, emotional stress, environmental disturbances, medication, illness, or pain.

One full sleep cycle begins with stage N1. The sleeper then progresses through stages N2 and N3 (slow-wave sleep and deep sleep); followed by a return to stage N2. From stage N2, the sleeper slips into REM sleep. The end of the first REM sleep cycle is the conclusion of the first sleep cycle.

From REM sleep, the individual moves back to stage N2, and a new sleep cycle starts (Figure 17–10). The duration of each sleep cycle is about 90 to 110 minutes. The sleep cycles become longer as the sleeper becomes rested. Between four to six full cycles of sleep occur during a normal night's sleep.

The normal young adult moves from stages N1 to N3 in about 30 minutes. The sleeper usually remains in deep sleep stage N3 for about 20 or 30 minutes. During the next 20 or 30 minutes, the sleeper moves back to slow-wave stage N3, and then stage N2. The first REM sleep lasts for about 5 to 30 minutes. As the night progresses, REM sleep periods increase in duration and deep sleep (stage N3) decreases. If awakened during any stage, the sleeper must return to stage N1 sleep and proceed through all the stages. By morning, the majority of sleep is spent in stages N1, N2, and REM.

Figure 17–10

Normal sleep cycle. The sleeper progresses through stages N1, N2, and N3; followed by a return to stage N2. From stage N2 the sleeper moves into REM sleep. The end of REM sleep ends the first sleep cycle. From REM sleep, the sleeper moves back to stage N2, and a new sleep cycle begins.

© Cengage Learning 2013

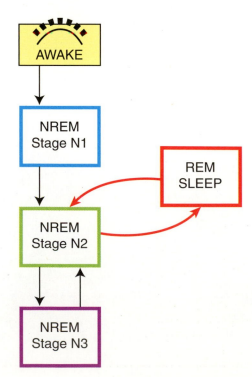

Older sleeping adults, in either stage N2 or N3 non-REM sleep, often bypass REM sleep altogether and awaken. Except for the older adult, changes in body position during sleep usually occur 20 to 40 times during the night. One or two awakenings are normal for the young adult. The number and duration of nocturnal awakenings tend to increase with age. The duration of non-REM and REM sleep varies with age. Figure 17–11 illustrates the normal sleep cycles of children, young adults, and older adults.

Figure 17–11

Normal sleep cycles of children, young adults, and older adults.

© Cengage Learning 2013

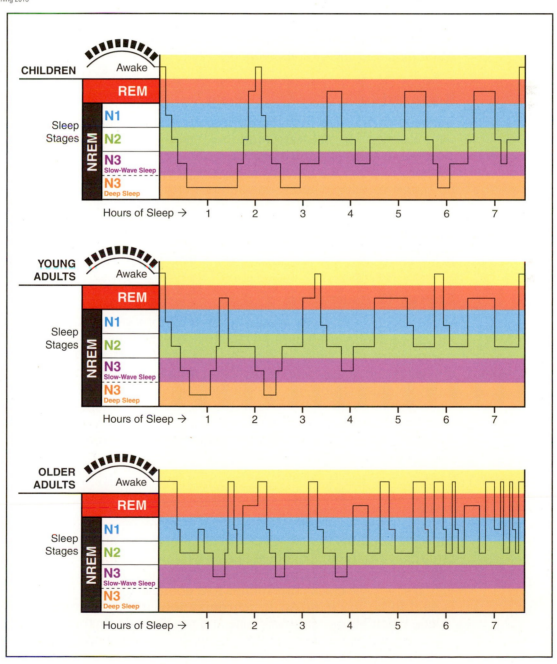

Functions of Sleep

In spite of the fact that sleep is essential for survival—right alongside food and water—the precise function of sleep is still unknown. Once considered a passive, dormant part of our daily lives, it is now known that the brain is very active during sleep. For example, during sleep, the cortical activity is depressed, but the brainstem continues to control such functions as respiration, heart rate, and blood pressure.

In addition, the lack of sleep has adverse affects on our physical and mental health in numerous ways that are just now beginning to be understood. For example, too little sleep leaves the individual drowsy and unable to concentrate. It also leads to impaired memory and physical performance and reduced ability to carry out basic mental functions. Extreme sleep deprivation can lead to depression, paranoia, hallucinations, and mood swings.

The two most widely accepted theories regarding the purpose of sleep are *restoration* and *energy conservation.*

Restoration

The most widely accepted theory of sleep function is that it provides the body with a period for restoration and recuperation. It is thought that non-REM, slow-wave sleep promotes physical growth and healing. This theory is further supported by the fact that slow-wave sleep coincides with the release of growth hormone in children and young adults. Furthermore, many of the body's cells also show increased production and reduced breakdown of proteins during deep sleep. REM sleep appears to play an important role in the restoration of the brain processes, such as attention span, learning and memory, emotional healing, and performing basic social skills.

Energy Conservation

Some suggest that sleep is an extension of homeostasis. In other words, the increased energy used during wakeful hours must be offset by the decreased energy consumed while asleep. This is based, in part, by the fact that the metabolic rate decreases 5 to 25 percent during non-REM, slow-wave sleep. The energy conservation theory is further supported by the fact that slow-wave sleep declines with age; that is, as the energy requirements decrease with age, the need to conserve energy also decreases. It is believed that the decreased need to conserve energy is directly reflected in the decreased slow-wave sleep seen in the older adult.

Circadian Rhythms

Biologic rhythms that occur at regular intervals of about 24 hours are called circadian rhythms. Examples of biorhythms include the sleep–wake cycles, changes in cortisol levels, and body temperature fluctuations. When an individual's biologic clock corresponds to a good sleep–wake pattern, the person is said to be in circadian synchronization. In other words, the person is asleep when his or her physiologic and psychologic rhythms are at their lowest level and awake when his or her physiologic and psychologic rhythms are at their highest level.

In fact, current publications that deal with many public policy and safety issues involving sleep, sleep deprivation, and sleep disorders strongly suggest that the number-one sleep-related problem affecting most people today is sleep debt. Sleep debt is based on the assumption that each person has a specific sleep requirement, an amount that must be obtained each night to maintain constant functioning. All amounts less than this specific sleep requirement constitute lost sleep, and the size of an individual's sleep debt is the total of all nights of lost sleep. A discussion of the relationship of circadian synchronization and normal sleep patterns throughout the average life span follows.

Normal Sleep Patterns

Sleep patterns are well established in the first few months of life and continue throughout life. With advancing age, regular sleep patterns gradually decrease. In general, the well-rested person awakens feeling refreshed, mentally alert, energized, and ready to meet the daily challenges of life. However, the normal sleep–wake pattern (circadian rhythm) varies significantly throughout life.

Newborns and Infants

The newborn sleeps about 16 to 17 hours a day. However, this total sleep time is usually divided into about seven fairly equal sleep periods throughout the day and night. Initially, the infant usually awakens every 3 or 4 hours, eats, and then goes back to sleep. About 50 percent of the sleep period is spent in non-REM (stages N1, N2, and N3), and about 50 percent is spent in REM. During the REM periods, the infant commonly exhibits a lot of activity, such as twitching movements, gurgles, and coughing. By 4 months, most infants sleep through the night and take short naps throughout the day. At the end of 1 year, most infants sleep about 14 hours a day and take one or two naps during daylight hours.

Toddlers and Preschoolers

Total sleep time declines from about 14 hours a day at age 2 to about 12 hours a day by the fifth year—primarily due to the elimination of the afternoon nap. Most preschoolers still need an afternoon nap. Getting the child to sleep, however, is a frequently reported problem. REM sleep decreases to about 30 percent. Slow-wave sleep is also high.

Children and Adolescents

School-age children sleep between 8 and 12 hours a day. As the child approaches 12 years of age, less sleep is usually required. About 20 percent is spent in REM sleep. Most adolescents need between 8 and 10 hours of sleep. About 20 percent is spent in REM sleep.

Young and Older Adults

The young adult usually requires between 6 and 8 hours of sleep a day. About 20 percent is spent in REM sleep. Stage N3 progressively decreases during this age, and the number of arousals from sleep increases. The **older adult** needs between 6 and 8 hours of sleep a day. About 20 to 25 percent is spent in REM sleep. Stage N3 is significantly reduced or absent. Older adults frequently require longer periods of time to fall asleep, awaken more frequently, take longer to fall back to sleep, often feel drowsy during the daytime, and take longer to adjust to changes in schedules.

Factors Affecting Sleep

A number of factors affect both the quality (i.e., appropriate amounts of REM and non-REM sleep) and the total time an individual sleeps. Table 17–3 provides an overview of factors affecting sleep.

Table 17–3	
Factors Affecting Sleep	
Age	Age is one of the most important factors affecting sleep.
Illness	Illnesses that cause pain and physical stress can disrupt sleep. Respiratory problems can disrupt a person's sleep. Elevated temperatures can cause reduction in Stage N3 sleep and REM sleep.
Environment	The environment can either enhance or hinder sleep. For example, a sudden noise change or light change in the environment can disrupt sleep. Too much or too little ventilation can affect sleep. Too warm or too cold environments can also affect sleep.
Fatigue	Moderate fatigue promotes restful sleep. The more fatigued an individual is, the shorter the first periods of REM sleep. As the sleeper becomes more rested, the REM sleep increases in duration.
Lifestyle	Frequent work shift changes (e.g., nights vs. days) disrupt sleep. Moderate exercise enhances sleep, whereas excessive exercise can delay sleep.
Emotional stress	Anxiety and depression can disrupt sleep.
Alcohol and stimulants	Excessive alcohol often disrupts sleep and may cause nightmares. Caffeine beverages stimulate the central nervous system and, thus, can interfere with sleep.
Diet	Both weight loss and weight gain are felt to affect sleep. Weight loss is usually associated with decreased sleep time, more arousals, and earlier awakenings. Weight gain is associated with an increased total sleep time, fewer arousals, and later awakenings.
Smoking	Smokers usually have more difficulty falling asleep, are easily aroused and often describe themselves as light sleepers. This is thought to be due to the stimulating effects of nicotine.
Motivation	Fatigue can often be overcome when a person desires to remain awake (e.g., a tired person watching a basketball game). However, when an individual is bored and unmotivated to stay awake, sleep usually rapidly ensues.
Medications	Hypnotics disrupt Stage N3, NREM sleep and suppress REM sleep. Beta-blockers may cause insomnia and nightmares. Narcotics suppress REM sleep and cause frequent arousals and drowsiness. Tranquilizers disrupt REM sleep.

Common Sleep Disorders

A basic understanding of common sleep disorders helps the health care practitioner gather and assess important clinical information. Sleep-related problems play an important role in a number of human disorders. For example, problems like an asthma attack tend to occur more often during the night and early morning, perhaps because of changes in hormones, heart rate, medication effect run-out, and other characteristics observed during sleep. The most common sleep disorders include insomnia, hypersomnia, narcolepsy, sleep apnea, periodic limb movement disorder (PLMD), and restless legs syndrome (RLS).

Insomnia

Insomnia is the most common sleep disorder. It is characterized by the inability to fall asleep or to remain asleep. It has been recently said that Americans are in the midst of an "insomnia epidemic"! Insomnia is classified as **transient insomnia** (lasting less than a week), **short-term insomnia** (lasting 1 to 3 weeks), or **chronic insomnia** (lasting longer than 3 weeks). Almost everyone suffers from transient insomnia at one time or another. Common causes of insomnia include changes in sleep environment, unpleasant room temperature, excessive noise, stressful events, jet lag, acute medical or surgical illnesses, ingestion of stimulant medications, and diet. Current research indicates that many insomniacs are hypermetabolic. Insomnia tends to increase with age and affects more women than men. Recent evidence suggests that hospitalized patients are generally sleep deprived, and many institutions are becoming involved in the "Quiet Hospital" noise abatement movement.

Hypersomnia

Hypersomnia is defined as periods of deep, long sleep, or sleep of excessive depth or abnormal duration. It is commonly caused by psychological rather than physical factors. The individual with hypersomnia is often described as being in a state of confusion on awakening or as having extreme drowsiness associated with lethargy. The differential diagnosis of hypersomnia includes sleep apnea, self-imposed sleep restriction, medication effects, periodic limb movement disorders, and circadian rhythm disorders.

Narcolepsy

Narcolepsy is a hereditary disorder characterized by sudden "sleep attacks" that often occur several times a day. The attacks last from several seconds to more than 30 minutes. Narcolepsy is classified as a hypersomnia. Individuals with narcolepsy may also experience *cataplexy* (loss of muscle tone and paralysis of voluntary muscles triggered by emotion), temporary paralysis when they awaken, and visual or auditory hallucinations at the onset or offset of sleep. The symptoms of narcolepsy begin in adolescence or young adulthood and persist throughout life. Nonhereditary narcolepsy symptoms may occur after cerebral trauma, in a condition called *post-traumatic narcolepsy*.

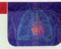

Clinical Connection—17-3

Clinical Signs and Symptoms of Obstructive Sleep Apnea

- Loud snoring, snorting, nocturnal choking
- Observed episodes of breathing cessation during sleep (>20 seconds long)
- Abrupt awakenings accompanied by shortness of breath
- Difficulty staying asleep (insomnia)
- Awakening with a dry mouth, sore throat, or headache

- Nausea
- Excessive daytime sleepiness (hypersomnia)
- Intellectual and personality changes, forgetfulness
- Moodiness, irritability, depression
- Nocturnal enuresis
- Sexual impotence

Sleep Apnea

Sleep apnea is a sleep disorder characterized by the temporary cessation or absence of breathing during sleep. Based on analyses of breathing patterns, the following three types of sleep apnea have been identified: obstructive sleep apnea, central sleep apnea, and mixed sleep apnea.

Obstructive sleep apnea is defined as the cessation of airflow through the nose and mouth with the persistence of diaphragmatic and intercostal muscle activities. Obstructive sleep apnea is the most common of the apneic syndromes affecting about 4 percent of U.S men and 2 percent of women. During an episode of obstructive sleep apnea, the sleeper attempts to inhale during a period in which the upper airway muscle tone is momentarily reduced or absent. The negative pressure generated during inspiration causes the pharynx to narrow and the tongue to be sucked back into the oropharygeal area.

The obstructive sleep apnea episode is characterized by loud snoring, followed by silence, during which the sleeper struggles to breathe against an obstructed airway. As the oxygen level falls, the sleeper works even harder to inhale, which in turn increases the upper airway negative pressure and further augments the airway obstruction. Often, the apneic episode ends only after an intense struggle, followed by a loud snorting. The sleeper then resumes snoring. In severe cases, the sleeper may suddenly awaken, sit up in bed, and gasp for air. This cycle may be repeated hundreds of times a night.

The frequent and intense struggles to breathe leave the person sleepy, irritable, or depressed during the day. In addition, because of the low oxygen concentrations associated with each apnea episode, the patient with sleep apnea is more likely to have morning headaches, a loss of interest in sex, a decline in mental (cognitive) function, high blood pressure, irregular heart rhythms, about two times the incidence of heart attacks, and two to three times the frequency of strokes. The obstructive sleep apnea patient is seven times more likely to have an automobile accident than the general population. In severe cases, obstructive sleep apnea may even lead to sudden death from respiratory failure during sleep. The incidence of sleep apnea in patients with strokes is between 60 and 80 percent.

Clinical Connection—17-4

The Therapeutic Effects of Continuous Positive Airway Pressure (CPAP) in Obstructive Sleep Apnea

The most common—and arguably the most effective—treatment for obstructive sleep apnea (OSA) is the use of a continuous positive airway pressure (CPAP) device. Nocturnal CPAP therapy is useful in preventing the collapse of the airway and is the standard treatment for most cases of OSA. CPAP is not indicated in pure central sleep apnea (Figure 17-12).

Figure 17–12

A. A patient on CPAP during a sleep study. **B.** An obstructive airway during inspiration. **C.** The therapeutic effects of positive pressure from a CPAP mask preventing airway obstruction.

Image A courtesy of Dr. George Burton. All images © Cengage Learning 2013

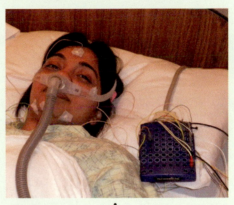

A

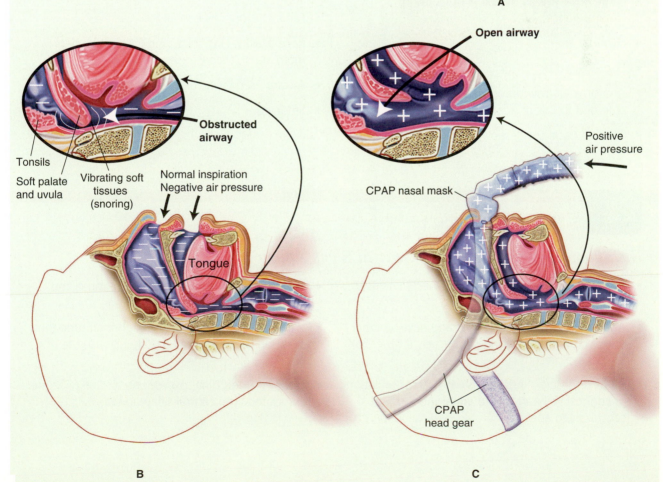

B

C

Central sleep apnea is characterized by the cessation of airflow with *no* respiratory efforts; that is, both the diaphragmatic and intercostals muscle activities are absent.

Mixed sleep apnea is characterized by an initial cessation of airflow with no respiratory effort (central apnea), followed by a period of upper airway obstruction (obstructive apnea).

It is estimated that approximately 18 million people in the United States have sleep apnea. However, most have not had the problem diagnosed. Common characteristics of sleep apnea include loud snoring, obesity, and excessive daytime sleepiness and fatigue. The disorder can easily be diagnosed at a sleep center that performs polysomnography. If sleep apnea is diagnosed, several treatments are available based on the type of sleep apnea the patient demonstrates.

Clinical Connection—17-5

Risk Factors Associated with Obstructive Sleep Apnea

- Male gender

- Excessive weight (obesity)

- Increasing age (especially older than 65)

- Large neck size (in males, >17inches in circumference)

- Hypertension

- Hypothyroidism

- Anatomic narrowing of upper airway (e.g., enlarged tonsils or adenoids)

- Chronic nasal congestion

- Diabetes

- Postmenopausal state

- Craniofacial abnormalities (e.g., retrognathia, Down's syndrome)

- Family history of sleep apnea

- Race (Blacks, Hispanics, and Pacific Islanders more at risk than Caucasians)

- Alcohol, sedatives, or tranquilizers

- Smoking

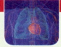

Clinical Connection—17-6

Risk Factors Associated with Central Sleep Apnea

- Male sex—males are more likely than females to develop central sleep apnea.

- Age—people over 65 years of age have a higher risk of central sleep apnea, especially if other risk factors are present.

- Heart disorders—individuals with atrial fibrillation or congestive heart failure are at more risk of central sleep apnea.

- Stroke or brain tumor—either can impair the brain's ability to regulate breathing.

- High altitude—sleeping at a higher altitude than a person is accustomed to can increase the risk of central sleep apnea.

- Opioids—morphine, oxycodone and codeine are associated with central sleep apnea.

Periodic Limb Movement Disorder

Periodic limb movement disorder (PLMD) is characterized by repetitive stereotyped movements of the leg muscles during sleep with a rhythmic pattern occurring about 30 seconds apart. PLMD occurs during non-REM sleep and usually stops when the patient awakens. Because the patient is not aware of the problem, the disorder is usually first reported by a family member. The incidence of PLMD increases with age. PLMD is often seen in patients with *restless legs syndrome.*

Clinical Connection—17-7

Management of Sleep Apnea

It is now known that many pathologic conditions are associated with sleep apnea, including hypoxemia, fragmented sleep, cardiac arrhythmias, and neurologic and psychiatric disorders. In general, the prognosis is more favorable for obstructive and mixed apnea than for central sleep apnea. The following provides an overview of the common therapeutic strategies used for obstructive and central sleep apnea and their effectiveness:

Common Therapeutic Modalities for Obstructive Sleep Apnea and Central Sleep Apnea

	Types of Apnea	
Therapy	**Obstructive Sleep Apnea**	**Central Sleep Apnea**
Mechanical ventilation		
• Continuous positive airway pressure (CPAP)	Therapeutic (100%)	Only fairly effective
• Mechanical ventilation	Short-term	Short-term
• Negative-pressure ventilation	Contraindicated	Therapeutic
• Adaptive servo-ventilation (variable positive airway pressure [VPAP])	Not indicated	Therapeutic
Oxygen Therapy	Rarely therapeutic, but is used in addition to CPAP in severe cases	Sometimes therapeutic
Surgical		
• Tracheostomy	Therapeutic (100%)	Not indicated
• Palatopharyngoplasty	Occasionally therapeutic	Not indicated
• Mandibular advancement	Occasionally therapeutic	Not indicated
Medical devices (e.g., mandibular advancement devices)	Possibly indicated	Not indicated
Phrenic nerve pacemaker	Not indicated	Experimental
Carbonic anhydrase inhibitor drugs—acetazolamide	Contraindicated	Possibly indicated

Restless Legs Syndrome

Restless legs syndrome (RLS) is characterized as intense unpleasant feelings described as crawling, prickling, tingling, burning, painful, aching, cramping, knifelike, or itching sensations. These crawling sensations occur mostly between the knees and ankles, causing a strong urge to move the legs to relieve the feelings. Motor restlessness is noted mostly in the legs but is occasionally reported in the arms.

RLS is emerging as one of the most common sleep disorders. Although it may occur at any age, it is most common among the elderly. Iron deficiency anemia is often present. The disorder causes a constant leg movement during the day and insomnia during the night. RLS may be exacerbated during pregnancy or by caffeine, diabetes, or renal insufficiency.

Normal Cardiopulmonary Physiology During Sleep

In spite of the fact that the complete purpose of sleep is not known, a significant amount of scientific knowledge is known about the physiologic differences between wakefulness periods and sleep periods. The following provides an overview of important physiologic changes that normally occur during sleep.

Autonomic Nervous System

In general, parasympathetic activity increases at sleep onset and continues throughout non-REM sleep. The parasympathetic tone continues to increase during the transition to REM sleep. This increased parasympathetic activity causes a number of autonomic nervous system changes throughout several areas of the body, including the musculoskeletal system, thermal regulation, renal function, genital function, gastrointestinal function, endocrine function, cardiovascular function, sleep-related arrhythmias, cerebral blood flow, and respiratory physiology.

Musculoskeletal System

The somatic skeletal muscles usually have their highest muscle tone during the wakeful state. The muscle tone decreases with sleep onset and throughout non-REM sleep. Muscle tone is at its lowest level during REM sleep. During REM sleep, neural impulses to most skeletal muscles stop, and a lack of muscle tone ensues. In essence, the sleeper is temporarily paralyzed. This is especially true for the muscles of the back, neck, arms, and legs and the posterior muscles of the pharynx, including the genioglossus muscle (which normally pulls the tongue down and forward), the infrahyoid muscle group, and the palatal muscle group. The partial paralysis may allow the tongue to fall back into the oral pharyngeal area during inspiration (i.e., negative-pressure phase). In severe cases, this condition can lead to obstructive sleep apnea.

Less affected are the muscles that move the eyes and the diaphragm. This explains, in part, why the sleeper does not physically act out a vivid dream during REM sleep—such as running from someone or swinging at a baseball. Instead, the sleeper only twitches or makes small movements. Sleepers with a malfunctioning REM system, on the other hand, thrash around in their sleep, oftentimes hitting their spouse or hurting themselves as they act out a dream (the so-called REM behavior disorder).

Thermal Regulation

The body temperature usually falls by 1°C to 2°C during non-REM sleep. During REM sleep, the body temperature tends to increase with cyclic variability.

Renal Function

Renal perfusion is decreased during non-REM sleep, resulting in decreased urine production. In addition, water reabsorption increases during non-REM sleep, causing a decrease in urine production. Urine production decreases even more during REM sleep.

Genital Function

There are few or no changes in the genital function during non-REM sleep. In men, REM sleep is associated with penile tumescence (erection). The erection usually occurs at the start of REM sleep and continues throughout the REM sleep phase. In most cases, the erection is lost at the end of REM sleep. Similar genital changes occur in the erectile tissue of women during REM sleep. The sleep-related erections develop as a result of the increased parasympathetic activity and local vasodilation that normally occurs during REM sleep.

Gastrointestinal Function

The effects of sleep on the gastrointestinal system are mainly caused by an increased parasympathetic activity, circadian rhythm factors, and central nervous system activity. During sleep, salivation and esophageal motility (swallowing) are markedly decreased. Gastric acid secretion follows a circadian rhythm, with the peak acid production occurring between 10:00 P.M. and 2:00 A.M. This circadian pattern is mediated by the vagus nerve. Colonic function is also decreased during sleep, which in turn results in a reduced colonic motility. When awakened in the morning, the colonic motility increases significantly.

Endocrine Function

Plasma growth hormone concentrations usually peak about 90 minutes after the onset of sleep, typically during stage N3. Patients with obstructive sleep apnea or narcolepsy commonly have a decreased correlation between sleep and growth hormone concentration. Adrenocorticotropic hormone (ACTH) and cortisol secretions follow a circadian pattern, which typically peaks during delta sleep (stage N3) between 4:00 A.M. and 8:00 A.M.

Cardiovascular Function

During non-REM sleep, the vagal nerve function provides relative autonomic stability. The heart rate and blood pressure variations during non-REM sleep follow a sinusoidal pattern—called "nocturnal dipping." That is, during a normal inspiration, the heart rate and blood pressure increase briefly in order to accommodate venous return and increased cardiac output. During expiration, the heart rate and blood pressure gradually decrease. This normal cardiovascular rhythm unevenness is a positive marker for good cardiac health.

Its absence is associated with increased age, abnormal vagus nerve function, or heart pathology. During REM sleep, the heart rate becomes variable with episodes of both increased and decreased rates. The heart rate may increase as much as 35 percent during REM sleep.

Sleep-Related Arrhythmias

During non-REM sleep, there is an increased activity of the vagal nerve—which causes a decreased heart rate, blood pressure, and cardiac metabolism. Collectively, these activities reduce the sleeper's risk for cardiac arrhythmia. However, the decreased blood pressure during non-REM sleep may lead to myocardial hypoperfusion. On the other hand, the surge of autonomic activity during REM sleep increases the heart rate and blood pressure and increases the risk for heart arrhythmias. Premature ventricular contractions (PVCs), paroxysmal atrial tachycardia, atrial fibrillation, nonsustained ventricular tachycardia, and even periods of cardiac asystole may be seen. In addition, the increased sympathetic activity during REM sleep results in a reduced oxygen supply-to-demand ratio, coronary vasoconstriction, and variation of both cardiac ventricular preload and afterload. Nocturnal angina (chest pain) is sometimes seen in patients with sleep apnea, as is orthopnea and paroxysmal nocturnal dyspnea, reflecting congestive heart failure.

Cerebral Blood Flow

During non-REM sleep, cerebral blood flow decreases. During REM sleep, cerebral blood flow increases. Spinal cord blood flow also increases during REM sleep. In addition, the cerebral blood flow is decreased during postsleep wakefulness when compared to presleep wakefulness. The cerebral metabolic rate increases during REM sleep.

Respiratory Physiology

As discussed in Chapter 9, the intrinsic rhythmicity of ventilation is coordinated by the medulla oblongata, which responds to neural impulses generated from the oxygen (P_{O_2})-sensitive peripheral chemoreceptors (located in the aorta and carotid arteries) and the carbon dioxide (P_{CO_2}) or H^+-sensitive central chemoreceptors (located in the medulla). The primary function of ventilation, therefore, is to maintain the P_{O_2} and P_{CO_2} within normal physiologic boundaries.

Although the precise mechanism is not known, the medulla's ability to respond to P_{O_2} and P_{CO_2} changes is reduced during non-REM sleep. This is especially true in regard to the medulla's ability to react to sudden changes in the P_{CO_2} level. In non-REM sleep, the respiratory rate decreases, causing the minute ventilation to fall as much as 0.5 to 1.5 L/min. It is suggested that the reduced minute ventilation is caused, in part, by (1) the decreased metabolic rate that occurs during sleep, (2) the reduced ability for the medulla to respond to ventilatory signals during sleep, (3) the decreased sensitivity of the P_{O_2} and P_{CO_2} chemoreceptors to send signals to the medulla during sleep, and (4) the increased airway resistance caused by reduced muscle tone in the upper airway. Figure 17–13 illustrates the normal ventilatory response to changing P_{CO_2} levels during non-REM and REM sleep. During REM sleep, the respiratory rate increases and decreases irregularly. This irregular respiratory pattern is thought to be secondary to brainstem respiratory neuron activity.

© Cengage Learning 2013

Figure 17–13

Normal ventilatory response to changing P_{CO_2} level during non-REM and REM sleep.

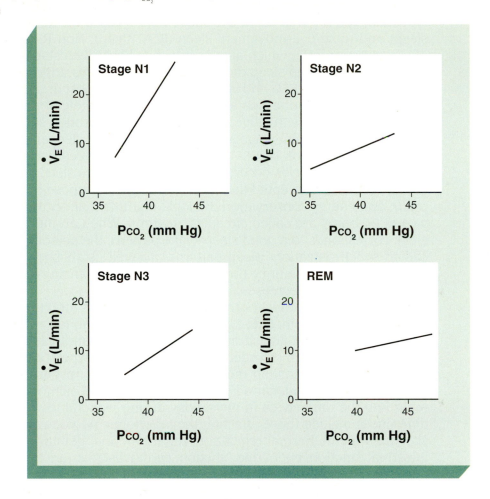

 Clinical Connection—17-8

Case Study—The Role of the Respiratory Therapist in Caring for the Obstructive Sleep Apnea Patient

In the **Clinical Application Section—Case 1** (page 550), the respiratory therapist is called to care for a 65-year-old man with obstructive sleep apnea. This case illustrates how patients with acute transient ischemic attacks and minor strokes are ideal candidates for CPAP therapy—especially if other co-morbidities such as obesity can be addressed. The role of the respiratory therapist in this case can be seen in the (1) initial assessment of the patient in the Emergency Department, (2) instructing the patient for his polysomnogram in the Sleep Disorders Center, and (3) the continued involvement in education of the patient and CPAP compliance monitoring once the patient was discharged.

Chapter Summary

Sleep is a naturally occurring state of partial unconsciousness. The two major types of sleep are non-rapid-eye-movement sleep (non-REM sleep or NREM sleep) and rapid-eye-movement sleep (REM sleep). Non-REM sleep consists of stages N1 and N2, which are described as light-sleep stages, and stage N3 is referred to as deep sleep or slow-wave sleep stages. REM sleep resembles wakefulness on the EEG and is the period in which most dreaming occurs and when there is temporary paralysis of most of the skeletal muscles. One full sleep cycle begins with stage N1 and progresses through stages N2 and N3; followed by a return to stage N2. From stage N2, the sleeper moves into REM sleep. The conclusion of REM sleep ends the first sleep cycle. Between four and six full sleep cycles occur during a normal night's sleep.

The two most accepted theories regarding the purpose of sleep are restoration and energy conservation. Biologic rhythms that occur at regular intervals of 24 hours are called circadian rhythms. When an individual's biologic clock corresponds to a good sleep–wake pattern, the person is said be in circadian synchronization. Sleep patterns are well established in the first few months of life and continue throughout life. With advancing age, regular sleep patterns gradually decrease.

Numerous facts affect both the quality of and the total time an individual sleeps. Such factors include age, illness, environment, fatigue, lifestyle, emotional stress, alcohol and stimulants, diet, smoking, motivation, and medications. Common sleep disorders include insomnia, hypersomnia, narcolepsy, sleep apnea, periodic limb movement disorder, and restless legs syndrome. Although not fully understood, a considerable amount of information is known regarding the differences in physiology during wakefulness and sleep. Such differences include those affecting the autonomic nervous system, musculoskeletal system, thermal regulation, renal function, genital function, gastrointestinal function, endocrine function, cardiovascular function, sleep-related arrhythmias, cerebral blood flow, and respiratory physiology.

Clinical connections associated with these topics include (1) the sleep disorder specialist—trends, education, and certification, (2) types of sleep studies, (3) clinical signs and symptoms associated with obstructive sleep apnea, (4) the therapeutic effects of continuous positive airway pressure in obstructive sleep apnea, (5) risk factors linked to obstructive sleep apnea, (6) risk factors linked to central sleep apnea, (7) management of sleep apnea, and (8) the role of the respiratory therapist in caring for the obstructive sleep apnea patient.

1   Clinical Application Case

A 65-year old man with a long history of insulin-dependent diabetes mellitus, hypertension, and a recent transient ischemic attack (TIA) came to the hospital Emergency Department with a history of slurred speech, left-sided weakness, and increasing somnolence. The respiratory therapist who first saw him found the following sleep history: the man got into bed around 11:00 P.M.; woke frequently during the night with gasping, choking, and snorting; and woke at 6:00 A.M. not feeling refreshed. His bed partner stated that he snored loudly and that he stopped breathing in his sleep many times each night. It was further noted that these events had gotten worse since the patient's TIAs.

His medications were aspirin (325 mg daily), metformin, and lisinopril. He did not smoke, abuse alcohol, or use caffeine. He was retired from work as an insurance executive. He fell asleep during the day when reading or watching television, but denied any sleep-related automobile accidents.

Physical examination revealed the following: height 5 feet 8 inches, weight 240 pounds, BMI = 36. Temperature 98.8°F, pulse 84, blood pressure 146/90, respiratory rate 16, Sp_{O_2} on room air awake 96 percent. HEENT examination (head, ears, eyes, nose, and throat) showed a class IV Mallampati configuration, with a low-lying soft palate, large uvula, and widened tonsillar pillars. There was "scalloping" of the edges of the tongue, suggesting an element of macroglossia. His neck circumference was 18 inches, and he was very jowly. Examination of his heart, lungs, and abdomen was normal. There was 2+ bilateral leg edema. Neurological examination showed mild weakness of the left arm and hand but was otherwise normal, except for what appeared to be some short-term memory loss. His Epworth Sleepiness Scale was 20/24.[4]

While the patient was in the Emergency Department, he fell asleep repeatedly and snored loudly. He was placed on a pulse oximeter and was found to frequently desaturate to an Sp_{O_2} of less than 75 percent. He was easily aroused, and a CT scan of the head was normal. He was discharged, and an outpatient nocturnal polysomnogram was scheduled for a few days later.

The polysomnogram was performed in the hospital's Sleep Disorders Center, where a respiratory therapist assisted in the initial setup and monitoring. The study showed that he had an Apnea-Hypopnea Index of 56 episodes per hour (normal ≤ 5/hr). The longest episode was 62 seconds long, and there were cyclical oxygen desaturations to a low 70 percent. All the events were obstructive in nature.

Once these results were known, a CPAP titration study was done the following night. This study showed that a CPAP pressure of 8.0 cm H_2O reduced the apnea-hypopnea index to 2.0/hr, and reduced the nadir—that is, the lowest point—of his oxygen saturation to 92 percent.

The respiratory therapist assisted in obtaining a comfortable CPAP mask for the patient, enrolled him in an AWAKE class for patients with sleep apnea, and monitored him there for CPAP compliance. The patient was also referred to the hospital's weight loss management program and did well thereafter. There had been no recurrence of cardiovascular or neurological events at his scheduled 2-year follow-up.

Discussion

Patients with acute TIA and minor stroke are ideal candidates for prevention of recurrent events—particularly if co-morbidities such as sleep apnea and obesity can be addressed. Long-term studies of the effect of CPAP in this setting are currently in process. The role of the respiratory therapist in this case can be seen in the (1) initial assessment of the patient in the Emergency Department, (2) instructing the patient for his polysomnogram in the Sleep Disorders Center, and (3) the continued involvement in education of the patient and CPAP compliance monitoring once the patient was discharged.

---

[4] The Epworth Sleepiness Scale is an eight-question assessment of daytime sleepiness in which the respondent rates how likely one is to fall asleep in a variety of situations. Scores less than 10 are normal, and scores higher than 10 may suggest the need for additional evaluation by a sleep specialist.

Review Questions

1. Which of the following is also known as paradoxic sleep?
   A. Stage N1 non-REM sleep
   B. Stage N2 non-REM sleep
   C. Stage N3 non-REM sleep
   D. Stage W (wake)
   E. REM sleep

2. Most sleep study epochs are
   A. 10 seconds in duration
   B. 20 seconds in duration
   C. 30 seconds in duration
   D. 60 seconds in duration

3. K complexes first appear in which of the following stages during one full sleep cycle?
   A. Stage N1
   B. Stage N2
   C. Stage N3
   D. REM

4. The newborn sleeps about how many total hours during a 24-hour period?
   A. 6 to 8 hours
   B. 8 to 12 hours
   C. 13 to 15 hours
   D. 16 to 17 hours

5. Which of the following is the most common sleep disorder?
   A. Insomnia
   B. Narcolepsy
   C. Sleep apnea
   D. Restless legs syndrome

6. Which of the following is characterized by prominent alpha waves (>50 percent)?
   A. Eyes open—wake
   B. Eyes closed—wake
   C. Stage N2 non-REM sleep
   D. REM sleep

7. Which of the following occupies the greatest proportion of the total sleep time?
   A. Stage N1 non-REM sleep
   B. Stage N2 non-REM sleep
   C. Stage N3 non-REM sleep
   D. REM sleep

8. Sleep spindles first appear in which of the following?
   A. Stage N1 non-REM sleep
   B. Stage N2 non-REM sleep
   C. Stage N3 non-REM sleep
   D. REM sleep

9. Vertex shape waves often appear toward the end of which of the following sleep stages?
   A. Stage N1 non-REM sleep
   B. Stage N2 non-REM sleep
   C. Stage N3 non-REM sleep
   D. REM sleep

10. Delta waves are associated with which of the following stages?
1. Stage N1 non-REM sleep
2. Stage N2 non-REM sleep
3. Stage N3 non-REM sleep
4. Stage wake
5. REM sleep
   A. 3 only
   B. 1 and 2 only
   C. 2 and 3 only
   D. 3 and 5 only

Directions: Match the type of waveform listed under column A to the graphic appearance of the waveform shown under column B.

COLUMN A   COLUMN B

1. _____ Delta waves   A.

2. _____ Alpha waves   B.

3. _____ K complex   C.

4. _____ Sleep spindles D.

5. _____ Beta waves   E.

Clinical Application Questions

1. On the Epworth Sleepiness Scale, scores less than _____ are normal, and scores higher than _____ may suggest the need for additional evaluation by a sleep specialist.

2. True _____ False _____ Patients with acute TIA and minor stroke are ideal candidates for prevention of recurrent events.

3. True _____ False _____ The respiratory care practitioner's role includes CPAP compliance monitoring.

The Cardiopulmonary System During Unusual Environmental Conditions

Chapter 18

Exercise and Its Effects on the Cardiopulmonary System

Objectives

By the end of this chapter, the student should be able to:

1. Describe the effects of exercise on the following components of the cardiopulmonary system:
   —Ventilation
   —Oxygen consumption
   —Arterial blood gases
   —Oxygen diffusion capacity
   —Alveolar-arterial oxygen tension difference
   —Circulation
     • Sympathetic discharge
     • Cardiac output
     • Arterial blood pressure
     • Pulmonary vascular pressures
     • Muscle capillaries
2. Describe the interrelationships among muscle work, oxygen consumption, and cardiac output.

3. Describe the effect of training on the heart and on cardiac output.
4. Describe the clinical connection associated with the general benefits of exercise.
5. Differentiate between stroke volume and heart rate in increasing the cardiac output.
6. Describe how body temperature and cutaneous blood flow relate to a number of symptoms collectively referred to as heat stroke.
7. List the benefits of pulmonary rehabilitation.
8. Complete the review questions at the end of this chapter.

Introduction

During heavy exercise, components of the cardiopulmonary system may be stressed close to their limit. Alveolar ventilation may increase as much as 20-fold, oxygen diffusion capacity as much as 3-fold, cardiac output as much as 6-fold, muscle blood flow as much as 25-fold, oxygen consumption as much as 20-fold, and heat production as much as 20-fold.

Muscle training can increase muscle size and strength 30 to 60 percent. The efficiency of intracellular metabolism may increase by 30 to 50 percent. The size of the heart chambers and the heart mass in elite athletes, such as marathon runners, may be increased by 40 percent. When the level of exercise is greater, however, than the ability of the cardiopulmonary system to provide a sufficient supply of oxygen to the muscles, anaerobic metabolism ensues. The point at which anaerobic metabolism develops is called the **anaerobic threshold**.

Ventilation

Control of Ventilation

The precise mechanism responsible for increased alveolar ventilation during exercise is not well understood. Exercise causes the body to consume a large amount of oxygen and, simultaneously, to produce a large amount of carbon dioxide. Alveolar ventilation increases so much, however, that the concentration of these gases in the body does not change significantly. In addition, no oxygen or carbon dioxide chemoreceptors have been identified on the venous side of circulation, or in the lungs, that could account for the increased alveolar ventilation during exercise. Thus, it is unlikely that the increased ventilation seen in exercise is caused by either of these gases.

It has been suggested that the increased ventilation is caused by neural impulses sent to the medulla by way of the following pathways (Figure 18–1):

1. The cerebral cortex sending signals to the exercising muscles may also send collateral signals to the medulla oblongata to increase the rate and depth of breathing.

2. Proprioceptors in the moving muscles, tendons, and joints transmit sensory signals via the spinal cord to the respiratory centers of the medulla.

3. The increase in body temperature during exercise also may contribute to increased ventilation.

Figure 18–1

Mechanisms by which exercise stimulates ventilation. **1.** Collateral fibers from the motor neurons travel to the medulla; **2.** sensory signals from the exercising limbs are sent to the medulla; **3.** the increase in body temperature during exercise may also increase ventilation.

© Cengage Learning 2013

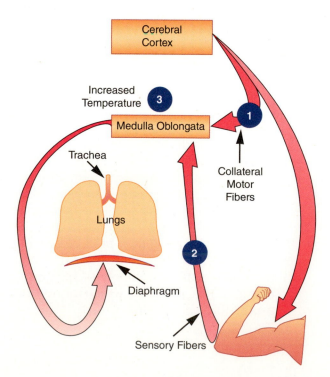

Alveolar Ventilation

During normal quiet breathing, an adult exchanges about 6 L of gas per minute. During strenuous exercise, this can increase to 120 L/min, a 20-fold increase. Depending on the intensity and duration of the exercise, alveolar ventilation must increase to (1) supply sufficient oxygen to the blood and (2) eliminate the excess carbon dioxide produced by the skeletal muscles. The increased alveolar ventilation is produced mainly by an increased depth of ventilation (increased tidal volume), rather than by an increased rate of ventilation. During very heavy exercise, however, both an increased depth and frequency of ventilation are seen. The tidal volume is usually about 60 percent of the vital capacity, and the respiratory rate may be as high as 30 breaths/min.

Three distinct consecutive breathing patterns are seen during mild and moderate exercise. The **first stage** is characterized by an increase in alveolar ventilation, within seconds after the onset of exercise. The **second stage** is typified by a slow, gradual further increase in alveolar ventilation developing during approximately the first 3 minutes of exercise. Alveolar ventilation during this period increases almost linearly with the amount of work performed. During the **third stage**, alveolar ventilation stabilizes. When an individual stops exercising, alveolar ventilation decreases abruptly (Figure 18–2).

During very heavy exercise, the steady-state third stage may not be seen. In fact, when approximately 60 to 70 percent of the maximal exercise level is reached during the linear second stage, alveolar ventilation increases proportionately more than the oxygen uptake. The additional stimulation is thought to be caused primarily by the accumulation of lactic acids in the blood after the anaerobic threshold has been reached. It is suggested that the H^+ ions generated by the lactic acids stimulate the peripheral chemoreceptors, which in turn send neural impulses to the medulla oblongata to increase alveolar ventilation (refer to Figure 9–8).

Figure 18–2

The relationship of exercise and ventilation. Note **A.** the abrupt increase in ventilation at the outset of exercise and **B.** the even larger, abrupt decrease in ventilation at the end of exercise.

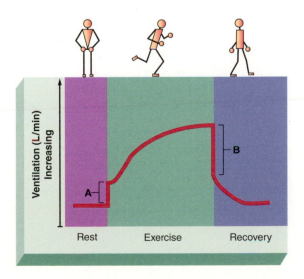

The maximum alveolar ventilation generated during heavy exercise under normal conditions is only about 50 to 65 percent of the maximum voluntary ventilation (also called maximum breathing capacity). This provides the athlete with an important reserve of alveolar ventilation, which may be required in such conditions as short bursts of increased exercise, exercise at high altitudes, or exercise during very hot and humid conditions. Because there is normally a large alveolar ventilatory reserve during exercise, it is not the limiting factor in the delivery of oxygen to the muscles during maximal muscular aerobic metabolism. As discussed later, the inability of the heart to pump sufficient blood to the working muscles is the major limiting factor.

Oxygen Consumption

At rest, normal oxygen consumption ($\dot{V}_{O_2}$) is about 250 mL/min. The skeletal muscles account for approximately 35 to 40 percent of the total $\dot{V}_{O_2}$. During exercise, the skeletal muscles may account for more than 95 percent of the $\dot{V}_{O_2}$. During heavy exercise, the $\dot{V}_{O_2}$ of an untrained person may be more than 3500 mL of O_2/min. The $\dot{V}_{O_2}$ of an elite athlete while running a marathon may be over 5000 mL O_2/min. Figure 18–3 shows the linear relationship between $\dot{V}_{O_2}$ and alveolar ventilation exercise intensity increases.

Figure 18–3

There is a linear relationship between oxygen consumption ($\dot{V}_{O_2}$) and alveolar ventilation as the intensity of exercise increases. Note that when the anaerobic threshold is reached during strenuous exercise, the linear relationship between $\dot{V}_{O_2}$ and alveolar ventilation will no longer exist. When the anaerobic threshold is reached, there will be an abrupt increase in alveolar ventilation with little or no increase in $\dot{V}_{O_2}$.

© Cengage Learning 2013

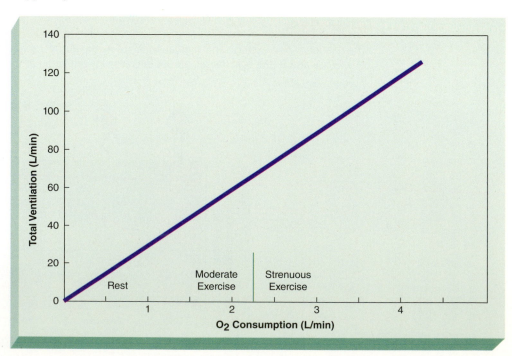

Arterial Blood Gas Levels During Exercise

No significant Pa_{O_2}, Pa_{CO_2}, or pH changes are seen between rest and approximately 60 to 70 percent of maximal $\dot{V}_{O_2}$. During very heavy exercise, however, when lactic acidosis is present, both the pH and Pa_{CO_2} decline. Although controversy exists, it is believed that arterial acidosis stimulates the carotid chemoreceptors, causing increased alveolar ventilation and promoting respiratory acid–base compensation. The Pa_{O_2} remains constant during mild, moderate, and heavy exercise (Figure 18–4).

Oxygen Diffusion Capacity

The oxygen diffusion capacity increases linearly in response to the increased oxygen consumption ($\dot{V}_{O_2}$) during exercise (Figure 18–5 on page 562). The oxygen diffusion capacity may increase as much as 3-fold during maximum exercise. It has been shown that the increased oxygen diffusion capacity results from the increased cardiac output during exercise. The increased cardiac output causes the intravascular pressure in the pulmonary artery and left atrium to increase, which in turn serves to (1) distend the pulmonary capillaries that are not fully dilated and (2) open, or recruit, closed pulmonary capillaries (refer to Figure 5–24). As more blood flows through the lungs, more alveolar-capillary units become available for gas exchange. This provides a greater surface area through which oxygen can diffuse into the pulmonary capillary blood.

Figure 18–4

The effect of oxygen consumption on Pa_{O_2} and Pa_{CO_2} as the intensity of exercise increases.

© Cengage Learning 2013

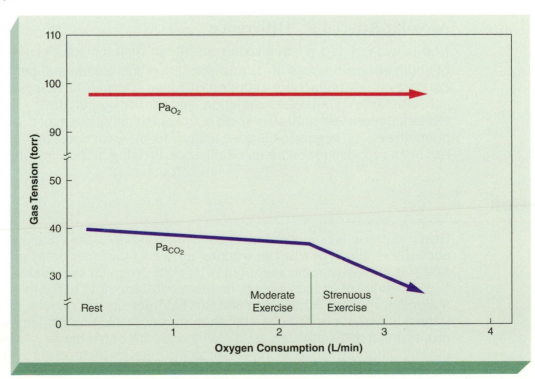

Figure 18–5

Oxygen diffusion capacity increases linearly in response to increased oxygen consumption as the intensity of exercise increases.

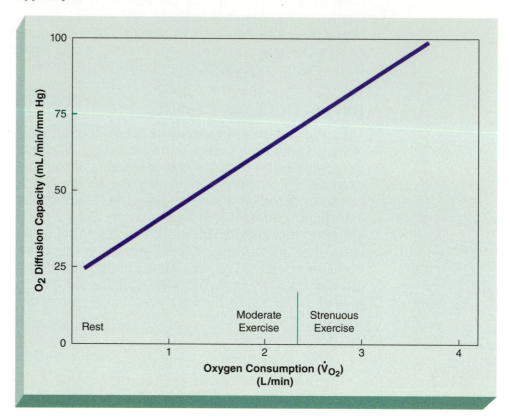

Alveolar-Arterial P_{O_2} Difference

Normally, there is a mean alveolar-arterial oxygen tension difference $P_{(A-a)O_2}$ of about 10 torr because of (1) mismatching of ventilation and perfusion and (2) right-to-left pulmonary shunting of blood. Despite increases in oxygen consumption ($\dot{V}_{O_2}$), alveolar ventilation, and cardiac output, the $P_{(A-a)O_2}$ remains essentially constant until 40 percent of the maximal $\dot{V}_{O_2}$ is reached; beyond this point, the $P_{(A-a)O_2}$ begins to increase (Figure 18–6). An average $P_{(A-a)O_2}$ of 33 torr has been reported for endurance runners exercising at their maximal $\dot{V}_{O_2}$.

Circulation

Heavy exercise is one of the most stressful conditions the circulatory system encounters. Blood flow to the working muscles may increase as much as 25-fold and the total cardiac output may increase as much as 8-fold.

The ability of an individual to increase cardiac output to the muscles is the major determinant of how long and to what intensity the exercise can be sustained. In fact, the speed of a marathon runner or swimmer is almost directly proportional to the athlete's ability to increase his or her cardiac output. Thus, the circulatory system is as important as the muscles themselves in setting the limits for exercise.

Figure 18–6

The alveolar-arterial oxygen tension difference $P_{(A-a)O_2}$ begins to increase when approximately 40 percent of the maximal $\dot{V}_{O_2}$ is exceeded.

© Cengage Learning 2013

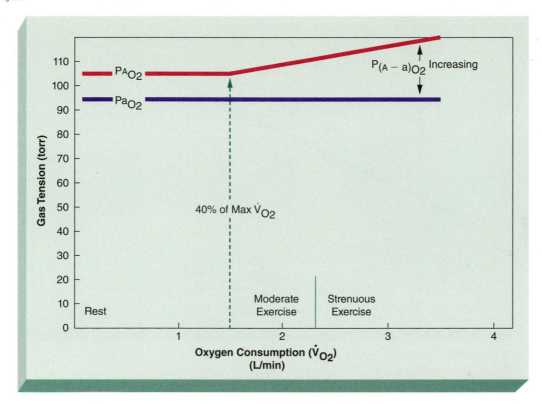

During exercise, three essential physiologic responses must occur in order for the circulatory system to supply the working muscles with an adequate amount of blood: (1) sympathetic discharge, (2) increase in cardiac output, and (3) increase in arterial blood pressure.

Sympathetic Discharge

At the onset of exercise, the brain transmits signals to the vasomotor center in the medulla oblongata to trigger a sympathetic discharge. This sympathetic discharge has two circulatory effects: (1) the heart is stimulated to increase its rate and strength of contraction, and (2) the blood vessels of the peripheral vascular system constrict, except for the blood vessels of the working muscles, which strongly dilate in response to local vasodilators in the muscles themselves. The net result is an increased blood supply to the working muscles while the blood flow to nonworking muscles is reduced. Note that vasoconstriction in the heart and brain does not occur during exercise, because both the heart and the brain are as important to exercise as the working muscles themselves.

Cardiac Output

The increased oxygen demands during exercise are met almost entirely by an increased cardiac output. Figure 18–7 on page 564 shows the linear relationship between the cardiac output and the intensity of exercise. The increased cardiac output during exercise results from (1) increased stroke volume, (2) increased heart rate, or (3) a combination of both.

Figure 18–7

A linear relationship exists between cardiac output and the intensity of exercise.

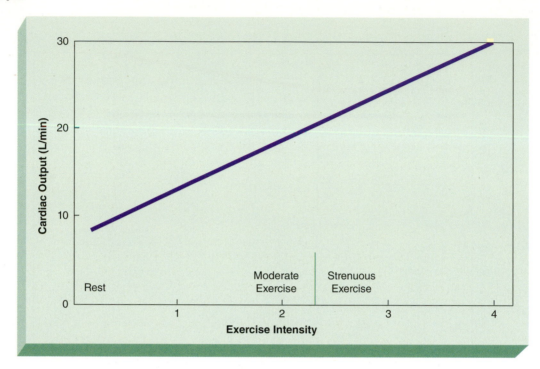

Increased Stroke Volume

The increased stroke volume during exercise is primarily due to vasodilation in the working muscles; that is, the vasodilation in the working muscles increases the venous return to the heart. The heart, in turn, pumps more oxygenated blood back to the working muscles. Thus, the degree of vasodilation in the working muscles directly influences the stroke volume; therefore, the greater the vasodilation in the working muscles, the greater the stroke volume and cardiac output. Another factor that facilitates an increased venous return during exercise is the sympathetic discharge. This causes a constriction of all venous blood reservoirs and forces more blood out of the veins and toward the heart.

As discussed in Chapter 5, the ability of the heart to accommodate the increased venous return and, subsequently, increase the cardiac output is due to the Frank-Starling curve (refer to Figure 5–22). When more venous blood returns to the heart, the heart chambers increase in size to accommodate the increased volume. As the heart chambers increase in size, the force of the heart muscle contractions increase, which in turn increases the stroke volume.

In addition to the Frank-Starling curve, the heart is also strongly stimulated by the sympathetic discharge. Increased sympathetic stimulation causes (1) increased heart rate (as high as 200 bpm) and (2) increased strength of contraction. The combined effect of these two mechanisms greatly increases the heart's ability to pump blood beyond what could be accomplished by the Frank-Starling curve alone.

Increased Heart Rate

An individual's maximum heart rate is estimated by the following formula:

Maximum heart rate = 220 − Age (in years)

Thus, the maximum heart rate for a 45-year-old person is about 175 (220 − 45 = 175).

Although the heart rate increases linearly with oxygen consumption, the magnitude of the change is influenced by the size of the stroke volume; that is, when the stroke volume decreases, the heart rate increases, and when the stroke volume increases, the heart rate decreases. The stroke volume, in turn, is influenced by (1) the individual's physical condition, (2) the specific muscles that are working, and (3) the distribution of blood flow. The body's ability to increase the heart rate and stroke volume during exercise progressively declines with age.

Arterial Blood Pressure

There is an increase in arterial blood pressure during exercise because of the (1) sympathetic discharge, (2) increased cardiac output, and (3) vasoconstriction of the blood vessels in the nonworking muscle areas. Depending on the physical condition of the individual, as well as the intensity and duration of the exercise, the systolic arterial blood pressure may increase as little as 20 mm Hg or as much as 80 mm Hg.

Pulmonary Vascular Pressures

As oxygen consumption and cardiac output increase during exercise, the systolic, diastolic, and mean pulmonary arterial and wedge pressures also increase linearly (Figure 18–8 on page 566). As discussed earlier, this mechanism enhances oxygen uptake by (1) distending the pulmonary capillaries and (2) opening closed pulmonary capillaries.

Muscle Capillaries

At rest, approximately only 20 to 25 percent of the muscle capillaries are dilated. During heavy exercise, all these capillaries dilate to facilitate the distribution of blood. This reduces the distance that oxygen and other nutrients must travel from the capillaries to the muscle fiber. At the same time, the blood vessels of the viscera and nonworking muscles constrict.

The dilation of the blood vessels in the working muscles is caused primarily by local vasodilators acting directly on the arterioles. The most important local vasodilator effect is the reduction of oxygen in the working muscles. It is suggested that a diminished oxygen concentration in the muscles causes vasodilation because either (1) the vessels are unable to maintain contraction at low oxygen levels or (2) low oxygen levels cause the release of vasodilator substances. The most likely vasodilator substance is *adenosine*. Other vasodilator substances include potassium ions, acetylcholine, adenosine triphosphate, lactic acids, and carbon dioxide. The precise role of each of these substances in increasing blood flow to working muscles is not known.

Figure 18–8

The systolic, diastolic, and mean pulmonary arterial and wedge pressures increase linearly as oxygen consumption and cardiac output increase.

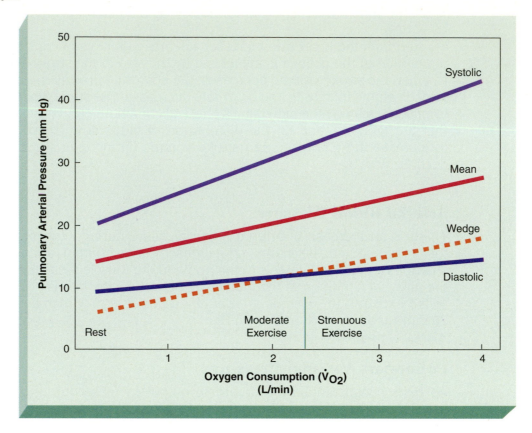

Finally, because the vasodilation of the major working muscle groups is greater than the vasoconstriction of the nonworking muscle groups, the overall peripheral vascular resistance decreases. This is why elite athletes can substantially increase their cardiac output with only a slight increase in their mean systemic arterial blood pressure. Untrained individuals have a high peripheral vascular resistance and, therefore, high arterial blood pressure in response to modest increases in cardiac output during exercise.

Interrelationships among Muscle Work, Oxygen Consumption, and Cardiac Output

Figure 18–9 shows that muscle work, oxygen consumption, and cardiac output are all related to each other. Increased muscle work increases oxygen consumption, and the increased oxygen consumption, in turn, dilates the intramuscular blood vessels. As the intramuscular blood vessels dilate, venous return increases, causing the cardiac output to rise. Marathon runners can have a cardiac output as great as 40 L/min. The maximum cardiac output of a young, untrained individual is less than 25 L/min.

Figure 18–9

Relationship among muscle work, oxygen consumption, and cardiac output.

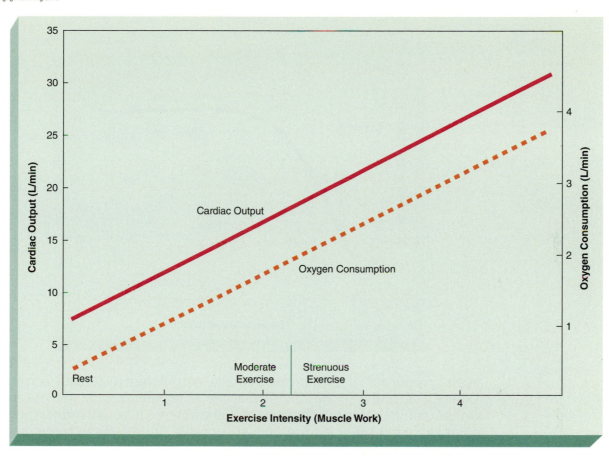

The Influence of Training on the Heart and Cardiac Output

The increased cardiac output seen in marathon runners results mainly from the fact that the heart chambers and heart mass increase as much as 40 percent. Cardiac enlargement and increased pumping ability occur only in the endurance type of athletic training and not in the sprint type of activity. The "athlete's heart" is an effective and physiologically sound heart. It should not be considered a pathologic heart. At rest, the cardiac output of the elite athlete is almost the same as that of the average untrained individual. The former, however, has a greater stroke volume and a reduced heart rate.

Stroke Volume versus Heart Rate in Increasing Cardiac Output

Figure 18–10 on page 568 shows the approximate changes that occur in stroke volume and heart rate as the cardiac output increases from about 5 to 30 L/min in a marathon runner. The stroke volume increases from about 100 mL to about 150 mL, an increase of about 50 percent. The heart rate increases from 50 to 180 beats/min, an increase of 260 percent. Thus, during very strenuous exercise, the increase in heart rate accounts for a much

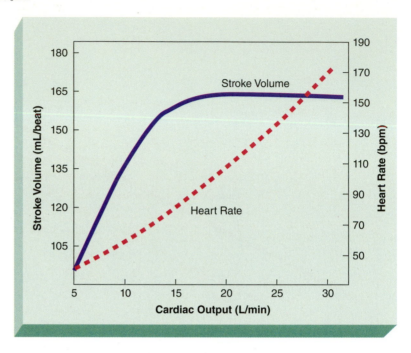

Figure 18–10

Approximate changes in stroke volume and heart rate that occur when the cardiac output increases from about 5 to 30 L/min in a marathon runner.

© Cengage Learning 2013

greater proportion of the increased cardiac output than the increase in stroke volume. In fact, the stroke volume reaches its maximum when the maximum cardiac output is at only approximately 50 percent. Thus, any further increase in cardiac output beyond the midway point is due solely to the increased heart rate.

At maximum exercise, cardiac output reaches about 90 percent of the maximum than can be achieved. Because maximum exercise taxes the respiratory system only about 65 percent of maximum, it can be seen that normally the cardiovascular system is a greater limiting factor on maximal

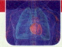

Clinical Connection—18-1

General Benefits of Exercise

In addtion to the well-documented cardipulmonary benefits associated with exercise, even a moderate about of exercise is strongly connected to the following benefits:

- Reduced stress

- Reduced weight

- Reduced symptoms of depression and anxiety

- Reduced risk of developing diabetes

- Reduced cholesterol levels

- Increased mood and energy

- Improved sleep

- Increased bone density

- The building and and maintenance of healthy muscles

- Improved quality of life

exercise than the respiratory system. Thus, the maximum performance that a marathon runner can achieve is directly related to the condition of the cardiovascular system. Any type of heart disease that reduces the heart's ability to pump blood will also decrease an individual's muscle power. This explains, in part, why a patient with congestive heart failure may have difficulty in generating enough muscle power to climb out of bed or to walk short distances.

Body Temperature/Cutaneous Blood Flow Relationship

During exercise, the body generates a tremendous amount of heat, and heat production may increase as much as 20-fold. Although some of the heat is stored in the body during exercise, most of the heat is dissipated through the skin. This requires a substantial increase in blood flow to the body surface. Nevertheless, even during normal temperature and humidity conditions, the body temperature may rise from its normal 98.6°F to 102°F to 103°F (37°C to 40°C) during endurance athletics.

When exercise is performed during very hot and humid conditions, or without adequately ventilated clothing, heat loss may be impaired, and an unusually large amount of blood may be distributed to the skin. During these conditions, the body temperature can easily rise to 106°F to 108°F (41°C to 42°C). As much as 5 to 10 pounds of body fluid can be lost in 1 hour. When this happens, a number of signs and symptoms may appear, which collectively are referred to as **heat stroke**. These signs and symptoms include:

- Profuse sweating, followed by no sweating
- Extreme weakness
- Muscle cramping
- Exhaustion
- Nausea
- Headache
- Dizziness
- Confusion
- Staggering gait
- Altered level of consciousness
- Unconsciousness
- Circulatory collapse

Heat stroke can be fatal if not treated immediately. Even when the individual stops exercising, the temperature does not readily return to normal, because (1) the temperature-regulating mechanism often fails at a very high temperature, and (2) the intracellular metabolism is much faster at higher temperatures, which in turn generates still more heat.

The primary treatment of heat stroke is to reduce the victim's body temperature as fast as possible. This is done by (1) spraying cool water on the victim's body, (2) continually sponging the victim with cool water, (3) blowing air over the body with a strong fan, or (4) a combination of all three measures.

Pulmonary Rehabilitation

Pulmonary rehabilitation is now a well-accepted, multidisciplinary health care service for patients with chronic obstructive lung disease (COPD). It provides patients with a process of developing and maintaining a desirable level of physical, social, and psychological well-being. The typical pulmonary rehabilitation team consists of a physician, nurse, respiratory therapist, physical therapist, psychologist or social worker, and dietitian. The primary goal of the program is to achieve and maintain the patient's maximum level of independence and functioning in the community. Table 18–1 provides an overview of the major components of a pulmonary rehabilitation program.

Table 18–1
Components of Pulmonary Rehabilitation

General Factors
- Patient and family education
- Nutrition instruction and weight control
- Avoidance of smoking and inhaled irritants
- Avoidance of infections (e.g., immunization)
- Proper living environment
- Proper hydration

Medications
- Bronchodilators
- Expectorants
- Antimicrobials
- Corticosteroids
- Cromolyn sodium/nedocromil sodium
- Leukotriene antagonists/inhibitors
- Diuretics
- Psychopharmacologic agents

Respiratory Therapy Modalities
- Aerosol therapy
- Oxygen therapy
- Home ventilators

Physical Therapy Modalities
- Relaxation training
- Breathing retraining
- Chest percussion and postural drainage
- Deliberate coughing and expectoration
- Exercise conditioning

Occupational Therapy
- Evaluate activities of daily living
- Outline energy-conserving maneuvers
- Psychosocial rehabilitation

Vocational Rehabilitation

Based on information from Hodgkin JE, Celli BR, Connors GL (2009). *Pulmonary Rehabilitation Guidelines to Success* (4th ed.). Mosby/Elsevier.

Pulmonary rehabilitation programs are commonly divided into the following three phases.

Phase I

This phase is the pretesting portion of the program. The patient performs a variety of tests such as pulmonary function studies, stress tests, and 6- to 12-minute walking tests. During this phase, the patient is also evaluated for any nutritional, psychological, lifestyle, and vocational needs.

Phase II

This phase also consists of patient and family education, group and individual counseling, and group discussion sessions. Educational topics include basic cardiopulmonary anatomy and physiology, breathing techniques, pulmonary hygiene, nutritional guidelines, medications, respiratory therapy equipment, and the importance of exercise. During this phase, the patient begins active range-of-motion exercises. Such exercises include work on the treadmill, air-dyne bike, arm ergometer, rowing machine, chest pulleys, and steps. The primary objective during this phase is the conditioning of the cardiovascular system (aerobic) and skeletal muscles. During the last portion of this phase, long-term graded exercises are emphasized, such as walking, walking/ jogging, stationary bicycling, and/or swimming.

Phase III

This phase consists of follow-up care and long-term maintenance. Components of this phase include efforts to modify risk factors (e.g., control of blood lipids, hypertension, obesity, smoking cessation) and the establishment of a routine program of physical activity. This phase should continue indefinitely. The patient commonly undergoes yearly evaluation, which includes graded exercise testing. Some patients may require more frequent evaluations.

Table 18–2 provides an overview of the benefits of pulmonary rehabilitation reported by the **Global Initiative on Chronic Obstructive Lung Disease (GOLD)** report.

Table 18–2
Benefits of Pulmonary Rehabilitation in COPD

- Exercise capacity is improved.
- Patient's perceived intensity of breathlessness is reduced.
- Health-related quality of life is improved.
- Number of hospitalizations and days in the hospital are reduced.
- Anxiety and depression associated with COPD are reduced.
- Strength and endurance training of the upper limbs improves arm function.
- Benefits extend well beyond the immediate period of training.
- Survival rate is improved.
- Respiratory muscle training is beneficial—especially when combined with general exercise training.
- Psychological intervention is helpful.

Chapter Summary

A basic knowledge of the effects of exercise on the cardiopulmonary systems is helpful to the respiratory therapist. Important topics regarding ventilation during exercise include the control of ventilation, alveolar ventilation, oxygen consumption, arterial blood gas values, increased oxygen diffusion capacity, and alveolar-arterial difference. In addition, exercise has a significant effect on circulation. Topics in this area include sympathetic discharge, cardiac output, arterial blood pressure, pulmonary vascular pressure, and the dilation of muscle capillaries. In addition, a basic understanding of the following should be mastered: the interrelationship among muscle work, oxygen consumption, and cardiac output; the influence of training on the heart and on cardiac output; and the relationship between body temperature and cutaneous blood flow. Finally, the respiratory therapist should know the primary components of the three phases of a pulmonary rehabilitation program. A clinical connection associated with these topics includes the general benefits of exercise.

Review Questions

1. During strenuous exercise, an adult's alveolar ventilation can increase as much as
    A. 10-fold
    B. 20-fold
    C. 30-fold
    D. 40-fold

2. The maximum alveolar ventilation generated during heavy exercise under normal conditions is about what percent of the maximum voluntary ventilation?
    A. 20–35 percent
    B. 30–45 percent
    C. 40–55 percent
    D. 50–65 percent

3. During heavy exercise, the total cardiac output may increase as much as
    A. 2-fold
    B. 4-fold
    C. 6-fold
    D. 8-fold

4. At the onset of exercise, sympathetic discharge causes the
    1. heart rate to decrease
    2. peripheral vascular system to constrict
    3. heart to increase its strength of contraction
    4. blood vessels of the working muscles to dilate
        A. 3 only
        B. 2 and 4 only
        C. 1 and 2 only
        D. 2, 3, and 4 only

5. During exercise, the stroke volume reaches its peak when the cardiac output is at about what percent of its maximum?
    A. 30 percent
    B. 40 percent
    C. 50 percent
    D. 60 percent

6. During exercise, heat production may increase as much as
    A. 10-fold
    B. 20-fold
    C. 30-fold
    D. 40-fold

7. During exercise, the oxygen consumption ($\dot{V}_{O_2}$) of the skeletal muscles may account for more than
    A. 65 percent of the total $\dot{V}_{O_2}$
    B. 75 percent of the total $\dot{V}_{O_2}$
    C. 85 percent of the total $\dot{V}_{O_2}$
    D. 95 percent of the total $\dot{V}_{O_2}$

8. During very heavy exercise, the
    1. pH increases
    2. Pa_{CO_2} decreases
    3. Pa_{O_2} remains constant
    4. pH decreases
    5. Pa_{CO_2} increases
        A. 1 and 2 only
        B. 4 and 5 only
        C. 2 and 4 only
        D. 2, 3, and 4 only

9. During maximum exercise, the oxygen diffusion capacity may increase as much as
    A. 3-fold
    B. 6-fold
    C. 9-fold
    D. 12-fold

10. During exercise, the $P_{(A-a)O_2}$ begins to increase when the oxygen consumption reaches about what percent of its maximum?
    A. 10 percent
    B. 20 percent
    C. 30 percent
    D. 40 percent

Chapter 19

High Altitude and Its Effects on the Cardiopulmonary System

Objectives

By the end of this chapter, the student should be able to:

1. Describe the effects of high altitude on the following components of the cardiopulmonary system:
   —Ventilation
   —Red blood cell production (polycythemia)
   —Acid–base status
   —Oxygen diffusion capacity
   —Alveolar-arterial oxygen tension difference
   —Ventilation-perfusion relationships
   —Cardiac output
   —Pulmonary vascular system
2. Describe the clinical connection associated with altitude training.

3. Describe other physiologic changes caused by high altitude, including:
   —Sleep disorders
   —Myoglobin concentration
   —Acute mountain sickness
   —High-altitude pulmonary edema
   —High-altitude cerebral edema
   —Chronic mountain sickness
4. Complete the review questions at the end of this chapter.

High Altitude

The effects of high altitude on the cardiopulmonary system are of interest because better understanding of long-term oxygen deprivation can be applied to the treatment of chronic hypoxia caused by lung disease. Nearly 30 million people live at altitudes greater than 2500 meters—mostly in the Rocky Mountains of North America, the Andes Mountains of South America, the Himalaya Mountains of south central Asia, and the Ethiopian Highlands of East Africa. In addition, many lowlanders travel to high altitudes for work and recreation. Unfortunately, these short-term high-altitude exposures also pose the hazards of acute altitude illnesses. The purpose of this chapter is to review both the normal responses and adaptive processes that occur in response to high altitude.

Under normal conditions, the barometric pressure—and P_{O_2}—progressively decreases with altitude (Figure 19–1 on page 576). At an altitude of 18,000 to 19,000 ft, the barometric pressure is about half the sea-level value of 760 mm Hg

The barometric pressure and the atmospheric P_{O_2} decrease linearly as altitude increases.

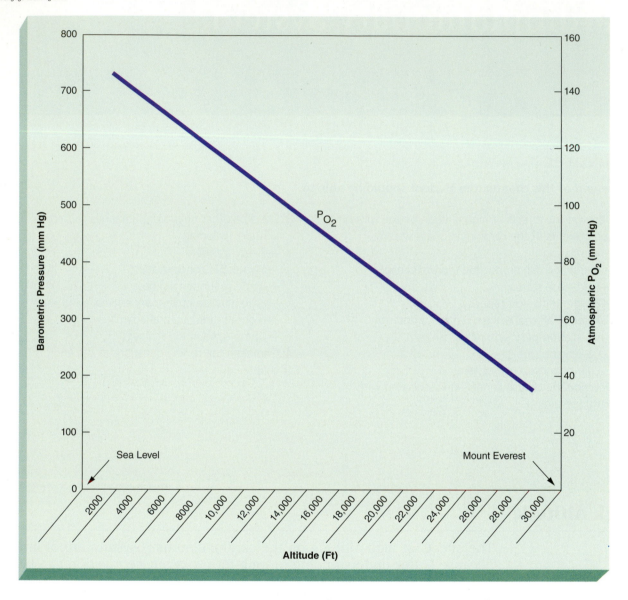

(380 mm Hg). The barometric pressure on the summit of Mount Everest (altitude: 29,028 ft) is about 250 mm Hg (the atmospheric P_{O_2} is about 43 mm Hg). At an altitude of about 65,000 ft, the barometric pressure falls below the pressure of water vapor, and tissue fluids begin to "boil" or "vaporize." Table 19–1 provides an overview of the altitude (in feet and meters), barometric pressure, and inspired P_{O_2} relationship.

When an individual who normally lives near sea level spends a period of time at high altitudes, a number of compensatory responses develop—a process known as acclimatization. For example, it is an interesting fact that after a period of acclimatization, an individual may reach the summit of Mount Everest without supplemental oxygen. However, when an individual is

Table 19-1

The Altitude, Barometric Pressure, and Inspired P_{O_2} Relationship

Altitude (meters)	Altitude (feet)	Barometric Pressure (torr)	Inspired P_{O_2} (torr)
0	0	760	159
1,000	3,280	674	141
2,000	6,560	596	125
3,000	9,840	526	110
4,000	13,120	463	97
5,000	16,400	405	85
6,000	19,680	354	79
8,000	26,240	268	56
8,848	29,028	253	43

© Cengage Learning 2013

Based on information from Luks AM, Schoene RB, High Altitude. In Murray & Nadel's Textbook of Respiratory Medicine, Editors: (5th ed.), Editors: Mason RJ, Broaddus CV, Saunders/Elsevier, 2010, pp 1651–1673.

suddenly exposed to the oxygen tension found at the summit of Mount Everest, a loss of consciousness occurs within minutes.

The following are some of the primary cardiopulmonary changes seen at high altitude.

Ventilation

One of the most prominent features of acclimatization is increased alveolar ventilation. As already mentioned, when an individual ascends above the earth's surface, the barometric pressure progressively decreases, and the atmospheric P_{O_2} declines. As the atmospheric P_{O_2} decreases, the individual's arterial oxygen pressure (Pa_{O_2}) also decreases. Eventually, the Pa_{O_2} will fall low enough (to about 60 torr) to stimulate the carotid and aortic bodies, known collectively as the **peripheral chemoreceptors** (refer to Figure 9–4).

When the peripheral chemoreceptors are stimulated, they transmit signals to the medulla to increase ventilation (refer to Figure 9–5). This response is called the **hypoxic ventilator response (HVR)**. The HVR works to minimize the drop in alveolar P_{O_2}. Because the peripheral chemoreceptors do not acclimate to a decreased oxygen concentration, increased alveolar ventilation will continue for the entire time the individual remains at the high altitude.

Pulmonary Function and Mechanics

As an individual ascends, the following changes occur in lung function as a result of acute hypoxic exposure: The vital capacity decreases within the first 24 hours. It is believed the causes of the reduced vital capacity include increased interstitial lung fluid—which in turn results in airway narrowing, air trapping, and delayed emptying of alveolar gas—pulmonary vascular engorgement, and decreased respiratory muscle strength. It is interesting to note that the peak expiratory flow rates are actually increased. It is believed that this lower airway resistance is due, in part, to the decreased air density, which works to offset any airway narrowing.

Unlike individuals exposed to acute hypoxic environments, long-term high-altitude residents have an increased vital capacity. Research shows a direct relationship to the vital capacity size and the length of time one resides at high altitudes—that is, the more time spent at high altitudes, the larger the vital capacity. People born and raised at high altitudes develop larger vital capacities than those who reside in high altitudes later in life.

Polycythemia

When an individual is subjected to a low concentration of oxygen for a prolonged period of time, the hormone *erythropoietin* from the kidneys stimulates the bone marrow to increase red blood cell (RBC) production. The increased hemoglobin available in polycythemia is an adaptive mechanism that increases the oxygen-carrying capacity of the blood. In fact, people who live at high altitudes often have a normal, or even above-normal, oxygen-carrying capacity, despite a chronically low Pa_{O_2} and oxygen saturation.

In lowlanders who ascend to high altitudes, the RBCs increase for about 6 weeks before the production rate levels off. As the level of RBCs increases, the plasma volume decreases. Thus, there is no significant change in the total circulating blood volume. After 6 weeks, an average hemoglobin concentration of 20.5 g/dL has been observed in mountain climbers who climbed to altitudes greater than 18,000 ft.

Acid–Base Status

Because of the increased ventilation generated by the peripheral chemoreceptors at high altitudes, the Pa_{CO_2} decreases, causing a secondary respiratory alkalosis. Over a 24- to 48-hour period, the renal system tries to offset the respiratory alkalosis by eliminating some of the excess bicarbonate. In spite of this mechanism, however, a mild respiratory alkalosis usually persists. In fact, even natives who have been at high altitudes for generations commonly have a mild respiratory alkalosis.

It is assumed that respiratory alkalosis may be advantageous for the transfer of oxygen across the alveolar-capillary membrane because alkalosis increases the affinity of hemoglobin for oxygen. In other words, the alkalosis enhances the loading of oxygen to the hemoglobin as desaturated blood passes through the alveolar-capillary system. It is also argued, however, that the increased affinity interferes with the unloading of oxygen at the cells.

There is both experimental and theoretical evidence that the increased oxygen affinity at high altitude is beneficial. This is further supported by the fact that a mild respiratory alkalosis usually persists in mountain climbers, high-altitude natives, and even in animals who live in low-oxygen environments. The alkalosis persists even after the kidneys should have had more than enough time to fully eliminate the excess bicarbonate.

Oxygen Diffusion Capacity

In response to short-term exposure to high altitude, there are a number of factors that limit oxygen diffusion. The decreased barometric pressure lowers the alveolar P_{O_2}—which in turn reduces the pressure gradient for diffusion. At altitudes greater than 2500 meters, even the estimated at-rest pulmonary capillary transit time of 0.75 second may not be adequate for end-capillary equilibration of oxygen to occur. This diffusion limitation is exacerbated during exercise because of the shortened transit time of blood moving through the alveolar-capillary system.

With long-term residence at high altitude, there is a remarkable change in the oxygen diffusion capacity, although the mechanism remains unclear. Individuals residing at high-altitude have a lower alveolar-arterial P_{O_2} difference, an increased diffusing capacity, and higher arterial P_{O_2} at rest and exercise. High-altitude natives have been shown to have an oxygen diffusion capacity that is about 20 to 25 percent greater than predicted, both during rest and exercise. The increased oxygen diffusion may be explained, in part, by the polycythemia that often develops at high altitudes. Increased numbers of red blood cells increase the diffusion capacity of oxygen (refer to Table 4–3).

The increased oxygen diffusion may also be explained by the larger lung volumes or capacities seen in high-altitude natives. It is suggested that the larger lungs provide an increased alveolar surface area and a larger capillary blood volume. This is further supported by studies that demonstrate that when animals are exposed to low-oxygen partial pressures during their active growth period, they develop larger lungs and greater diffusion capacity. On the other hand, animals exposed to high concentrations of oxygen during their active growth period develop smaller lungs than expected.

Alveolar-Arterial P_{O_2} Difference

During acute high altitude exposures, oxygen diffusion across the alveolar-capillary membrane is limited and this results in an increased **alveolar-arterial oxygen tension difference** ($P_{(A-a)O_2}$) Figure 19–2 on page 580 shows that under normal circumstances, there is ample time for oxygen to equilibrate between the alveoli and the end-capillary blood. In contrast, Figure 19–3 on page 581 shows the estimated time necessary for oxygen to equilibrate for a climber at rest on the summit of Mount Everest. Note that the pulmonary blood enters the alveolar-capillary system with a P_{O_2} of about 21 torr and slowly rises to about 28 torr. Thus, as the blood leaves the alveolar-capillary system, there is a large $P_{(A-a)O_2}$ characteristic of oxygen diffusion limitations. In other words, percentage-wise, only 80 percent of the P_{O_2} (Pa_{O_2} of 28 torr divided by a PA_{O_2} of 35 = 0.80) actually moved across the alveolar-capillary membrane. Twenty percent of the PA_{O_2} did not move across

Figure 19–2

Under normal resting conditions, blood moves through the alveolar-capillary membrane in about 0.75 second. The oxygen pressure P_{O_2} reaches equilibrium in about 0.25 second—one-third of the time available.

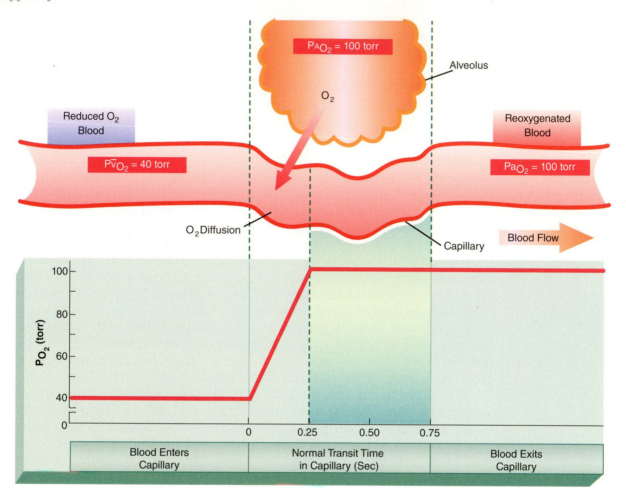

the alveolar-capillary membrane into the capillary blood. At high altitude, the $P_{(A-a)O_2}$ is further increased (1) during exercise—because of the increased cardiac output—and (2) in individuals with alveolar thickening caused by interstitial lung disease.

Ventilation-Perfusion Relationships

At high altitude, the increased ventilation is matched by increased cardiac output and pulmonary perfusion. In addition, the acute alveolar hypoxia activates hypoxic pulmonary vasoconstriction (HPV), which in turn increases pulmonary vascular resistance. These mechanisms cause the redistribution of pulmonary blood flow to areas of the lung that are not as well perused at sea level—thus, improving the overall ventilation-perfusion ratio and optimizing gas exchange.

Cardiac Output

During acute exposure to a hypoxic environment, the cardiac output during both rest and exercise increases, which in turn increases the oxygen delivery

Figure 19–3

Estimated time necessary for oxygen diffusion for a climber at rest on the summit of Mount Everest. As the blood leaves the alveolar-capillary system, there is a large alveolar-arterial oxygen tension difference $P_{(A-a)O_2}$.

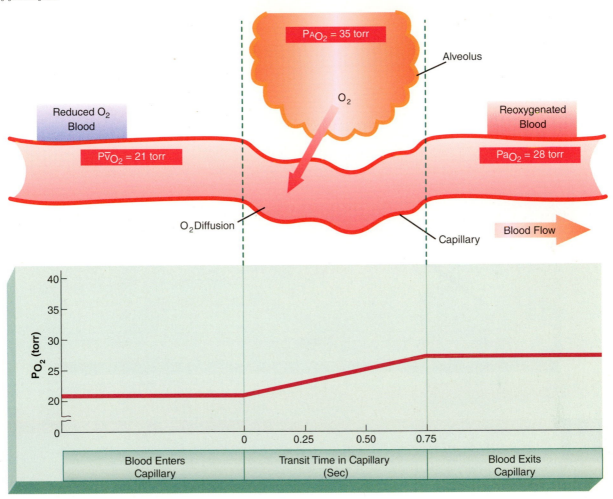

to the peripheral cells. In individuals who have acclimatized to high altitude, however, and in high altitude natives, increased cardiac output is not seen. Cardiac output and oxygen uptake are the same as at sea level. The precise reason for the return of the cardiac output and oxygen uptake to sea level values is unknown. It has been suggested that the polycythemia that develops in well-acclimatized subjects may play a role.

Pulmonary Vascular System

As an individual ascends from the earth's surface, pulmonary hypertension progressively increases as a result of *hypoxic pulmonary vasoconstriction*. A linear relationship exists between the degree of ascent and the degree of pulmonary vasoconstriction and hypertension (Figure 19–4 on page 582). The exact mechanism of this phenomenon is unclear. It is known, however, that it is the partial pressure of oxygen in the alveoli, not the partial pressure of arterial oxygen, that chiefly controls this response.

Figure 19–4

Pulmonary hypertension increases linearly as altitude increases.

© Cengage Learning 2013

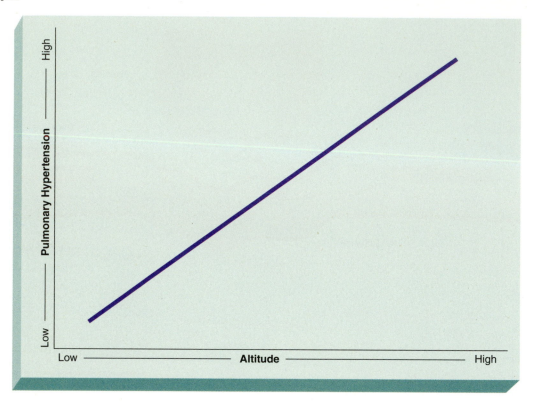

Clinical Connection—19-1

Altitude Training

Some endurance athletes practice altitude training for several weeks before an event. Proponents claim that this type of training environment—that is, a low, partial-pressure oxygen environment—increases the athlete's hemoglobin and, therefore, gives the athlete a competitive advantage. The benefits of altitude training, however, have not been conclusive. For example, many elite endurance athletes who have relocated to train at high altitudes did not realize any significant improvements after returning to sea level. In part, the rationale for no measurable benefits was this: in comparing athletes' performances at sea level, the athletes were unable to attain the same maximum speeds and power output at high altitudes.

Today, altitude training can be simulated—that is, "bringing the mountain to the athlete"—through the use of an oxygen-depleted tent (altitude simulation tent); an altitude simulation room; or a mask-based hypoxicator system, where the barometric pressure is maintained at a constantly low level.[1] A key question that has emerged regarding any form of altitude training is what "dose" of hypoxic exposure is required to see a benefit in sea-level performance. In general, the most recent data suggest that athletes need to reside at 2000 to 2500 meters for more than 4 weeks for more than 22 hours per day in order to derive physiologic benefits.

---

[1] It should be noted that many of the devices used for altitude training do not have FDA approval.

Other Physiologic Changes

Sleep Disorders

During the first few days at high altitude, lowlanders frequently awaken during the night and complain that they do not feel refreshed when they awake in the morning. When sleeping, they commonly demonstrate breathing that waxes and wanes with apneic periods of 10- to 15-second duration (Cheyne-Stokes respiration). The arterial oxygen saturation (Sa_{O_2}) fluctuates accordingly.

Myoglobin Concentration

The concentration of myoglobin in skeletal muscles is increased in high-altitude natives, and studies of this group have shown a high concentration of myoglobin in the diaphragm, the adductor muscles of the leg, the pectoral muscles, and the myocardium. Myoglobin enhances the transfer of oxygen between the capillary blood and peripheral cells, buffers regional P_{O_2} differences, and provides an oxygen storage compartment for short periods of very severe oxygen deprivation.

Acute Mountain Sickness

Newcomers to high altitude frequently experience what is known as **acute mountain sickness**, which is characterized by headache, fatigue, dizziness, palpitation, nausea, loss of appetite, and insomnia. Symptoms usually do not occur until 6 to 12 hours after an individual ascends to a high altitude. The symptoms are generally most severe on the second or third day after ascent. Acclimatization is usually complete by the fourth or fifth day.

The precise cause of acute mountain sickness is not known. It is suggested that the primary cause is hypoxia, complicated by the hypocapnia and respiratory alkalosis associated with high altitude. It may also be linked to a fluid imbalance, because pulmonary edema, cerebral edema, and peripheral edema are commonly associated with acute and chronic mountain sickness.

Sensitivity to acute mountain sickness varies greatly among individuals. Being physically fit is no guarantee of immunity. Younger people appear to be more at risk. In some cases, descent to a lower altitude may be the only way to reduce the symptoms.

High-Altitude Pulmonary Edema

High-altitude pulmonary edema is sometimes seen in individuals with acute mountain sickness. A typical scenario is as follows: A lowlander rapidly ascends to a high altitude and is very active during the trip or upon arrival. Initially, the lowlander demonstrates shortness of breath, fatigue, and a dry cough. Physical signs include tachypnea, tachycardia, and crackles at the lung bases. Orthopnea (see page 135) is commonly present at this time. In severe cases, the lowlander may cough up large amounts of pink, frothy sputum. Death may occur.

The exact cause of high-altitude pulmonary edema is not fully understood. It may be associated with the pulmonary vasoconstriction that occurs in response to the alveolar hypoxia. It may also be associated with an increased permeability of the pulmonary capillaries. The best treatment of high-altitude pulmonary edema is rapid descent. Oxygen therapy should be administered.

High-Altitude Cerebral Edema

High-altitude cerebral edema is a serious complication of acute mountain sickness. It is characterized by photophobia, ataxia, hallucinations, clouding of consciousness, coma, and possibly death. The precise cause of high-altitude cerebral edema is unclear. It is suggested that it may be linked to the increased cerebral vasodilation and blood flow that result from hypoxia. Oxygen therapy should be administered if available.

Chronic Mountain Sickness

Chronic mountain sickness (also known as Monge's disease) is sometimes seen in long-term residents at high altitude. It is characterized by fatigue, reduced exercise tolerance, headache, dizziness, somnolence, loss of mental acuity, marked polycythemia, and severe hypoxemia. The severe oxygen desaturation and polycythemia cause a cyanotic appearance. A hematocrit of 83 percent and hemoglobin concentrations as high as 28 g/dL have been reported. As a result of the high hematocrit, the viscosity of the blood is significantly increased. Right ventricular hypertrophy is common.

Chapter Summary

A basic knowledge of the effects of high altitude on the cardiopulmonary system can enhance the respiratory care practitioner's understanding of how chronic oxygen deprivation can be applied to the treatment of chronic hypoxia caused by lung disease. Major cardiopulmonary changes seen after a period of acclimatization at high altitude include increased ventilation, polycythemia, acid–base balance changes, an increased oxygen diffusion capacity, an increased alveolar-arterial P_{O_2} difference, and an overall improved ventilation-perfusion ratio. Long-term exposure to high altitude does not change an individual's cardiac output but does cause pulmonary hypertension. Finally, high altitudes disrupt normal sleep patterns; increase myoglobin in the skeletal muscles; and can cause acute or chronic mountain sickness, pulmonary edema, and cerebral edema. The clinical connection associated with these topics discusses altitude training.

Review Questions

1. The barometric pressure is about half the sea-level value of 760 torr at an altitude of
   A. 4,000–5,000 ft
   B. 9,000–10,000 ft
   C. 14,000–15,000 ft
   D. 18,000–19,000 ft

2. The oxygen diffusion capacity of high-altitude natives is about
   A. 5–10 percent greater than predicted
   B. 10–15 percent greater than predicted
   C. 15–20 percent greater than predicted
   D. 20–25 percent greater than predicted

3. Acute mountain sickness is characterized by
    1. sleep disorders
    2. headache
    3. dizziness
    4. palpitation
    5. loss of appetite
        A. 1 and 3 only
        B. 2 and 4 only
        C. 1, 4, and 5 only
        D. 1, 2, 3, 4, and 5

4. The symptoms of acute mountain sickness are generally most severe on the
    A. first or second day after ascent
    B. second or third day after ascent
    C. third or fourth day after ascent
    D. fourth or fifth day after ascent

5. When an individual is subjected to a high altitude for a prolonged period of time, which of the following is(are) seen?
    1. An increased red blood cell production
    2. A decreased Pa_{CO_2}
    3. An increased $P_{(A-a)O_2}$
    4. A decreased alveolar ventilation
        A. 1 and 3 only
        B. 2 and 4 only
        C. 3 and 4 only
        D. 1, 2, and 3 only

6. At high altitude, the overall ventilation perfusion ratio improves.   True _____   False _____

7. In individuals who have acclimatized to a high altitude, an increased cardiac output is seen.   True _____   False _____

8. There is a linear relationship between the degree of ascent and the degree of pulmonary vasoconstriction and hypertension.   True _____   False _____

9. Natives who have been at high altitudes for generations commonly demonstrate a mild respiratory alkalosis.   True _____   False _____

10. The concentration of myoglobin in skeletal muscles is decreased in high-altitude natives.   True _____   False _____

Chapter 20

High-Pressure Environments and Their Effects on the Cardiopulmonary System

Objectives

By the end of this chapter, the student should be able to:

1. Describe the following effects of a high-pressure environment on the cardiopulmonary system:
   —Breath-hold diving
   —The CO_2–O_2 paradox
   —The mammalian diving reflex
   —Decompression sickness
   —Barotrauma
   —Hyperbaric medicine

2. Describe the clinical connection associated with the Guinness world record for breath-holding.
3. Describe the clinical connection associated with glossopharyngeal insufflation.
4. Complete the review questions at the end of this chapter.

High-pressure environments have a profound effect on the cardiopulmonary system. Such environments are encountered in recreational scuba diving, deep sea diving, and hyperbaric medicine. The effects of high-pressure environments on the cardiopulmonary system are typically studied in (1) actual dives in the sea; (2) hyperbaric chambers, where the subject is exposed to mixtures of compressed gases (known as "simulated dry dives"); and (3) a water-filled hyperbaric chamber that can simulate any depth by adjusting the gas pressure above the water (known as "simulated wet dives").

Diving

Because water is incompressible, the pressure increases linearly with depth. For every 33 feet (10 meters) below the surface, the pressure increases 1.0 atmosphere (760 mm Hg). Thus, the total pressure at a depth of 33 feet is 2 atmospheres (1520 mm Hg)—1.0 atmosphere (1 atm) owing to the water column and 1.0 atmosphere pressure owing to the gaseous atmosphere above the water. At 66 feet (20 meters) below the surface, the pressure is 3.0 atmospheres (2280 mm Hg) (Figure 20–1 on page 588).

As an individual descends into water, the lung is compressed according to Boyle's law:

$$P_1 \times V_1 = P_2 \times V_2$$

Figure 20–1

Pressure increases linearly with depth. For every 33 feet (10 meters) below sea level, the pressure increases 1.0 atmosphere (atm). The depth in feet below sea water is referred as *feet of sea water* (FSW).

© Cengage Learning 2013

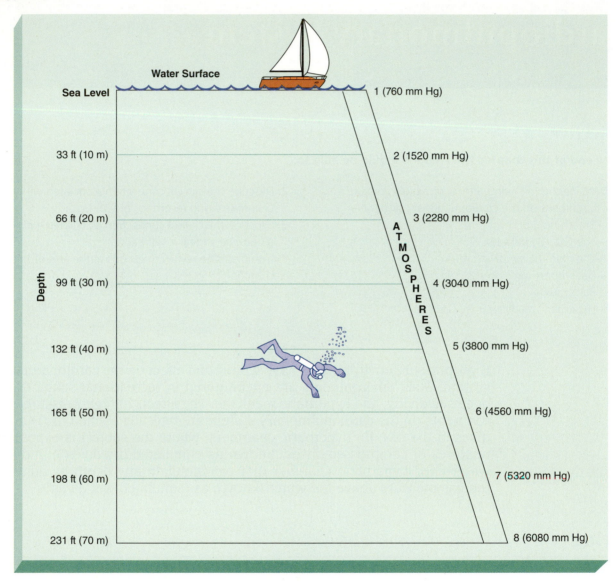

where P_1 = the pressure prior to the dive, V_1 = the lung volume prior to the dive, P_2 = the pressure generated at a specific water depth, and V_2 = the lung volume at that water depth.

Thus, if an individual fully inhales to a total lung capacity of 6 L at sea level, and dives to a depth of 33 feet, the lungs will be compressed to about 3 L:

$$V_2 = \frac{P_1 \times V_1}{P_2}$$

$$= \frac{1 \times 6}{2}$$

$$= 3 \text{ L}$$

At 66 feet, the lungs would be compressed to about 2 L. At 99 feet, the lungs would be compressed to about 1.5 L.

Boyle's law can also be used to calculate the pressure within a diver's lungs at a specific depth. For example, when the previously mentioned diver descends from sea level to a depth of 33 feet (compressing the lung volume from 6 to 3 L), the pressure within the diver's lungs will increase from 760 mm Hg to about 1520 mm Hg:

$$P_2 = \frac{P_1 \times V_1}{V_2}$$

$$= \frac{760 \times 6}{3}$$

$$= 1520 \text{ mm Hg}$$

At 66 feet, the pressure within a diver's lungs will be about 2280 mm Hg. At 99 feet, the pressure will be about 3040 mm Hg.

Breath-Hold Diving

Breath-hold diving is the simplest and most popular form of diving. The maximum duration of a breath-hold dive is a function of (1) the diver's metabolic rate and (2) the diver's ability to store and transport O_2 and CO_2. A delicate balance exists between the diver's O_2 and CO_2 levels during a breath-hold dive. For example, the P_{CO_2} must not rise too rapidly and reach the so-called

Clinical Connection—20-1

Guinness World Record for Breath-Holding

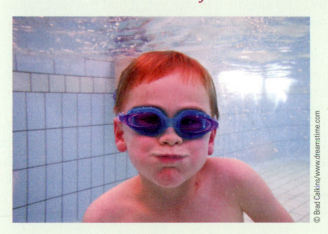

© Brad Calkins/www.dreamstime.com

On April 30, 2008, magician David Blaine set the world record for the longest breath-holding, by holding his breath for 17 minutes and 4.4 seconds, during a live telecast of *The Oprah Winfrey Show*

in Chicago.[1] Blaine spent 23 minutes inhaling pure oxygen, packing his lungs with extra oxygen just before the breathing tubes were removed in a sphere filled with 1800 gallons of water. Up to 30 minutes of so-called oxygen hyperventilation is allowed under the Guinness guidelines.

The reader is challenged to consider the following: assuming an average total lung capacity, approximately how much oxygen did Mr. Blaine have in his lungs for the record breath-hold? (Remember from Chapter 6 that the average person consumes about 250 mL of oxygen per minute.) How fast was his heart rate during this event? What was the impact of a rapid heart rate on Mr. Blaine's oxygen consumption? What were his Pa_{CO_2} and pH levels at the end of this event?

[1] http://www.oprah.com/oprahshow/David-Blaines-World-Record-Video

respiratory drive **breaking point** (generally about 55 torr) before the diver returns to the surface. On the other hand, the diver's P_{CO_2} must rise fast enough (relative to the decrease in O_2) to alert the diver of the need to return to the surface before hypoxia-induced loss of consciousness occurs.

Voluntary hyperventilation can prolong the duration of a breath-hold dive. Hyperventilation reduces the diver's CO_2 stores and, therefore, increases the time before the CO_2 stores are replenished and the breaking point is reached. Note, however, that hyperventilation prior to a breath-hold dive can be dangerous. The diver's oxygen stores may fall to a critically low level before the CO_2 breaking point is reached. Should this happen, the diver could lose consciousness before reaching the surface and drown.

The CO_2–O_2 Paradox

When an individual breath-hold dives to a great depth, a so-called paradoxical reversal occurs in the flow of CO_2 and O_2 between the alveoli and the pulmonary capillary blood. This **CO_2–O_2 paradox** is caused by the pressure changes that develop around the diver's body during the dive. The CO_2 paradox occurs as the diver descends, and the O_2 paradox occurs as the diver ascends.

The reason for the CO_2 paradox is as follows: As the diver descends, the lungs are compressed and the pressure in the lungs increases. In fact, the gas pressure in the lungs is about doubled when the diver reaches a depth of 33 feet (2 atm). Thus, assuming a normal $P_{A_{O_2}}$ of about 100 torr and $P_{A_{CO_2}}$ of about 40 torr, at a depth of 33 feet the $P_{A_{O_2}}$ will be about 200 torr and the $P_{A_{CO_2}}$ will be about 80 torr.

In view of these pressure increases, it can be seen that as a diver progressively descends, a CO_2 paradox will occur when the $P_{A_{CO_2}}$ becomes greater than the $P\bar{v}_{CO_2}$ of the pulmonary capillary blood (normally about 46 torr). In other words, the CO_2 in the alveoli will move into the pulmonary capillary blood. As the diver returns to the surface, the alveolar air expands, causing the $P_{A_{CO_2}}$ to decrease. When this happens, the CO_2 from the pulmonary capillary blood will again move into the alveoli. It is suggested that this mechanism might work to relieve the respiratory CO_2 drive (breaking point) as the diver moves toward the surface.

The reason for the O_2 paradox is as follows: Like the $P_{A_{CO_2}}$, the $P_{A_{O_2}}$ increases as the diver descends, causing more O_2 to move from the alveoli into the pulmonary capillary blood. This mechanism provides more dissolved O_2 for tissue metabolism. However, this physiologic advantage is lost as the diver returns to the surface and the lungs expand and the $P_{A_{O_2}}$ decreases. If a good portion of the O_2 is taken up from the lungs during descent, the $P_{A_{O_2}}$ decline during ascent may be significant. In fact, $P_{A_{O_2}}$ the can fall below the $P\bar{v}_{O_2}$ of the pulmonary capillary blood. When this happens, the O_2 paradox occurs. That is, the O_2 in the pulmonary capillary blood moves into the alveoli. The fall in $P_{A_{O_2}}$ as a diver returns to the surface is also known as the **hypoxia of ascent**.

The Mammalian Diving Reflex

The **mammalian diving reflex** (also known as *diving reflex* or *diving response*) consists of bradycardia, decreased cardiac output, lactate accumulation in underperfused muscles, and peripheral vasoconstriction elicited during a breath-hold deep dive. The mammalian diving reflex is a set of physiologic reflexes that acts as the first line of defense against hypoxia. The diving reflex may partially explain the survival of numerous near-drowning cases in cold water after submersion lasting more than 40 minutes. It is suggested that the peripheral vasoconstriction elicited during a deep dive conserves oxygen for the heart and central nervous system by shunting blood away from less vital tissues.

Decompression Sickness

During a deep dive, the dissolved nitrogen in the diver's blood will move into body tissues. The amount of dissolved gas that enters the tissues is a function of (1) the solubility of the gas in the tissues, (2) the partial pressure of the gas, and (3) the hydrostatic pressure in the tissue.

During ascent (decompression), the pressure around the diver's body falls, reducing the hydrostatic pressure in the tissues and, therefore, the ability of the tissues to hold inert gases. When the decompression is performed at an appropriately slow rate, the gases leaving the tissues will be transported (in their dissolved state) by the venous blood to the lungs and exhaled. When the decompression is conducted too rapidly, the gases will be released from the tissue as bubbles. Depending on the size, number, and location of the bubbles, they can cause a number of signs and symptoms, collectively referred to as decompression sickness. Decompression sickness includes, but is not limited to, joint pains (the bends), chest pain and coughing (the chokes), paresthesia and paralysis (spinal cord involvement), circulatory failure and, in severe cases, death.

Barotrauma

While diving, the increased pressure can cause tissue injury in the lungs, middle ear, paranasal sinuses, and gastrointestinal tract. Middle-ear barotrauma is the most common diving-related disorder encountered by divers. Barotrauma can occur in the alveoli distal to a blocked airway, in a paranasal sinus with an obstructed orifice, in a small pocket of air left between a tooth filling and the base of the tooth, or in the air space within a diving mask (mask squeeze). Facial edema, ecchymoses (bluish discoloration of an area of skin), and conjunctival hemorrhages are often observed after diving. Gastrointestinal barotrauma may also occur when air enters the stomach as a result of

Clinical Connection—20-2

Glossopharyngeal Insufflation

Glossopharyngeal insufflation (GI)—also called **lung packing** or **buccal pumping**—is a technique used by competitive breath-hold divers to enhance their diving performance. The breath-hold diver uses the oropharyngeal musculature to pump boluses of air into the lungs to increase the volume above his or her normal total lung capacity. Breath-hold divers use GI to help prevent lung compression at great water depth and to increase the volume of oxygen in the lungs—thus, increasing breath-hold time. Although the experienced breath-hold diver can increase their lung volumes by up to 3 L, this maneuver is associated with hypotension, decreased cardiac output, pulmonary barotrauma, and pneumomediastinum.

a faulty breathing apparatus or by swallowing air. On ascent, the expanding gas can distend the stomach or intestine. In severe cases, the distention of the stomach may cause the stomach to rupture and pneumoperitoneum (air in the peritoneal cavity of the abdomen).

Hyperbaric Medicine

The administration of oxygen at increased ambient pressures is now being used routinely to treat a variety of pathologic conditions. Clinically, this therapy is referred to as hyperbaric medicine and is accomplished by means of a compression chamber (also called a hyperbaric chamber). Most of the therapeutic benefits of hyperbaric oxygenation are associated with the increased oxygen delivery to the tissues.

As discussed in Chapter 6, hemoglobin is about 97 percent saturated with oxygen at a normal arterial P_{O_2} of 80 to 100 torr. Very little additional O_2 can be combined with hemoglobin once this saturation level is reached. However, the quantity of dissolved O_2 will continue to rise linearly as the Pa_{O_2} increases. Approximately 0.3 mL of O_2 physically dissolves in each 100 mL of blood for every Pa_{O_2} increase of 100 torr (Figure 20–2).

Figure 20–2

The quantity of dissolved O_2 increases linearly as the Pa_{O_2} increases. About 0.3 mL of O_2 physically dissolves in each 100 mL of blood for every 100 mm Hg increase in Pa_{O_2}.

© Cengage Learning 2013

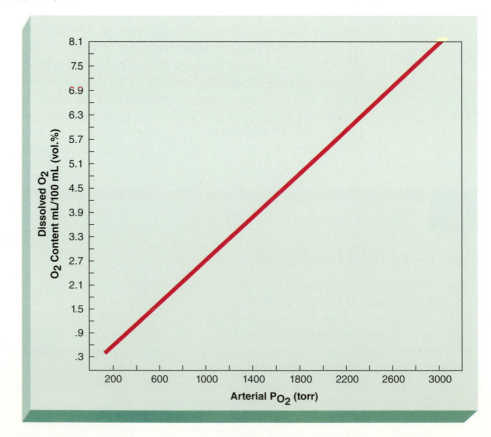

Indications for Hyperbaric Oxygenation

As shown in Table 20–1, the administration of hyperbaric oxygen is now indicated for a number of clinical conditions. Hyperbaric oxygen has long been useful in the treatment of diseases such as decompression sickness and gas embolism. Regardless of the cause of the bubbles, hyperbaric oxygen is effective in reducing bubble size, accelerating bubble resolution, and maintaining tissue oxygenation.

Hyperbaric oxygen is used empirically to enhance wound healing in conditions associated with ischemic hypoxia. Clinically, such conditions include radiation necrosis of bone or soft tissue, diabetic microangiopathy, compromised skin grafts, crush wounds, acute traumatic ischemias, and thermal burns. It appears that hyperbaric oxygen not only increases tissue oxygenation in these conditions, but increases capillary density as well.

Clinical evidence supports the use of hyperbaric oxygen for the treatment of anaerobic infections, including clostridial myonecrosis (gas gangrene), a variety of necrotizing soft-tissue infections, and chronic refractory osteomyelitis. Hyperbaric oxygen added to surgery and antibiotics in the treatment of clostridial myonecrosis increases tissue salvage and decreases mortality.

Hyperbaric oxygen is effective in the treatment of carbon monoxide poisoning. Carbon monoxide poisoning, which is caused by all sources of combustion (such as defective indoor heaters, automobile exhaust systems, or smoke inhalation), is the leading cause of death by poisoning in the United States. The severity of intoxication is a function of both the level and duration of carbon monoxide exposure. The administration of hyperbaric oxygen (1) increases the physically dissolved O_2 in the arterial blood by as much as

Table 20–1
Indications for Hyperbaric Oxygenation
Gas Disorders • Decompression sickness • Gas embolism
Vascular Disorders • Radiation necrosis • Diabetic microangiopathy • Nonhealing skin grafts • Crush injuries • Acute traumatic ischemias • Thermal burns
Infections • Clostridial gangrene • Necrotizing soft-tissue infections (flesh-eating bacteria) • Refractory osteomyelitis
Oxygen Transport Disorders • Carbon monoxide (CO) poisoning • Severe anemia or blood loss

5 vol% O_2, (2) increases the pressure gradient for driving oxygen into ischemic tissues, and (3) reduces the half-life of **carboxyhemoglobin** (CO_{Hb}). The CO_{Hb} half-life when a victim is breathing room air at 1 atm is approximately 5 hours. That is, a CO_{Hb} of 20 percent will decrease to about 10 percent in 5 hours and 5 percent after another 5 hours. Breathing 100 percent oxygen at 1 atm reduces the CO_{Hb} half-life to less than 1 hour.

Chapter Summary

High-pressure environments have a profound effect on the cardiopulmonary system. Important topics in this area include scuba diving, breath-hold diving, the CO_2–O_2 paradox, the mammalian diving reflex, barotrauma, and decompression sickness. Currently, the administration of hyperbaric oxygen is being used routinely to treat a variety of pathologic conditions, including gas diseases (e.g., decompression sickness), vascular insufficiency states (e.g., compromised skin grafts, thermal burns), infections (e.g., clostridial myonecrosis), and defects in oxygen transport (e.g., carbon monoxide poisoning). Clinical connections associated with these topics include the world record for breath-holding and glossopharyngeal insufflation.

Review Questions

1. At what depth below the water surface does the pressure increase to 3.0 atm?
   A. 33 feet
   B. 66 feet
   C. 99 feet
   D. 132 feet

2. If an individual fully inhales to a total lung capacity of 4.5 L at sea level (760 mm Hg) and dives to a depth of 66 feet, the lungs will be compressed to about
   A. 1.0 L
   B. 1.5 L
   C. 2.0 L
   D. 2.5 L

3. At sea level, a diver has the following:
   - Lung volume: 6 L
   - Pressure within the lungs: 755 mm Hg

   If this individual dives to a depth of 99 feet and compresses the lung volume to 2 L, what will be the pressure within the diver's lungs?

   A. 960 mm Hg
   B. 1420 mm Hg
   C. 1765 mm Hg
   D. 2265 mm Hg

4. The diving reflex consists of
1. tachycardia
2. decreased cardiac output
3. bradycardia
4. peripheral vasoconstriction
    A. 2 only
    B. 3 and 4 only
    C. 1 and 3 only
    D. 2, 3, and 4 only

5. The half-life of carboxyhemoglobin (CO_{Hb}) when a victim is breathing room air at 1 atm is approximately
    A. 2 hours
    B. 3 hours
    C. 4 hours
    D. 5 hours

6. Hyperventilation prior to a breath-hold dive can be dangerous.
True _____ False _____

7. The fall in $P_{A_{O_2}}$ as a diver returns to the surface is known as the hypoxia of ascent.
True _____ False _____

8. Chest pain and coughing caused by decompression sickness is known as the bends.
True _____ False _____

9. The so-called P_{CO_2} respiratory drive breaking point during a dive is about 55 torr.
True _____ False _____

10. Approximately 0.3 mL of O_2 is physically dissolved in each 100 mL of blood for every Pa_{O_2} increase of 100 torr.
True _____ False _____

Glossary

A

Abduct to draw away from the median plane of the body or from one of its parts.

Absolute shunt the sum of the anatomic and capillary shunts is referred to as *true* or *absolute shunt*. Absolute shunting is refractory to oxygen therapy.

Acclimatization physiologic or psychologic adjustment to a new environment.

Acetylcholine a chemical found in most organs and tissues. Acetylcholine plays an important role in the transmission of parasympathetic nerve impulses at the synapses.

Acid a compound that yields hydrogen ions when dissociated in aqueous solution (Arrhenius definition) or acts as a hydrogen ion donor (Brønsted definition) or acts as an electron pair acceptor (Lewis definition). Acids turn blue litmus red, have a sour taste, and react with bases to form salts. Acids have chemical properties essentially the opposite to those of bases.

Acidemia a decrease in the arterial blood pH below 7.35. The hydrogen ion concentration of the blood increases as reflected by a lowering of serum pH values.

Acidosis (*adj. acidotic*) an abnormal increase in hydrogen ion concentration in the body, resulting from an accumulation of an acid or the loss of a base. It is indicated by a blood pH below the normal range (7.35 to 7.45). The various forms of acidosis are named for their cause; for example, renal tubular acidosis results from failure of the kidney to secrete hydrogen ions or reabsorb bicarbonate ions, respiratory acidosis results from respiratory retention of CO_2, and diabetic acidosis results from an accumulation of ketones associated with lack of insulin. Treatment depends on diagnosis of the underlying abnormality and concurrent correction of the acid–base imbalance. Compare **alkalosis**.

Acinus (*pl. acini*) any small saclike structure, particularly one found in a gland. A subdivision of the lung consisting of the tissue distal to a terminal bronchiole.

Acromion process lateral portion of the spine of the scapula that forms the point of the shoulder. It articulates with the clavicle and gives attachment to the deltoid and trapezius muscles.

Action potential an electrical impulse consisting of a self-propagating series of polarizations and depolarizations, transmitted across the plasma membranes of a nerve fiber during the transmission of a nerve impulse and across the plasma membranes of a muscle cell during contraction or other activity. In the absence of an impulse, the inside is electrically negative and the outside is positive (the resting potential). During the passage of an impulse at any point on the nerve fiber, the inside becomes positive and the outside, negative. Also called *action current*.

Acute beginning abruptly with marked intensity or sharpness, then subsiding after a relatively short period. Compare **chronic**.

Acute alveolar hyperventilation a condition marked by low levels of carbon dioxide, and a high pH in the blood, due to breathing excessively. Also called respiratory alkalosis.

Acute epiglottitis a severe, rapidly progressing bacterial infection of the upper respiratory tract that occurs in young children, primarily between 2 and 7 years of age. It is characterized by sore throat, croupy stridor, and inflamed epiglottis, which may cause sudden respiratory obstruction and possibly death. The infection is generally caused by *Haemophilus influenzae*, type B, although streptococci may occasionally be the causative agent. Transmission occurs by infection with airborne particles or contact with infected secretions. The diagnosis is made by bacteriologic identification of *H. influenzae*, type B, in a specimen taken from the upper respiratory tract or in the blood. A lateral X-ray film of the neck shows an enlarged epiglottis and distention of the hypopharynx, which distinguishes the condition from croup. Direct visualization of the inflamed, cherry-red epiglottis by depression of the tongue or indirect laryngoscopy is also diagnostic but may produce total acute obstruction and should be attempted only by trained personnel with equipment to establish an airway or to provide respiratory resuscitation, if necessary. Compare **croup**.

Acute respiratory distress syndrome a severe pulmonary congestion characterized by diffuse injury to alveolar-capillary membranes. Fulminating sepsis, especially when gram-negative bacteria are involved, is the most common cause. ARDS may occur after trauma; near-drowning; aspiration of gastric acid; paraquat ingestion; inhalation of corrosive chemicals, such as chlorine, ammonia, or phosgene; or the use of certain drugs, including barbiturates, chlordiazepoxide, heroin, methadone hydrochloride, propoxyphene hydrochloride, and salicylates. Other causes include diabetic ketoacidosis, fungal infections, high altitude, pancreatitis, tuberculosis, and uremia. Also called adult respiratory distress syndrome, congestive atelectasis, hemorrhagic lung, noncardiogenic pulmonary edema, pump lung, shock lung, stiff lung, wet lung.

Acute ventilatory failure with partial renal compensation a condition marked by high levels of carbon dioxide and a low pH in the blood resulting from hypoventilation, which is partly corrected by the retention of HCO_3^- via the renal system and/or the administration of HCO_3^-.

Adenoid one of two masses of lymphatic tissue situated on the posterior wall of the nasopharynx behind the posterior nares. During childhood these masses often swell and block the passage of air from the nasal cavity into the pharynx, preventing the child from breathing through the nose. Also called pharyngeal tonsils.

Adrenergic nerve fibers that, when stimulated, release epinephrine at their endings. Adrenergic fibers include nearly all sympathetic postganglionic fibers except those innervating sweat glands.

Afferent carrying impulses toward a center.

Afferent nerves nerves that carry impulses from the periphery to the central nervous system.

Affinity attraction between two substances that, when united, form new substances (i.e., oxygen and hemoglobin form oxyhemoglobin).

Agranulocyte any leukocyte that does not contain predominant cytoplasmic granules, such as a monocyte or lymphocyte.

Air trapping the prevention of gas from leaving the alveoli during exhalation. This is usually caused by airway closure during exhalation.

Airway resistance a measure of the impedance to airflow through the bronchopulmonary system. Calculated by the pressure difference between the mouth and alveoli divided by flow rate.

Alkalemia an increase in the arterial blood pH above 7.45 due to a decrease in the hydrogen ion concentration or an increase in hydroxyl ions.

Alkalosis an abnormal condition of body fluids, characterized by a tendency toward a blood pH level greater than 7.45, for example, from an excess of alkaline bicarbonate or a deficiency of acid. Respiratory alkalosis may be caused by hyperventilation, resulting from an excess loss of carbon dioxide and a carbonic acid deficit. Metabolic alkalosis may result from an excess intake or retention of bicarbonate, loss of gastric acid in vomiting, potassium depletion, or any stimulus that increases the rate of sodium-hydrogen exchange. When a buffer system, such as carbon dioxide retention or bicarbonate excretion, prevents a shift in pH, it is labeled compensating alkalosis. Treatment of uncompensated alkalosis involves correction of dehydration and various ionic deficits to restore the normal acid-base balance in which the ratio of carbonic acid to bicarbonate is 20:1. Compare **acidosis**.

Allergen any substance that causes an allergic reaction. It may or may not be a protein.

Allergy a hypersensitive reaction to common, often intrinsically harmless substances, most of which are environmental.

Alpha receptor any of the postulated adrenergic components of receptor tissues that respond to norepinephrine and to various blocking agents. The activation of the alpha receptors causes such physiologic responses as increased peripheral vascular resistance, dilation of the pupils, and contraction of pilomotor muscles. Also called *alpha-adrenergic receptor*. Compare **beta receptor**.

Alveolar hyperventilation with partial renal compensation a condition marked by low levels of carbon dioxide and a high pH in the blood due to hyperventilation, which is partly corrected by the excretion of HCO_3^- via the renal system.

Alveolar sac an air sac at one of the terminal cavities of lung tissue.

Alveolus a small outpouching of walls of alveolar space through which gas exchange between alveolar air and pulmonary capillary blood takes place. The term is often used interchangeably with acinus. See also **alveolar sac**, **pulmonary alveolus**.

Amniocentesis an obstetric procedure in which a small amount of amniotic fluid is removed for laboratory analysis. It is usually performed between the sixteenth and twentieth weeks of gestation to aid in the diagnosis of fetal abnormalities, especially genetic disorders.

Amniotic fluid liquid produced by the fetal membranes and the fetus; it surrounds the fetus throughout pregnancy, usually totaling about 1000 mL at term.

Anaerobic threshold the point at which the level of exercise is greater than the ability of the cardiopulmonary system to provide a sufficient supply of oxygen to the muscles, causing anaerobic metabolism to ensue.

Analogous similar in function but having a different origin or structure.

Anastomosis joining of vessels, either naturally or surgically, to allow flow to other structures.

Anatomic shunt an anatomic shunt (also called a *true shunt*) exists when blood flows from the right side of the heart to the left side without coming in contact with an alveolus for gas exchange. In the healthy lung, there is a normal anatomic shunt of about 3 percent of the cardiac output. This normal shunting is caused by nonoxygenated blood completely bypassing the alveoli and entering (1) the pulmonary vascular system by means of the bronchial venous drainage and (2) the left atrium by way of the thebesian veins. Common abnormalities that cause anatomic shunting include congenital heart disease, intrapulmonary fistula, and vascular lung tumors.

Anemia disorder characterized by a decrease in hemoglobin in the blood to levels below the normal range.

Anemic hypoxia a type of hypoxia in which the oxygen tension in the arterial blood is normal, but the oxygen-carrying capacity of the blood is inadequate. This form of hypoxia may develop from (1) a low amount of hemoglobin in the blood or (2) a deficiency in the ability of hemoglobin to carry oxygen, such as carbon monoxide poisoning.

Angiogram an x-ray film of an artery injected with a radiopaque contrast medium.

Anoxia an abnormal condition characterized by a local or systemic lack of oxygen in body tissues. It may result from an inadequate supply of oxygen to the respiratory system, an inability of the blood to carry oxygen to the tissues, or a failure of the tissues to absorb the oxygen from the blood.

Anterior indicating the front of a structure or body surface relative to other body parts.

Antibody protein substance that develops in response to and interacts with an antigen. The antigen–antibody reaction forms the basis of immunity.

Antigen substance that induces the formation of antibodies that interact specifically with it. The antigen-antibody reaction forms the basis for immunity.

Antitrypsin inhibitor of trypsin; may be deficient in persons with emphysema.

Aorta the main trunk of the systemic arterial circulation, comprising four parts: the ascending aorta, the arch of the aorta, the thoracic portion of the descending aorta, and the abdominal portion of the descending aorta.

Aortic arch the proximal one of the four portions of the aorta, giving rise to three arterial branches called the innominate (brachiocephalic), left common carotid, and left subclavian arteries. The arch rises at the level of the border of the second sternocostal articulation of the right side, passes to the left in front of the trachea, bends dorsally, and becomes the descending aorta. Also called the arch of the aorta.

Aperture opening or hole in an object or anatomic structure.

Apex top end or tip of a structure.

Apnea complete absence of spontaneous ventilation.

Apneustic center a portion of the pontine respiratory centers that influences the respiratory components of the medulla. If unrestrained, the apneustic center continually sends neural impulses to the ventral respiratory group and dorsal respiratory group in the medulla.

Arrhythmia any deviation from the normal pattern of the heartbeat.

Arterial pertaining to one artery or a network of arteries.

Arterial-venous oxygen content difference the difference between the oxygen content of arterial blood (Ca_{O_2}) and the oxygen content of venous blood (Cv_{O_2}).

Arteriogram the reconstruction of blood vessels damaged by disease or injury, often performed by inflating a balloon within the vessel lumen at the site of narrowing to reconstitute flow.

Arteriole the smallest of the arteries. Blood flowing from the heart is pumped through the arteries, to the arterioles, to the capillaries, into the veins, and retuned to the heart. The muscular walls of the arterioles constrict and dilate in response to both local factors and neurochemical stimuli; thus, arterioles play a significant role in peripheral vascular resistance and in regulation of blood pressure.

Arteriosclerosis a common arterial disorder characterized by thickening, loss of elasticity, and calcification of arterial walls, resulting in a decreased blood supply.

Arteriovenous shunt a passageway, artificial or natural, that allows blood to flow from an artery to a vein without going through a capillary network.

Artery one of the large blood vessels carrying blood in a direction away from the heart.

Asphyxia severe hypoxia leading to hypoxemia and hypercapnia, loss of consciousness, and, if not corrected, death. Some of the more common causes of asphyxia are drowning, electrical shock, aspiration of vomitus, lodging of a foreign body in the respiratory tract, inhalation of toxic gas or smoke, and poisoning. Oxygen and artificial ventilation are promptly administered to prevent damage to the brain. The underlying cause is then treated.

Aspiration (1) drawing in or out by suction. (2) the act of withdrawing a fluid, such as mucus or serum, from the body by a suction device. See also **aspiration pneumonia**.

Aspiration pneumonia an inflammatory condition of the lungs and bronchi caused by the inhalation of foreign material or acidic vomitus.

Asthma a respiratory disorder characterized by recurring episodes of paroxysmal dyspnea, wheezing on expiration and/or inspiration caused by constriction of the bronchi, coughing, and viscous mucoid bronchial secretions. The episodes may be precipitated by inhalation of allergens or pollutants, infection, cold air, vigorous exercise, or emotional stress. Treatment may include elimination of the causative agent, hyposensitization, aerosol or oral bronchodilators, beta-adrenergic drugs, methylxanthines, cromolyn, leukotriene inhibitors, and short- or long-term use of corticosteroids.

Ataxia an abnormal condition characterized by impaired ability to coordinate movement.

Atelectasis an abnormal condition character-ized by the collapse of alveoli, preventing the respiratory exchange of carbon dioxide and oxygen in a part of the lungs. Symptoms may include diminished breath sounds or aspiratory crackles, a mediastinal shift toward the side of the collapse, fever, and increasing dyspnea. The condition may be caused by obstruction of the major airways and bronchioles, by compression of the lungs as a result of fluid or air in the pleu-ral space, or by pressure from a tumor outside the lung. Loss of functional lung tissue may sec-ondarily cause increased heart rate, blood pres-sure, and respiratory rate. Secretions retained in the collapsed alveoli are rich in nutrients for bacterial growth, a condition often leading to stasis pneumonia in critically ill patients.

Atherosclerosis a common arterial disorder characterized by yellowish plaques of choles-terol, lipids, and cellular debris in the medial layer of the walls of the large and medium-sized arteries.

Atmospheric pressure pressure of the air on the earth at mean sea level; approximately 760 mm Hg (14.7 pounds per square inch).

Atria a chamber or cavity, such as the right and left atria of the heart or the nasal cavity.

Atrium (*pl. atria*) a chamber or cavity, such as the right and left atria of the heart or the nasal cavity.

Augment to enlarge or increase in size, amount, or degree; make bigger.

Automaticity the unique ability of the cells in the sinoatrial node of the heart to generate an action potential without being stimulated.

B

Bacteriuria the presence of bacteria in the urine.

Balloon angioplasty a method of dilating or opening an obstructed blood vessel by threading a small, balloon-tipped catheter into the vessel. The balloon is inflated to compress arteriosclerotic lesions against the walls of the vessel, leaving a larger lumen, through which blood can pass. It is used in treating arteriosclerotic heart disease.

Baroreceptor one of the pressure-sensitive nerve endings in the walls of the atria of the heart, the aortic arch, and the carotid sinuses. Baroreceptors stimulate central reflex mechanisms that allow physiologic adjustment and adaptation to changes in blood pressure via changes in heart rate, vasodilation, or va-soconstriction. Baroreceptors are essential for homeostasis. Also called *pressoreceptor*.

Basal pertaining to the fundamental or the basic, as basal anesthesia, which produces the first stage of unconsciousness, and the basal metabolic rate, which indicates the lowest met-abolic rate; basal membrane.

Base a chemical compound that increases the concentration of hydroxide ions in aqueous solution.

Basophil a type of white blood cell that has a granular nucleus stained with basic dyes. These cells represent 1 percent or less of the total white blood cell count. Normal range: 0 to 0.75 percent of leukocyte differential.

Beta receptor any one of the postulated adrenergic (sympathetic fibers of autonomic nervous system) components of receptor tissues that respond to epinephrine and such blocking agents as propranolol. Activation of beta receptors causes various physiologic reactions such as relaxation of the bronchial muscles and an increase in the rate and force of cardiac contraction. Also called *beta-adrenergic receptor*. Compare **alpha receptor**.

Bicarbonate (HCO_3^-) an anion of carbonic acid in which only one of the hydrogen atoms has been removed, as in sodium bicarbonate ($NaHCO_3$).

Bicuspid valve the bicuspid valve is situated between the left atrium and the left ventricle and is the only valve with two rather than three cusps. The bicuspid valve allows blood to flow from the left atrium into the left ven-tricle but prevents blood from flowing back into the atrium. Ventricular contractions in systole forces the blood against the valve, closing the two cusps and assuring the flow of blood from the ventricle into the aorta. Also called the *mitral valve.*

Bifurcation a separation into two branches; the point of forking.

Biot's breathing short episodes of rapid, uniformly deep inspirations, followed by 10 to 30 seconds of apnea.

Blood the liquid pumped by the heart through all the arteries, veins, and capillaries. The blood is composed of a clear yellow fluid, called plasma, and the formed elements, and a series of cell types with different functions. The major function of the blood is to transport oxygen and nutrients to the cells and to remove carbon dioxide and other waste products from the cells for detoxification and elimination. Adults normally have a total blood volume of 7% to 8% of body weight, or 70 mL/kg of body weight for men and about 65 mL/kg for women. Blood is pumped through the body at a speed of about 30 cm/second, with a complete circulation time of 20 seconds.

Blood-brain barrier membrane between the circulating blood and the brain that prevents or slows the passage of some drugs and other chemical compounds, radioactive ions, and disease-causing organisms such as viruses from the blood into the central nervous system.

Blood doping the administration of blood, red blood cells, or related blood products to an athlete to enhance performance, often preceded by the withdrawal of blood so that training continues in a blood-depleted state.

Bohr effect as the PCO_2 level increases (increased H^+ concentration), the oxyhemoglobin saturation decreases, shifting the oxyhemoglobin dissociation curve to the right, whereas decreasing PCO_2 levels (decreased H^+ concentration) shift the curve to the left. The effect of PCO_2 and pH on the oxyhemoglobin curve is known as the Bohr effect.

Bolus intravenous bolus, a relatively large dose of medication administered into a vein in a short period, usually within 1 to 30 minutes.

Bradycardia a slow heartbeat marked by a pulse rate below 60 beats per minute in an adult.

Bradykinin a peptide produced by activation of the kinin system in a variety of inflammatory conditions. It is an extremely potent vasodilator; it also increases vascular permeability, stimulates pain receptors, and causes contraction of a variety of extravascular smooth muscles.

Bronchiectasis an abnormal condition of the bronchial tree characterized by irreversible dilation and destruction of the bronchial walls. The condition is sometimes congenital but is more often a result of bronchial infection or of obstruction by a tumor or an aspirated foreign body. Symptoms include a constant cough producing copious purulent sputum; hemoptysis; chronic sinusitis; clubbing of fingers; and persistent moist, coarse crackles. Some of the complications of bronchiectasis are pneumonia, lung abscess, empyema, brain abscess, and amyloidosis. Treatment includes frequent postural drainage, expectorants, antibiotics, and, rarely, surgical resection of the affected part of the lungs.

Bronchitis acute or chronic inflammation of the mucous membranes of the tracheobronchial tree. Caused by the spread of upper respiratory viral or sometimes bacterial infections to the bronchi, it is often observed with or after childhood infections, such as measles, whooping cough, diphtheria, and typhoid fever.

Bronchoconstriction a narrowing of the lumen of the bronchi restricting airflow to and from the lungs. See also **bronchospasm**.

Bronchodilator a substance, especially a drug, that relaxes contractions of the smooth muscle of the bronchioles to improve ventilation to the lungs. Pharmacologic bronchodilators are prescribed to improve aeration in asthma, bronchiectasis, bronchitis, and emphysema. Commonly used bronchodilators include albuterol, terbutaline, and various derivatives and combinations of these drugs. The adverse effects vary, depending on the particular class of bronchodilating drug. In general, bronchodilators are given with caution to people with impaired cardiac function. Nervousness, irritability, gastritis, or palpitations of the heart may occur.

Bronchospasm an excessive and prolonged contraction of the smooth muscle of the bronchi and bronchioles, resulting in an acute narrowing and obstruction of the respiratory airway. The contractions may be localized or general and may be cased by irritation or injury to the respiratory mucosa, infections, or allergies. A cough with generalized wheezing usually indicates the condition. Bronchospasm is a chief characteristic of asthma and bronchitis. Treatment includes the use of active bronchodilators, catecholamines, corticosteroids, or methylxanthines and preventive drugs such as cromolyn sodium. Also called **bronchoconstriction**.

Buffer a substance or group of substances that tends to control the hydrogen ion concentration in a solution by reacting with hydrogen ions of an acid added to the system and releasing hydrogen ions to a base added to the system. Buffers minimize significant changes of pH in a chemical system. Among the functions carried out by buffer systems in the body is maintenance of the acid–base balance of the blood and of the proper pH in kidney tubules.

C

Calcification process in which organic tissue becomes hardened by the deposition of lime salts in the tissue.

Calculus a pathologic stone formed of mineral salts. Calculi are usually found within hollow organs or ducts.

Caliber the inside diameter of a tube, commonly given in millimeters and fractions of an inch.

Canalicular pertaining to a small channel or canal.

Capacitance vessels the veins differ from the arteries in that they are capable of holding a large amount of blood with very little pressure change. Because of this unique feature, the veins are called capacitance vessels.

Capillary shunt a capillary shunt exists when blood flows from the right side of the heart to the left side without coming in contact with ventilated alveoli for gas exchange. Capillary shunting is commonly caused by (1) alveolar collapse or atelectasis, (2) alveolar fluid accumulation, or (3) alveolar consolidation.

Capillary stasis stagnation of normal flow of fluids or blood in capillaries.

Capnography the process of continuously recording the level of carbon dioxide in expired air. The percentage of carbon dioxide at the end of expiration can be estimated and gives a close approximation of the alveolar carbon dioxide concentration. The process, which requires the use of infrared spectroscopy, is used to monitor critically ill patients and in pulmonary function testing. The data are typically recorded automatically on a strip of graph paper on a bedside patient monitor

Carbon dioxide (CO_2) colorless, odorless, incombustible gas formed during respiration and combustion.

Carboxyhemoglobin a compound produced by the exposure of hemoglobin to carbon monoxide. Carbon monoxide from the environment is inhaled into the lungs, absorbed through the alveoli, and bound to hemoglobin in the blood, blocking the sites for oxygen transport. Oxygen levels decrease, and hypoxia and anoxia may result.

Cardiac output (CO) the total volume of blood discharged from the ventricles per minute.

Cardiac tamponade compression of the heart produced by the accumulation of blood or other fluid in the pericardial sac. Also called cardiac compression, pericardial tamponade.

Carotid sinus massage firm rubbing at the bifurcation of the carotid artery at the angle of the jaw. It creates an elevation of blood pressure in the carotid sinus that results in reflex slowing of atrioventricular conduction and sinus rate. The technique may be used to reduce the heart rate in tachyarrhythmia.

Cartilage dense, firm, compact connective tissue capable of withstanding considerable pressure and tension. Located in the tracheobronchial tree, all true joints, the outer ear, and the movable sections of the ribs.

Catecholamines biologically active amines that behave as epinephrine and norepinephrine.

Central venous pressure (CVP) pressure within the superior vena cava, which reflects the pressure under which the blood is returned to the right atrium.

Cerebrospinal fluid (CSF) fluid cushion that protects the brain and spinal cord from shock.

C-fibers an extensive network of free nerve endings located in the small conducting airways, blood vessels, and interstitial tissues between the pulmonary capillaries and alveolar walls. The C-fibers near the alveolar capillaries are called juxtapulmonary-capillary receptors, or J-receptors. These receptors react to certain chemicals and to mechanical stimulation. When stimulated, a reflex response triggers a rapid, shallow breathing pattern.

Chemoreceptor sense organ or sensory nerve ending, located outside the central nervous system, which is stimulated by and reacts to chemical stimuli.

Cheyne-Stokes respiration 10 to 30 seconds of apnea, followed by a gradual increase in the volume and frequency of breathing, followed by a gradual decrease in the volume of breathing until another period of apnea occurs.

Chloride shift during carbon dioxide transport, as HCO_3^- moves out of the red blood cells, the Cl^- (which has been liberated from the NaCl compound) moves into the red blood to maintain electric neutrality. This movement is known as the chloride shift or the *Hamburger phenomenon*.

Chordae tendineae the strands of tendon that anchor the cusps of the mitral and tricuspid valves to the papillary muscles of the ventricles of the heart, preventing prolapse of the valves into the atria during ventricular contraction.

Chronic persisting for a long period, often for the remainder of a person's lifetime. Compare **acute**.

Chronic alveolar hyperventilation with complete renal compensation a condition marked by low levels of carbon dioxide in the blood resulting from hyperventilation and a normal pH, which has been corrected by the excretion of HCO_3^- via the renal system. Also called chronic alveolar hyperventilation.

Chronic bronchitis a very common, debilitating pulmonary disease, characterized by greatly increased production of mucus by the glands of the trachea and bronchi and resulting in a cough with expectoration for at least 3 months of the year for more than 2 consecutive years.

Chronic obstructive pulmonary disease (COPD) a progressive and irreversible condition characterized by diminished inspiratory and expiratory capacity of the lungs. The condition is aggravated by cigarette smoking and air pollution. COPDs include asthma, chronic bronchiectasis, chronic bronchitis, and emphysema.

Chronic ventilatory failure with complete renal compensation a condition marked by high levels of carbon dioxide in the blood resulting from hypoventilation and a normal pH, which has been corrected by the retention of HCO_3^- via the renal system and/or the administration of HCO_3^-. Also called chronic ventilatory failure.

Cilia small, hairlike projections on the surface of specific epithelial cells. In the bronchi they propel mucus and foreign particles in a whiplike movement toward the throat.

Circulatory hypoxia a form of hypoxia in which the arterial blood reaching the tissue cells has a normal oxygen tension and content, but the amount of blood—and, therefore, the amount of oxygen—is not adequate to meet tissue needs.

Clinical manifestations symptoms or signs demonstrated by a patient.

Colloid a state of matter composed of single large molecules or aggregations of smaller molecules of solids, liquids, or gases, in a continuous medium (dispersal medium), which also may be a solid, liquid, or gas.

Combined metabolic and respiratory alkalosis a blood pH above 7.45 caused by both a low carbon dioxide level and a high bicarbonate level. Also called metabolic and respiratory alkalosis.

Complete blood cell count a determination of the number of red and white blood cells per cubic millimeter of blood. A CBC is one of the most routinely performed tests in a clinical laboratory and one of the most valuable screening and diagnostic techniques. Most laboratories use an electronic counter for reporting numbers of red and white blood cells and platelets. Examining a stained slide of blood yields useful information about red cell morphologic characteristics and types of white blood cells (WBCs). The normal red blood cell (RBC) count in adult males is 4.7 to 6.1 million/ mm^3. In adult females the normal RBC is 4.2 to 5.4 million/mm^3. Each type of white blood cell can be represented as a percentage of the total number of white cells observed. This is called a differential count. The normal adult WBC count is 5000 to 10,000/cm^3. Electronic blood counters also automatically determine hemoglobin or hematocrit and include this value in the CBC.

Composition makeup; what something is made of.

Compromise a blending of the qualities of two different things; an unfavorable change.

Concave a hollow surface, like the inside of a bowl.

Conception the union of sperm and ovum.

Conductivity the ability of the heart cells to transmit electrical current from cell to cell throughout the entire conductive system.

Congenital existing at and usually before birth; referring to conditions that are present at birth, regardless of their cause.

Congestion an abnormal accumulation of fluid in an organ or body area. The fluid is often mucus, but it may be bile or blood.

Congestive heart failure (CHF) an abnormal condition that reflects impaired cardiac pumping. Its causes include myocardial infarction, ischemic heart disease, and cardiomyopathy. Failure of the ventricles to eject blood efficiently results in volume overload, ventricular dilation, and elevated intracardiac pressure. Increased pressure in the left side of the heart causes pulmonary congestion; increased pressure in the right side causes systemic venous congestion and peripheral edema.

Consolidation the combining of separate parts into a single whole; a state of solidification;

(in medicine) the process of becoming solid, as when lungs become firm and inelastic in pneumonia.

Constriction an abnormal closing or reduction in the size of an opening or passage of the body, as in vasoconstriction of a blood vessel.

Contiguous being in actual contact; touching along a boundary or at a point.

continuous positive airway pressure (CPAP) a method of noninvasive or invasive ventilation assisted by a flow of air delivered at a constant pressure throughout the respiratory cycle. It is performed for patients who can initiate their own respirations but who are not able to maintain adequate arterial oxygen levels without assistance. CPAP may be given through a ventilator and endotracheal tube, through a nasal cannula, or into a hood over the patient's head. Respiratory distress syndrome in the newborn and sleep apnea are often treated with CPAP. Also called constant positive airway pressure, continuous positive pressure breathing.

Contractility the ability of muscle tissue to contract when its thick (myosin) and thin (actin) filaments slide past each other.

Contusion injury in which the skin is not broken; a bruise.

Convex having a rounded, somewhat elevated surface, resembling a segment of the external surface of a sphere.

Cor pulmonale failure of the right ventricle resulting from disorders of the lungs or pulmonary vessels.

coronary angiography the x-ray visualization of the internal anatomy of the heart and blood vessels after the intravascular introduction of radiopaque contrast medium. The procedure is used as a diagnostic aid in myocardial infarction, vascular occlusion, calcified atherosclerotic plaques, cerebrovascular insult, portal hypertension, renal neoplasms, renal artery stenosis as a causative factor in hypertension, pulmonary emboli, and congenital and acquired lesions of pulmonary vessels. The contrast medium may be injected into an artery or vein or introduced into a catheter inserted in a peripheral artery and threaded through the vessel to a visceral site. Because the iodine in the contrast medium may cause a marked allergic reaction in some patients and may lead to death in severe cases, testing for hypersensitivity is indicated before the radiopaque substance is used. Because iodinated contrast agents are nephrotoxic, renal function also must be determined before angiography. After the procedure the patient is monitored for signs of bleeding at the puncture site, and bed rest for a number of hours is indicated.

coronary bypass open heart surgery in which a prosthesis or a section of a vein is grafted from the aorta onto one of the coronary arteries, bypassing a narrowing or blockage in the coronary artery. The operation is performed in coronary artery disease to improve the blood supply to the heart muscle and to relieve anginal pain. Coronary arteriography pinpoints the areas of obstruction before surgery. Under general anesthesia and with the use of a cardiopulmonary bypass machine, one end of a 15- to 20-cm prosthesis or a segment of saphenous vein from the patient's leg is grafted to the ascending aorta. The other end is sutured to the clogged coronary artery at a point distal to the stoppage. The internal mammary artery may also be used as graft tissue. Usually double or triple grafts are done for multiple areas of blockage. After surgery, close observation in an intensive care unit is essential to ensure adequate ventilation and cardiac output. The systolic blood pressure is not allowed to drop significantly below the preoperative baseline, nor is it allowed to rise significantly, because hypertension can rupture a graft site. Arrhythmias are treated with medications or by electrical cardioversion. The patient is usually discharged within 5 to 8 days, unless complications occur.

Coronary sinus the wide venous channel, about 2.25 cm long, situated in the coronary sulcus and covered by muscular fibers from the left atrium. Through a single semilunar valve it drains five coronary veins: the great cardiac vein, the small cardiac vein, the middle cardiac vein, the posterior vein of the left ventricle, and the oblique vein of the left atrium.

Corpuscle any small, rounded body; an encapsulated sensory nerve ending.

Cortex the outer layer of an organ.

Cotyledons the visible segments on the maternal surface of the placenta. A typical placenta may have 15 to 28 cotyledons, each consisting of fetal vessels, chorionic villi, and intervillous space.

Crackle a common, abnormal respiratory sound consisting of discontinuous bubbling noises heard on auscultation of the chest during inspiration. Fine crackles have a popping sound produced by air entering distal bronchioles or alveoli that contain serous secretions, as in congestive heart failure, pneumonia, or early tuberculosis. Coarse crackles may originate in the larger bronchi have a lower pitch. Crackles are not cleared by coughing. Formerly called *rales*. Compare **rhonchus, wheeze**.

Creatinine a substance formed from the metabolism of creatine, commonly found in blood, urine, and muscle tissue.

Croup an acute viral infection of the upper and lower respiratory tract that occurs primarily in infants and young children 3 months to 3 years of age after an upper respiratory tract infection. It is characterized by hoarseness; irritability; fever; a distinctive harsh, brassy cough; persistent stridor during inspiration; and dyspnea and tachypnea, resulting from obstruction of the larynx. Cyanosis or pallor occurs in severe cases. The most common causative agents are the parainfluenza viruses, especially type 1, followed by the respiratory syncytial viruses and influenza A and B viruses. Also called *angina trachealis, exudative angina, laryngostasis*. Compare **acute epiglottitis**.

croup syndrome an abnormal high-pitched musical sound caused by an obstruction in the trachea or larynx. It is usually heard during inspiration. Stridor may indicate several neoplastic or inflammatory conditions, including glottic edema, asthma, diphtheria, laryngospasm, and papilloma.

Cystic fibrosis an inherited autosomal-recessive disorder of the exocrine glands, causing those glands to produce abnormally thick secretions of mucus, elevation of sweat electrolytes, increased organic and enzymatic constituents of saliva, and overactivity of the autonomic nervous system. The glands most affected are those in the pancreas and respiratory system and the sweat glands. Cystic fibrosis is usually recognized in infancy or early childhood, chiefly among Caucasians. The earliest manifestation is meconium ileus, an obstruction of the small bowel by viscid stool. Other early signs are a chronic cough; frequent, foul-smelling stools; and persistent upper respiratory infections. The most reliable diagnostic tool is the sweat test, which shows elevations of levels of both sodium and chloride. Because there is no known cure, treatment is directed at prevention of respiratory infections, which are the most frequent cause of death. Mucolytic agents and bronchodilators are used to help liquefy the thick, tenacious mucus. Physical therapy measures, such as postural drainage and breathing exercises, can also dislodge secretions. Broad-spectrum antibiotics may be used prophylactically.

D

Dead space ventilation volume of gas that is ventilated, but not physiologically effective. There are three types of dead space ventilation: *Anatomic dead space*—the volume of gas in the conducting airways: the nose, mouth, pharynx, larynx, and lower airways down to, but not including, the respiratory bronchioles. *Alveolar dead space*—alveoli that are ventilated, but not perfused with blood. *Physiologic dead space*—the sum of the anatomic dead space and alveolar dead space.

Deciliter (dL) one-tenth of a liter; 100 mL.

Defensin a peptide with natural antibiotic activity found within human neutrophils. Three types of defensins have been identified, each consisting of a chain of about 30 amino acids. Similar molecules occur in white blood cells of other animal species. They show activity toward viruses and fungi, in addition to bacteria.

Density mass of a substance per unit of volume (g/cm³).

Deoxyhemoglobin hemoglobin not bound with oxygen. Also called *reduced hemoglobin*.

Deoxyribonucleic acid (DNA) a large, double-stranded, helical molecule that is the carrier of genetic information. In eukaryotic cells, it is found principally in the chromosomes of the nucleus. DNA is composed of four kinds of serially repeating nucleotide bases: adenine, cytosine, guanine, and thymine. Genetic information is coded in the sequence of the nucleotides. Also called *desoxyribonucleic acid*.

Depolarize to reduce to a nonpolarized condition; to reduce the amount of electrical charge between oppositely charged particles (ions).

Desquamation the process in which the cornified layer of the epidermis is sloughed in fine scales.

Determinant an element that identifies or determines the nature of something or that fixes or conditions an outcome.

Diabetes a general term referring to a variety of disorders characterized by excessive urination (polyuria), as in diabetes mellitus and diabetes insipidus.

Diagnostic pertaining to the use of scientific and skillful methods to establish the cause and nature of a sick person's disease.

Diapedesis the passage of red or white blood corpuscles through the walls of the vessels that contain them without damage to the vessels.

Diastole normal period in the heart cycle during which the muscle fibers lengthen, the heart dilates, and the chambers fill with blood.

Diastolic pressure the minimum level of blood pressure measured between contractions of the heart. It may vary with age, gender, body weight, emotional state, and other factors.

Differentiate to separate according to differences.

Diffusion the movement of gas molecules from an area of relatively high concentration of gas to one of low concentration. Different gases each move according to their own individual partial pressure gradients. Diffusion continues until all the gases in the two areas are in equilibrium.

Digitation a finger-like projection.

Distal away from or being the farthest from any point of reference.

Dorsal pertaining to the back or to the posterior portion of a body.

Driving pressure pressure difference between two areas in any vessel or airway.

Ductus arteriosus vessel between the left pulmonary artery and the aorta that bypasses the lungs in the fetus.

Dyspnea difficulty in breathing, of which the individual is aware.

E

Ectopic foci an area of the heart that produces abnormal beats. Ectopic foci may occur in both healthy and diseased hearts and are usually associated with irritation of a small area of myocardial tissue. They are produced in association with myocardial ischemia, drug (catecholamine) effects, emotional stress, and stimulation by foreign objects, including pacemaker catheters.

Edema a local or generalized condition in which the body tissues contain an excessive amount of extracellular fluid.

Efferent carrying away from a central organ or section.

Efferent nerves nerves that carry impulses from the brain or spinal cord to the periphery.

Elastance the natural ability of matter to respond directly to force and to return to its original resting position or shape after the external force no longer exists. In pulmonary physiology, elastance is defined as the change in pressure per change in volume.

Electrocardiogram (ECG) record of the electrical activity of the heart.

Electrolyte an element or compound that, when melted or dissolved in water or other solvent, dissociates into ions and is able to conduct an electric current.

Elongation the condition or process of being extended.

Embryonic pertaining to the early stages (i.e., first 3 months) of fetal development.

Emphysema an abnormal condition of the pulmonary system, characterized by overinflation and destructive changes in alveolar walls. It results in a loss of lung elasticity and decreased gas exchange. See also **pulmonary emphysema**.

Empyema an accumulation of pus in the pleural space, as a result of bacterial infection, such as pleurisy or tuberculosis. It is usually removed by surgical incision, aspiration, and drainage. Antibiotics, usually penicillin or vancomycin, are administered to combat the underlying infection. Oxygen therapy may also be administered.

End-expiration the portion of a ventilatory cycle at which expiration stops.

End-inspiration the portion of a ventilatory cycle at which inspiration stops.

Endocardium the lining of the heart chambers, containing small blood vessels and a few bundles of smooth muscle. It is continuous with the endothelium of the great blood vessels.

Endothelium the layer of epithelial cells, originating from the mesoderm, that lines the cavities of the heart, the blood and lymph vessels, and the serous cavities of the body.

Endotracheal within the trachea.

Endotracheal intubation the management of the patient with an airway catheter inserted through the mouth or nose into the trachea. An endotracheal tube may be used to maintain a patent airway, to prevent aspiration or material from the digestive tract in the unconscious or paralyzed patient, to permit suctioning of tracheobronchial secretions, or to administer positive-pressure ventilation that cannot be given effectively by a mask. Endotracheal tubes may be made of rubber or plastic and usually have an inflatable cuff to maintain a closed system with the ventilator.

Endotracheal tube a large-bore catheter inserted through the mouth or nose and into the trachea to a point above the bifurcation of the trachea. It is used for delivering oxygen under pressure when ventilation must be totally controlled and in general anesthetic procedures. See also **endotracheal intubation**.

Eosinophil a cell or cellular structure that stains readily with the acid stain eosin; specifically, a granular leukocyte. Normal range: 1 to 4 percent of leukocyte differential.

Epicardium one of the three layers of tissue that form the heart wall. It is composed of a single sheet of squamous epithelial cells overlying delicate connective tissue. Epicardium is the visceral portion (visceral layer) of the serous pericardium and folds back on itself to form the parietal portion of the serous pericardium.

Epinephrine one of two active hormones (the other is norepinephrine) secreted by the adrenal medulla.

Epistaxis bleeding from the nose. Also called *nosebleed*.

Equilibrium condition in which one or more forces are evenly balanced by opposite forces.

Erythrocyte a mature red blood cell (RBC).

Erythropoiesis the process of erythrocyte production involving the maturation of a nucleated precursor into a hemoglobin-filled nucleus-free erythrocyte that is regulated by erythropoietin, a hormone produced by the kidney.

Esophagus the esophagus (or oesophagus) is an organ in vertebrates which consists of a muscular tube through which food passes from the pharynx to the stomach. During swallowing, food passes from the mouth through the pharynx into the esophagus and travels via peristalsis to the stomach. The word esophagus is derived from the Latin œsophagus, which derives from the Greek word oisophagos, lit. "entrance for eating." In humans the esophagus is continuous with the laryngeal part of the pharynx at the level of the C6 vertebra. The esophagus passes through posterior mediastinum in thorax and enters abdomen through a hole in the diaphragm at the level of the tenth thoracic vertebrae (T10). It is usually about 25–30 cm long depending on individual height.

It is divided into cervical, thoracic and abdominal parts. Due to the inferior pharyngeal constrictor muscle, the entry to the esophagus opens only when swallowing or vomiting.

Ethmoid bone the very light, sievelike, and spongy bone at the base of the cranium, also forming the roof and most of the walls of the superior part of the nasal cavity. It consists of four parts: a horizontal plate, a perpendicular plate, and two lateral labyrinths.

Etiology study of the cause of disease.

Eupnea normal, spontaneous breathing.

Excitability the ability of a cell to reach its threshold potential and respond to a stimulus or irritation. The lower the stimulus needed to activate a cell, the more excitable the cell; conversely, the greater the stimulus needed, the less excitable the cell.

Excretion elimination of waste products from the body.

Excursion the extent of movement from a central position or axis.

Expectoration clearing the lungs by coughing up and spitting out matter.

Expiratory reserve volume (ERV) the maximum volume of air that can be exhaled after a normal tidal volume exhalation.

External respiration gas exchange between the pulmonary capillaries and the alveoli.

Extra-alveolar pertaining to the area outside of the alveoli.

Extracellular outside a cell or in the cavities or spaces between cell layers or groups of cells.

Extravascular outside a vessel.

F

Fascia the fibrous connective membrane of the body that may be separated from other specifically organized structures, such as the tendons, the aponeuroses, and the ligaments, and that covers, supports, and separates muscles.

Fertilization the union of sperm and ovum.

Fetus the developing human *in utero* from the third month to birth.

FEV$_1$ forced expiratory volume in one second.

Fibrin whitish, filamentous protein formed by the action of thrombin on fibrinogen.

Fibroelastic composed of fibrous and elastic tissue.

Fibrosis the repair and replacement of inflamed tissues or organs by connective tissues. The process results in the replacement of normal cells by fibroblasts (and eventually, the replacement of normal organ tissue by scar tissue).

Fissure cleft or groove on the surface of an organ, often marking the division of the organ into parts, such as the lobes of the lung.

Fistula abnormal passage or communication, usually between two internal organs or leading from an internal organ to the surface of the body.

Flail chest a thorax in which multiple rib fractures cause instability in part of the chest wall and paradoxical breathing, with the lung underlying the injured areas moving in on inspiration and bulging on expiration. If it is uncorrected, hypoxia will result.

Flex to contract, as a muscle; to increase the angle of a joint.

Foramen ovale an opening in the septum between the right and the left atria in the fetal heart. This opening provides a bypass for blood that would otherwise flow to the fetal lungs. After birth the foramen ovale functionally closes when the newborn takes the first breath and full circulation through the lungs begins.

Forced vital capacity the maximum volume of gas that can be forcibly and rapidly exhaled after a full inspiration.

Frank-Starling curve a graphic illustration that shows the relationship between the degree of myocardial stretch and cardiac output.

Friction rub a dry, grating sound heard with a stethoscope during auscultation. It is a normal finding when heard over the liver and splenic areas. A friction rub auscultated over the pericardial area is suggestive of pericarditis; a rub over the pleural area may be a sign of lung disease.

Functional residual capacity (FRC) the volume of air remaining in the lungs after a normal exhalation.

Functionally according to its proper use or action; working as it should.

FVC the maximum volume of gas that can be forcibly and rapidly exhaled after a full inspiration.

G

Gastrointestinal tract the route taken by food from the stomach to the rectum.

Generation the process of forming a new organism or part of an organism in the airways; a sequential, numbered branch off the trachea.

Gestation the period of time from the fertilization of the ovum until birth.

Glomerulonephritis inflammation of the glomerulus in the nephron of the kidney.

Glomerulus a tuft or cluster; a structure composed of blood vessels or nerve fibers, such as a *renal glomerulus.*

Glossopharyngeal nerve the ninth cranial nerve.

Glottis the glottis is defined as the combination of the vocal folds (vocal cords) and the space in between the folds (the rima glottidis).

Glycoprotein any of a class of conjugated proteins consisting of a compound of a protein with a carbohydrate group.

Goblet cell one of many specialized epithelial cells that secrete mucus and form glands of the epithelium of the stomach, the intestine, and parts of the respiratory tract.

Gradient a slope or grade; a difference in values between two points.

Gram percent (g%) the number of grams of a substance in 100 mL of fluid.

Granulocyte a type of leukocyte characterized by the presence of cytoplasmic granules.

Gravity the universal effect of the attraction between any body of matter and any planetary body. The force of the attraction depends on the relative masses of the bodies and on the inverse of the square of the distance between them.

Gravity dependent a phrase used to describe the natural tendency of blood, which is a relatively heavy substance, to move to the portion of the body, or portion of the organ, that is closest to the ground.

H

Haldane effect the phenomenon in which deoxygenated blood enhances the loading of carbon dioxide and the oxygenation of blood enhances the unloading of carbon dioxide during carbon dioxide transport.

Hamburger phenomenon see **chloride shift**.

Heart the muscular cone-shaped hollow organ, about the size of a clenched fist, that pumps blood throughout the body and beats normally about 70 times per minute by coordinated nerve impulses and muscular contractions. Enclosed in pericardium, it rests on the diaphragm between the lower borders of the lungs, occupying the middle of the mediastinum. It is covered ventrally by the sternum and the adjoining parts of the third to the sixth costal cartilages. The organ is about 12 cm long, 8 cm wide at its broadest part, and 6 cm thick. The weight of the heart in men averages between 280 and 340 g and in women, between 230 and 280 g. The layers of the heart, starting from the outside, are the epicardium, the myocardium, and the endocardium. The chambers include two ventricles with thick muscular walls, making up the bulk of the organ, and two atria with thin muscular walls. A septum separates the ventricles and extends between the atria (interatrial septum), dividing the heart into the right and the left sides. The left side of the heart pumps oxygenated blood into the aorta and on to all parts of the body. The right side receives deoxygenated blood from the vena cava and pumps it into the pulmonary arteries. The valves of the heart include the tricuspid valve, the bicuspid (mitral) valve, the semilunar aortic valve, and the semilunar pulmonary valve. The sinoatrial node in the right atrium of the heart (under the control of the medulla oblongata in the brainstem) initiates the cardiac impulse, causing the atria to contract. The atrioventricular (AV) node near the septal wall of the right atrium spreads the impulse over the AV bundle (bundle of His) and its branches, causing the ventricles to contract. Both atria contract simultaneously, followed quickly by the simultaneous contraction of the ventricles. The sinoatrial node of the heartbeat sets the rate. Other factors affecting the heartbeat are emotion, exercise, hormones, temperature, pain, and stress.

Hematocrit volume of erythrocytes packed by centrifugation in a given volume of blood; is expressed as the percentage of total blood volume that consists of erythrocytes.

Hemodynamics the study of the physical aspects of blood circulation, including cardiac function and peripheral vascular physiologic characteristics.

Hemoglobin a complex protein-iron compound in the blood that carries oxygen to the cells from the lungs and carbon dioxide away from the cells to the lungs. Each erythrocyte contains 200 to 300 molecules of hemoglobin.

Hemolysis the breakdown of red blood cells and the release of hemoglobin.

Heparin a polysaccharide produced by the mast cells of the liver and by basophil leukocytes that inhibits coagulation by preventing conversion of prothrombin to thrombin. It also inhibits coagulation by preventing liberation of thromboplastin from blood platelets.

Histamine a substance that is normally present in the body and exerts a pharmacologic action when released from injured cells. It is produced from the amino acid *histidine*.

Histotoxic hypoxia a type of hypoxia that develops in any condition that impairs the ability of tissue cells to utilize oxygen.

Homeostasis a physiologic state resulting from a dynamic equilibrium maintained by monitoring processes and altered effector activity, incorporating negative feedback pathways.

Hormone a substance originating in an organ or gland that is conveyed through the body to another part of the body, which it stimulates by chemical action to increased functional activity and/or increased secretion.

Hydrostatic pertaining to the pressure of liquids in equilibrium and the pressure exerted on liquids.

Hydrous containing water, usually chemically combined.

Hyperbaric oxygen therapy (HBOT) the administration of oxygen at greater than normal atmospheric pressure. The procedure is performed in specially designed chambers that permit the delivery of 100% oxygen at atmospheric pressure that is three times normal. The technique is used to overcome the natural limit of oxygen solubility in blood, which is about 0.3 mL of oxygen per 100 mL of blood. In hyperbaric oxygenation, dissolved oxygen can be increased to almost 6 mL per 100 mL and the P_{O_2} in blood may be nearly 2000 mm Hg at 3 atmospheres absolute. Hyperbaric oxygenation has been used to treat carbon monoxide poisoning, air embolism, smoke inhalation, acute cyanide poisoning, decompression sickness, wounds, clostridial myonecrosis, and certain cases of blood loss or anemia in which increased oxygen transport may compensate in part for hemoglobin deficiency. Factors limiting the usefulness of hyperbaric oxygenation include the hazards of fire and explosive decompression, pulmonary damage and neurologic toxicity at high atmospheric pressures, cardiovascular debility of the patient, and the need to interrupt treatments repeatedly because exposures at maximum atmospheric pressures must be limited to 90 minutes. Also called hyperbaric oxygen.

Hypercapnia greater than normal amount of carbon dioxide in the blood. Also called *hypercarbia.*

Hyperchloremia an excessive level of chloride in the blood that results in acidosis.

Hyperinflation distention by air, gas, or liquid, as in the hyperinflation of the alveoli.

Hyperkalemia increased amount of potassium in the blood.

Hyperpnea increased depth (volume) of breathing, with or without an increased frequency.

Hypersecretion substance or fluid produced by cells or glands in an excessive amount or more than normal.

Hypersensitivity an abnormal condition characterized by an exaggerated response of the immune system to an antigen.

Hypertension higher than normal blood pressure.

Hyperthermia higher than normal body temperature.

Hyperventilation pulmonary ventilation rate greater than that metabolically necessary for gas exchange, resulting from an increased respiration rate, an increased tidal volume, or both. Hyperventilation causes an excessive intake of oxygen and elimination of carbon dioxide and may cause hyperoxygenenation. Hypocapnia and respiratory alkalosis then occur, leading to dizziness, faintness, numbness of the fingers and toes, possibly syncope, and psychomotor impairment. Causes of hyperventilation include asthma or early emphysema; increased metabolic rate caused by exercise, fever, hyperthyroidism, or infection; lesions of the central nervous system, as in cerebral thrombosis, encephalitis, head injuries, or meningitis; hypoxia or metabolic acidosis; use of hormones and drugs, such as epINEPHrine, progesterone, and salicylates; difficulties with mechanical respirators; and psychogenic factors, such as acute anxiety or pain. Compare hypoventilation.

Hypochloremia a decreased amount of chloride in the blood.

Hypokalemia a decreased amount of potassium in the blood.

Hypoperfusion deficiency of blood coursing through the vessels of the circulatory system.

Hypothalamus portion of the brain that controls certain metabolic activities.

Hypoventilation an abnormal condition of the respiratory system that occurs when the volume of air that enters the alveoli and takes part in gas exchange is not adequate for the body's metabolic needs. It is characterized by cyanosis, polycythemia, increased Pa_{CO_2}, and generalized decreased respiratory function. Hypoventilation may be caused by an uneven distribution of inspired air (as in bronchitis), obesity, neuromuscular or skeletal disease affecting the thorax, decreased response of the respiratory center to carbon dioxide, or a reduced amount of functional lung tissue, as in atelectasis, emphysema, and pleural effusion. The results of hypoventilation are hypoxia, hypercapnia, pulmonary hypertension with cor pulmonale, and respiratory acidosis. Treatment includes weight reduction in cases of obesity, artificial respiration, and possibly tracheostomy.

Hypoxemia an abnormal deficiency in the concentration of oxygen in arterial blood. Symptoms of acute hypoxemia are cyanosis, restlessness, stupor, coma, Cheyne-Stokes respiration, apnea, increased blood pressure, tachycardia, and an initial increase in cardiac output that later falls, producing hypotension and ventricular fibrillation or asystole.

Hypoxia inadequate oxygen tension at the cellular level, characterized by tachycardia, hypertension, peripheral vasoconstriction, dizziness, and mental confusion.

I

Iatrogenic pneumothorax a condition in which air or gas is present in the pleural cavity as a result of mechanical ventilation, tracheostomy tube placement, or other therapeutic intervention.

Iliac crest long curved upper margin of the hip bone.

Immaturity the state of being not fully developed or ripened.

Immunoglobulin one of a family of closely related but not identical proteins that are capable of acting as antibodies.

Immunologic mechanism reaction of the body to substances that are foreign or are interpreted by the body as foreign.

Impede to slow down; to stand in the way of; to fight against.

Inferior vena cava (IVC) venous trunk for the lower extremities and the pelvic and abdominal viscera.

Inflammation the protective response of body tissues to irritation or injury. Inflammation may be acute or chronic; its cardinal signs are redness, heat, swelling, and pain, often accompanied by loss of function. The process begins with a transitory vasoconstriction, then is followed by a brief increase in vascular permeability. The second stage is prolonged and consists of sustained increase in vascular permeability, exudation of fluids from the vessels, clustering of leukocytes along the vessels walls, phagocytosis of microorganisms, deposition of fibrin in the vessel, disposal of the accumulated debris by macrophages, and finally migration of fibroblast to the area and development of new, normal cells. The severity, timing, and local character of any particular inflammatory response depend on the cause, the area affected, and the condition of the host. Histamine, kinins, and various other substances mediate the inflammatory process.

Inguinal ligament a fibrous band formed by the inferior border of the aponeurosis of the external oblique that extends from the anterior superior iliac spine to the pubic tubercle.

Inhibitory repressive; tending to restrain a function.

Innervation the distribution or supply of nerve fibers or nerve impulses to a body part.

Insomnia chronic inability to sleep or to remain asleep throughout the night; wakefulness; sleeplessness. Insomnia may be the symptom of a psychiatric disorder.

Inspiratory capacity the volume of air that can be inhaled after a normal exhalation.

Inspiratory reserve volume (IRV) the maximum volume of air that can be inhaled after a normal tidal volume inhalation.

Inspiratory stridor stridor is a high pitched wheezing sound resulting from turbulent air flow in the upper airway. Stridor is a physical sign which is produced by narrow or obstructed airway path. It can be inspiratory, expiratory or biphasic. Inspiratory stridor is common.

Interatrial septum the partition or wall that separates the right and left atrium of the heart.

Internal respiration gas exchange between the systemic capillaries and the cells.

Interstitial placed or lying between; pertaining to the interstices or spaces within an organ or tissue.

Interventricular septum the partition or wall that separates the right and left ventricles of the heart.

Intra prefix meaning within.

Intra-alveolar within the alveoli.

Intrapleural within the pleura.

Intrapulmonary within the lungs.

Intrarenal within the kidneys.

Intratubular within a tube.

Intrinsic an intrinsic property is an essential or inherent property of a system or of a material itself or within. It is independent of how much of the material is present and is independent of the form the material, e.g., one large piece or a collection of smaller pieces. Intrinsic properties are dependent mainly on the chemical composition or structure of the material.

Intubation passage of a tube into a body aperture; specifically, the insertion of a breathing tube through the mouth or nose or into the trachea to ensure a patent airway for the delivery of anesthetic gases and oxygen or both. Kinds of intubation include **endotracheal intubation** and *nasotracheal intubation*.

Inverse opposite in order, nature, or effect; as one variable increases, the other decreases.

Ion atom, group of atoms, or molecule that has acquired a net electrical charge by gaining or losing electrons.

Ischemia decreased blood supply to a body organ or part.

Isobar a line on a map, chart, or nomogram connecting areas of equal pressure.

K

Ketoacidosis acidosis accompanied by an accumulation of ketones in the body, resulting from extensive breakdown of fats because of faulty carbohydrate metabolism. It occurs primarily as a complication of diabetes mellitus and is characterized by a fruity odor of acetone on the breath, mental confusion, dyspnea, nausea, vomiting, dehydration, weight loss, and, if untreated, coma.

Kussmaul breathing abnormally deep, very rapid sighing respirations characteristic of diabetic ketoacidosis.

L

Lactic acid acid formed in muscles during activity by the breakdown of sugar without oxygen.

Laryngitis an inflammation of the larynx. It causes hoarse voice or the complete loss of the voice because of irritation to the vocal folds (vocal cords). Dysphonia is the medical term for a vocal disorder, of which laryngitis is one cause. Laryngitis is categorized as acute if it lasts less than a few days. Otherwise it is categorized as chronic, and may last over 3 weeks. The chronic form of disease occurs mostly in middle age and is much more common in men than women.

Laryngopharynx the laryngopharynx or hypopharynx (Latin: pars laryngea pharyngis) is the caudal part of the pharynx; it is the part of the throat that connects to the esophagus. It lies inferior to the epiglottis and extends to the location where this common pathway diverges into the respiratory (larynx) and digestive (esophagus) pathways. At that point, the laryngopharynx is continuous with the esophagus posteriorly. The esophagus conducts food and fluids to the stomach; air enters the larynx anteriorly. During swallowing, food has the "right of way", and air passage temporarily stops. Corresponding roughly to the area located between the 4th and 6th cervical vertebrae, the superior boundary of the laryngopharynx is at the level of the hyoid bone. The laryngopharynx includes three major sites: the pyriform sinus, postcricoid area, and the posterior pharyngeal wall. Like the oropharynx above it, the laryngopharynx serves as a passageway for food and air and is lined with a stratified squamous epithelium. It is innervated by the pharyngeal plexus.

Laryngotracheobronchitis laryngotracheobronchitis (or croup) is a respiratory condition that is usually triggered by an acute viral infection of the upper airway. The infection leads to swelling inside the throat, which interferes with normal breathing and produces the classical symptoms of a "barking" cough, stridor, and hoarseness. It may produce mild, moderate, or severe symptoms, which often worsen at night. It is often treated with a single dose of oral steroids; occasionally epinephrine is used in more severe cases. Hospitalization is rarely required.

Larynx the organ of voice that is part of the upper airway passage connecting the pharynx with the trachea. It accounts for a large bump in the neck called the Adam's apple and is larger in men than in omen, although it remains the same size in men and women until puberty. The larynx forms the caudal portion of the anterior wall of the pharynx and is lined with mucous membrane that is continous with that of the pahrynx and the trachea. The larynx exends vertically to the fourth, fifth, and sixth cervical vertebrae and is somewhat higher in the female and during childhood. It is composed of three single cartilages and three paired cartilages, all connected together by ligaments and moved by various muscles. The single cartilages are the thyroid, cricoid, and epiglottis. The paired cartilages are the arytenoid, corniculate, and cuneiform, which support the vocal folds.

Leukocyte a white blood cell, one of the formed elements of the circulating blood system. Five types of leukocytes are classified by the presence or absence of granules in the cytoplasm of the cell. Normal range: 5000 to 10,000/mm³. The agranulocytes are lymphocytes and monocytes. The granulocytes are neutrophils, basophils, and eosinophils. Also called *leucocyte, white blood cell,* and *white corpuscle.*

Leukocytosis an abnormal increase in the number of circulating white blood cells. An increase often accompanies bacterial, but not usually viral, infections. The normal range is 5000 to 10,000/mm³. Leukemia may be associated with a white blood cell count as high as 500,000 to 1 million per cubic millimeter of blood, the increase being either equally or disproportionately distributed among all types.

Kinds of leukocytosis include *basophilia, eosinophilia,* and *neutrophilia.*

Ligamentum nuchae upward continuation of the supraspinous ligament, extending from the seventh cervical vertebra to the occipital bone.

Lingual tonsil a mass of lymphoid follicles near the root of the tongue. Each follicle forms a rounded eminence containing a small opening leading into a funnel-shaped cavity surrounded by lymphoid tissue.

Linea alba "white line" of connective tissue in the middle of the abdomen from sternum to pubis.

Linear response a response or output that is directly proportional to the input.

Lipid any of numerous fats generally insoluble in water that constitute one of the principal structural materials of cells.

Lobar pertaining to a lobe, such as the lobes of the lung.

Lower airways the lower airways consist of the following tracheobronchial tree components below the larynx: trachea, main stem bronchi, lobar bronchi, semental bronchi, and subsegmental bronchi.

Lumen inner open space of a tubular organ, such as a blood vessel or intestine.

Lung capacities two or more lung volumes.

Lung compliance a measure of the ease of expansion of the lungs and thorax. It is determined by pulmonary volume and elasticity. A high degree of compliance indicates a loss of elastic recoil of the lungs, as in old age or emphysema. Decreased compliance means a greater change in pressure is needed for a given change in volume, as in atelectasis, edema, fibrosis, pneumonia, or absence of surfactant. Dyspnea on exertion is the main symptom of diminished lung compliance.

Lymphocyte small agranulocytic leukocytes originating from fetal stem cells and developing in the bone marrow. Lymphocytes normally comprise 25 percent of the total white blood cell count but increase in number in response to infection. Two forms occur: B cells and T cells. B cells circulate in an immature form and synthesize antibodies for insertion into their own cytoplasmic membranes. T cells are lymphocytes that have circulated through the thymus gland and have differentiated to become thymocytes. When exposed to an antigen, they divide rapidly and produce large numbers of new T cells sensitized to that antigen.

M

Macrophage any phagocytic cell of the reticuloendothelial system, including specialized Kupffer's cells in the liver, lungs, spleen, and histocyte in loose connective tissue.

Magnitude pertaining to size.

Malar pertaining to the cheek or cheekbones.

Malformation deformity; abnormal shape or structure, especially congenital.

Mastoid process projection of the posterior portion of the temporal bone; gives attachment to the sternocleidomastoid, splenius capitis, and longissimus capitis muscles.

Maxilla one of a pair of large bones (often referred to as one bone) that form the upper jaw and teeth, consisting of a pyramidal body and four processes: the zygomatic, frontal, alveolar, and palatine.

Maxillary pertaining to the upper jawbone.

Mean occupying a middle position; being near the average.

Mechanical relating to physical properties.

Mechanoreceptor receptor that receives mechanical stimuli such as pressure from sound or touch.

Medial pertaining to the middle.

Mediastinum a part of the thoracic cavity in the middle of the thorax, between the pleural sacs containing the two lungs. It extends from the sternum to the vertebral column and contains all the thoracic viscera except the lungs. It is enclosed in a thick extension of the thoracic subserous fascia and is divided into the cranial part and the caudal part.

Mediated between two parts or sides.

Medulla oblongata a bulbous continuation of the spinal cord just above the foramen magnum and separated from the pons by a horizontal groove. It is one of three parts of the brainstem and mainly contains white substance with some mixture of gray substance. The medulla contains the cardiac, vasomotor, and respiratory centers of the brain; medullary injury or disease often proves fatal.

Mesoderm the middle of the three cell layers of the developing embryo, which lies between the ectoderm and endoderm.

Metabolic acidosis acidosis in which excess acid is added to the body fluids or bicarbonate is lost from them. Metabolis acidosis is indicated by a blood pH below 7.35 and a normal carbon dioxide level (35 to 45 torr).

metabolic alkalosis alkalosis in which excess bicarbonate is added to the body fluids or acid is lost from them. Metabolic alkalosis is indicated by a blood pH above 7.45 and a normal carbon dioxide level (35 to 45 torr).

metabolic and respiratory acidosis a blood pH below 7.35 caused by both a high carbon dioxide level and a low bicarbonate level. Also called combined metabolic and respiraory acidosis.

Metabolism sum of all physical and chemical changes that take place within an organism; all energy and material transformations that occur within living cells.

Microvilli minute cylindrical processes on the free surface of a cell (especially cells of the proximal convoluted renal tubule and those of the intestinal epithelium), which increase the surface area of the cell.

Mild hypoxemia an arterial oxgen pressure (Pa_{O_2}) between 60 and 80 mm Hg.

Mitral valve see **bicuspid valve**.

Moderate hypoxemia an arterial oxgen pressure (Pa_{O_2}) between 40 and 60 mm Hg.

Molecular weight weight of a molecule attained by adding the atomic weight of its constituent atoms.

Monocyte a large, mononuclear leukocyte normally found in lymph nodes, spleen, bone marrow, and loose connective tissue. Normal range: 3 to 7 percent of leukocyte differential.

Motor nerve a nerve consisting of efferent fibers that conduct impulses from the brain or the spinal cord to one of the muscles or organs.

Mucous pertaining to or resembling mucus; secreting mucus.

Mucus the viscous, slippery secretions of mucous membranes and glands, containing mucin, white blood cells, water, inorganic salts, and exfoliated cells.

Myelin a lipoproteinaceous substance constituting the sheaths of various nerve fibers throughout the body and enveloping the axis of myelinated nerves. It is largely composed of phospholipids and protein, which gives the fibers a white, creamy color. It is largely composed of fat, giving the fibers a white, creamy color.

Myocardial infarction necrosis of a portion of cardiac muscle caused by an obstruction in a coronary artery resulting from atherosclerosis, a thrombus, or a spasm. Also called heart attack.

Myocardium a thick contractile middle layer of uniquely constructed and arranged muscle cells that forms the bulk of the heart wall. The myocardium contains a minimum of other tissue, except blood vessels, and is covered interiorly by the endocardium. The contractile tissue of the myocardium is composed of fibers with the characteristic cross-striations of muscular tissue. The fibers are about one third as large in diameter as those of skeletal muscle and contain more sarcoplasm. They branch frequently and are interconnected to form a network that is continuous except where the bundles and the laminae are attached at their origins and insertions into the fibrous trigone of the heart. Myocardial muscle contains less connective tissue than does skeletal muscle. Specially modified fibers of myocardial muscle constitute the conduction system of the heart, including the sinoatrial node, the atrioventricular (AV) node, the AV bundle, and the Purkinje fibers. Most of the myocardial fibers function to contract the heart. The metabolic processes of the myocardium are almost exclusively aerobic. Many key enzymatic reactions of the heart, such as the citric acid cycle and oxidative phosphorylation, take place in the highly concentrated myocardial sarcosomes. The process of oxidative phosphorylation produces adenosine triphosphate (ATP), the immediate energy source for myocardial contraction. Oxygen, which significantly affects ATP production and contractibility, is a critical metabolic component of the myocardium, which consumes from 6.5 to 10 mL/100 g of tissue per minute. Without this oxygen supply, myocardial contractions decrease in a few minutes. The myocardium maintains a relatively constant level of glycogen in the form of sarcoplasmic granule.

Myoepithelial cells spindle-shaped cells found around sweat, mammary, and salivary glands. The myoepithelial cells are contractile and resemble smooth muscle cells.

Myoglobin a ferrous globin complex consisting of one heme group and one globin polypeptide chain. It is responsible for the red pigment seen in skeletal muscle.

N

Nares the pairs of anterior and posterior openings to the nasal cavity that allow the passage of air to the pharynx and ultimately the lungs during respiration.

Nasal septum the partition dividing the nostrils. It is composed of bone and cartilage covered by mucous membrane.

Necrosis localized tissue death that occurs in groups of cells in response to disease or injury.

Neoplasm any abnormal growth of new tissue, benign or malignant. Also called *tumor*.

Neuropathy any abnormal condition characterized by inflammation and degeneration of the peripheral nerves.

Neutrophil a polymorphonuclear, granular leukocyte that stains easily with neutral dyes. The nucleus stains dark blue and contains three to five lobes connected by slender threads of chromatin. The cytoplasm contains fine, inconspicuous granules. Neutrophils are the circulating white blood cells essential for phagocytosis and proteolysis by which bacteria, cellular debris, and solid particles are removed and destroyed. Normal range: 57 to 67 percent of leukocyte differential.

Nomogram a graph consisting of several lines or curves (usually parallel) graduated for different variables in such a way that a straight line cutting the three lines gives the related values of the three variables.

Nonlinear having or being a response or output that is not directly proportional to the input.

Norepinephrine one of two active hormones (the other is epinephrine) secreted by the adrenal medulla. It is chiefly a vasoconstrictor and has little effect on cardiac output.

Nose the structure that protrudes from the anterior part of the face and seves as a passagway for air to and from the lungs. The nose filers the air, warming, moistening, and chemcally examining it for impurities that might irritate the mucous lining of the respiratory tract. The nose also contains receptor cells for smell, and it aids the faculty of speech. It consists of an internal and an external part. The external part, which protudes from the face, is considerably smaller than the internal part, whcih lies over the roof of the mouth. The hollow interior part is separated into a right and a left cavity by a septum. Each cavity is divided into the superior, middle and inferior meati by the projection of nasal conchae. The external part of the nose is perforated by two nostrils (anterior nares), and the internal part by two posterior nares. The pairs of sinuses that drain into the nose are the frontal, maxillary, ethmoidal, and sphenoidal sinuses. Ciliated mucous membrane lines the nose, closely abhering to the periosteum. The mucous membrane is continous withthe skin through the nares and with the mucous membrane of the nasal part of the pharynx through the choanae. The mucous membrane contains the olfactory cells that form the olfactory nerve that enters the cranium.

Nostrils the ends of the nostrils that open anteriorly into the nasal cavity and allow the inhalation and the exhalation of air. Each is an oval opening that measures about 1.5 cm anteroposteriorly and about 1 cm in diameter. The anterior nares connect with the nasal fossae. Also called anterior nares.

O

Obstructive lung disorder obstructive respiratory disease is the result of a reduction of airway size that impedes air flow. The obstruction may result from bronchospasm, edema of the bronchial mucosa, or excessive bronchial secretions. Obstructive disease is characterized by reduced expiratory flow rates and increased total lung capacity. Acute obstructive respiratory diseases include asthma, bronchitis, and bronchiectasis; chronic obstructive diseases include emphysema, chronic bronchitis, or combined emphysema and chronic bronchitis. Patients with obstructive diseases may have acute respiratory failure from any respiratory stress, such as infections or general anesthesia.

Occipital referring to the back part or bone of the head.

Occlude to close, obstruct, or join together.

Olfactory pertaining to the sense of smell.

Oncotic pressure the osmotic pressure of a colloid in solution, such as when there is a higher concentration of protein in the plasma on one side of a cell membrane than in the neighboring interstitial fluid.

Open pneumothorax the presence of air or gas in the chest as a result of an open wound in the chest wall.

Oral cavity [L, oralis, pertaining to the mough, cavum, cavity], the space within the mouth, containing the tongue and teeth.

Orthopnea a condition in which an individual is able to breathe most comfortably only in the upright position.

Osmosis the movement of a pure solvent such as water through a differentially permeable membrane from a solution that has a lower solute concentration to one that has a higher solute concentration. The membrane is impermeable to the solute but is permeable to the solvent. The rate of osmosis depends on the concentration of solute, the temperature of the solution, the electrical charge of the solute, and the difference between the osmotic pressures exerted by the solutions. Movement across the membrane continues until the concentrations of the solutions equalize.

Osmotic pressure pressure that develops when two solutions with different concentrations of solutes are separated by a semipermeable membrane.

Otitis media an inflammation or infection of the middle ear, common in early childhood. Acute otitis media is most often caused by Haemophilus influenzae, Moraxella catarrhalis, or Streptococcus pneumoniae. Chronic otitis media is usually caused by gram-negative bacteria such as Proteus, Klebsiella, and Pseudomonas. Allergy, Mycoplasma, and several viruses also may be causative factors. Otitis media is often preceded by an upper respiratory infection.

Oxygen consumption the amount of oxygen in milliliters per minute that the body requires for normal aerobic metabolism; normally about 250 mL/min.

Oxygen content total amount of oxygen in the blood.

Oxygen extraction ratio the amount of oxygen extracted by the peripheral tissues divided by the amount of oxygen delivered to the peripheral cells. Normally, about 25 percent. Also known as *oxygen coefficient ratio* or *oxygen utilization ratio*.

Oxygen toxicity a condition of oxygen overdosage that can result in pathologic tissue changes, such as retinopathy of prematurity or bronchopulmonary dysplasia. It can also decrease CO_2 drive to breathe.

Oxyhemoglobin the product of combining hemoglobin with oxygen. The loosely bound complex dissociates easily when the concentration of oxygen is low.

P

Palatine bones one of a pair of bones of the skull, forming the posterior part of the hard palate, part of the nasal cavity, and the floor of the orbit of the eie. It resembles a letter L and consists of horizontal and vertical parts and three processes.

Palatine tonsils palatine tonsil, one of a pair of almond-shaped masses of lymphoid tissue between the palatoglossal and palatopharyngeal arches on each side of the fauces.

Pallor an unnatural paleness or absence of color in the skin.

Papillitis an abnormal condition characterized by the inflammation of a papilla.

Paradoxic pertaining to a person, situation, statement, or act that may appear to have inconsistent or contradictory qualities or that may be true but appears to be absurd or unbelievable. Also paradoxical.

Parasympathetic nervous system a division of the autonomic nervous system that is mediated by the release of acetylcholine and primarily involves the protection, conservation, and restoration of body resources.

Parenchyma essential parts of an organ that are concerned with its function.

Parietal layer pertaining to the outer wall of a cavity or organ.

Paroxysmal concerning the sudden, periodic attack or recurrence of symptoms of a disease.

Parturition the action or process of giving birth to offspring.

Pathogen any agent causing disease, especially a microorganism.

Peak flow meter an instrument for measuring the flow of air in the early part of forced expiration.

Perfusion passing of blood or fluid through a vascular bed.

Peribronchial located around the bronchi.

Pericarditis inflammation of the pericardium associated with trauma, malignant neoplastic disease, infection, uremia, myocardial infarction, collagen disease, or unknown causes.

Pericardium a fibroserous sac that surrounds the heart and the roots of the great vessels.

Peripheral airways small bronchioles on the outer sections of the lung.

Peristalsis a progressive wave movement that occurs involuntarily in hollow tubes of the body, especially the intestines.

Perivascular located around a vessel, especially a blood vessel.

Permeable capable of allowing the passage of fluids or substances in solution.

Persistent pulmonary hypertension of the neonate (PPHN) an elevated pulmonary vascular resistance in the newborn caused by a low P_{O_2} level. The infant's ductus arteriosus remains open as a result of this condition.

pH symbol for the logarithm of the reciprocal of the hydrogen ion concentration. The abbreviation for potential hydrogen, a scale representing the relative acidity of a solution in which a value of 7.0 is neutral, below 7.0 is acid, and above 7.0 is alkaline.

Phalanges the bones of the fingers and toes.

Pharyngotympanic (auditory) tubes a tube lined with mucous membrane that joins the nasopharynx and the middle ear cavity. It is normally closed but opens during yawning, chewing, and swallowing to allow equalization of the air pressure in the middle ear with atmospheric pressure.

Pharynx the throat, a tubular structure about 13 cm long that extends from the base of the skull to the esophagus and is situated immediately in front of the cervical vertebrae. The pharynx serves as a passageway for the respiratory and digestive tracts and changes shape to allow the formation of various vowel sounds. The pharybnx is composed of muscle, is lined with mucous membrane, and is divided into the nasopharynx, the oropharynx, and the laryngopharynx. It contains the opeings of the right and left auditory tubes, the openings of the two posterior nares, the fauces, the opening into the larynx, and the opening into the esophagus. It also contains the pharyngeal tonsils, the palatien tonsils, and the lingual tonsils. Also called throat.

Phosphate a salt of phosphoric acid. Phosphates are extremely important in living cells, particularly in the storage and use of energy and the transmission of genetic information within a cell and from one cell to another.

Photophobia abnormal sensitivity of the eyes to light.

Pituitary gland an endocrine gland suspended beneath the brain in the pituitary fossa of the sphenoid bone, supplying numerous hormones that govern many vital processes.

Plasma the watery straw-colored fluid part of the lymph and the blood in which the leukocytes, erythrocytes, and platelets are suspended. Plasma is made up of water, electrolytes, proteins, glucose, fats, bilirubin, and gases and is essential for carrying the cellular elements of the blood through the circulation, transporting nutrients, maintaining the acid-base balance of the body, and transporting wastes from the tissues. Plasma and interstitial fluid correspond closely in content and concentration of proteins; therefore, plasma is important in maintaining the osmotic pressure and the exchange of fluids and electrolytes between the capillaries and the tissues.

Platelet the smallest cells in the blood. They are formed in the red bone marrow and some are stored in the spleen. Platelets are disk shaped, contain no hemoglobin, and are essential for the coagulation of blood and in maintenance of hemostasis. Normally, between 140,000 and 340,000/mm³.

Pleura (*pl. pleurae*) a delicate serous membrane enclosing the lung, composed of a single layer of flattened mesothelial cells resting on a delicate membrane of connective tissue. Beneath the membrane is a stroma of collagenous tissue containing yellow elastic fibers. The pleura divides into the visceral pleura, which covers the lungs, dipping into the fissures between the lobes, and the parietal pleura, which lines the chest wall, covers the diaphragm, and reflects over the structures of the mediastinum. The parietal and visceral pleurae are separated from each other by a small amount of fluid that acts as a lubricant as the lungs expand and contract during respiration. See also **pleural space**.

Pleural effusion an abnormal accumulation of fluid in the intrapleural spaces of the lungs. It is characterized by chest pain, dyspnea, adventitious lung sounds, and nonproductive cough. The fluid is an exudate or a transudate from inflamed pleural surfaces and may be aspirated or surgically drained. An exudate may result from pulmonary infarction, trauma, tumor, or infection, such as tuberculosis. The specific cause of the exudate is treated. Treatment of the effusion may include the administration of corticosteroids, diuretics, or vasodilators; oxygen therapy; intermittent positive-pressure breathing; or thoracentesis or use of a mobile system such as the Pleurx catheter.

Pleural space the potential space between the visceral and parietal layers of the pleurae. The space contains a small amount of fluid that acts as a lubricant, allowing the pleurae to slide smoothly over each other as the lungs expand and contract with respiration.

Pleurisy inflammation of the parietal pleura of the lungs. It is characterized by dyspnea and stabbing pain, leading to restriction of ordinary breathing with spasm of the chest on the affected side. A pleural friction rub may be heard on auscultation. Simple pleurisy with undetectable exudate is called fibrinous or dry pleurisy. Pleural effusion indicates extensive inflammation with considerable amounts of exudate in the pleural spaces. Common causes of pleurisy include bronchial carcinoma, lung or chest wall abscess, pneumonia, pulmonary infarction, and tuberculosis. The condition may result in permanent adhesions between the pleura and adjacent surfaces. Treatment consists of pain relief and therapy for the primary disease.

Pneumothorax a collection of air or gas in the pleural space, causing the lung to collapse.

Point of maximal intensity (PMI) the place where the apical pulse is palpated as strongest, often in the fifth intercostal space of the thorax, just medial to the left midclavicular line.

Polycythemia an increase in the number of erythrocytes in the blood caused by chronic hypoxemia secondary to pulmonary disease, heart disease, or prolonged exposure to high altitudes, or it may be idiopathic.

Polymer a compound formed by combining or linking a number of monomers, or small molecules. A polymer may be composed of many units of more than one type of monomer (a copolymer) or of many units of the same monomer (homopolymer).

Polysomography The polygraphic recording during sleep of multiple physiologic variables, both directly and indirectly related to the state and stages of sleep, to assess possible sleep disorders.

Pontine respiratory group a portion of the pontine respiratory centers that influences the respiratory components of the medulla. Neural impulses from the pneumotaxic center simultaneously cause (1) the depth of breathing to decrease and (2) the rate of breathing to increase by almost an equal amount. Some investigators believe the pneumotaxic center is closely related to the so-called panting center in animals such as dogs.

Posterior back part of something; toward the back.

Postural drainage drainage from the affected parts of the lungs are selected. Pillows and raised sections of the hospital bed are used to support or elevate parts of the body. The procedure is begun with the patient level, and the head is gradually lowered to a full Trendelenburg's position. Inhalation through the nose and exhalation through the mouth are encouraged. Simultaneously the nurse or other health care provider may use cupping and vibration over the affected area of the lungs to dislodge and mobilize secretions. The person is then helped to a position conducive to coughing and is asked to breathe deeply at least three times and to cough at least twice.

Premature ventricular complex (PVC) an arrhythmia characterized by ventricular depolarization occurring earlier than expected. It appears on the electrocardiogram as an early wide QRS complex without a preceding related P wave. PVCs may occur occasionally in a regular pattern or as several in sequence. They may be idiopathic or caused by stress, electrolyte imbalance, ischemia, hypoxemia, hypercapnia, ventricular enlargement, or a toxic reaction to drugs. Isolated PVCs are not clinically significant in healthy individuals, but they may produce decreased cardiac output in people with heart disease, and frequent PVCs may be a precursor of ventricular tachycardia or fibrillation.

Prerenal pertaining to the area in front of the kidney; pertaining to events occurring before reaching the kidney.

Pressoreceptor see **baroreceptor**.

Pressure a force, or stress, applied to a surface by a fluid or an object, usually measured in units of mass per unit of area, such as pounds per square inch.

Prognosis a prediction of the probable outcome of a disease based on the conditions of the person and the usual course of the disease as observed in similar situations.

Proliferate increasing or spreading at a rapid rate; the process or result of rapid reproduction.

Prostaglandins a group of fatty acid derivatives present in many organs that affect the cardiovascular system and smooth muscle and stimulate the uterus to contract.

Prostate a gland in males that surrounds the neck of the bladder and the deepest part of the urethra and produces a fluid that becomes part of semen.

Prostatic hypertrophy enlargement of the prostate gland.

Proximal nearest the point of attachment, center of the body, or point of reference.

Pubic symphysis junction of the pubic bones, composed of fibrocartilage.

Pulmonary pertaining to the lungs or the respiratory system.

Pulmonary alveolus one of the numerous terminal air sacs in the lungs where oxygen and carbon dioxide are exchanged.

Pulmonary congestion an excessive accumulation of fluid in the lungs, usually associated with either an inflammation or congestive heart failure.

Pulmonary edema the accumulation of extravascular fluid in lung tissues and alveoli, caused most commonly by congestive heart failure. Serous fluid is pushed through the pulmonary capillaries into alveoli and quickly enters bronchioles and bronchi. The condition also may occur in barbiturate and opiate poisoning, diffuse infections, hemorrhagic pancreatitis, and renal failure or after a stroke, skull fracture, near-drowning, inhalation of irritating gases, and rapid administration of whole blood, plasma, serum albumin, or IV fluids.

Pulmonary embolus the blockage of a pulmonary artery by fat, air, tumor tissue, or a thrombus that usually arises from a peripheral vein (most frequently one of the deep veins of the legs). Predisposing factors include an alteration of blood constituents with increased coagulation, damage to blood vessel walls, and stagnation or immobilization, especially when associated with pregnancy and childbirth, congestive heart failure, polycythemia, or surgery. Pulmonary embolism is difficult to distinguish from myocardial infarction and pneumonia. It is characterized by dyspnea, anxiety, sudden chest pain, shock, and cyanosis. Pulmonary infarction, which often occurs within 24 hours after the formation of a pulmonary embolus, is further characterized by pleural effusion, hemoptysis, leukocytosis, fever, tachycardia, atrial arrhythmias, and striking distension of the neck veins. Analysis of blood gases reveals arterial hypoxia and hypocapnia. Pulmonary embolism is detected by chest radiographic films, pulmonary angiography, and radioscanning of the lung fields. Two thirds of patients with a massive pulmonary embolus die within 2 hours. Initial resuscitative measures include external cardiac massage, oxygen, vasopressor drugs, embolectomy, and correction of acidosis. The formation of further emboli is prevented by the use of anticoagulants, sometimes the use of streptokinase or urokinase, and also surgical intervention. Ambulation, exercise, and use of sequential compression devices on the lower extremities also are recommended for prevention. A vena cava filter may be inserted if pulmonary emboli recur.

Pulmonary emphysema a chronic obstructive disease of the lungs, marked by an overdistention of the alveoli and destruction of the supporting alveolar structure. See also **emphysema.**

Pulmonary shunting that portion of the cardiac output that enters the left side of the heart without exchanging gases with alveolar gases.

Pulmonary surfactant one of certain lipoproteins that reduce the surface tension of pulmonary fluids, allowing the exchange of gases in the alveoli of the lungs and contributing to the elasticity of pulmonary tissue. **See also surfactant**

Pulmonary vascular resistance (PVR) pressure loss, per unit of blood flow, from the pulmonary artery to the left ventricle. The resistance in the pulmonary vascular bed against which the right ventricle must eject blood.

Pulse oximeter a device that measures the amount of saturated hemoglobin in the tissue capillaries by transmitting a beam of light through the tissue to a receiver. This noninvasive method of measuring the saturated hemoglobin is a useful screening tool for determining basic respiratory function. This cliplike device may be used on either the earlobe or the fingertip. As the amount of saturated hemoglobin alters the wavelengths of the transmitted light, analysis of the received light is translated into a percentage of oxygen saturation (SO_2) of the blood.

Pyelonephritis a diffuse pyogenic infection of the pelvis and parenchyma of the kidney.

R

Rales see **crackle**.

Red blood cells mature red blood cell (also called erythrocytes); a biconcave disk about 7 μm in diameter that contains hemoglobin confined within a lipoid membrane. It is the major cellular element of the circulating blood and transports oxygen as its principal function. The number of cells per cubic millimeter of blood is usually maintained between 4.5 and 5.5 million in men and between 4.2 and 4.8 million in women. It varies with age, activity, and environmental conditions. For example, an increase to a level of 8 million/mm³ can normally occur at over 10,000 feet above sea level. An erythrocyte normally lives for 110 to 120 days, when it is removed from the bloodstream and broken down by the reticuloendothelial system. New erythrocytes are produced at a rate of slightly more than 1% a day; thus a constant level is usually maintained. Acute blood loss, hemolytic anemia, or chronic oxygen deprivation may cause erythrocyte production to increase greatly. Erythrocytes originate in the marrow of the long bones. Maturation proceeds from a stem cell (promegaloblast) through the pronormoblast stage to the normoblast, the last stage before the mature adult cell develops.

Reflex an involuntary response to a stimulus.

Relative shunt a capillary shunt exists when blood flows from the right side of the heart to the left side without coming in contact with ventilated alveoli for gas exchange. Capillary shunting is commonly caused by (1) alveolar collapse or atelectasis, (2) alveolar fluid accumulation, or (3) alveolar consolidation. **See also Shunt-like effect**

Renal pertaining to the kidneys.

Renal dysplasia abnormal development of tissue in the kidneys.

Residual volume (RV) the amount of air remaining in the lungs after a maximal exhalation.

Resonance quality of the sound heard on percussion of a hollow structure such as the chest or abdomen.

Respiration the molecular exchange of oxygen and carbon dioxide within the body's tissue. Compare **ventilation**.

Respiratory acidosis a condition marked by high levels of carbon dioxide, and a low pH in the blood, due to hypventilation. Also called respiratory acidosis.

Respiratory distress syndrome an acute lung disease of the newborn, characterized by airless alveoli, inelastic lungs, a respiration rate greater than 60 breaths per minute, nasal flaring, intercostal and subcostal retractions, grunting on expiration, and peripheral edema. The condition occurs most often in premature babies. It is caused by a deficiency of pulmonary surfactant, resulting in overdistended alveoli and at times hyaline membrane formation, alveolar hemorrhage, severe right-to-left shunting of blood, increased pulmonary resistance, decreased cardiac output, and severe hypoxemia. The disease is self-limited; the infant dies in 3 to 5 days or completely recovers with no aftereffects. Treatment includes measures to correct shock, acidosis, and hypoxemia and use of continuous positive airway pressure to prevent alveolar collapse. Also called hyaline membrane disease, idiopathic respiratory distress syndrome. Compare adult respiratory distress syndrome.

Resting membrane potential (RMP) the transmembrane voltage that exists when the heart muscle is at rest.

Restrictive lung disorder restrictive respiratory disease is caused by conditions that limit lung expansion, such as fibrothorax, obesity, a neuromuscular disorder, kyphosis, scoliosis, spondylitis, or surgical removal of lung tissue. Pregnancy causes a self-limiting restrictive disease in the third trimester. Characteristics of restrictive respiratory disease are decreased forced expired vital capacity and total lung capacity, with increased work of breathing and inefficient exchange of gases. Acute restrictive conditions are the most common pulmonary cause of acute respiratory failure. Infectious diseases include pneumonia and tuberculosis.ucus. Physical therapy measures, such as postural drainage and breathing exercises, can also dislodge secretions. Broad-spectrum antibiotics may be used prophylactically.

Rhinitis inflammation of the mucous membranes of the nose, usually accompanied by swelling of the mucosa and a nasal discharge.

Rhonchus (*pl. rhonchi*) an abnormal sound heard on auscultation of an airway obstructed by thick secretions, muscular spasm, neoplasm, or external pressure. The continuous rumbling sound is more pronounced during expiration and characteristically clears on coughing, whereas gurgles do not.

Rima glottidis also called rima glottidis, true glottis. a slitlike opening between the true vocal cords (plica vocalis).

S

Semipermeable permitting diffusion or flow of some liquids or solutes but preventing the transmission of others, usually in reference to a membrane.

Septal cartilage a flat plate of cartilage in the lower anterior part of the nasal septum. Also called nsal cartilage.

Septic pertaining to infection or contamination.

Septicemia systemic infection in which pathogens are present in the circulating blood, having spread from an infection in any part of the body. It is diagnosed by culture of the blood and is vigorously treated with antibiotics. Characteristically septicemia causes fever, chill, hypotension, prostration, pain,

headache, nausea, or diarrhea. Also called *blood poisoning*.

Septum wall dividing two cavities.

Serotonin a potent vasoconstrictor that is present in platelets, gastrointestinal mucosa, mast cells, and carcinoid tumors.

Serum clear watery fluid, especially that moistening surfaces of serous membranes or exuded inflammation of any of those membranes; the fluid portion of the blood obtained after removal of the fibrin clot and blood cells; sometimes used as a synonym for antiserum.

Shunt to turn away from; to divert; an abnormal passage to divert flow from one route to another.

Shunt-like effect pulmonary capillary perfusion in excess of alveolar ventilation; commonly seen in patients with chronic obstructive lung disorders and alveolar-capillary diffusion defects. Also called *relative shunt*.

Sign an objective finding as perceived by an examiner, such as fever, a rash, or the whisper heard over the chest in pleural effusion. Many signs accompany symptoms; for example, erythema and a maculopapular rash are often seen with pruritus. Compare **symptom**.

Sinusitis an inflammation of one or more paranasal sinuses.

Slow vital capacity (SVC) the maximum volume of air that can be slowly exhaled after a maximal inspiration.

Smooth muscle muscle tissue that lacks cross-striations on its fibers, is involuntary in action, and is found principally in visceral organs.

Soft palate the structue composed of mucous membrane, muscular fibers, and mucous glands, suspended from the posterior border of the hard palate forming the roof of the mouth. When the soft palate rises, as in swallowing and in sucking, it separates the nasal cavity and the nasopharynx from the posterior part of the oral cavity and the oral part of the pharynx. The posterior border of the soft palate hangs like a curtain between the mouth and the pharynx. Suspended from it is the conical, pendulous, palatine uvula. Arching laterally from the base of the uvula are the two curved musculomembranous pillars of the fauces.

Somatic nerve nerve that innervates somatic structures, that is, those constituting the body wall and extremities.

Somnolence the condition of being sleepy or drowsy.

Spasm involuntary sudden movement or convulsive muscular contraction.

Sputum substance expelled by coughing or clearing the throat that may contain a variety of materials from the respiratory tract, including one or more of the following: cellular debris, mucus, blood, pus, caseous material, and microorganisms.

Stasis stagnation of normal flow of fluids, as of the blood, urine, or intestinal mechanism. A disorder in which the normal flow of a fluid through a vessel of the body is slowed or halted.

Stent a rod or threadlike device for supporting tubular structures during surgical anastomosis or for holding arteries open during angioplasty.

Stroke volume amount of blood ejected by the ventricle at each beat.

Subcutaneous under the skin.

Sulfonamide one of a large group of synthetic, bacteriostatic drugs that are effective in treating infections caused by many gram-negative and gram-positive microorganisms.

Superior situated above or oriented toward a higher place, as the head is superior to the torso.

Superior vena cava venous trunk draining blood from the head, neck, upper extremities, and chest.

Surfactant an agent, such as soap or detergent, dissolved in water to reduce its surface tension or the tension at the interface between the water and another liquid. Certain lipoproteins reduce the surface tension of pulmonary fluids, allowing the exchange of gases in the alveoli of the lungs and contributing to the elasticity of the pulmonary tissue. Also called *pulmonary surfactant*.

Sympathetic nervous system a division of the autonomic nervous system that accelerates the heart rate, constricts blood vessels, and raises blood pressure.

Sympathomimetic producing effects resembling those resulting from stimulation of the sympathetic nervous system.

Symptom a subjective indication of a disease or a change in condition as perceived by the patient. For example, the halo symptom of glaucoma is seen by the patient as colored rings around a single light source. Many symptoms are accompanied by objective signs, such as pruritus, which is often reported with erythema and a maculopapular eruption on the skin. Some symptoms may be objectively confirmed, such as numbness of the body part, which may be confirmed by absence of response to a pin prick. Compare **sign**.

Systemic pertaining to the whole body rather than to one of its parts.

Systemic reaction whole body response to a stimulus.

Systemic system the general blood circulation of the body, not including the lungs.

Systole that part of the heart cycle in which the heart is in contraction.

Systolic pressure maximum blood pressure; occurs during contraction of the ventricle.

T

Tachycardia an abnormal circulatory condition in which the myocardium contracts regularly but at a rate of greater than 100 beats per minute.

Tachypnea a rapid rate of breathing.

Tension pneumothorax the presence of air in the pleural space when pleural pressure exceeds alveolar pressure, caused by a rupture through the chest wall or lung parenchyma associated with the valvular opening. Air passes through the valve during coughing but cannot escape on exhalation. Unrelieved pneumothorax can lead to respiratory arrest.

The barometric pressure (PB) the pressure exerted by the weight of the atmosphere. The average atmospheric pressure at sea level is approximately 14.7 pounds per square inch. With increasing altitude the pressure decreases: at 30,000 feet, approximately the height of Mt. Everest, the air pressure is 4.3 pounds per square inch. Also called atmospheric pressure.

Thoracentesis the surgical perforation of the chest wall and pleural space with a needle to aspirate fluid for diagnostic or therapeutic purposes or to remove a specimen for biopsy. The procedure is usually performed using local anesthesia, with the patient in an upright position. Thoracentesis may be used to aspirate fluid to treat pleural effusion or to collect fluid samples for culture or examination. Also called thoracocentesis.

Thoracolumbar relating to the thoracic and lumbar portions of the vertebral column.

Thrombocyte combining form meaning "platelet": *thrombocytopenia, thrombocytosis.*

Tidal volume the volume of air that normally moves into and out of the lungs in one quiet breath; the measured inspired or expired volume of gas moved in one breath.

Tone that state of a body or any of its organs or parts in which the functions are healthy and normal.

Tongue the principal organ of the sense of taste that also assists in the mastication and deglutition of food. It is located in the floor of the mouth within the curve of the mandible. Its root is connected to the hyoid bone posteriorly. It is also connected to the epiglottis, soft palate, and pharynx. The apex of the tongue rests anteriorly against the lingual surfaces of the lower incisors. The mucous membrane connecting the tongue to the mandible reflects over the floor of the mouth to the lingual surface of the gingiva and in the midline of the floor is raised into a vertical fold. The dorsum of the tongue is divided into symmetric halves by a median sulcus, which ends posteriorly in the foramen cecum. A shallow sulcus terminalis runs from this foramen laterally and forward on either side to the margin of the organ. From the sulcus the anterior two thirds of the tongue are covered with papillae. The posterior third is smoother and contains numerous mucous glands and lymph follicles. The use of the tongue as an organ of speech is not anatomic but a secondary acquired characteristic.

Total lung capacity the maximum amount of air that the lung can accommodate.

Total oxygen delivery the total amount of oxygen delivered or transported to the peripheral tissues.

Transairway pressure the barometric pressure difference between the mouth pressure and the alveolar pressure.

Transmural pressure the pressure difference that occurs across the airway wall.

Transrespiratory pressure (Prs) the difference between the barometric (atmospheric) pressure (PB) and the alveolar pressure (Palv). Also called transairway pressure.

Transient passing especially quickly into and out of existence; passing through or by a place with only a brief stay.

Transpulmonary pressure the difference between the alveolar pressure and the pleural pressure.

Transthoracic pressure the difference between the alveolar pressure and the body surface pressure.

Tricuspid valve a valve with three main cusps situated between the right atrium and right ventricle of the heart. The tricuspid valve includes the ventral, dorsal, and medial cusps. The cusps are composed of strong fibrous tissue and are anchored to the papillary muscles of the right ventricle by several tendons. As the right and left ventricles relax during the diastolic phase of the heartbeat, the tricuspid valve opens, allowing blood to flow into the ventricle. In the systolic phase of the heartbeat, both blood-filled ventricles contract, pumping out their contents, while the tricuspid and mitral valves close to prevent any backflow.

Trimester one of the three periods of approximately 3 months into which pregnancy is divided.

True shunt see **absolute shunt**.

U

Unilateral renal agenesis failure of one of the kidneys to develop.

Upper airway the upper airways consist of the nose, oral cavity, pharynx, and larynx.

Uvula an opening in the arch connects the mouth with the oropharynx; the uvula is suspended from the middle of the posterior border of the arch.

V

Vagus nerve the tenth cranial nerve. It is a mixed nerve, having motor and sensory functions and a wider distribution than any of the other cranial nerves.

Vallecula epiglottica a furrow between the glossoepiglottic folds of each side of the posterior oropharynx. Also called (informal) vallecula.

Vascular relating to or containing blood vessels.

Vascular system the circulatory network composed of two major subdivisions: the systemic system and the pulmonary system.

Vasoconstriction decrease in the caliber of blood vessels.

Vasodilation widening of blood vessels, especially the small arteries and arterioles.

Vasomotor tone the state of vascular contraction.

Vein any one of the many vessels that convey blood from the capillaries as part of the pulmonary venous system, the systemic venous network, and the portal venous complex. Most of the veins of the body are systemic veins that convey blood from the whole body (except the lungs) to the right atrium of the heart. Each vein is a macroscopic structure enclosed in three layers of different kinds of tissue homologous with the layers of the heart. The outer tunica adventitia of each vein is homologous with the epicardium, the tunica media with the myocardium, and the tunica intima with the endocardium. Deep veins course through the more internal parts of the body, and superficial veins lie near the surface, where many of them are visible through the skin. Veins have thinner coatings and are less elastic than arteries and collapse when cut. They also contain semilunar valves at various intervals to control the direction of the blood flow back to the heart.

Venous pertaining to a vein or veins.

Venous admixture the mixing of shunted, non-reoxygenated blood with reoxygenated blood distal to the alveoli.

Venous return the amount of blood returning to the atria of the heart.

Ventilation the mechanical movement of air into and out of the lungs in a cyclic fashion. It is the mechanism by which oxygen is carried from the atmosphere to the alveoli and by which carbon dioxide is carried from the lungs to the atmosphere. Compare respiration.

Ventilation-perfusion ratio the relationship of the overall alveolar ventilation (L/min) to the overall pulmonary blood flow (L/min). The normal ventilation-perfusion ratio is 4:5, or 0.8.

Ventral pertaining to the anterior portion or front of the body.

Ventricle either of two lower chambers of the heart.

Venule any one of the small blood vessels that gather blood from the capillary plexuses and anastomose to form the veins.

Vestibule a space or a cavity that serves as the entrance to a passageway, such as the vestbule of the ear.

Viscera (*sing. viscus*) the internal organs enclosed within a body cavity, including the abdominal, thoracic, pelvic, and endocrine organs.

Viscosity stickiness or gumminess; internal friction resistance offered by a fluid to change of form or relative position of its particles due to attraction of molecules to each other.

Viscous sticky; gummy; gelatinous.

Vital capacity the maximum volume of air that can be exhaled after a maximal inspiration.

Volume percent (vol%) the number of milliliters (mL) of a substance contained in 100 mL of another substance. For example, under normal conditions there are about 20 mL of oxygen in every 100 mL of arterial blood—or 20 vol% oxygen.

Vomer the plow-shaped bone forming the posterior and inferior part of the nasal septum and having two surfaces and four borders.

W

Wenckebach phenomenon named for Karel F. Wenckebach, Dutch-Austrian physician (1864–1940), a form of second-degree atrioventricular block with a progressive beat-to-beat prolongation of the PR interval, finally resulting in a nonconducting P wave. At this point the sequence recurs and is referred to as Wenckebach periodicity. Also called *Mobitz I* and *type I AV block.*

Wheeze a form of rhonchi characterized by a high-pitched or low-pitched musical quality. It is caused by a high-velocity flow of air passing through a narrowed airway and is heard during both inspiration and expiration. It may be caused by bronchospasm, inflammation, or obstruction of the airway by a tumor or foreign body. Wheezes are associated with asthma and chronic bronchitis. Unilateral wheezes are characteristic of bronchogenic carcinoma, foreign bodies, and inflammatory lesions. In asthma expiratory wheezing is more common, although inspiratory and expiratory wheezes are heard. Compare **crackle**, **rhonchus**.

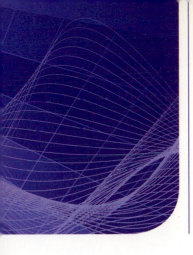

Appendix I

Symbols and Abbreviations

The symbols and abbreviations listed below are commonly used in respiratory physiology.

Primary Symbols

Gas Symbols

P	Pressure
V	Gas volume
$\dot{V}$	Gas volume per unit of time, or flow
F	Fractional concentration of gas

Blood Symbols

Q	Blood volume
$\dot{Q}$	Blood flow
C	Content in blood
S	Saturation

Secondary Symbols

Gas Symbols

I	Inspired
E	Expired
A	Alveolar
T	Tidal
D	Dead space

Blood Symbols

a	Arterial
c	Capillary
v	Venous
$\bar{v}$	Mixed venous

Abbreviations

Lung Volume

VC	Vital capacity
IC	Inspiratory capacity
IRV	Inspiratory reserve volume
ERV	Expiratory reserve volume
FRC	Functional residual capacity
RV	Residual volume
TLC	Total lung capacity

continued

continued

RV/TLC(%)	Residual volume to total lung capacity ratio, expressed as a percentage
V_T	Tidal volume
$\dot{V}_A$	Alveolar ventilation
V_D	Dead space ventilation
V_L	Actual lung volume

Spirometry

FVC	Forced vital capacity with maximally forced expiratory effort
FEV_T	Forced expiratory volume timed
$FEF_{200-1200}$	Average rate of airflow between 200–1200 mL of the FVC
$FEF_{25\%-75\%}$	Forced expiratory flow during the middle half of the FVC (formerly called the maximal midexpiratory flow or MMF)
PEFR	Maximum flow rate that can be achieved
$\dot{V}_{max\,x}$	Forced expiratory flow related to the actual volume of the lungs as denoted by subscript x, which refers to the amount of lung volume remaining when measurement is made
MVV	Maximal voluntary ventilation as the volume of air expired in a specified interval

Mechanics

C_L	Lung compliance; volume change per unit of pressure change
R_{aw}	Airway resistance; pressure per unit of flow

Diffusion

DL_{CO}	Diffusing capacity of carbon monoxide (CO)

Blood Gases

PA_{O_2}	Alveolar oxygen tension
Pc_{O_2}	Pulmonary capillary oxygen tension
Pa_{O_2}	Arterial oxygen tension
$P\bar{v}_{O_2}$	Mixed venous oxygen tension
PA_{CO_2}	Alveolar carbon dioxide tension
Pc_{CO_2}	Pulmonary capillary carbon dioxide tension
Pa_{CO_2}	Arterial carbon dioxide tension
Sa_{O_2}	Arterial oxygen saturation
$S\bar{v}_{O_2}$	Mixed venous oxygen saturation
pH	Negative logarithm of the H^+ concentration used as a positive number
HCO_3^-	Plasma bicarbonate concentration
mEq/L	The number of grams of solute dissolved in a normal solution
Ca_{O_2}	Oxygen content of arterial blood

Cc_{O_2}	Oxygen content of capillary blood
$C\bar{v}_{O_2}$	Oxygen content of mixed venous blood
$\dot{V}/\dot{Q}$	Ventilation-perfusion ratio
$\dot{Q}s/\dot{Q}_T$	Shunt fraction
$\dot{Q}_T$	Total cardiac output

Oxygen Transport Studies

$C(a - \bar{v})_{O_2}$	Arterial-venous oxygen content difference
$\dot{V}_{O_2}$	Oxygen consumption (oxygen uptake)
O_2ER	Oxygen extraction ratio
D_{O_2}	Total oxygen delivery

Hemodynamic Measurement Abbreviations

Direct Measurements

CVP	Central venous pressure
RAP	Right atrial pressure
$\overline{PAP}$	Mean pulmonary artery pressure
PCWP	Pulmonary capillary wedge pressure
PAW	Pulmonary artery wedge
PAO	Pulmonary artery occlusion
CO	Cardiac output

Indirect Measurements

SV	Stroke volume
SVI	Stroke volume index
CI	Cardiac index
RVSWI	Right ventricular stroke work index
LVSWI	Left ventricular stroke work index
PVR	Pulmonary vascular resistance
SVR	Systemic vascular resistance

Metric Measurement Abbreviations

Linear Measurements

m	meter
cm	centimeter ($m \times 10^{-2}$)
mm	millimeter ($m \times 10^{-3}$)
μm	micrometer ($m \times 10^{-6}$)

Volume Measurements

L	liter
dL	deciliter (1×10^{-1})
mL	milliliter (1×10^{-3})
μL	microliter (1×10^{-6})
nL	nanoliter (1×10^{-9})

Weight Measurements

g	gram
mg	milligram ($g \times 10^{-3}$)
μg	microgram ($g \times 10^{-6}$)
ng	nanogram ($g \times 10^{-9}$)

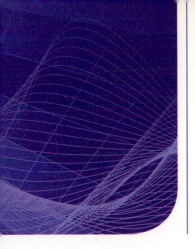

Units of Measurement

Metric Length

Meter	Centimeter	Millimeter	Micrometer	Nanometer
1	100	1000	1,000,000	1,000,000,000
.01	1	10	10,000	10,000,000
.001	.1	1	1000	1,000,000
.000001	.0001	.001	1	1000
.000000001	.0000001	.000001	.001	1

Metric Volumes

Liter	Centiliter	Milliliter	Microliter	Nanoliter
1	100	1000	1,000,000	1,000,000,000
.01	1	10	10,000	10,000,000
.001	.1	1	1000	1,000,000
.000001	.0001	.001	1	1000
.000000001	.0000001	.000001	.001	1

Metric Weight

Grams	Centigrams	Milligrams	Micrograms	Nanograms
1	100	1000	1,000,000	1,000,000,000
.01	1	10	10,000	10,000,000
.001	.1	1	1000	1,000,000
.000001	.0001	.001	1	1000
.000000001	.0000001	.000001	.001	1

Weight Conversions
(Metric and Avoirdupois)

Grams	Kilograms	Ounces	Pounds
1	.001	.0353	.0022
1000	1	35.3	2.2
28.35	.02835	1	$\frac{1}{16}$
454.5	.4545	16	1

Weight Conversions
(Metric and Apothecary)

Grams	Milligrams	Grains	Drams	Ounces	Pounds
1	1000	15.4	.2577	.0322	.00268
.001	1	.0154	.00026	.0000322	.00000268
.0648	64.8	1	$\frac{1}{60}$	$\frac{1}{480}$	$\frac{1}{5760}$
3.888	3888	60	1	$\frac{1}{8}$	$\frac{1}{96}$
31.1	31104	480	8	1	$\frac{1}{12}$
373.25	373248	5760	96	12	1

Approximate Household
Measurement Equivalents (Volume)

	1 tsp =	5 mL
	1 tbsp = 3 tsp =	15 mL
	1 fl oz = 2 tbsp = 6 tsp =	30 mL
1 cup =	8 fl oz =	240 mL
1 pt = 2 cups =	16 fl oz =	480 mL
1 qt = 2 pt = 4 cups =	32 fl oz =	960 mL
1 gal = 4 qt = 8 pt = 16 cups =	128 fl oz =	3840 mL

Weight

Metric	Approximate Apothecary Equivalents
Grams	**Grains**
.0002	$\frac{1}{300}$
.0003	$\frac{1}{200}$
.0004	$\frac{1}{150}$
.0005	$\frac{1}{120}$
.0006	$\frac{1}{100}$
.001	$\frac{1}{60}$
.002	$\frac{1}{30}$
.005	$\frac{1}{12}$
.010	$\frac{1}{6}$
.015	$\frac{1}{4}$
.025	$\frac{3}{8}$
.030	$\frac{1}{2}$
.050	$\frac{3}{4}$
.060	1
.100	$1\frac{1}{2}$
.120	2
.200	3
.300	5
.500	$7\frac{1}{2}$
.600	10
1	15
2	30
4	60

Liquid Measure

Metric	Approximate Apothecary Equivalents
Milliliters	
1000	1 quart
750	$1\frac{1}{2}$ pints
500	1 pint
250	8 fluid ounces
200	7 fluid ounces
100	$3\frac{1}{2}$ fluid ounces
50	$1\frac{3}{4}$ fluid ounces

continued

Liquid Measure (Continued)

Metric	Approximate Apothecary Equivalents
Milliliters	
30	1 fluid ounce
15	4 fluid drams
10	$2\frac{1}{2}$ fluid drams
8	2 fluid drams
5	$1\frac{1}{4}$ fluid drams
4	1 fluid dram
3	45 minims
2	30 minims
1	15 minims
0.75	12 minims
0.6	10 minims
0.5	8 minims
0.3	5 minims
0.25	4 minims
0.2	3 minims
0.1	$1\frac{1}{2}$ minims
0.06	1 minim
0.05	$\frac{3}{4}$ minim
0.03	$\frac{1}{2}$ minim

Volume Conversions (Metric and Apothecary)

Milliliters	Minims	Fluid Drams	Fluid Ounces	Pints
1	16.2	.27	.0333	.0021
.0616	1	$\frac{1}{60}$	$\frac{1}{480}$	$\frac{1}{7680}$
3.697	60	1	$\frac{1}{8}$	$\frac{1}{128}$
29.58	480	8	1	$\frac{1}{16}$
473.2	7680	128	16	1

Liters	Gallons	Quarts	Fluid Ounces	Pints
1	.2642	1.057	33.824	2.114
3.785	1	4	128	8
.946	$\frac{1}{4}$	1	32	2
.473	$\frac{1}{8}$	$\frac{1}{2}$	16	1
.0296	$\frac{1}{128}$	$\frac{1}{32}$	1	$\frac{1}{16}$

Length Conversions (Metric and English System)

Unit	Millimeters	Centimeters	Inches	Feet	Yards	Meters
1 Å =	$\frac{1}{10,000,000}$	$\frac{1}{100,000,000}$	$\frac{1}{254,000,000,000}$	$\frac{1}{3,050,000,000}$	$\frac{1}{9,140,000,000}$	$\frac{1}{10,000,000,000}$
1 nm =	$\frac{1}{1,000,000}$	$\frac{1}{10,000,000}$	$\frac{1}{25,400,000}$	$\frac{1}{305,000,000}$	$\frac{1}{914,000,000}$	$\frac{1}{1,000,000,000}$
1 μm =	$\frac{1}{1000}$	$\frac{1}{10,000}$	$\frac{1}{25,400}$	$\frac{1}{305,000}$	$\frac{1}{914,000}$	$\frac{1}{1,000,000}$
1 mm =	1.0	0.1	0.03937	0.00328	0.0011	0.001
1 cm =	10.0	1.0	0.3937	0.03281	0.0109	0.01
1 in. =	25.4	2.54	1.0	0.0833	0.0278	0.0254
1 ft =	304.8	30.48	12.0	1.0	0.333	0.3048
1 yd =	914.40	91.44	36.0	3.0	1.0	0.9144
1 m =	1000.0	100.0	39.37	3.2808	1.0936	1.0

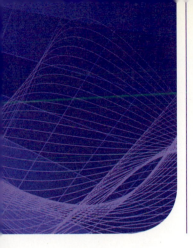

Appendix III

Poiseuille's Law

Poiseuille's Law for Flow Rearranged to a Simple Proportionality

$\dot{V} \simeq \Delta P r^4$, or rewritten as $\dfrac{\dot{V}}{r^4} \simeq \Delta P$.

When ΔP remains constant, then

$$\frac{\dot{V}_1}{r_1^{\,4}} \simeq \frac{\dot{V}_2}{r_2^{\,4}}$$

Example 1. If the radius (r_1) is decreased to one-half its previous radius $\left(r_2 = \frac{1}{2}r_1\right)$, then

$$\frac{\dot{V}_1}{r_1^{\,4}} \simeq \frac{\dot{V}_2}{\left(\frac{1}{2}r_1\right)^4}$$

$$\frac{\dot{V}_1}{r_1^{\,4}} \simeq \frac{\dot{V}_2}{\left(\frac{1}{16}r_1\right)^4}$$

$$(r_1^{\,4})\frac{\dot{V}_1}{r_1^{\,4}} \simeq (r_1^{\,4})\frac{\dot{V}_2}{\left(\frac{1}{16}\right)r_1^{\,4}}$$

$$\dot{V}_1 \simeq \frac{\dot{V}_2}{\frac{1}{16}}$$

$$\left(\frac{1}{16}\right)\dot{V}_1 \simeq \left(\frac{1}{16}\right)\frac{\dot{V}_2}{\frac{1}{16}}$$

$$\left(\frac{1}{16}\right)\dot{V}_1 \simeq \dot{V}_2$$

and gas flow $(\dot{V}_1)$ is reduced to $\frac{1}{16}$ its original flow rate $\left[\dot{V}_2 \simeq \left(\frac{1}{16}\right)\dot{V}_1\right]$.

Example 2. If the radius (r_1) is decreased by 16% $(r_2 = r_1 - 0.16r_1 = 0.84r_1)$, then

$$\frac{\dot{V}_1}{r_1^{\,4}} \simeq \frac{\dot{V}_2}{r_2^{\,4}}$$

$$\frac{\dot{V}_1}{r_1^{\,4}} \simeq \frac{\dot{V}_2}{(0.84r_1)^4}$$

$$\dot{V}_2 \simeq \frac{(0.84r_1)^4\,\dot{V}_1}{r_1^{\,4}}$$

639

$$\dot{V}_2 \simeq \frac{0.4979 \, r_1^4 \, \dot{V}_1}{r_1^4}$$

$$\dot{V}_2 \simeq \tfrac{1}{2}\dot{V}_1$$

and the flow rate ($\dot{V}_1$) would decrease to one-half the original flow rate ($\dot{V}_2 \simeq \tfrac{1}{2}\dot{V}_1$).

Poiseuille's Law for Pressure Rearranged to a Simple Proportionality

$P \simeq \dfrac{\dot{V}}{r^4}$, or rewritten as $P \cdot r^4 \simeq \dot{V}$

when $\dot{V}$ remains constant, then

$$P_1 \cdot r_1^4 \simeq P_2 \cdot r_2^4$$

Example 1. If the radius (r_1) is reduced to one-half its original radius $\left[r_2 = \left(\tfrac{1}{2}\right)r_1\right]$, then

$$P_1 \cdot r_1^4 \simeq P_2 \cdot r_2^4$$

$$P_1 \cdot r_1^4 \simeq P_2\left[\left(\tfrac{1}{2}\right)r_1\right]^4$$

$$P_1 \cdot r_1^4 \simeq P_2 \cdot \left(\tfrac{1}{16}\right)r_1^4$$

$$\frac{P_1 \cdot r_1^4}{r_1^4} \simeq \frac{P_2 \cdot \left(\tfrac{1}{16}\right)r_1^4}{r_1^4}$$

$$P_1 \simeq P_2 \cdot \left(\tfrac{1}{16}\right)$$

$$16\,P_1 \simeq 16 \cdot P_2 \cdot \left(\tfrac{1}{16}\right)$$

$$16\,P_1 \simeq P_2$$

and the pressure (P_1) will increase to 16 times its original level ($P_2 \simeq 16 \cdot P_1$).

Example 2. If the radius (r_1) is decreased by 16% ($r_2 = r_1 - 0.16r_1 = 0.84r_1$), then

$$P_1 \cdot r_1^4 \simeq P_2 \cdot r_2^4$$

$$P_1 \cdot r_1^4 \simeq P_2(0.4979)r_1^4$$

$$\frac{P_1 r_1^4}{(0.4979)r_1^4} = P_2$$

$$2\,P_1 = P_2$$

and the pressure (P_1) would increase to twice its original pressure ($P_2 \simeq 2 \cdot P_1$).

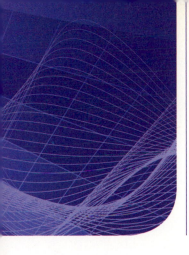

Appendix IV

DuBois Body Surface Chart

Directions

To find body surface of a patient, locate the height in inches (or centimeters) on Scale I and the weight in pounds (or kilograms) on Scale II and place a straight-edge (ruler) between these two points which will intersect Scale III at the patient's surface area.

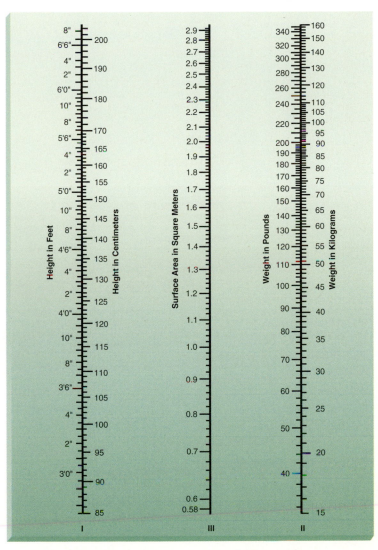

Adapted from DuBois and Eugene F. *Basal Metabolism in Health and Disease*. Philadelphia: Lea and Febiger, 1924.

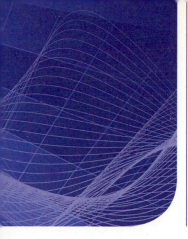

Appendix V

Cardiopulmonary Profile

A representative example of a cardiopulmonary profile sheet used to monitor the critically ill patient. Refer to Chapters 5, 6, and 7 for explanations of the various components presented in this sample cardiopulmonary profile. Areas shaded in pink represent normal ranges.

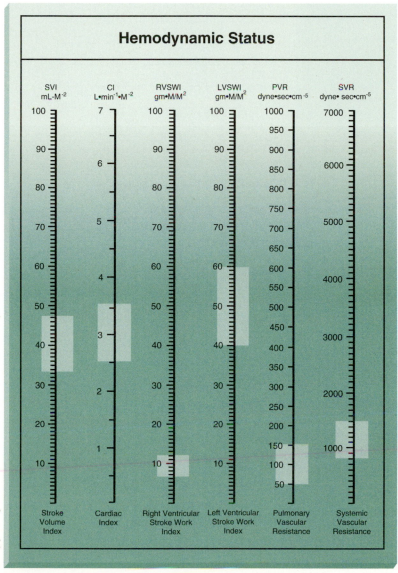

Hemodynamic Status

SVI mL-M^{-2}	CI L•min^{-1}•M^{-2}	RVSWI gm•M/M^2	LVSWI gm•M/M^2	PVR dyne•sec•cm^{-5}	SVR dyne• sec•cm^{-5}
Stroke Volume Index	Cardiac Index	Right Ventricular Stroke Work Index	Left Ventricular Stroke Work Index	Pulmonary Vascular Resistance	Systemic Vascular Resistance

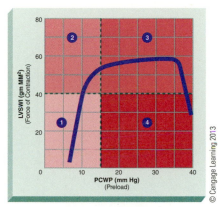

Quadrant 1: Hypovolemia
Quadrant 2: Optimal Function
Quadrant 3: Hypervolemia
Quadrant 4: Cardiac Failure

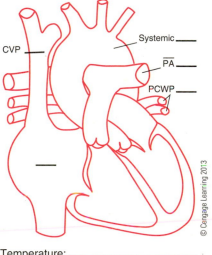

Temperature: _____

Heart Rate: _____

Cardiac Output: _____

Medications: _____

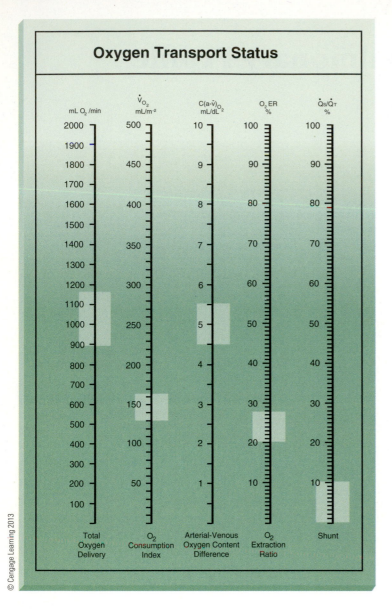

Oxygen Transport Status

mL O_2 /min	$\dot{V}_{O_2}$ mL/m^{-2}	$C(a\text{-}\bar{v})_{O_2}$ mL/dL^{-2}	O_2 ER %	$\dot{Q}_S/\dot{Q}_T$ %
2000	500	10	100	100
1900				
1800	450	9	90	90
1700				
1600	400	8	80	80
1500				
1400	350	7	70	70
1300				
1200	300	6	60	60
1100				
1000	250	5	50	50
900				
800	200	4	40	40
700				
600	150	3	30	30
500				
400	100	2	20	20
300				
200	50	1	10	10
100				

Total Oxygen Delivery | O_2 Consumption Index | Arterial-Venous Oxygen Content Difference | O_2 Extraction Ratio | Shunt

© Cengage Learning 2013

Blood Gas Values

pH _____

Pa_{CO_2} _____

HCO_3^- _____

Pa_{O_2} _____ $P\bar{v}_{O_2}$ _____

Sa_{O_2} _____% $S\bar{v}_{O_2}$ _____%

FI_{O_2} _____   Hb _____

Mode(s) of Ventilatory

Support: _____

_____

_____

_____

_____

_____

Shaded areas represent normal ranges.

Patient's Name _____

Date _____

Time _____

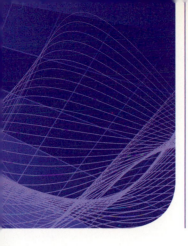

Appendix VI

$P_{CO_2}/HCO_3^-/pH$ Nomogram

Nomogram — Slide 1

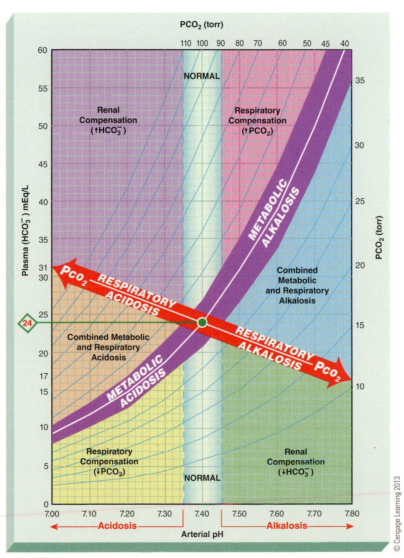

© Cengage Learning 2013

Cut out the above two-sided nomogram and have it laminated for use as a handy, pocket-sized reference tool. Refer to Chapter 7 on how to use the nomogram in the clinical setting.

Nomogram — Slide 2

pH, PCO_2, HCO_3 RELATIONSHIP

$PaCO_2$		pH	HCO_3
100	≈	7.10	30
80	≈	7.20	28
60	≈	7.30	26
40	≈	7.40	24
30	≈	7.50	22
20	≈	7.60	20
10	≈	7.70	18

EX: ACUTE CHANGES ON CVF

AVF on CVF		CVF Baseline		AAH on CVF
		pH		
7.21	←	7.39	→	7.53
		$PaCO_2$		
110	←	76	→	51
		HCO_3		
43	←	41	→	37
		PaO_2		
34	←	61	→	46

CVF: Chronic ventilatory failure
AVF: Acute ventilatory failure
AAH: Acute alveolar hyperventilation

PaO_2 & SaO_2 RELATIONSHIP

	PaO_2	SaO_2
Normal	97	97
Range	>80–100	>95
Hypoxemia	<80	<95
Mild	60–80	90–95
Moderate	40–60	75–90
Severe	<40	<75

PaO_2 & SaO_2 RELATIONSHIP

PO_2 30 ≈ 60% saturated
PO_2 40 ≈ 75% saturated
PO_2 50 ≈ 85% saturated
PO_2 60 ≈ 90% saturated

FIO_2 & PaO_2 RELATIONSHIP

FIO_2		PaO_2
0.30	≈	150
0.40	≈	200
0.50	≈	250
0.80	≈	400
1.00	≈	500

O_2 TRANSPORT

	Normal Values
DO_2	1000 ml O_2/min
$\dot{V}O_2$	250 ml O_2/min
$C(a-\bar{v})O_2$	5 vol%
O_2ER	25%
$S\bar{v}O_2$	75%

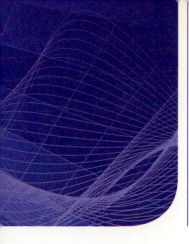

Appendix VII

Calculating Heart Rate by Counting the Number of Large ECG Squares

Distance between Two QRS Complexes (no. of large squares)	Estimated Heart Rate (per min)
1	300
1½	200
2	150
2½	125
3	100
3½	85
4	75
4½	65
5	60
5½	55
6	50
6½	45

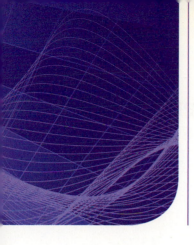

Answers to Review Questions in Text

The Anatomy and Physiology of the Respiratory System

Chapter 1

1. A	8. D	15. D
2. D	9. D	16. A
3. A	10. B	17. B
4. B	11. C	18. C
5. A	12. C	19. B
6. D	13. C	20. A
7. A	14. A	

Ventilation

Chapter 2

1. A	12. D
2. A	13. D
3. D	14. 6375 mL
4. D	15. Part I: 79 mL/cm H_2O
5. C	Part II: 70 mL/cm H_2O
6. C	Part III: decreasing
7. B	16. D
8. B	17. C
9. D	18. A
10. B	19. D
11. A	20. A

Clinical Application Questions

Case 1

1. Caved inward
2. Partially collapsed; decreased
3. Positive pressure; moved outward; resting level

Case 2

1. Low
2. Large; little or no
3. Tracheobronchial tree constriction; excessive airway secretions
4. Longer; long
5. Decreases

Pulmonary Function Measurements

Chapter 3

1. D	5. C	9. B
2. B	6. B	10. B
3. D	7. D	11. A
4. D	8. B	

Clinical Application Questions

Case 1

1. Personal best PEFR

2. Effort-independent flow; dynamic compression; equal pressure point

3. Closer to the alveoli

Case 2

1. FVC; FEV_1; $FEF_{200-1200}$; PEFR

2. VC; RV; FRC

3. Increased; increased

The Diffusion of Pulmonary Gases

Chapter 4

1. C	5. B	9. A
2. B	6. C	10. B
3. A	7. C	
4. D	8. D	

Clinical Application Questions

Case 1

1. Also increase

2. Decreased

3. $P_{A_{O_2}}$; P_1

4. Pressure at the level of the alveoli; $F_{I_{O_2}}$ to 0.4

Case 2

1. Thickness

2. P_A (P_1)

3. T (thickness)

4. Increased oxygen concentration (P_1)

The Anatomy and Physiology of the Circulatory System

Chapter 5

1. D	6. D	11. B
2. C	7. B	12. D
3. B	8. B	13. D
4. C	9. B	14. D
5. A	10. A	15. A

Clinical Application Questions

Case 1

1. Baroreceptors; decreased

2. Blood pressure (78/42 mm Hg)

3. Decreases

4. (1) Lowering the patient's head and elevating her legs, which used the effects of gravity to move blood to the patient's lungs; (2) replacing the volume of blood lost by administering Ringer's lactated solution through the patient's intravenous tube

Case 2

1. High blood pressure of 214/106 mm Hg

2. Rales; rhonchi

3. Decreased Pa_{O_2} of 48 torr

4. Distended neck veins and peripheral edema

5. Afterloads

Oxygen and Carbon Dioxide Transport

Chapter 6

1. A	5. B	9. D
2. C	6. D	10. D
3. C	7. D	
4. B	8. C	

11. Case Study: Automobile Collision Victim

Based on the questions asked and the information provided, the patient's $P_{A_{O_2}}$, $C_{C_{O_2}}$, and $C\bar{v}_{O_2}$ should first be calculated.

$$P_{A_{O_2}} = (BP - P_{H_2O}) F_{I_{O_2}} - Pa_{CO_2} (1.25)$$
$$= (745 - 47) \, 0.50 - 38 \, (1.25)$$
$$= (698) \, 0.50 - 47.5$$
$$= 349 - 47.5$$

Answer = 301.5 mm Hg

$$C_{C_{O_2}} = (Hb \times 1.34) + P_{A_{O_2}} \times 0.003$$
$$= (11 \times 1.34) + 301.5 \times 0.003$$
$$= 14.74 + 0.904$$

Answer = 15.64 vol% O_2

$$Ca_{O_2} = (Hb \times 1.34 \times Sa_{O_2}) + (Pa_{O_2} \times 0.003)$$
$$= (11 \times 1.34 \times 0.90) + (60 \times 0.003)$$
$$= 13.266 + 0.18$$

Answer = 13.446 vol% O_2

$$C\bar{v}_{O_2} = (Hb \times 1.34 \times S\bar{v}_{O_2}) + (P\bar{v}_{O_2} \times 0.003)$$
$$= (11 \times 1.34 \times 0.65) + (35 \times 0.003)$$
$$= 9.581 + 0.105$$

Answer = 9.686 vol% O_2

With the above information and the data provided in the question, the following can now be calculated:

A. Total oxygen = $\dot{Q}_T \times Ca_{O_2} \times 10$
Delivery = $6 \, L \times 13.446$ vol% $\times 10$
$= 806.76$ mL $O_{2/min}$

Answer: 806.76 mL O_2/min

B. Arterial-venous oxygen content difference $C(a - \bar{v})_{O_2}$
$$C(a - \bar{v})_{O_2} = Ca_{O_2} - C\bar{v}_{O_2}$$
$$= 13.446 - 9.686$$
$$= 3.760 \text{ vol% } O_2$$
Answer: 3.76 vol% O_2

C. Intrapulmonary shunting ($\dot{Q}_S/\dot{Q}_T$)

$$(\dot{Q}_S/\dot{Q}_T) = \frac{C_{C_{O_2}} - Ca_{O_2}}{C_{C_{O_2}} - C\bar{v}_{O_2}}$$

$$= \frac{15.644 - 13.446}{15.664 - 9.686}$$

$$= \frac{2.198}{5.958}$$

$$= 0.368\%$$
Answer: 36.8%

D. Oxygen consumption ($\dot{V}_{O_2}$)
$$\dot{V}_{O_2} = \dot{Q}_T \, [C(a - \bar{v})_{O_2} \times 10]$$
$$= 6L \times 3.760 \times 10$$
$$= 225.6 \text{ mL } O_2/min$$
Answer: 225.6 mL O_2/min

E. Oxygen extraction ratio = $\dfrac{Ca_{O_2} - C\bar{v}_{O_2}}{Ca_{O_2}}$

$$= \frac{13.446 - 9.686}{13.446}$$

$$= \frac{3.760}{13.446}$$

$$= 0.279$$

Answer: 27.9%

Clinical Application Questions

Case 1

1. Unconscious, cyanotic, and hypotensive, and her skin was cool and damp to the touch

2. D_{O_2}, O_2ER

3. 68%

Case 2

1. Decreased; increased

2. Increased; increased; decreased

3. Right

4. Lower

Acid–Base Balance and Regulation

Chapter 7

1. D	12. B
2. B	13. 9 mEq/L
3. A	14. Both metabolic and respiratory acidosis
4. C	
5. D	15. Acute alveolar hyperventilation with partial renal compensation, or partially compensated respiratory alkalosis
6. D	
7. D	
8. D	
9. D	
10. B	
11. A	

Clinical Application Questions

Case 1

1. Impaired
2. Left
3. Cherry red
4. Increased the total oxygen delivery
5. (1) Low Pa_{CO_2}; (2) loss of stomach acid
6. Decreased Pa_{CO_2}

Case 2

1. Acids
2. Low Pa_{O_2} (38 torr), which produces lactic acids
3. Aggressive ventilation
4. Higher

Ventilation-Perfusion Relationships

Chapter 8

1. D	3. D	5. B
2. C	4. D	

Clinical Application Questions

Case 1

1. Ineffective
2. Wasted or dead space
3. Decreased; decreased

Case 2

1. Low
2. Fall
3. A. decreased; B. increased; C. decreased; D. increased; E. decreased

Control of Ventilation

Chapter 9

1. C	3. D	5. D
2. B	4. A	6. D

7. D	9. D
8. C	10. B

Clinical Application Questions

Case 1

1. True
2. False
3. Peripheral chemoreceptors
4. Decreases
5. An increased Pa_{CO_2} level, the formation of H^+, and the stimulation of the central chemoreceptors, which, in turn, increases the individual's ventilatory rate

Case 2

1. Ketone acids
2. Peripheral chemoreceptors
3. No
4. The decreased Pa_{CO_2} worked to offset the patient's acidic pH level caused by the increased ketone acids.

Fetal Development and the Cardiopulmonary System

Chapter 10

1. B	5. A	9. D
2. B	6. B	10. D
3. A	7. D	
4. D	8. D	

Clinical Application Questions

Case 1

1. 28th
2. Infant respiratory distress syndrome (IRDS)
3. Interstitial edema; intra-alveolar edema; intra-alveolar hemorrhage; alveolar consolidation; intra-alveolar hyaline membrane formation; atelectasis

4. All the conditions listed in answer No. 3 cause the alveolar-capillary membrane's thickness to increase.

5. Cyanosis, increased respiratory rate and heart rate, and decreased Pa_{O_2}; nasal flaring, intercostal retractions, exhalation grunting, bilateral crackles, and ground-glass appearance and air bronchogram on the chest X-ray

6. Because the baby's Pa_{O_2} was less than 45 torr shortly after he was born, the ductus arteriosus remained patent. As the infant's Pa_{O_2} increased, the ductus arteriosus closed and the signs and symptoms associated with PPHN disappeared.

Case 2

1. The ability of the fetus to absorb oxygen, nutrients, and other substances and excrete carbon dioxide and other wastes was interrupted. Complete separation brings about immediate death of the fetus.

2. Abdominal pain, uterine tenderness, uterine contraction, and hemorrhage

3. Shock and death can occur in minutes; cesarean section

Aging and the Cardiopulmonary System

Chapter 11

1. D	5. D	9. D
2. D	6. C	10. C
3. D	7. D	
4. B	8. D	

Electrophysiology of the Heart

Chapter 12

1. A	5. B	9. B
2. C	6. B	10. D
3. C	7. D	
4. A	8. A	

The Standard 12-ECG Lead System

Chapter 13

1. D	5. B	9. A
2. A	6. B	10. D
3. D	7. C	
4. D	8. C	

ECG Interpretation

Chapter 14

1. QRS duration: *0.06 second* QT duration: *0.40 second*

   Ventricular rate and rhythm: *86/min*

   Atrial rate and rhythm: *86/min*

   PR interval: *0.16 second*

   Interpretation: *sinus rhythm 86/min with one PAC (6th complex)*

2. QRS duration: *0.08 second* QT duration: *cannot determine*

   Ventricular rate and rhythm: *75–150/min*

   Atrial rate and rhythm: *cannot determine*

   PR interval: *none*

   Interpretation: *atrial fibrillation, ventricular rate 75–150/min*

3. QRS duration: *0.10 second* QT duration: *0.44 second*

   Ventricular rate and rhythm: *50/min regular*

   Atrial rate and rhythm: *50/min regular*

   PR interval: *0.16–0.20 second*

   Interpretation: *sinus bradycardia at 40/min*

4. QRS duration: *0.40–0.10 second* QT duration: *cannot determine*

   Ventricular rate and rhythm: *86–100/min*

   Atrial rate and rhythm: *300*

   PR interval: *none*

   Interpretation: *atrial flutter, ventricular rate 86–100/min*

5. QRS duration: *0.08 second* QT duration: *0.36 second*

   Ventricular rate and rhythm: *86/min*

   Atrial rate and rhythm: *75/min*

   PR interval: *0.24 second*

   Interpretation: *first-degree AV block*

6. QRS duration: *0.12 second* QT duration: *0.32 second*

   Ventricular rate and rhythm: *168/min regular*

   Atrial rate and rhythm: *cannot determine*

   PR interval: *cannot determine*

   Interpretation: *ventricular tachycardia at 168/min*

7. QRS duration: *0.08 second* QT duration: *0.28 second*

   Ventricular rate and rhythm: *150/min regular*

   Atrial rate and rhythm: *150/min regular*

   PR interval: *0.16 second*

   Interpretation: *sinus tachycardia at 150/min*

8. QRS duration: *cannot determine* QT duration: *cannot determine*

   Ventricular rate and rhythm: *cannot determine*

   Atrial rate and rhythm: *cannot determine*

   PR interval: *cannot determine*

   Interpretation: *ventricular fibrillation*

9. QRS duration: *0.08 second* QT duration: *0.38 second*

   Ventricular rate and rhythm: *60/min*

   Atrial rate and rhythm: *60/min*

   PR interval: *0.16 second*

   Interpretation: *sinus ventricular rate at 60/min with a PAC (last complex)*

10. QRS duration: *0.06 second* QT duration: *0.32 second*

    Ventricular rate and rhythm: *125/regular*

    Atrial rate and rhythm: *125/regular*

    PR interval: *0.16 second*

    Interpretation: *sinus tachycardia at 125/min with frequent uniform PVCs*

Hemodynamic Measurements

Chapter 15

1. F	6. G	11. D
2. E	7. J	12. D
3. A	8. B	13. D
4. K	9. D	14. D
5. D	10. I	15. A

Clinical Application Questions

Case 1

1. The SVR (peripheral vascular resistance) to increase

2. Nitroprusside is a vasodilator. It was used to reduce the patient's afterload.

3. As the patient's SVR decreased in response to the nitroprusside, the left ventricular afterload also decreased. This action in turn allowed blood to be more readily ejected from the left ventricle.

Case 2

1. 5 cm H_2O was the PEEP level that produced the least depression of cardiac output and the maximum total oxygen delivery.

2. Profile 1:
   $Ca_{O_2} = (Hb \times 1.34 \times Sa_{O_2}) + (Pa_{O_2} \times 0.003)$
   $= (15 \times 1.35 \times 0.91) + (57 \times 0.003)$
   $= (20.1 \times 0.91) = 0.17$
   $= 18.29 + 0.17$
   $= 18.46$

Profile 2:
$$Ca_{O_2} = (Hb \times 1.34 \times Sa_{O_2}) + (Pa_{O_2} \times 0.003)$$
$$= (15 \times 1.35 \times 0.9) + (61 \times 0.003)$$
$$= (20.1 \times 0.91) = 0.18$$
$$= 18.09 + 0.18$$
$$= 18.27$$

Profile 1:
$$D_{O_2} = \dot{Q}_T \times (Ca_{O_2} \times 10)$$
$$= 3.83 \times (18.46 \times 10)$$
$$= 3.83 \times 184.6$$
$$= 707 \text{ mL } O_2/min$$

Profile 2:
$$D_{O_2} = \dot{Q}_T \times (Ca_{O_2} \times 10)$$
$$= 3.1 \times (18.27 \times 10)$$
$$= 3.1 \times 182.7$$
$$= 566 \text{ mL } O_2/min$$

A PEEP of 5 cm H_2O resulted in a D_{O_2} of 707 mL O_2/min. A PEEP of 10 cm H_2O resulted in a D_{O_2} of 566 mL O_2/min. The "best PEEP" in this case was 5 cm H_2O, which resulted in a D_{O_2} that was 141 mL O_2/min more than the PEEP of 10 cm H_2O.

Renal Failure and Its Effects on the Cardiopulmonary System

Chapter 16

1. D	5. C	9. B
2. B	6. D	10. D
3. B	7. D	
4. D	8. B	

Clinical Application Questions

Case 1

1. The patient's left ventricular failure (a prerenal abnormality)

2. A sharp reduction in urine output

3. Because of increased H^+ and K^+ ion levels and the loss of HCO_3^-

4. Fluid accumulation in the patient's lungs and extremities, causing swelling in the patient's ankles, hands, and eyelids; white fluffy patches visible on the patient's chest X-ray; Pa_{O_2} of 64 torr

Case 2

1. Hypovolemia

2. Inflammation of the tracheobronchial tree, bronchospasm, excessive bronchial secretions and mucous plugging, decreased mucosal ciliary transport mechanism, atelectasis, alveolar edema, and frothy secretions

3. White fluffy densities throughout both fields (X-ray), and the low Pa_{O_2} of 47 torr

Sleep Physiology and Its Relationship to the Cardiopulmonary System

Chapter 17

1. E	5. A	9. A
2. C	6. B	10. A
3. B	7. B	
4. D	8. B	

Matching

1. D	3. A	5. C
2. E	4. B	

Clinical Application Questions

Case 1

1. 10, 10	3. True
2. True	

Exercise and Its Effects on the Cardiopulmonary System

Chapter 18

1. B	5. C	9. A
2. D	6. B	10. D
3. D	7. D	
4. D	8. D	

High Altitude and Its Effects on the Cardiopulmonary System

Chapter 19

1. D	5. D	9. True
2. D	6. True	10. False
3. D	7. False	
4. B	8. True	

High-Pressure Environments and Their Effects on the Cardiopulmonary System

Chapter 20

1. C	5. D	9. True
2. B	6. True	10. True
3. D	7. True	
4. D	8. False	

Bibliography

General Anatomy and Physiology

Applegate E (2011). *The Anatomy and Physiology Learning System* (4th ed.). Philadelphia, PA: Saunders/Elsevier.

Colbert BJ, Ankney J, Lee KT (2010). *Anatomy and Physiology for Health Professionals* (2nd ed). Upper Saddle River, NJ: Prentice Hall.

Drake RL, Vogl WA, Mitchell AWM (2010). *Gray's Anatomy for Students* (2nd ed.). Philadelphia, PA: Churchill/Livingstone/Elsevier.

Marieb EN, Hoehn K (2010). *Human Anatomy and Physiology* (8th ed.). Redwood City, CA: Pearson-Benjamin Cummings.

Martini FH, Nath JL (2008). *Fundamentals of Anatomy and Physiology* (7th ed.). Redwood City, CA: Pearson-Benjamin Cummings.

Mason RJ, Broaddus CV, Martin TR, King TE, Schraufnagel DE, Murray JF, Nadel JA (Eds.) (2010). *Murray and Nadel's Textbook of Respiratory Medicine* (5th ed.). Philadelphia, PA: Saunders/Elsevier.

Netter FH (2010). *Atlas of Human Anatomy* (5th ed.). Philadephia, PA: Saunders/Elsevier.

Patton KT, Thibodeau GA (2008). *Structure & Function of the Body* (13th ed). St. Louis, MO: Mosby/Elsevier.

Patton KT, Thibodeau GA (2010). *Anatomy & Physiology* (7th ed.). St. Louis, MO: Mosby/Elsevier.

Saladin KS (2009). *Anatomy and Physiology: The Unity of Form and Function* (5th ed.). New York: McGraw-Hill.

Seeley RR, Stephens TD, Tate P (2006). *Anatomy and Physiology* (7th ed.). New York: McGraw-Hill.

Shier DN, Butler JL, Lewis R (2009). *Hole's Human Anatomy Physiology* (12th ed.). New York: McGraw-Hill.

Solomon EP (2008). *Introduction to Human Anatomy and Physiology* (3rd ed.). Philadelphia, PA: Saunders/Elsevier.

Standring S (2009). *Gray's Anatomy—The Anatomic Basis of Clinical Practice* (40th ed.). Philadelphia, PA: Churchill/Livingstone/Elsevier

Tortora GJ, Nielsen M (2008). *Principles of Anatomy and Physiology* (11th ed.). New York: John Wiley Sons.

Cardiopulmonary Anatomy and Physiology

Beachey W (2007). *Respiratory Care Anatomy and Physiology: Foundations for Clinical Practice* (2nd ed.) St. Louis, MO: Mosby/Elsevier.

Comroe JH (1974). *Physiology of Respiration* (2nd ed.). Chicago: Year Book Medical Publishers.

Conover MH, Zalis EG (2003). *Understanding Electrocardiography* (8th ed.). St. Louis, MO: Mosby/Elsevier.

Cottrell, GP (2001). *Cardiopulmonary Anatomy and Physiology for Respiratory Care Practitioners*. Philadelphia, PA: FA Davis.

Hicks GH (2000). *Cardiopulmonary Anatomy and Physiology.* Philadelphia, PA: Saunders/Elsevier.

Lewis KM, Handal KA (2000). *Sensible ECG Analysis.* Clifton Park, NY: Delmar, Cengage Learning.

Levitzky MG (2007). (Lange Pulmonary Physiology) *Pulmonary Physiology* (7th ed.). New York: McGraw-Hill Health Professions Division.

Murray JF (1986). *The Normal Lung* (2nd ed.). Philadelphia, PA: Saunders/Elsevier.

Murray JG, Nadel JA (2005). *Textbook of Respiratory Medicine* (4th ed.). Philadelphia, PA: Saunders/Elsevier.

Slonim NB, Hamilton LH (1987). *Respiratory Physiology* (5th ed.). St. Louis, MO: Mosby/Elsevier.

West JB (2008). *Respiratory Physiology: The Essentials* (8th ed.). Philadelphia, PA: Lippincott Williams and Wilkins.

Hemodynamics

Darovic GO (2002). *Hemodynamic Monitoring: Invasive and Noninvasive Clinical Applications* (3rd ed.) Philadelphia, PA: Saunders/Elsevier.

Darovic GO (2004). *Handbook of Hemodynamic Monitoring,* (2nd ed.) Philadelphia, PA: Saunders/Elsevier.

Fawcett JAD (2006). *Hemodynamic Monitoring Made Easy.* St. Louis, MO: Bailliere Tindall.

Hodges RK, Garrett K, Chernecky CC, Schumacher L (2005). *Real World Nursing Survival Guide: Hemodynamic Monitoring,* Philadelphia, PA: Saunders/Elsevier.

Leeper B (2006). *Monitoring and Hemodynamics: An Issue of Critical Care Nursing Clinics.* Philadelphia, PA: Saunders/Elsevier.

Siegel M (2007). *Monitoring in the Intensive Care Unit: An Issue of Critical Care Clinics.* Philadelphia, PA: Saunders/Elsevier.

Pulmonary Function Testing

Ferguson GT et al. (2000). Office spirometry for lung health assessment in adults: A consensus statement from the National Lung Health Education Program, *Chest* 117(4):1146.

Hansen JE, Sun X-G, Wasserman K (2007). Spirometric criteria for airway obstruction. *Chest* 131:349–355; doi:10.1378.

Hyatt RE, Scanlon PD (2002). *Interpretation of pulmonary Function Tests: A Practical Guide* (2nd ed.). Philadelphia, PA: JB Lippincott.

Madama VC (1998). *Pulmonary Function Testing and Cardiopulmonary Stress Testing* (2nd ed.). Albany, NY: Delmar.

Ruppel GL (2009). *Manual of Pulmonary Function Testing* (9th ed.). St. Louis, MO: Mosby/Elsevier.

Arterial Blood Gases

Hennessey IA, Japp AG (2007). *Arterial Blood Gases Made Easy.* Philadelphia, PA: Churchill Livingstone/Elsevier.

Malley WJ (2005). *Clinical Blood Gases: Applications and Intervention* (2nd ed.). Philadelphia, PA: Saunders/Elsevier.

Martin L (1999). *All You Really Need to Know to Interpret Arterial Blood Gases* (2nd ed.). Baltimore: Williams and Wilkins.

Shapiro BA, Peruzzi WT, Kozlowska-Templin R (1994). *Clinical Application of Blood Gases* (5th ed.). St. Louis, MO: Mosby/Elsevier.

Selected Oxygenation Topics

Cane RD et al. (1988). Unreliability of oxygen tension-based indices in reflecting intrapulmonary shunting in critically ill patients. *Crit Care Med* 16:1243.

Hess D, Kacmarek RM (1993). Techniques and devices for monitoring oxygenation. *Respir Care* 38(6): 646.

Kandel G, Aberman A (1993). Mixed venous oxygen saturation: Its role in the assessment of the critically ill patient. *Arch Intern Med* 143:1400.

Nelson LD (1993). Assessment of oxygenation: Oxygenation indices. *Respir Care* 38(6):631.

Nelson LD, Rutherford EJ (1992). Monitoring mixed venous oxygen. *Respir Care* 37(2):154.

Rasanen J et al. (1987). Oxygen tension and oxyhemoglobin saturations in the assessment of pulmonary gas exchange. *Crit Care Med* 15:1058.

Schafroth Torok S, Leuppi JD, Baty F, Tamm M, Chhajed PN (2008). Combined oximetry-cutaneous capnography in patients assessed for long-term oxygen therapy. *Chest* 133:1421–1425.

Selected Hypoxic-Drive Topics

Aubier M et al. (1980). Effects of the administration of oxygen on ventilation and blood gases in patients with chronic obstructive pulmonary disease during acute respiratory failure. *Am Rev Respir Dis* 122:747.

Cullen JH, Kaemmerlen JT (1967). Effect of oxygen administration at low rates of flow in hypercapic patients. *Am Rev Respir Dis* 95:116.

Dunn WF, Nelson SB, Hubmayr RD (1991). Oxygen-induced hypercapnia in obstructive pulmonary disease. *Am Rev Respir Dis* 144:526.

French W (2000). Hypoxic-drive theory revisited. *RT/J Respir Care Practitioners*, 2:84–85.

Sassoon CS, Hassell KT, Mahutte CK (1987). Hyperoxic-induced hypercapnia in stable chronic obstructive pulmonary disease. *Am Rev Respir Dis* 135:907.

Respiratory Pharmacology

Colbert BJ, Kennedy BL (2008). *Integrated Cardiopulmonary Pharmacology* (2nd ed.). Upper Saddle River, NJ: Pearson Education.

Downie G, Mackenzie J, Williams A, Hind C (2008). *Pharmacology and Medicines Management for Nurses* (4th ed.). Philadelphia, PA: Churchill Livingstone.

Gardenhir DS (2009). *Rau's respiratory care pharmacology* (9th ed.). St. Louis, MO: Mosby.

Lehne RA (2010). *Pharmacology for Nursing Care* (7th ed.). Philadelphia, PA: Saunders/Elsevier.

Lilley LL, Harrington S, Snyder P, Snyder JS (2007). *Pharmacology and the Nursing Process* (5th ed.). St. Louis, MO: Mosby/Elsevier.

Sleep Physiology

Aaron S, Vandenheeur K, Hebert P, et al. (2005). Outpatient oral prednisone after emergency treatment of chronic obstructive pulmonary disease. *N Engl J Med* 348:2618–2625.

Aloia MS, Stanchina M, Arnedt JT, Malhotra A, Millman RP (2005). Treatment adherence and outcomes in flexible vs standard continuous positive airway pressure therapy. *Chest* 127:2085–2093.

Antic NA, Buchan C, Esterman A, et al. (2009). A randomized controlled trial of nurse-led care for symptomatic moderate-severe obstructive sleep apnea. *Am J Respir Crit Care Med* 179:5001–508.

Baldwin CM, Griffith KA, Nieto FJ, O'Connor GT, Walsleben JA, Redline S (2001). The association of sleep-disordered breathing and sleep symptoms with quality of life in the Sleep Heart Health Study. *Sleep* 24:96–105.

Baltzan MA, Kassissia I, Elkholi O, Palayew M, Dabrusin R, Wolkove N (2006). Prevalence of persistent sleep apnea in patients treated with continuous positive airway pressure. *Sleep* 29:557–563.

Berry RB, Patel PB (2006). Effect of zolpidem on the efficacy of continuous positive airway pressure as treatment for obstructive sleep apnea. *Sleep* 29:1052–1060.

Boyer S, Kapur V (2002). Obstructive sleep apnea: Its relevance in the care of diabetic patients. *Clinical Diabetes* 20(3):126–131.

Campos-Rodriguez F, Pena-Grinan N, Reyes-Nunez N, et al. (2005). Mortality in obstructive sleep apnea-hypopnea patients treated with positive airway pressure. *Chest* 128:624–633.

Chesson AL Jr, Ferber RA, Fry JM, et al. (1997). The indications for polysomnography and related procedures. *Sleep* 20:423–487.

Collop NA, Anderson WM, Boehlecke B, et al. (2007). Clincal guidelines for the use of unattended portable monitors in the diagnosis of obstructive sleep apnea in adult patients. *J Clin Sleep Med* 3:1–16.

Engleman HM, Wild MR (2003). Improving CPAP use by patients with the sleep apnoea/hypopnoea syndrome (SAHS). *Sleep Med Rev* 7:81–99.

Flegal KM, Carroll MD, Ogden CL, Johnson CL (2002). Prevalence and trends in obesity among US adults, 1999–2000. *JAMA* 288:1723–1727.

Flemons WW, Douglas NJ, Kuna ST, Rodenstein DO, Wheatley J (2004). Access to diagnosis and treatment of patients with suspected sleep apnea. *Am J Respir Crit Care Med* 169:668–672.

Flemons WW, Littner MR, Rowley JA, Gay P, Anderson WM, Hudgel American College of Chest Physicians, American Thoracic Society (2003). Home diagnosis of sleep apnea: A systematic review of the literature. *Chest* 124:1543–1579.

Gay P, Weaver T, Loube D, Iber C (2006). Evaluation of positive airway pressure treatment for sleep related breathing disorders in adults: A review of the positive airway pressure task force of the Standards of Practice Committee of the American Academy of Sleep Medicine. *Sleep* 29:381–401.

Giles TL, Lasserson TJ, Smith BH, et al. (2006). Continuous positive airways pressure for obstructive sleep apnea. *Cochran Database Syst Rev.* 3:CD001106.

Goodwin JL, Kaemingk KL, Fegosi RF, et al. (2003). Clinical outcomes associated with sleep-disordered breathing in Caucasian and Hispanic children—the Tucson Children's Assessment of Sleep Apnea study (TuCASA). *Sleep* 26:587–591.

Iber C, Ancoli-Israel S, Chesson A, Quan SF, American Academy of Sleep Medicine (2007). *The AASM Manual for the Scoring of Sleep and Associated Events: Rules, Terminology and Technical Specifications* (2nd ed.). Westchester, IL: American Academy of Sleep Medicine.

Jokic R, Klimaszewski A, Sridhar G, Fitzpatrick MF (1998). Continuous positive airway pressure requirement during the first month of treatment in patients with severe obstructive sleep apnea. *Chest* 114:1061–1069.

Kaneko Y, Floras JS, Usui K, et al. (2003). Cardiovascular effects of continuous positive airway pressure in patients with heart failure and obstructive sleep apnea. *N Engl J Med* 348(13):1233–1241.

Kessler R, Weitzenblum E, Chaouat A, et al. (2003). Evaluation of unattended automated titration to determine therapeutic continuous positive airway pressure in patients with obstructive sleep apnea. *Chest* 123(3):704–710.

Kribbs NB, Pack AI, Kline LR, et al. (1993). Objective measurement of patterns of nasal CPAP use by patients with obstructive sleep apnea. *Am Rev Respir Dis* 147:887–895.

Kryger MH (2010). *Atlas of Clinical Sleep Medicine.* Philadelphia, PA: Saunders/Elsevier.

Kushida CA, Littner MR, Hirshkowitz M, et al. (2006). Practice parameters for the use of continuous and bilevel positive airway pressure devices to treat adult patients with sleep-related breathing disorders. *Sleep* 29:375–380.

Kushida CA, Littner MR, Morgenthaler T, et al. (2005). Practice parameters for the indications for polysomnography and related procedures: An update for 2005. *Sleep* 28:499–521.

Littner MR, Kushida C, Wise M, et al. (2005). Practice parameters for clinical use of the multiple sleep latency test and the maintenance of wakefulness test. *Sleep* 28:113–121.

Lloberes P, Ballester E, Montserrat JM, et al. (1996). Comparison of manual and automatic CPAP titration in patients with sleep apnea/hypopnea syndrome. *Am J Respir Crit Care Med* 154(6 pt 1):1755–1758.

Mansfield DR, Gollogly NC, Kaye DM, et al. (2004). Controlled trial of continuous positive airway pressure in obstructive sleep apnea and heart failure. *Am J Respir Crit Care Med* 169(3):361–366.

Marin JM, Carrizo SJ, Vicente E, Agusti AG (2005). Long-term cardiovascular outcomes in men with obstructive sleep apnoea-hypopnoea with or without treatment with continuous positive airway pressure: An observational study. *Lancet* 365:1046–1053.

Masa JF, Jimenez A, Duran J, et al. (2004). Alternative methods of titrating continuous positive airway pressure: A large multicenter study. *Am J Respir Crit Care Med* 170(11):1218–1224.

Massie CA, Hart RW (2003). Clinical outcomes related to interface type in patients with obstructive sleep apnea/hypopnea syndrome who are using continuous positive airway pressure. *Chest* 123:1112–1118.

Mokhlesi B, Tulaimat A (2007). Recent advances in obesity hypoventilation syndrome. *Chest* 132:1322–1336.

Montgomery-Downs HE, O'Brien LM, Gulliver TE, Goval D (2006). Polysomnographic characteristic in normal preschool and early school-aged children. *Pediatrics* 117:741–753.

Morgenthaler TL, et al. (2008). Practice parameters for the use of autotitrating continuous positive airway pressure devices for titrating pressures and treating adult patients with obstructive sleep apnea syndrome: An update for 2007. *Sleep* 31(1):141–147.

Morgenthaler TI, Kagramanov V, Hanak V, Decker PA (2006). Complex sleep apnea syndrome: Is it a unique clinical syndrome? *Sleep* 29:1203–1209.

Mulloy E, McNicholas WT (1996). Ventilation and gas exchange during sleep and exercise in patients with severe COPD. *Chest* 109:387–394.

Nilius G, Happel A, Domanski U, Ruhle KH (2006). Pressure-relief continuous positive airway pressure vs constant continuous positive airway pressure: A comparison of efficacy and compliance. *Chest* 130:1018–1024.

Nussbaumer Y, Bloch KE, Genser T, Thunheer R (2006). Equivalence of autoadjusted and constant continuous positive airway pressure in home treatment of sleep apnea. *Chest* 129:638–643.

Pack AL (2004). Sleep-disordered breathing: Access is the issue. *Am J Respir Crit Care Med* 169:666–667.

Parthasarathy S, Habib M, Quan SF (2005). How are automatic positive airway pressure and related devices prescribed by sleep physicians? A web-based survey. *J Clin Sleep Med* 1:27–34.

Patel SR, White DP, Malhotra A, Stanchina ML, Ayas NT (2003). Continuous positive airway pressure therapy for treating sleepiness in a diverse population with obstructive sleep apnea: Results of a meta-analysis. *Arch Intern Med* 163:565–571.

Peppard PE, Young T, Palta M, Skatrud J (2000). Prospective study of association between sleep-disordered breathing and hypertension. *N Eng J Med* 342:1378–1384.

Polysomnography Task Force, American Sleep Disorders Association Standards of Practice Committe (1997). Practice parameters for the indications for polysomnography and related procedures. *Sleep* 20:406–422.

Positive Airway Pressure Titration Task Force of the American Academy of Sleep Medicine. (2008). Clinical guidelines for the manual titration of positive airway pressure in patients with obstructive sleep apnea. *J Clin Sleep Med* 4(2):157.

Rosen IM, Manaker S (2008). Sleeping at Home, *Chest* 134:682; doi:10.1378/chest.08-1799.

Sanders MH, Costantino JP, Strollo PJ, Studnicki K, Atwood CW (2000). The impact of split-night polysomnography for diagnosis and positive pressure therapy titration on treatment acceptance and adherence in sleep apnea/hypopnea. *Sleep* 23:17–24.

Sanders MH, Newman AB, Haggerty CL, et al. (2003). Sleep and sleep-disordered breathing in adults with predominantly mild obstructive airway disease. *Am J Respir Crit Care Med* 167:7–14.

Senn O, Brack T, Russi EW, Bloch KE (2006). A continuous positive airway pressure trial as a novel approach to the diagnosis of the obstructive sleep apnea syndrome. *Chest* 129(1):67–75.

Series F (2000). Accuracy of an unattended home CPAP titration in the treatment of obstructive sleep apnea. *Am J Respir Crit Care Med* 162:94–97.

Silva RS, Truksinas V, de Mello-Fujita L, et al. (2008). An orientation session improves objective sleep quality and mask acceptance during positive airway pressure titration. *Sleep Breath* 12:85–89.

Sin DD, Mayer I, Man GC, Ghahary A, Pawluk L (2000). Can continuous positive airway pressure therapy improve the general health status of patients with obstructive sleep apnea? A clinical effectiveness study. *Chest* 122:1679–1685.

Standards of Practice Committee of the American Academy of Sleep Medicine. (2006). Practice parameters for the medical therapy of obstructive sleep apnea. *Sleep* 29(8):1031–1035.

Uong EC, Epperson M, Bathon SA, Jeffe DB (2007). Adherence to nasal positive airway pressure therapy among school-aged children and adolescents with obstructive sleep apnea syndrome. *Pediatrics* 120:e1203-1211.

Weaver TE, Kribbs NB, Pack AI, et al. (1997). Night-to-night variability in CPAP use over the first three months of treatment. *Sleep* 20:278–283.

Weaver TE, Maislin G, Dinges DF, Bioxham T, et. al. (2007). Relationship between hours of CPAP use and achieving normal levels of sleepiness and daily function. *Sleep* 30(6):711–719.

Yaggi HK, Concato J, Kernan WN, Lichtman JH, Brass LOM, Mohsenin V (2005). Obstructive sleep apnea as a risk factor for stroke and death. *N Engl J Med* 353:2034–2041.

Young T, Palta M, Dempsey J, Skatrud J, Weber S, Badr S (1993). The occurrence of sleep-disordered breathing among middle-aged adults. *N Engl J Med* 328:1230–1235.

Young T, Skatrud J, Peppard PE (2004). Risk factors for obstructive sleep apnea in adults. *JAMA* 291(16):2013–2016.

Pathophysiology

Copstead LE, Banasik JL (2005). *Pathophysiology* (3rd ed.). St. Louis, MO: Elsevier Saunders.

Damjanov I (2006). *Pathology for the Health Profession* (3rd ed.). Philadelphia, PA: Saunders/Elsevier.

Gould BE (2011). *Pathophysiology for Health Profession* (4th ed.). Philadelphia, PA: Saunders/Elsevier.

Huether SE, McCance KL (2008). *Understanding Pathophysiology* (4th ed.). St. Louis, MO: Elsevier/Mosby.

Kumar V, Abbas A, Fausto N, Aster J (2010). *Robbins' & Cotran's Pathologic Basis of Disease* (8th ed.). Philadelphia, PA: Saunders/Elsevier.

McCance KL, Huether SE (2006). *Pathophysiology: The Biologic Basis for Disease in Adults and Children* (5th ed.). St. Louis, MO: Elsevier/Mosby.

Porth CM, Matfin G (2008). *Essentials of Pathophysiology: Concepts of Altered Health States* (8th ed.).Philadelphia, PA: JB Lippincott/Williams and Wilkins.

Price SA, Wilson LM (2003). *Pathophysiology: Clinical Concepts of Disease Processes* (6th ed.). St. Louis, MO: Mosby/Elsevier.

Pulmonary Disorders

Albert RK, Spiro SG, Jett JR (2008). *Clinical Respiratory Medicine* (3rd ed.). St. Louis, MO: Mosby/Elsevier.

Crapo JD, Glassroth JL, Karlinsky JB, King TE (2003). *Baum's Textbook of Pulmonary Diseases* (7th ed.). Philadelphia, PA: JB Lippincott.

DesJardins TR, Burton GG (2011). *Clinical Manifestations and Assessment of Respiratory Disease* (6th ed.). St. Louis, MO: Mosby/Elsevier.

Fishman AP, Elias JA, Fishman JA, Grippi MA, Senior RM, Pack AI (Eds.) (2008). *Fishman's Pulmonary Diseases and Disorders* (4th ed.). New York: McGraw-Hill.

Fraser RS, Colman NC, Nestor ML, Pare PD (2005). *Synopsis of Diseases of the Chest* (3rd ed.). Philadelphia, PA: Saunders/Elsevier.

Fraser RS, Muller NL, Colman N, Pare PD (1999). *Diagnosis of Diseases of the Chest* (Volumes I through IV) (4th ed.) Philadelphia, PA: Saunders/Elsevier.

George RB, Light RW, Matthay MA, Matthay RA (2000). *Chest Medicine—Essentials of Pulmonary and Critical Care Medicine* (4th ed.). Philadelphia, PA: JB Lippincott.

Gibson J, Geddes D, Costabel U, Sterk P, Corrin B (2003). *Respiratory Medicine* (3rd ed.). Philadelphia, PA: Saunders/Elsevier.

Murray JF, Nadel JA (2005). *Textbook of Respiratory Medicine* (4th ed.). Philadelphia, PA: Saunders/Elsevier.

Weinberger SE, Cockrill BA, Mandel J (2008). *Principles of Pulmonary Medicine* (5th ed.). Philadelphia, PA: Sauders/Elsevier.

West JB (2007). *Pulmonary Pathophysiology: The Essentials* (7th ed.). Baltimore: Williams and Wilkins.

Wilkins RL, Dexter JR, Gold PM (2007). *Respiratory Disease—A Case Study Approach to Patient Care* (3rd ed.). Philadelphia, PA: FA Davis.

Cardiopulmonary Anatomy and Physiology of the Fetus and the Newborn

Barnhart SL, Czervinske MP (2003). *Perinatal and Pediatric Respiratory Care* (2nd ed.) Philadelphia, PA: Saunders/Elsevier.

Fanaroff AA, Martin RJ, Walsh MC (2011). *Fanaroff and Marin's Neonatal-Perinatal Medicine: Diseases of the Fetus and Infant* (9th ed.). Philadelphia, PA: Saunders/Elsevier.

Feischer GR, Ludwig S (2010). *Textbook of Pediatric Emergency Medicine* (6th ed.). Philadelphia, PA: Lippincott/Williams and Wilkins.

Kilegman RM, Stanton BMD, St. Gem J, Behrman RE (2011). *Nelson Textbook of Pediatrics* (19th ed.). Philadelphia, PA: Saunders/Elsevier.

MacDonald M, Mullett M, Seshia M (2005). *Avery's Neonatology Pathophysiology and Management of the Newborn* (6th ed.). Philadelphia, PA: JB Lippincott.

Taeusch WH, Ballard RA, Gleason CA (2005). *Avery's Diseases of the Newborn* (8th ed.). Philadelphia, PA: Elsevier/Saunders.

Taussig LM, Landau LL (2008). *Pediatric Respiratory Medicine* (2nd ed.). St. Louis, MO: Mosby/Elsevier.

Turcios NL, Fink RJ (2009) *Pulmonary Manifestations of Pediatric Disease.* Philadelphia, PA: Saunders/Elsevier.

Verklan TM, Walden M (2004). *Core Curriculum for Neonatal Intensive Care Nursing* (3rd ed.). Philadelphia, PA: Elsevier/Saunders.

Walsh BK, Czervinske MP, DiBlasi RM (2010). *Perinatal and Pediatric Respiratory Care* (3rd ed.). Philadelphia, PA: Saunders/Elsevier.

Aging and the Cardiopulmonary System

Beers MH (2005). *The Merck Manual of Health and Aging.* Whitehouse Station, NJ: Merck Company.

Beers MH, Jones TV, et al. (Eds.) (2005). *The Merck Manual of Geriatrics.* Whitehouse Station, NJ: Merck Company.

Cardus J, Burgos R, et al. (1997). Increase in pulmonary ventilation-perfusion inequality with age in healthy individuals. *Am J Resp Crit Care Med* 56(2):648–653.

Cerveri I, Zoia MC, et al. (1995). Reference values of arterial oxygen tension in the middle aged and elderly. *Am J Resp Crit Care Med* 152(3):934–941.

Cristian A (2006). *Geriatric Rehabilitation, An Issue of Clinics in Geriatric Medicine.* Philadelphia, PA: Saunders/Elsevier.

Derstine JB, Drayton Hargrove S (2001). *Comprehensive Rehabilitation Nursing.* Philadelphia, PA: Saunders/Elsevier.

Fillit H (2010). Brocklehurst's Textbook of Geriatric Medicine and Gerontology (7th ed.). Philadelphia, PA: Saunders/Elsevier.

Frownfelter D, Dean E (2006). *Cardiovascular and Pulmonary Physical Therapy* (4th ed.). St. Louis, MO: Mosby/Elsevier.

Hazzard WR et al. (Eds.) (2003). *Principles of Geriatric Medicine and Gerontology.* New York: McGraw-Hill.

Hoeman S (2007). *Rehabilitation Nursing.* St. Louis, MO: Mosby/Elsevier.

Jensen M, Molton I (2010). *Aging with a Physical Disability, An Issue of Physical Medicine and Rehabilitation Clinics.* Philadelphia, PA: Saunders/Elsevier.

Malley WJ (2005). *Clinical Blood Gases: Applications and Intervention* (2nd ed.). Philadelphia, PA: Saunders/Elsevier.

Martinson IM, Widmer AG, Portillo C (2002). *Home Health Care Nursing* (2nd ed.). Philadelphia, PA: Saunders/Elsevier.

Oxyenham H, Sharpe N (2003). Cardiovascular aging and heart failure. *Euro J Heart Failure* 5:427–434.

Exercise and Its Effects on the Cardiopulmonary System

Bell C (2008). *Cardiovascular Physiology in Exercise and Sport.* Philadelphia, PA: Churchill Livingstone/Elsevier.

Buckley J (2008). *Exercise Physiology in Special Populations.* Philadelphia, PA: Churchill Livingstone/Elsevier.

Costill DL, Wilmore JH (2005). *Physiology of Sport and Exercise* (3rd ed.). Champaign, IL: Human Kinetics Publishers.

Cuppert M, Walsh K (2005). *General Medical Conditions in the Athlete.* St. Louis, MO: Mosby/Elsevier.

Froelicher VF, Myers JN (2006). *Exercise and the Heart* (5th ed.). Philadelphia, PA: Saunders/Elsevier.

Hodgkin JE, Celli BR, Connors GL (2009). *Pulmonary Rehabilitation Guidelines to Success* (4th ed.). St. Louis, MO: Mosby/Elsevier.

Katch FI, Katch VL, Mcardle W (2006). *Essentials of Exercise Physiology.* Philadelphia, PA: Lippincott Williams and Wilkins.

Myers JN (1996). *Essentials of Cardiopulmonary Exercise Testing.* Champaign, IL: Human Kinetics Publishers.

Reilly T, Waterhouse J (2005). *Sport Exercise and Environmental Physiology.* New York: Churchill Livingstone/Elsevier.

Robergs RA, Keteyian SJ (2002). *Fundamentals of Exercise Physiology.* New York: McGraw-Hill.

Whyte G, Spurway N, MacLaren D (2006). *The Physiology of Training.* New York: Churchill Livingstone.

Woolf-May K (2006). *Exercise Prescription—The Physiological Foundation.* Philadelphia, PA: Churchill Livingstone/Elsevier.

High Altitude and Its Effects on the Cardiopulmonary System

Auerbach P (2001). *Wilderness Medicine: Management of Wilderness and Environmental Emergencies* (4th ed.). St. Louis, MO: Mosby/Elsevier.

Beidleman BA, Muza SR, Fulco CS, et al. (2003). Intermittent altitude exposures improve muscular performance at 4,300 m. *J Appl Physiol* 95:1824–1832.

Chapman RF, Stray-Gundersen J, Levine BD (1998). Individual variation in response to altitude training. *J Appl Physiol* 85:1448–1456.

Deboeck G, Moraine JJ, Naeije R (2005). Respiratory muscle strength may explain hypoxia-induced decreased vital capacity. *Med Sci Sports Exerc* 37:754–758.

Hornbein TF, Schoene RB (Eds.) (2001). *High Altitude: An Exploration of Human Adaptation* (*Lung Biology in Health and Disease,* Vol 161, pp. 139–174). New York: Marcel Dekker.

Jaeger JJ, Sylvester JT, Cymerman A, et al. (1979). Evidence for increased intrathoracic fluid volume in man at high altitude. *J Appl Physiol* 47:670–676.

Levine BD, Stray-Gundersen J (2006). Dose-response of altitude training. How much altitude is enough? *Adv Exp Med Biol* 588:233–247.

Loeppky JA, Icenogle MV, Maes D, et al. (2005). Early fluid retention and severe acute mountain sickness. *J Appl Physiol* 98:591–597.

Luks AM, Schoene RB, Schoene RB, Swenson ER (2010). High altitude. In Mason RJ, Broaddus CV (Eds.), *Murray & Nadel's Textbook of Respiratory Medicine* (5th ed., pp. 1651–1673). Philadelphia, PA: Saunders/Elsevier.

Singh I, Khanna PK, Srivastava MC, et al. Acute mountain sickness. N Engl J Med 280: 175–184.

Smith CA, Dempsey JA, Hornbein TF (2000). Control of breathing at high altitude. In Ward MP, Milledge JS, West JB (Eds.), *High Altitude Medicine and Physiology* (3rd ed.). London: Arnold.

Welsh CH, Wagner PD, Reeves JT, et al. (1993). Operation Everest II: Spirometric and radiographic changes in acclimatized humans at simulated high altitudes. *Am Rev Respir Dis* 147:1239–1244.

West JB, Schoene RB, Milledge JS (2007). *High Altitude Medicine and Physiology* (4th ed). London: Hodder Arnold.

West JB: Highlife (1998). *A History of High Altitude Physiology and Medicine.* Oxford, UK: Oxford University Press.

High-Pressure Environments and Their Effect on the Cardiopulmonary System

Bove AA, Davis JC (2004). *Diving Medicine* (4th ed.). Philadelphia, PA: Saunders/Elsevier.

Kindwall E, Whelan H (2008). *Hyperbaric Medicine Practice* (3rd ed.). Flagstaff, AZ: Best Publishing Company.

Luks AM, Schoene RB, Swenson ER (2010). Diving medicine. In Mason RJ, Broaddus CV (Eds.), *Murray & Nadel's Textbook of Respiratory Medicine* (5th ed., pp. 1674–1690). Philadelphia, PA: Saunders/Elsevier.

Neubauer RA (2004). *Textbook of Hyperbaric Medicine.* Göttingen, Germany: Hogrefe Huber Pub.

Neuman JS, Thom SR (2008). *Physiology and Medicine of Hyperbaric Oxygen Therapy.* Philadelphia, PA: Saunders/Elsevier.

Fundamentals of Respiratory Care

Hess DR, MacIntyre NR, Galvin WF, Adams AB, Saposnick AB (2002). *Respiratory Care—Principles and Practice*. Philadelphia, PA: Saunders/Elsevier.

Kacmarek RM, Dimas S (2005). *Essentials of Respiratory Care* (4th ed.). St. Louis, MO: Mosby/Elsevier.

Wilkins RL, Stoller JK, Kacmarek RM (2009). *Egan's Fundamentals of Respiratory Care* (9th ed.). St. Louis, MO: Mosby/Elsevier.

Respiratory Care Equipment

Branson RD, Hess DR, Chatburn RL (1998). *Respiratory Care Equipment* (2nd ed.). Philadelphia, PA: JB Lippincott.

Cairo JM, Pilbean SP (2010). *Mosby's Respiratory Equipment* (8th ed.). St. Louis, MO: Mosby/Elsevier.

White GC (2005). *Equipment Theory for Respiratory Care* (4th ed.). Clifton Park, NY: Delmar, Cengage Learning.

Mechanical Ventilation

Chang DW (2006). *Clinical Application of Mechanical Ventilation* (3rd. ed.). Clifton Park, NY: Delmar, Cengage Learning.

Dupuis YG (1992). *Ventilators: Theory and Clinical Applications* (2nd ed.). St. Louis, MO: Mosby/Elsevier.

Hess DR, Kacmarek RM (2002). *Essentials of Mechanical Ventilation* (2nd ed.). New York: McGraw-Hill.

MacIntyre NR, Branson RD (2009). *Mechanical Ventilation* (2nd ed.). Philadelphia, PA: Saunders/Elsevier.

Pilbeam SP, Cairo JM (2006). *Mechanical Ventilation: Physiological and Clinical Applications* (4th ed.). St. Louis, MO: Mosby/Elsevier.

Medical Dictionaries

Dorland's Illustrated Medical Dictionary (30th ed.). (2003). Philadelphia, PA: Saunders/Elsevier.

Mosby's Dictionary of Medicine, Nursing & Health Professions (8th ed.) (2009). St. Louis, MO: Mosby/Elsevier.

Websites of Interest

American Association for Respiratory Care: www.aarc.org

American Association of Respiratory Care—Clinical Practice Guidelines: www.aarc.org/resources/cpgs_guidelines_statements/

American Cancer Society: www.cancer.org

American College of Cardiology Resource Center: www.acc.org

American College of Chest Physician: www.chestnet.org/

American Lung Association: www.lungusa.org

American Heart Association: www.americanheart.org

American Medical Association: http://www .ama-assn.org/

American Sleep Apnea Association: www.sleepapnea.org

American Thoracic Society: www.thoracic.org/

Centers for Disease Control and Prevention: www.cdc.gov

Center for Drug Evaluation and Research: www.fda.gov/cder/

FDA Approved Drug Products: www.accessdata .fda.gov/scripts/cder/drugsatfda/

Global Initiative for Asthma (GINA): http://www.ginasthma.org/

Global Initiative for Chronic Obstructive Lung Disease (GOLD): http://www.goldcopd.org

Health Information: www.medlineplus.gov

Journal of American Medical Association: www.jama.com

Lung cancer.org: www.lungcancer.org/

Mayo Clinic: www.mayoclinic.com

Medicine: www.emedicine.com

National Board for Respiratory Care: www.nbrc.org

National Heart, Lung, and Blood Institute (Lung Disease Information): www.nhlbi.nih.gov/ health/prof/lung/index.htm#asthma

National Library of Medicine: www.nlm.nih.gov

NHLBI-NAEPP Asthma Management Guidelines EPR-3: www.nhlbi.nih.gov/guidelines/ asthma/asthgdln.pdf

United States Pharmacopeia: www.usp.org/

Web MD Health: www.my.webmed.com

World Health Organization: www.who.int

Index

669